WeightWatchers®

Complete Food Companion®

Over 18,400 foods!
Over 5,700 new items!
Now with Filling Foods!

table of contents

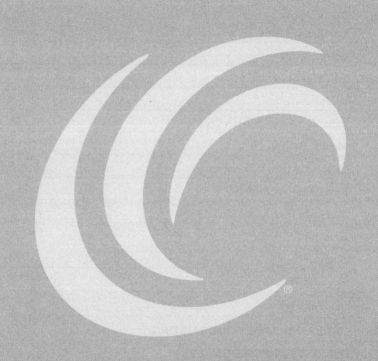

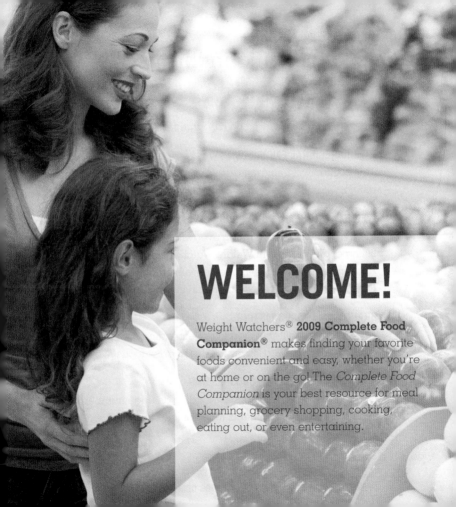

WELCOME!

Weight Watchers® **2009 Complete Food Companion**® makes finding your favorite foods convenient and easy, whether you're at home or on the go! The *Complete Food Companion* is your best resource for meal planning, grocery shopping, cooking, eating out, or even entertaining.

What you'll find in this book:

- **COMPLETE A-Z FOOD LIST**
  Use this general listing as a resource for finding **POINTS**® values.

- **ETHNIC/REGIONAL FAVORITES**
  This section will help make staying on the plan easier while eating out at local eateries or family gatherings.

- **WEIGHT WATCHERS® FOOD PRODUCTS LISTING**
  Menu planning is easier than ever with this comprehensive listing of all the current Weight Watchers food products. And since everything is in one convenient place, finding the **POINTS** values you're looking for is a snap.

- **BRAND NAME FOODS LISTING**
  Containing more items than ever before, finding the **POINTS** values of your favorite supermarket foods is easy.

- **INDEX TO BRAND NAME FOODS LISTING**
  Looking for a specific product? Finding its page number is a "piece of cake" with this index of food types.

A word about the food listings:

- Just about every food you can think of is included, and all listings include **POINTS** values.

- **POINTS** values in the *Complete Food Companion* were calculated by nutritionists at Weight Watchers International, Inc. using the most current calorie, fat, and fiber information available from manufacturers and the United States Department of Agriculture (USDA).

Product formulations and nutrition information may change during the year, so it's a good idea to continue to use nutrition labels and your **POINTSfinder®** slide or your **POINTS** calculator occasionally to check the **POINTS** values of foods.

How to use this book:

This *Complete Food Companion*® is organized to make finding your favorite foods easier. Following are some search tips to help you make the most of this valuable guide.

General Search Tips:

COMPLETE A-Z FOOD LIST

- ***POINTS*®** values for foods in this listing are based on an average of several brands or homemade recipes.
- ***POINTS*** values for foods in this listing may be different than the values for foods listed by brand name.
  - For example: Beef stew is listed with different ***POINTS*** values in the Complete A-Z Food List than in the Brand Name Foods Listing because the A-Z list uses an average of several brands, while the Brand Name Listing uses values specific to each brand.

BRAND NAME FOODS LISTING

- Foods in this section are listed by major category (also seen in table of contents), then by food type (also seen in index), then by brand name and, finally, by specific product.

- For example, in the major category of Condiments,
  Sauces & Gravies, the food type "Mayonnaise" is followed
  by numerous brands of mayonnaise, and under each
  brand is a list of specific products.

INDEX TO BRAND NAME FOODS LISTING

- For quick searches, use the index, which alphabetically lists
  foods by type and gives the exact page number where all the
  brands of that food type are listed.

Searching for Foods:

- Use the Complete A-Z Food List to easily find **POINTS** values
  of non-branded food items.
- Use the Brand Name Foods Listing to compare **POINTS** values
  of different brands.
- Use the Index to Brand Name Foods Listing to help find the
  brand name foods you are looking for faster.

As you can see, the lists in this guide were developed to give you
the best information possible. You can depend on them. The **Weight
Watchers® Complete Food Companion®** is a great tool to assist
you in your weight-loss goals!

For my lifestyle

THE BETTER EGG.

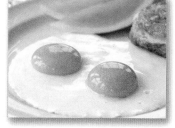

You're taking care of yourself. Watching what you eat. So why not enjoy the better egg…Eggland's Best.

EBs are the better-tasting eggs. They have more of the delicious, farm-fresh taste your family loves.

No wonder they were rated "America's Best Tasting Egg" by American Culinary ChefsBest™ for the 6th year in a row.

EBs are better nutritionally, too.

Compared to ordinary eggs, EBs provide:

- 10 times more vitamin E
- 3 times more Omega 3 (100 mg)
- 25% less saturated fat
- 19% less cholesterol;
  175 mg
  (58% DV) vs.
  215 mg
  (71% DV)

EBs are available in Large, Extra Large, Jumbo, Organic, Cage Free, and Brown varieties.

EBs also provide 200 mcg of lutein, a nutrient that's essential for good eye health. Plus, they're 100% natural, and produced without hormones, antibiotics, or steroids.

The "EB" stamp on every egg tells you you're getting eggs of the absolute highest quality.

So why settle for ordinary eggs when you can have the best? Eggland's Best.

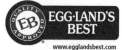

QUALITY APPROVED EB

EGG·LAND'S BEST

www.egglandsbest.com

**Better taste. Better nutrition.
Better eggs.**

The ChefsBest™ Award for Best Taste is awarded to the brand rated highest overall among leading brands by independent professional chefs.

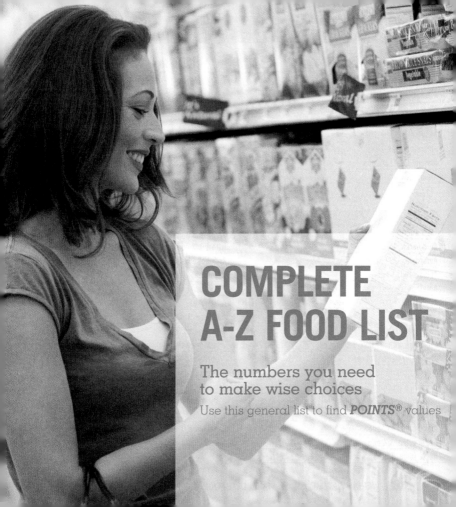

COMPLETE A-Z FOOD LIST

The numbers you need
to make wise choices

Use this general list to find *POINTS*® values

◈ | (POINTS VALUE)

A

All-fruit spread (spreadable fruit), 1 1/2 Tbsp	1
Allspice, ground, 1 tsp	0
Almond butter, 1 tsp	1
Almond float, 1/2 cup	2
Almonds	
1 cup sliced	13
1 cup whole	19
1 Tbsp sliced	1
23 nuts	4
Aloo palak, 1 cup	3
Ambrosia, 1/2 cup	2
Anise seed, 1 tsp	0
Antelope, cooked, 1 oz	1
Apple	
baked, 1 large	7
caramel, 1 large	9
◆ cooked, without skin, 1 cup sliced	1 (2)
dried, 1/4 cup (3/4 oz)	1
◆ fresh, 1 large (3 1/4" diameter)	2 (2)
◆ fresh, 1 medium (2 3/4" diameter)	1 (2)
◆ fresh, 1 small (2 1/2" diameter)	1 (2)
Apple brown Betty, 1 cup	5
Apple cider, 1/2 cup	1
Apple crisp, 3/4 cup	8
Apple juice, 1/2 cup	1

Apple kuchen, 1 piece (3" square)	10
Apple streusel, 1/2 cup	4
◆ **Applesauce,** unsweetened, 1 cup	2
Apricots	
◆ canned or frozen, unsweetened, 1 cup	2 (2)
dried, 6 halves (3/4 oz)	1
◆ fresh, 3 medium (3/4 oz)	1 (2)
Armadillo, cooked, 1 oz	1
◆ **Arrowhead,** cooked or raw, 1 medium	0
Arrowroot powder, 1 tsp	0
Arroz con gandules, 1 cup	8
Arroz con pollo, 3 oz chicken with 1 1/2 cup rice	13
Artichoke hearts	
◆ canned, without oil, 1/2 cup	0
◆ cooked, 1 cup	1
Artichokes	
◆ cooked, 1 medium	0
marinated, 1/2 cup	3
◆ raw, frozen, 1 package (9 oz)	1
stuffed, 1	14
◆ **Arugula,** 1 cup	0
Asparagus	
◆ cooked or raw, 1 cup or 12 spears	0
◆ raw, frozen, 1 package (10 oz)	1
Aspartame, 1 packet	0
◆ **Avocado,** 1/4 medium (2 oz)	2

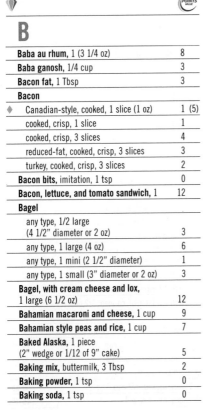

	POINTS VALUE

B

Baba au rhum, 1 (3 1/4 oz)	8
Baba ganosh, 1/4 cup	3
Bacon fat, 1 Tbsp	3
Bacon	
◆ Canadian-style, cooked, 1 slice (1 oz)	1 (5)
cooked, crisp, 1 slice	1
cooked, crisp, 3 slices	4
reduced-fat, cooked, crisp, 3 slices	3
turkey, cooked, crisp, 3 slices	2
Bacon bits, imitation, 1 tsp	0
Bacon, lettuce, and tomato sandwich, 1	12
Bagel	
any type, 1/2 large (4 1/2" diameter or 2 oz)	3
any type, 1 large (4 oz)	6
any type, 1 mini (2 1/2" diameter)	1
any type, 1 small (3" diameter or 2 oz)	3
Bagel, with cream cheese and lox, 1 large (6 1/2 oz)	12
Bahamian macaroni and cheese, 1 cup	9
Bahamian style peas and rice, 1 cup	7
Baked Alaska, 1 piece (2" wedge or 1/12 of 9" cake)	5
Baking mix, buttermilk, 3 Tbsp	2
Baking powder, 1 tsp	0
Baking soda, 1 tsp	0

	POINTS VALUE
Baklava	
1 piece (2" square)	4
store-bought, 1 piece (2 oz)	5
◆ **Bamboo shoots,** cooked or raw, 1 cup	0
Banana	
◆ 1 cup sliced	2 (2)
◆ 1 extra large (9" or larger)	2 (2)
◆ 1 large (8 to 8 7/8" long)	2 (2)
◆ 1 medium (7 to 7 7/8" long)	2 (2)
◆ 1 small (6 to 6 7/8" long)	1 (2)
Banana bread, with or without nuts, 1 slice (5 x 3/4")	5
Banana chips, 1 oz	3
Banana split, 3 scoops (1 1/2 cups) ice cream, 1 banana, 3 Tbsp syrup, and 1/2 cup whipped cream	19
Bananas Foster, 2 scoops (1 cup) ice cream with 1/2 banana and 1/3 cup sauce	16
Barley	
◆ cooked, 1 cup	3 (6)
◆ uncooked, 1/4 cup	3 (6)
Basil, fresh or dried, 1 tsp	0
Bay leaf, 1 leaf or 1 Tbsp	0
Bean and lentil stew (Dal maharani), 1 cup	6
Bean curd	
aburage (fried bean curd), 1 piece (0.49 oz)	1
agedashi tofu, fried, 1/2 block (1 1/2" x 2")	6

Bean curd (con't)	POINTS VALUE
bean curd skin, 1 skin (25" x 26")	1
Beans	
baked, 1/2 cup	5
baked, canned, 1/2 cup	2
baked, deli, 1/2 cup	3
baked, fast-food, 1 serving (6 oz)	4
baked, vegetarian, canned, 1/2 cup	2
black, and rice, 1 cup	4
black, canned, 1/2 cup	1 (5)
black, cooked, 1/2 cup	2 (5)
black, dry, 1 pound	31 (5)
black, refried, canned, 1/2 cup	1
black, refried, low-fat or fat-free, canned, 1/2 cup	1
black, with rice mix, prepared according to package directions, 1 cup	4
cannellini, canned, 1/2 cup	1 (5)
cranberry (roman), cooked, 1 cup	4 (5)
fava (broadbeans), cooked or canned, 1 cup	3 (5)
French, cooked, 1 cup	4
garbanzo, canned, 1 cup	5 (5)
garbanzo, cooked, 1/2 cup	2 (5)
garbanzo, dry, 1 pound	35 (5)
great northern, canned, 1 cup	5 (5)
great northern, dry, 1 cup	12 (5)
green, cooked, 1 cup	0
kidney, canned, 1 cup	3 (5)

	POINTS VALUE
kidney, cooked, 1/2 cup	1 (5)
kidney, dry, 1 pound	30 (5)
lima, canned, 1 cup	3 (5)
lima, cooked, 1/2 cup	1 (5)
lima, dry, 1 pound	30 (5)
mung, cooked, 1 cup	3 (5)
mung, dry, 1 cup	14 (5)
navy, canned, 1 cup	5 (5)
navy, cooked, 1/2 cup	2 (5)
navy, dry, 1 pound	30 (5)
pink, cooked, 1 cup	4 (5)
pink, dry, 1 cup	14 (5)
pinto, canned, 1 cup	3 (5)
pinto, cooked, 1/2 cup	2 (5)
pinto, dry, 1 pound	31 (5)
red, and rice, 1 cup	5
red, with rice mix, prepared according to package directions, 1 cup	5
refried, 1/2 cup	3
refried, canned, 1/2 cup	2
refried, fat-free, canned, 1/2 cup	2 (5)
refried, with sausage, canned, 1/2 cup	5
small white, cooked, 1 cup	4 (5)
small white, dry, 1 cup	14 (5)
snap, canned, 1/2 cup	0
snap, cooked, 1 cup	0
soy, cooked, 1/2 cup	3 (5)
soy, dry, 1 pound	45 (5)

	POINTS VALUE
◆ soy, green, cooked, 1 cup	5 (5)
◆ soy, green, raw, 1 cup	8 (5)
◆ soy, roasted, 1 cup	19 (5)
◆ soy, sprouted, cooked or raw, 1 cup	2 (5)
◆ wax, cooked, 1 cup	0
◆ white, cooked, 1/2 cup	2 (5)
◆ white, dry, 1 pound	30 (5)
◆ yellow, cooked, 1 cup	4 (5)
◆ yellow, dry, 1 cup	13 (5)
Beans and franks, 1 cup	11
Bear, cooked, 1 oz	2
Beaver, cooked, 1 oz	1
Beef	
◆ brain, cooked, 2 oz	4 (5)
◆ brain, raw, 1 oz	1 (5)
brisket, cooked, 3 oz	9
brisket, lean, trimmed, cooked, 3 oz	3
brisket, lean, trimmed, raw, 1 oz	1
brisket, raw, 1 oz	2
chuck, arm pot roast, cooked, 3 oz	7
chuck, arm pot roast, trimmed, cooked, 3 oz	6
chuck, blade roast, trimmed, cooked, 3 oz	7
corned, cooked, 3 oz	6
corned, raw, 1 oz	1
cube steak, cooked, 3 oz	5
◆ cube steak, trimmed, cooked, 2 oz	3 (5)
◆ cube steak, trimmed, cooked, 3 oz	4 (5)

	POINTS VALUE
◆ filet mignon, trimmed, cooked, 1 small (4 oz)	6 (5)
◆ filet mignon, trimmed, cooked, 3 oz	4 (5)
◆ filet mignon, trimmed, raw, 3 oz	3 (5)
◆ flank, lean, cooked, 3 oz	5 (5)
◆ flank, lean, cooked, 1 slice (2 oz)	2 (5)
flank, cooked, 1 slice (2 oz)	3
flank, cooked, 3 oz	5
◆ heart, cooked or raw, 1 oz	1 (5)
KC strip, cooked, 1 small (4 oz)	7
KC strip, cooked, 3 oz	5
◆ KC strip, trimmed, cooked, 1 small (4 oz)	5 (5)
◆ KC strip, trimmed, cooked, 3 oz	4 (5)
◆ KC strip, trimmed, raw, 3 oz	4 (5)
◆ kidney, cooked or raw, 1 oz	1 (5)
◆ lean (other than those listed here), cooked (round or loin cuts with all visible fat trimmed), 1 slice or 1/2 cup cubed or shredded (2 oz)	3 (5)
◆ liver, cooked, 1/2 cup or 1 slice (2 oz)	2 (5)
◆ liver, raw, 1 oz	1 (5)
◆ New York steak, cooked, 1 small (4 oz)	8
New York steak, cooked, 3 oz	6
◆ New York steak, trimmed, cooked, 1 small (4 oz)	6 (5)
◆ New York steak, trimmed, cooked, 3 oz	4 (5)
◆ New York steak, trimmed, raw, 3 oz	5 (5)
porterhouse steak, cooked, 3 oz	7
◆ porterhouse steak, trimmed, cooked, 3 oz	6 (5)

Beef (con't)	POINTS VALUE
regular (other than those listed here), cooked, 1 slice or 1/2 cup cubed or shredded (2 oz)	5
rib eye, trimmed, cooked, 3 oz	5
rib, large end, cooked, 3 oz	7
rib, small end, trimmed, cooked, 3 oz	5
rib, whole (ribs 6-12), lean and fat, raw, 1 oz	2
◆ round, lean only, cooked, 3 oz	4 (5)
◆ round, lean only, raw, 1 oz	1 (5)
◆ round, steak or roast, trimmed, cooked, 3 oz	4 (5)
round, steak or roast, cooked, 3 oz	5
rump roast, trimmed, cooked, 1 slice (2 oz)	2
rump roast, trimmed, cooked, 3 oz	3
shortribs, cooked, 3 oz	11
shortribs, lean only, cooked, 3 oz	6
sirloin, cooked, 3 oz	5
◆ sirloin, trimmed, cooked, 1 slice (2 oz)	3 (5)
◆ sirloin, trimmed, cooked, 3 oz	4 (5)
steak, lean, cooked (round or loin cuts with all visible fat trimmed), 1 small (4 oz)	5 (5)
steak, regular, cooked, 1 small (4 oz)	10
strip sirloin, cooked, 1 small (4 oz)	7
strip sirloin, cooked, 3 oz	5
◆ strip sirloin, trimmed, cooked, 3 oz	4 (5)
◆ strip sirloin, trimmed, cooked, 1 small (4 oz)	5 (5)

	POINTS VALUE
◆ strip sirloin, trimmed, raw, 3 oz	4 (5)
T-bone steak, cooked, 3 oz	7
T-bone steak, cooked, 1 small (4 oz)	9
◆ T-bone steak, trimmed, cooked, 3 oz	5 (5)
◆ T-bone steak, trimmed, cooked, 1 small (4 oz)	7 (5)
◆ T-bone steak, trimmed, raw, 3 oz	5 (5)
tenderloin, cooked, 1 slice (2 oz)	5
tenderloin, cooked, 3 oz	7
◆ tenderloin, trimmed, cooked, 1 slice (2 oz)	3 (5)
◆ tenderloin, trimmed, cooked, 3 oz	4 (5)
◆ tenderloin, trimmed, raw, 3 oz	3 (5)
◆ tongue, cooked, 1 oz	2 (5)
◆ tongue, raw, 1 oz	2 (5)
Beef and broccoli	
1 cup	4
frozen, 1 cup	5
Beef Bourguignon, 1 1/2 cups	20
Beef goulash, 1 cup	8
Beef masala, 1 cup	5
Beef stew	
1 cup	5
canned, 1 cup	6
frozen, 1 cup	3
Beef Stroganoff with noodles, 1 cup stroganoff with 1 cup noodles	15
Beef Wellington, 1 slice (3 1/2 x 2 1/2 x 1 1/2")	12
Beef, frozen, with barbecue sauce, 1/4 cup	3

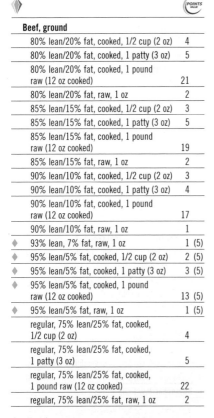

	POINTS VALUE
Beef, ground	
80% lean/20% fat, cooked, 1/2 cup (2 oz)	4
80% lean/20% fat, cooked, 1 patty (3 oz)	5
80% lean/20% fat, cooked, 1 pound raw (12 oz cooked)	21
80% lean/20% fat, raw, 1 oz	2
85% lean/15% fat, cooked, 1/2 cup (2 oz)	3
85% lean/15% fat, cooked, 1 patty (3 oz)	5
85% lean/15% fat, cooked, 1 pound raw (12 oz cooked)	19
85% lean/15% fat, raw, 1 oz	2
90% lean/10% fat, cooked, 1/2 cup (2 oz)	3
90% lean/10% fat, cooked, 1 patty (3 oz)	4
90% lean/10% fat, cooked, 1 pound raw (12 oz cooked)	17
90% lean/10% fat, raw, 1 oz	1
◆ 93% lean, 7% fat, raw, 1 oz	1 (5)
◆ 95% lean/5% fat, cooked, 1/2 cup (2 oz)	2 (5)
◆ 95% lean/5% fat, cooked, 1 patty (3 oz)	3 (5)
◆ 95% lean/5% fat, cooked, 1 pound raw (12 oz cooked)	13 (5)
◆ 95% lean/5% fat, raw, 1 oz	1 (5)
regular, 75% lean/25% fat, cooked, 1/2 cup (2 oz)	4
regular, 75% lean/25% fat, cooked, 1 patty (3 oz)	5
regular, 75% lean/25% fat, cooked, 1 pound raw (12 oz cooked)	22
regular, 75% lean/25% fat, raw, 1 oz	2

	POINTS VALUE
Beef jerky or stick, 1 oz	3
Beef patty, country-fried, store-bought, 1 (4 oz)	8
Beef stir-fry, with garlic or black bean sauce, 1 cup	8
Beef, orange-ginger, 1 cup	11
Beef, roast, open-faced sandwich with gravy, 6 oz	9
Beef, sliced, with gravy	
canned, 1/2 cup	6
frozen, 2 slices with gravy (4 3/4 oz)	2
Beef, sweet and sour, 1 cup	12
Beefalo, cooked, 1 oz	1
Beer	
light, 1 can or bottle (12 fl oz)	2
non-alcoholic, 1 can or bottle 12 fl oz	1
regular, 1 can or bottle (12 fl oz)	3
Beets	
◆ canned, 1 cup whole	0
◆ cooked, 1 cup	1
pickled, 1/2 cup	1
◆ raw, 1 cup	0
Beignet	
1 (2")	2
from mix, prepared, 1	3
Benny cake, 1 piece (2" x 3")	3
Berries	
◆ mixed, 1 cup	1
◆ wheat, raw, 1/4 cup	2

7

	POINTS VALUE
Beverage mix, sweet and sour, 1/2 cup	2
Bhuna gosht, 1 cup	8
Bialy, 1 (3 oz)	5
Biryani, chicken, 1 cup	9
Biscotti	
chocolate, 1 regular, 2 small, or 8 mini (1 oz)	3
fat-free, 1 regular, 2 small, or 8 mini (1 oz)	2
plain, 1 regular, 2 small, or 8 mini (1 oz)	3
Biscuit	
1 small (2" diameter)	3
cheese, 1 (2" diameter)	5
refrigerated, baked, 1 small (2 1/2" diameter) or 1/2 large (1 oz)	2
Biscuit mix, buttermilk, dry, reduced fat, 1 serving (1/4-1/3 cup)	3
Bison, lean, all visible fat trimmed, cooked, 3 oz	3
Bistec de palomilla (Cuban fried steak), 1 steak	10
♦ **Bittermelon (balsam-pear pods),** cooked or raw, 1 cup	0
Black Russian, 1	5
♦ **Blackberries,** 1 cup	1 (2)
Blanquette of veal, 2 cups	13
Blintz	
cheese, 1 (4 3/4 oz)	5
cheese, frozen, 1 (2 1/4 oz)	2
fruit, frozen, 1 (2 1/4 oz)	2
potato, frozen, 1 (2 1/4 oz)	2
Blood pudding (blood sausage), 1 oz	3
Bloody Mary, 1	2
Blueberries	
♦ 1 cup	1 (2)
canned, heavy syrup, 1 cup	4
♦ **Boar,** raw, 1 oz	1
Bok choy	
♦ raw, 1 cup	0
♦ raw, 1 head	1
Bologna	
beef or pork, 1 slice (1 oz)	2
turkey, 1 slice (1 oz)	1
Borscht	
1 cup with 2 Tbsp sour cream	4
♦ low-calorie, store-bought, 1 cup	0
♦ store-bought, 1 cup	2
Boston brown bread, 1 slice (3 3/4 x 1/2")	2
Boudin, store-bought, 2 oz	2
Bouillabaisse, 2 cups	7
Bouillon	
♦ any type except court, 1 cup	0
♦ court, 1 cup	3
♦ cube, beef, chicken, or vegetable, 1/2 cube	0
♦ granules, beef, 1 tsp	0
♦ **Boysenberries,** 1 cup	1 (2)

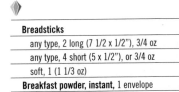

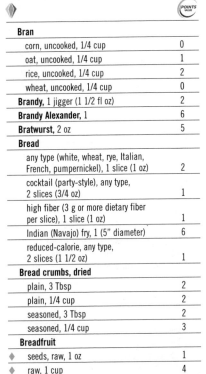

	POINTS VALUE
Bran	
corn, uncooked, 1/4 cup	0
oat, uncooked, 1/4 cup	1
rice, uncooked, 1/4 cup	2
wheat, uncooked, 1/4 cup	0
Brandy, 1 jigger (1 1/2 fl oz)	2
Brandy Alexander, 1	6
Bratwurst, 2 oz	5
Bread	
any type (white, wheat, rye, Italian, French, pumpernickel), 1 slice (1 oz)	2
cocktail (party-style), any type, 2 slices (3/4 oz)	1
high fiber (3 g or more dietary fiber per slice), 1 slice (1 oz)	1
Indian (Navajo) fry, 1 (5" diameter)	6
reduced-calorie, any type, 2 slices (1 1/2 oz)	1
Bread crumbs, dried	
plain, 3 Tbsp	2
plain, 1/4 cup	2
seasoned, 3 Tbsp	2
seasoned, 1/4 cup	3
Breadfruit	
◆ seeds, raw, 1 oz	1
◆ raw, 1 cup	4

	POINTS VALUE
Breadsticks	
any type, 2 long (7 1/2 x 1/2"), 3/4 oz	2
any type, 4 short (5 x 1/2"), or 3/4 oz	2
soft, 1 (1 1/3 oz)	2
Breakfast powder, instant, 1 envelope	3
Brioche, 1 slice (1 oz)	3
Broccoli rice casserole, 1 cup	5
Broccoli stir fry, 1 cup	3
Broccoli, cooked or raw, 1 cup	0
◆ **Broth, any type,** 1 cup	0
Broth, beef with tomato juice, 1 cup	2
Brownie	
1 (2" square)	5
fat-free, store-bought, 1 (1 1/2 oz)	2
low-fat, store-bought, 1 (1 1/2 oz)	3
Brunswick stew, 1 1/2 cups	5
Bruschetta, 1 slice (3 oz)	3
Brussels sprouts	
◆ cooked or raw, 1 cup	0
◆ frozen, cooked, 1 cup	1
◆ frozen, raw, 1 package (10 oz)	1
Bubble & squeak, 1 cup	3
◆ **Buckwheat,** 1 cup	11 (6)
Buffalo wings	
3 (4 1/2 oz)	9
frozen (prepared without fat), 3 (3 oz)	4
◆ **Buffalo, water,** cooked or raw, 1 oz	1 (5)

◆	POINTS VALUE
Bulgur	
◆ cooked, 1 cup	2 (6)
◆ uncooked, 1/4 cup	2 (6)
Burgoo, 1 cup	4
Burrito	
bean, 1 large (8")	8
bean, 1 small (6")	5
bean and cheese, reduced-fat, store-bought, 1 (5 1/2 oz)	5
bean and cheese, store-bought, 1	6
bean, fast food, 1	7
beef and bean, store-bought, 1 (5 oz)	8
beef and cheese, 1 large (8")	8
beef and cheese, 1 small (6")	5
beef or chicken and cheese, reduced-fat, store-bought, 1 small or 1/2 large (4 oz)	4
breakfast (egg, cheese and bacon, ham, or sausage), store-bought, 1 (3 1/2 oz)	5
chicken and cheese, 1 large (8")	7
chicken and cheese, 1 small (6")	5
chicken, store-bought, 1 (5 oz)	6
vegetable, 1 large (made with 10" tortilla)	10
vegetable, 1 small (made with 6" tortilla)	5
Butter	
light, 2 tsp	1
light, 1 Tbsp	2

◆	POINTS VALUE
regular, 1 tsp	1
regular, 1 cup	48
whipped, 1 tsp	1
whipped, 1 Tbsp	2
Butter chicken, 1 cup	8

C

Cabbage	
◆ all varieties, cooked or raw, 1 cup	0
stuffed, 2 (2 x 2 1/2")	6
Cajun seasoning, 1/4 tsp	0
Cake	
angel food, 1 slice (1/16 of 10" tube)	2
carrot, with cream cheese icing, 1/12 of 9" layer cake, or 3" square	16
fat-free, store-bought, 1 slice (3 1/2 oz)	4
pineapple upside-down, 2 1/2" square	5
pineapple upside-down, 1/8 of 10" skillet cake	10
pound, 1 slice (5" x 3" x 1")	8
snack, creme-filled, store-bought, 2 (2 1/4 oz)	6
sugar-free, store-bought, 1 slice (2 1/2 oz)	5
with icing, 1/12 of 9" layer cake or 3" square	12
with icing, store-bought, 3 oz	7
Cake mix, light, prepared, without icing, 1/12 of 9" cake	4

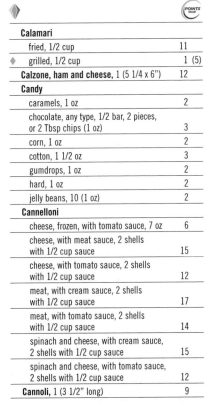

	POINTS VALUE
Calamari	
fried, 1/2 cup	11
◆ grilled, 1/2 cup	1 (5)
Calzone, ham and cheese, 1 (5 1/4 x 6")	12
Candy	
caramels, 1 oz	2
chocolate, any type, 1/2 bar, 2 pieces, or 2 Tbsp chips (1 oz)	3
corn, 1 oz	2
cotton, 1 1/2 oz	3
gumdrops, 1 oz	2
hard, 1 oz	2
jelly beans, 10 (1 oz)	2
Cannelloni	
cheese, frozen, with tomato sauce, 7 oz	6
cheese, with meat sauce, 2 shells with 1/2 cup sauce	15
cheese, with tomato sauce, 2 shells with 1/2 cup sauce	12
meat, with cream sauce, 2 shells with 1/2 cup sauce	17
meat, with tomato sauce, 2 shells with 1/2 cup sauce	14
spinach and cheese, with cream sauce, 2 shells with 1/2 cup sauce	15
spinach and cheese, with tomato sauce, 2 shells with 1/2 cup sauce	12
Cannoli, 1 (3 1/2" long)	9

	POINTS VALUE
Cantaloupe	
◆ 10 balls or 1 cup	1 (2)
◆ 1/4 large (6 1/2" diameter)	1 (2)
◆ 1 medium (5" diameter)	3 (2)
◆ 1 small	2 (2)
Capers, 1 Tbsp	0
Capon, cooked, with skin, without bone, 1 oz	2
Caponata (eggplant appetizer)	
1/4 cup	1
store-bought, 1/4 cup	2
Cappuccino	
◆ made with fat-free milk, 1 small (8 fl oz)	1
◆ made with fat-free milk, 1 tall (12 fl oz)	2
◆ made with fat-free milk, 1 grande (16 fl oz)	2
made with low-fat milk, 1 small (8 fl oz)	2
made with low-fat milk, 1 tall (12 fl oz)	3
made with low-fat milk, 1 grande (16 fl oz)	3
made with whole milk, 1 small (8 fl oz)	2
made with whole milk, 1 tall (12 fl oz)	3
made with whole milk, 1 grande (16 fl oz)	4
ready-made, from machine, any flavor, 1 cup	2
Cappuccino mix, any flavor, 4 tsp	2
Caraway seeds, 1 Tbsp	0
Cardamom, ground, 1 tsp	0

	POINTS VALUE
Cardoon, 1 cup	0
Caribou, cooked, 1 oz	1
Carne asada, 4 oz	10
Carne guisado (Cuban beef stew), 1 cup	5
Carnitas, 1 cup	9
Carob, without sugar, 1 tsp	0
Carrots	
cooked, 1 cup	1
raw, 1 cup, 1 large, or 10 baby	0
Carrots and parsnips, 1 cup	4
Casaba melon, 1 cup	1 (2)
Cashew butter, 1 Tbsp	2
Cashew chicken, 3 oz chicken with 1/3 cup sauce	7
Cashews, 14 (1 oz)	4
Cassava, raw, 1 cup	6
Cassoulet, 1 cup	11
Cauliflower, cooked or raw, 1 cup	0
Cavatelli with sausage & broccoli, 1 cup	5
Caviar (fish roe)	
any type, 1 oz	2 (5)
spread, store-bought, 2 Tbsp	3
Celeriac	
cooked, 1 cup	0
uncooked, 1 cup	1
Celery seed, 1 tsp	0
Celery, cooked or raw, 1 cup	0

	POINTS VALUE
Cereal bar	
fat-free, 1 (1 1/2 oz)	2
regular, 1 (1 1/4 oz)	3
Cereal, hot	
cream of rice, cooked, 1 cup	3
cream of wheat, cooked, 1 cup	2
farina, cooked, 1 cup	2
farina, uncooked, 1/4 cup	3
grits, corn, cooked, 1 cup	3
grits, corn, uncooked, 1/4 cup	3
grits, corn, yellow, quick, uncooked, 1 cup	11
in a cup, 1 (2 oz)	4
oatmeal, cooked, 1 cup	2
oatmeal, instant, flavored, 1 packet	3
oatmeal, instant, unflavored, 1 packet	2
oatmeal, uncooked, 1/4 cup	1
oatmeal, uncooked, 1 cup	5
whole wheat hot natural cereal, cooked, 1 cup	2
whole wheat hot natural cereal, uncooked, 1 cup	6
Cereal, granola	
1/2 cup	4
homemade, 1/2 cup	6
low-fat, 1/2 cup	3
Cereal, ready-to-eat	
any type other than those listed here, 1 cup	2

Food	POINTS VALUE
bran flakes, 3/4 cup	1
bran flakes, 1 cup	2
fortified, 1 cup	2
frosted, 1 cup	3
nuggets, 1/2 cup	3
puffed, 1 cup	1
raisin bran, 3/4 cup	2
raisin bran, 1 cup	3
shredded wheat, 1 biscuit	1
Ceviche, 1/2 cup	2
Challah bread, 1 slice (5" x 3" x 3/4")	2
Chalupa (pork & bean dish), 1 cup	6
Champagne, 1/2 cup	2
Chana dal, 1 cup	4
Channa masala, 1 cup	7
Chao tom (shrimp mousse over sugar cane), 4 pieces (1 1/2" each)	2
Chapati, 1 piece (5" diameter)	2
Char shiu bao (roast pork bun), 1 (2 oz)	4
Chard, Swiss, cooked or raw, 1 cup	0
Cheese ball, store-bought, 2 Tbsp	3
Cheese puffs, hot, 2 (1/2 oz each)	2
Cheese sandwich	
restaurant-type, grilled, 1 (4 oz)	13
with bacon, grilled, 1 (4 3/4 oz)	16
Cheese spread	
American, process, 2 Tbsp	2
pasteurized process, American, 1 oz	2

Food	POINTS VALUE
Cheese sticks, breaded, prepared without fat, store-bought, 2 (1 oz)	3
Cheese straws, 2 (2" long each)	2
Cheese twists or balls, 1 1/2 cups	4
Cheese, blue, 1/4 cup (crumbled)	3
Cheese, brie, 1 oz	3
Cheese, camembert, 1 wedge (1.33 oz)	3
Cheese, Cheddar	
1 slice (1 oz)	3
fat-free, shredded, 1/4 cup	1
fat-free, shredded, 1 Tbsp	0
Cheese, colby, 1 slice (1 oz)	3
Cheese, cottage	
fat-free, 1 cup	3
fat-free, with fruit, 1 cup	4
low-fat (1%), 1 cup	3
low-fat (1%), with fruit, 1 cup	5
reduced-fat (2%), 1 cup	4
regular (4%), 1 cup	5
regular, with fruit, 1 cup	6
Cheese, cream	
fat-free, 1/4 cup	1
fat-free, 8 oz	5
light, 1 Tbsp	1
regular, 1 Tbsp	1
regular, 8 oz	22
soy, 2 Tbsp	2
whipped, 1 Tbsp	1

	POINTS VALUE
Cheese, feta, 1/4 cup (crumbled) or 1 1/3 oz	3
Cheese, fontina	
1 cup diced	14
1 cup shredded	11
1 slice (1 oz)	3
Cheese, goat	
hard type, 1 oz	3
semisoft type, 1 cup	12
semisoft type, 1 oz	3
semisoft type, 1 Tbsp	1
soft type, 1 oz	2
soft type, 1 Tbsp	1
Cheese, gorgonzola, 1 oz	3
Cheese, gouda, 1 oz	3
Cheese, gruyere, 1 oz	3
Cheese, hard or semisoft, fat-free	
◆ 1 cube (1"), 3 Tbsp grated, or 4 Tbsp shredded (1 oz)	1
◆ 1 slice (3/4 oz)	1
Cheese, hard or semisoft, low-fat	
1 cube (1"), 3 Tbsp grated, or 4 Tbsp shredded (1 oz)	2
1 slice (3/4 oz)	1
Cheese, hard or semisoft, regular (except soy)	
1 cube (1"), 3 Tbsp grated, or 4 Tbsp shredded (1 oz)	3
1 slice (3/4 oz)	2
Cheese, havarti, 1 oz	3

	POINTS VALUE
Cheese, Mexican	
queso anejo, 1 cup (crumbled)	13
queso asadero, 1 cup (shredded)	11
queso chihuahua, 1 cup (shredded)	11
Cheese, Monterey, 1 slice (1 oz)	3
Cheese, mozzarella	
◆ fat-free, shredded, 1 Tbsp	0
◆ fat-free, shredded, 1/4 cup	1
part skim, 1 oz	2
whole milk, 1 cup shredded	8
Cheese, muenster, 1 slice (1 oz)	3
Cheese, Neufchatel, 1 Tbsp (1/2 oz)	1
Cheese, Parmesan	
2 Tbsp grated	1
1/4 cup grated	3
1 cup grated	12
1 oz	3
Cheese, pasteurized process, Swiss, 1 oz	2
◆ **Cheese, pot,** 1 cup	3
Cheese, provolone, 1 slice (1 oz)	3
Cheese, ricotta	
◆ fat-free, 1/2 cup	2
part-skim, 1/2 cup	4
whole milk, 1/2 cup	6
whole milk, 1 cup	11
Cheese, Romano, 1 oz	3
Cheese, Roquefort, 1 oz	3
Cheese, Swiss, 1 cup shredded	11

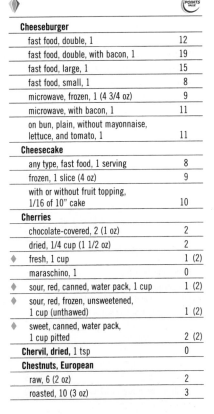

	POINTS VALUE
Cheeseburger	
fast food, double, 1	12
fast food, double, with bacon, 1	19
fast food, large, 1	15
fast food, small, 1	8
microwave, frozen, 1 (4 3/4 oz)	9
microwave, with bacon, 1	11
on bun, plain, without mayonnaise, lettuce, and tomato, 1	11
Cheesecake	
any type, fast food, 1 serving	8
frozen, 1 slice (4 oz)	9
with or without fruit topping, 1/16 of 10" cake	10
Cherries	
chocolate-covered, 2 (1 oz)	2
dried, 1/4 cup (1 1/2 oz)	2
fresh, 1 cup	1 (2)
maraschino, 1	0
sour, red, canned, water pack, 1 cup	1 (2)
sour, red, frozen, unsweetened, 1 cup (unthawed)	1 (2)
sweet, canned, water pack, 1 cup pitted	2 (2)
Chervil, dried, 1 tsp	0
Chestnuts, European	
raw, 6 (2 oz)	2
roasted, 10 (3 oz)	3

	POINTS VALUE
Chicken a la king, 1 cup	12
Chicken adobo, 1 thigh (4 oz)	6
Chicken and broccoli, 1 cup	2
Chicken and dumplings	
canned, 1 cup	5
cooked, with skin, 3 oz chicken with 2 dumplings	8
cooked, without skin, 3 oz chicken with 2 dumplings	7
frozen, 1 cup	7
Chicken and meatball fricassee, 2 cups	9
Chicken asopao, 1 cup with 1 piece chicken	8
Chicken back, without skin and bone, roasted or stewed, 1/2 back	2 (5)
Chicken breast	
barbecued, with skin and bone, 1 (4 1/2 oz)	6
cooked, without skin and bone, 1 cup chopped or diced	5 (5)
cooked, without skin and bone, 1 (3 oz)	3 (5)
cooked, without skin (with bone), 1 (4 1/2 oz)	3 (5)
cooked, with skin, without bone, 1 (3 oz)	4
cooked, with skin and bone, 1 (4 1/2 oz)	5
fillet, breaded, frozen, prepared without fat, 3 oz	4
fillet, grilled, 1 (3 oz)	3 (5)
five spice, with skin and bone, 1 (4 1/2 oz)	7

15

COMPLETE A-Z FOOD LIST

	POINTS VALUE
Chicken breast (con't)	
fried, with skin and bone, 1 (4 1/2 oz)	11
fried, with skin, without bone, 1	10
frozen, stuffed with long grain and wild rice, 1 (6 oz)	8
grilled, on bun, 1	9
patty, breaded, fat-free, prepared without fat, 1 (2 1/2 oz)	2
raw, without skin and bone, 1/2 breast (4 oz)	3 (5)
stuffed with vegetables and cheese, frozen, 1 (6 oz)	8
Chicken cacciatore, 1/2 breast or 1 thigh and leg (6 1/2 oz)	10
Chicken cordon bleu	
1 piece (5 1/2 oz)	13
frozen, 1 (6 1/4 oz)	10
Chicken cutlet, pan-fried, 4 oz	7
Chicken drumstick	
barbecued, with skin and bone, 1 (1 1/2 oz)	2
cooked, with skin and bone, 1 (1 1/2 oz)	2
cooked, without skin and bone, 1 (1 oz)	1 (5)
cooked, without skin (with bone), 1 (1 1/2 oz)	1 (5)
fried, with skin and bone, 1 (1 1/2 oz)	5
fried, with skin, fast food, 1	4
stewed, without skin and bone, 1	2
Chicken giblets, cooked, 1/2 cup chopped or diced	3 (5)

	POINTS VALUE
Chicken gizzard, cooked, 1 oz	1 (5)
Chicken heart, cooked, 1 oz	1 (5)
Chicken hekka, 1 cup	6
Chicken in barbecue sauce, frozen, 1/4 cup	3
Chicken in the pot, without skin, 2 cups	10
Chicken jalfrezi, 1 cup	6
Chicken Kiev	
1 (4 x 8")	18
frozen, 1 (6 oz)	13
Chicken leg	
five spice, 1 leg (thigh and drumstick, with skin and bone)	9
roasted, without skin and bone, 1 leg	4
roasted, with skin and bone, 1 leg	4
stewed, without skin and bone, 1 leg	4
Chicken liver, cooked, 1/2 cup (2 oz)	2 (5)
Chicken marsala, 4 oz chicken without bone, with sauce	15
Chicken mole, 1 cup	8
Chicken neck, simmered, without skin and bone, 1/2 neck	1 (5)
Chicken paprika, 1 breast or thigh with 1/2 cup sauce	7
Chicken parmigiana	
patty, store-bought, 1 patty with sauce (5 oz)	6
without sauce, 5 1/2 oz	8
with sauce, 5 oz with 1/2 cup sauce	10

Food	POINTS VALUE
Chicken patty, fried, frozen, 1 (2 1/2 oz)	4
Chicken pilaf (Kotta pilafi)	
1 cup	8
1 chicken breast with 1 cup pilaf	11
Chicken salad sandwich	
on reduced-calorie bread, 1 (5 1/4 oz)	8
on regular bread, 1 (5 1/4 oz)	9
Chicken sandwich, grilled, fast food, 1	7
Chicken sausage, cooked, 1 1/2 oz	2
Chicken stew, canned, 1 cup	4
Chicken stir-fry	
prepared without fat, 1 cup	3
with garlic or black bean sauce, 1 cup	7
Chicken subgum chow mein, 1 cup	4
Chicken tetrazzini, 1 1/2 cups	14
Chicken thigh	
barbecued, with skin and bone, 1 (1 oz)	5
cooked, with skin and bone, 1 (3 oz)	4
cooked, with skin, without bone, 1 (2 oz)	4
◆ cooked, without skin and bone, 1 (2 oz)	3 (5)
◆ cooked, without skin (with bone), 1 (3 oz)	3 (5)
fried, with skin and bone, 1 (3 oz)	7
fried, with skin, fast food, 1	8
◆ stewed, without skin and bone, 1 (2.4 oz)	3
Chicken tikka, 4 oz	5
Chicken wing	
cooked, with skin and bone, 1 (1 1/2 oz)	3
fried, with skin, fast food, 1	6
◆ raw, without skin, 1 (1 1/2 oz)	1 (5)

Food	POINTS VALUE
◆ roasted, without skin and bone, 1 (1 1/2 oz)	1
◆ stewed, without skin and bone, 1 (1 1/2 oz)	1
Chicken with cashews, 1 cup	9
Chicken, blackened, 1 breast (3 oz)	7
Chicken, broiler or fryer	
roasted, with skin (without bone), 1/2 (10 1/2 oz)	18
◆ roasted, without skin and bone, 1/2 (8 1/2 oz)	11 (5)
Chicken, canned, 1/2 cup (4 oz)	4 (5)
Chicken, dark meat	
◆ cooked, without skin and bone, 1/2 cup cubed or shredded	3 (5)
◆ cooked, without skin and bone, 1 slice (2 oz)	3 (5)
◆ raw, without skin and bone, 1 pound	15 (5)
◆ roasted, without skin and bone, 1/2 chicken (6.4 oz)	7 (5)
Chicken, fried	
frozen, 3 oz	7
skinless, frozen, 3 oz	5
Chicken, ground	
◆ 93% lean/7% fat, cooked, 3 oz	4 (5)
◆ 93% lean/7% fat, raw, 4 oz	4 (5)
◆ breast, raw, 4 oz	3 (5)
◆ cooked, 1/2 cup	3 (5)
◆ cooked, 1 patty (3 oz)	5 (5)

17

Chicken, ground (con't) — POINTS VALUE

cooked, 12 oz (1 pound raw)	20 (5)
cooked, 1 pound	26 (5)
raw, 4 oz	5
Chicken, light meat	
cooked, without skin and bone, 1 slice (2 oz)	2 (5)
cooked, without skin and bone, 1/2 cup cubed or shredded	2 (5)
roasted, without skin and bone, 1 cup chopped or diced	5 (5)
cooked, without skin and bone, 12 oz (1 pound raw)	12 (5)
Chicken, roasted, without skin and bone, 1 cup chopped or diced	6
Chicken, stewed, without skin and bone, 1 cup	6
Chicken, nugget-style, fried, 6 pieces (2 x 3/4" each)	8
fried, fast food, 6	8
pieces, frozen, 6 (2 x 3/4" each)	6
pieces, frozen, fat-free, 3 (3 oz)	2
Chicken, sesame, 1 cup	9
Chicken, sweet and sour, 1 cup	10
Chicory (curly endive), 1 cup	0
Chicory roots, raw, 1 root	1
Chicory, witloof, raw, 1/2 cup	0
Chiffon pie, 1/8 of 9" one-crust pie	9
Chile beef (Neua pad prik), 1 cup	6

	POINTS VALUE
Chili	
bean, in a cup, 1 (2 oz)	3
low-fat, canned, 1 cup	5
turkey, with beans, canned, 1 cup	4
turkey, without beans, canned, 1 cup	3
vegetarian, low-fat or fat-free, canned, 1 cup	3
with beans, canned, 1 cup	6
without beans, canned, 1 cup	11
without beans, frozen, 1 cup	12
Chili con carne	
with beans, 1 cup	8
without beans, 1 cup	8
Chili con queso	
1/4 cup	5
canned, 1/4 cup	2
frozen, 1/4 cup	5
Chili dog on roll, 1	10
Chili fish (Macher jhol), 1 fillet (6 oz)	12
Chili mac, canned, 1 cup	5
Chili powder, 1 tsp	0
Chili rellenos, beef and cheese, without sauce, 2	18
Chilies, chopped green, 1/2 cup	0
Chimichanga	
beef, 1 (3 x 3 1/2")	11
beef or chicken, with beans, frozen, 1 (6 1/2 oz)	8
chicken, 1 (3 x 3 1/2")	9

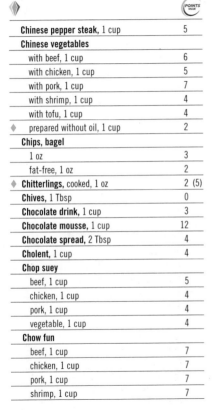

	POINTS VALUE
Chinese pepper steak, 1 cup	5
Chinese vegetables	
with beef, 1 cup	6
with chicken, 1 cup	5
with pork, 1 cup	7
with shrimp, 1 cup	4
with tofu, 1 cup	4
prepared without oil, 1 cup	2
Chips, bagel	
1 oz	3
fat-free, 1 oz	2
Chitterlings, cooked, 1 oz	2 (5)
Chives, 1 Tbsp	0
Chocolate drink, 1 cup	3
Chocolate mousse, 1 cup	12
Chocolate spread, 2 Tbsp	4
Cholent, 1 cup	4
Chop suey	
beef, 1 cup	5
chicken, 1 cup	4
pork, 1 cup	4
vegetable, 1 cup	4
Chow fun	
beef, 1 cup	7
chicken, 1 cup	7
pork, 1 cup	7
shrimp, 1 cup	7

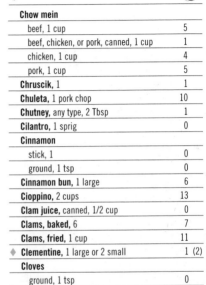

	POINTS VALUE
Chow mein	
beef, 1 cup	5
beef, chicken, or pork, canned, 1 cup	1
chicken, 1 cup	4
pork, 1 cup	5
Chruscik, 1	1
Chuleta, 1 pork chop	10
Chutney, any type, 2 Tbsp	1
Cilantro, 1 sprig	0
Cinnamon	
stick, 1	0
ground, 1 tsp	0
Cinnamon bun, 1 large	6
Cioppino, 2 cups	13
Clam juice, canned, 1/2 cup	0
Clams, baked, 6	7
Clams, fried, 1 cup	11
Clementine, 1 large or 2 small	1 (2)
Cloves	
ground, 1 tsp	0
whole, 1 Tbsp	0
Club sandwich, 1 (8 3/4 oz)	15
Club soda, 1 can or bottle (12 fl oz)	0
Cobbler, fruit,	
any type, 1 cup	10
frozen, 4 1/2 oz	6

COMPLETE A-Z FOOD LIST

	POINTS VALUE
Cocoa, hot, instant	
fat-free, sugar-free, 1 envelope (17 g)	1
fat-free, sugar-free, 1 Tbsp	0
fat-free, sugar-free, prepared, 6 fl oz	1
regular, prepared, 6 fl oz (1 oz packet with 6 fl oz water)	2
Cocoa, unsweetened, 3 Tbsp	0
Coconut cream, canned, 1/4 cup	15
Coconut custard pie, 1/8 of 9" one-crust pie	9
Coconut meat	
dried, without sugar, 1 oz	4
raw, 1 cup shredded	7
Coconut milk	
canned, 1/4 cup	3
light, 1/4 cup	1
Coconut rice	
Indian, 1 cup	5
Thai, 1 cup	8
Coconut shrimp, 4 jumbo	16
Coconut, packaged, shredded	
1 tsp	0
1 cup	8
Coffee	
black, without sugar, 1 cup	0
decaffeinated, black, without sugar, 1 cup	0

	POINTS VALUE
espresso, brewed, 1 fl oz	0
instant, decaffeinated, 1 tsp (rounded)	0
instant, decaffeinated, prepared with water, 1 cup	0
instant, regular, powder, 1 tsp dry	0
regular, prepared with water, 6 fl oz	0
Coffee cake	
3" square, or 1/12 of 9" tube	8
fat-free, store-bought, 2 oz	3
store-bought, 2 oz	6
Coffee drink	
Jamaican, store-bought, 1 cup	2
with milk, canned, 1	4
Coffee mix, flavored, sugar-free or with sugar, prepared, 1 cup	1
Coffee substitute or cereal beverage	
powder, 1 tsp	0
prepared with water, 1 cup	0
Cognac, 1 jigger (1 1/2 fl oz)	2
Colcannon, 1 cup	7
Coleslaw	
1/2 cup	4
◆ mix (shredded cabbage and carrots), packaged, 1 cup	0
◆ **Collards,** cooked or raw, 1 cup	0
Conch, cracked, 1 (6" long x 3")	9

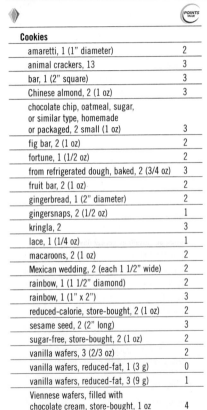

	POINTS VALUE
Cookies	
amaretti, 1 (1" diameter)	2
animal crackers, 13	3
bar, 1 (2" square)	3
Chinese almond, 2 (1 oz)	3
chocolate chip, oatmeal, sugar, or similar type, homemade or packaged, 2 small (1 oz)	3
fig bar, 2 (1 oz)	2
fortune, 1 (1/2 oz)	2
from refrigerated dough, baked, 2 (3/4 oz)	3
fruit bar, 2 (1 oz)	2
gingerbread, 1 (2" diameter)	2
gingersnaps, 2 (1/2 oz)	1
kringla, 2	3
lace, 1 (1/4 oz)	1
macaroons, 2 (1 oz)	2
Mexican wedding, 2 (each 1 1/2" wide)	2
rainbow, 1 (1 1/2" diamond)	2
rainbow, 1 (1" x 2")	3
reduced-calorie, store-bought, 2 (1 oz)	2
sesame seed, 2 (2" long)	3
sugar-free, store-bought, 2 (1 oz)	2
vanilla wafers, 3 (2/3 oz)	2
vanilla wafers, reduced-fat, 1 (3 g)	0
vanilla wafers, reduced-fat, 3 (9 g)	1
Viennese wafers, filled with chocolate cream, store-bought, 1 oz	4

	POINTS VALUE
Cooking spray, all varieties, 5 sprays	0
Coq au vin, 2 cups	13
Coquilles St. Jacques, 2 shells (13 2/3 oz)	8
Coriander	
leaf or seed, dried, 1 tsp	0
raw, 1/4 cup	0
Corn	
baby (ears), 1 cup	1 (6)
breaded, prepared without fat, 6 (3 oz)	4
cream-style, 1 cup	3
kernels, cooked, 1 cup	2 (6)
Corn cake, sweet, 1/2 cup	8
Corn casserole, 1/2 cup	8
Corn chips, 1 oz (10 large or 30 small)	4
Corn dog, 1 (2 3/4 oz)	5
Corn flake crumbs, 1/2 cup	3
Corn nuts, 1/2 cup	4
Corn on the cob	
1 large (8")	2 (6)
1 medium (7")	1 (6)
1 small (5 1/2")	1 (6)
Corn on the grill, with butter, 1	4
Corn pudding, home-prepared, 1 cup	7
Cornbread	
1 piece (2" square)	3
Mexican, 1 piece (1/12 of 10" round or 3 1/3 oz)	7
dressing, 1 cup	8

21

	POINTS VALUE
Corned beef, canned, 1 slice (2 oz)	4
Cornish hen	
cooked, with skin, 1/2 (4 1/2 oz)	9
cooked, without skin, 1/2 (3 3/4 oz)	3 (5)
Cornmeal	
cooked, 1 cup	2 (6)
dry, 1 tsp	0 (6)
dry, 2 Tbsp	1 (6)
dry, 1 cup	8 (6)
mix, self-rising, 2 Tbsp (3/4 oz)	1 (6)
yellow, dry, 1 cup	9 (6)
Cornstarch	
2 Tbsp	1
1 cup	10
Cosmopolitan, 1	4
Couscous (semolina)	
cooked, 1 cup	3
in a cup, 1 (2 oz)	4
uncooked, 1/4 cup	3
Couscous, whole-wheat	
cooked, 1 cup	3 (6)
uncooked, 1 tsp	0 (6)
uncooked, 1 Tbsp	1 (6)
uncooked, 1/4 cup	3 (6)
Cowpeas	
cooked, 1/2 cup	1 (5)
cooked, 1 cup	3 (5)
uncooked, 1 cup	11 (5)

	POINTS VALUE
Crab cakes, 2 (2 1/4 oz each, or 3" round)	4
Crab puffs, 6 (1 1/2" rounds)	5
Crab Rangoon	
1 large (4 1/2") or 5 mini	5
frozen, 8 (5 1/4 oz)	11
Crab, deviled, 1/2 cup	4
Crabapple, 1 cup (slices)	2 (2)
Cracker meal, 1/4 cup	2
Crackers	
any type (other than those listed here), 1 oz	3
cheese squares, mini, reduced-fat, 1 oz	3
cheese squares, mini, regular, 1 oz	3
fat-free, 7 (3/4 oz)	1
graham, 2 small (2 1/2" square)	1
graham, chocolate-coated, 2 (2 1/2" square)	3
graham, mini, any variety, 3/4 oz	2
oyster, 1 cup	4
saltines, 4	1
saltines, 6	2
snack, 1 oz	3
snack, with filling (cheese, wheat, rye, toast, or wafer crackers with cheese, peanut butter, or cream cheese filling), 6 (1 1/2 oz)	5
Cranberries	
dried, 1/4 cup	2
fresh, 1 1/2 cups (5 oz)	1 (2)

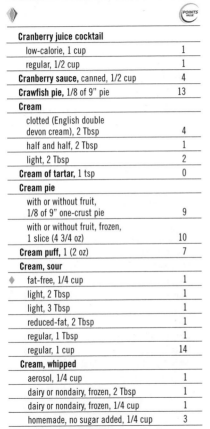

	POINTS VALUE
Cranberry juice cocktail	
low-calorie, 1 cup	1
regular, 1/2 cup	1
Cranberry sauce, canned, 1/2 cup	4
Crawfish pie, 1/8 of 9" pie	13
Cream	
clotted (English double devon cream), 2 Tbsp	4
half and half, 2 Tbsp	1
light, 2 Tbsp	2
Cream of tartar, 1 tsp	0
Cream pie	
with or without fruit, 1/8 of 9" one-crust pie	9
with or without fruit, frozen, 1 slice (4 3/4 oz)	10
Cream puff, 1 (2 oz)	7
Cream, sour	
♦ fat-free, 1/4 cup	1
light, 2 Tbsp	1
light, 3 Tbsp	1
reduced-fat, 2 Tbsp	1
regular, 1 Tbsp	1
regular, 1 cup	14
Cream, whipped	
aerosol, 1/4 cup	1
dairy or nondairy, frozen, 2 Tbsp	1
dairy or nondairy, frozen, 1/4 cup	1
homemade, no sugar added, 1/4 cup	3

	POINTS VALUE
Cream, whipping	
heavy, 2 Tbsp	3
heavy, 1/2 cup	12
light, 2 Tbsp	3
Creamed chipped beef, 1 cup	11
Creamed chipped chicken, 1 cup	11
Creamed chipped turkey, 1 cup	11
Creamer	
fat-free, 1 Tbsp	0
fat-free, 1/4 cup	1
fat-free, liquid, flavored, 2 Tbsp	1
nondairy, liquid, 2 Tbsp	1
nondairy, powder, 1 Tbsp	1
Creme brulee, 3/4 cup	11
Creme caramel, 1 cup	7
Creme fraiche, 2 Tbsp	3
Creole seasoning, 1/4 tsp	0
Creole	
chicken, without rice, 1 cup	6
shrimp, store-bought, 1 cup	5
shrimp, without rice, 1 cup	4
Crepes	
1 (6" diameter)	2
chicken, 2 (10 1/2 oz)	12
seafood, 2 (11 oz)	11
Suzette, 2 (4 3/4 oz)	10
♦ **Cress, garden,** cooked or raw, 1 cup	1

	POINTS VALUE
Crispbreads	
1 (3/4 oz)	1
5 thin (3/4 oz)	1
Croissant	
chocolate filled, 1 (5" long)	6
plain, 1 (5" long)	5
Croque monsieur, 1 (6 1/2 oz)	11
Croquettes	
beef, 2 (2 1/2 oz each)	10
chicken, 2 (2 1/2 oz each)	9
Croutons	
homemade, 1/2 cup	3
packaged, fat-free, 1/2 cup	2
packaged, regular, 1/2 cup	3
Cruller	
1	6
French, glazed, 1 (3" diameter)	4
glazed, 1 (4" diameter)	6
glazed, 1 long (approximately 5 1/4 x 2 1/2 x 1 1/2" high)	9
Crumbs, graham cracker, 2 Tbsp (1/2 oz)	1
Crumpet, 1 (3" diameter)	3
Cuban sandwich, 1/2 (6 1/2" x 3" x 4")	11
Cucumber	
1 cup	0
English, 1/2 cup	0
English, 1 medium	1

	POINTS VALUE
Cumin seeds, 1 tsp	0
Cupcake, creme-filled, store-bought, 1 (1 3/4 oz)	4
Currants	
dried, 1/4 cup (1 1/2 oz)	2
fresh, 1 cup	1 (2)
fresh, 1 1/2 cups	1 (2)
Curry	
African, fish, 1/2 cup	6
African, shrimp, 1/2 cup	6
beef, 1 cup	10
Bengali fish, 1 fillet (4 1/2 oz) and 1 cup vegetables	10
chicken, 1 cup	10
green chicken (Gaeng Kheow Wan Gai), 1 cup	7
lamb, 1 cup	10
Curry goat, 4 oz	5
Curry paste	
green, 1/4 cup	1
panang, 1/4 cup	1
red, 1/4 cup	1
Curry powder, 1 tsp	0
Custard, 1 cup	8
Custard pie, 1/8 of 9" one-crust pie	8

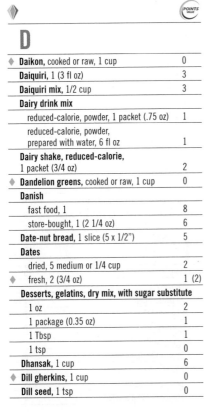

	POINTS VALUE
D	
◆ **Daikon,** cooked or raw, 1 cup	0
Daiquiri, 1 (3 fl oz)	3
Daiquiri mix, 1/2 cup	3
Dairy drink mix	
reduced-calorie, powder, 1 packet (.75 oz)	1
reduced-calorie, powder, prepared with water, 6 fl oz	1
Dairy shake, reduced-calorie, 1 packet (3/4 oz)	2
◆ **Dandelion greens,** cooked or raw, 1 cup	0
Danish	
fast food, 1	8
store-bought, 1 (2 1/4 oz)	6
Date-nut bread, 1 slice (5 x 1/2")	5
Dates	
dried, 5 medium or 1/4 cup	2
◆ fresh, 2 (3/4 oz)	1 (2)
Desserts, gelatins, dry mix, with sugar substitute	
1 oz	2
1 package (0.35 oz)	1
1 Tbsp	1
1 tsp	0
Dhansak, 1 cup	6
◆ **Dill gherkins,** 1 cup	0
Dill seed, 1 tsp	0

	POINTS VALUE
Dill	
fresh, 1 cup	0
weed, dried, 1 tsp	0
weed, fresh, 1 cup	0
Dim sum	
bean curd roll with shrimp and vegetables, 1 (5" long x 2" wide)	2
bean curd roll with vegetables, 1 (5" long x 1.5" wide)	2
sesame seed balls, 1 (3" x 3")	5
Dip	
any type other than those listed here, 2 Tbsp	2
artichoke, baked, 1/4 cup	6
◆ bean, fat-free, 1/2 cup	1
◆ black bean, fat-free, 2 Tbsp	0
spinach, 1/4 cup	5
Dolma	
4 (3 1/2 oz)	4
store-bought, 4 (3 1/2 oz)	3
Donair, 4 oz meat with onion, tomato and 2 Tbsp sauce	14
Donair sauce, 2 Tbsp	2
Doro wat, 1 cup	7
Doughnut	
any type other than those listed here, store-bought, 1 (2 oz)	5
cake-type, 1 (3 1/2" diameter)	6

Doughnut (con't) — POINTS VALUE

cake-type, with icing, 1 (3 1/2" diameter)	7
holes, yeast, glazed, 2 (1 oz)	3
mini, chocolate-covered, store-bought, 3-4 doughnuts (2 oz)	7
mini, powdered, sugar-covered, store-bought, 3-4 doughnuts (2 oz)	6
with creme filling, 1 (3 1/2 x 2 1/2" oval)	8
yeast, glazed, 1 (4" diameter)	6
yeast, with jelly filling, 1 (3 1/2 x 2 1/2" oval)	7
Dressing, salad, creamy	
fat-free, 2 Tbsp	1
reduced-calorie, reduced-fat, or light, 2 Tbsp	2
regular, 2 Tbsp	4
Dressing, salad, Italian-type (not creamy)	
fat-free, 2 Tbsp	0
reduced-calorie, reduced-fat, or light, 2 Tbsp	1
regular, 2 Tbsp	4
Dressing, salad, ginger, 2 Tbsp	2
Drink mix, fruit powdered, prepared, 1 cup (8 fl oz)	2
Duck a l'orange, 1/4 duck with 2 Tbsp sauce	13
Duck with fruit sauce, 1/4 duck with skin and 1/2 cup sauce	13

POINTS VALUE

Duck, domestic	
cooked, with skin, 1/4	13
◆ cooked, without skin, 1/4 (4 oz)	5
◆ cooked, without skin, 2 oz	3
Duck, tea smoked, 2 oz	3
Dumplings	
beef or pork, fried, 4 (6 1/2 oz)	6
beef or pork, steamed, 4 (5 3/4 oz)	6
chicken, fried, 4 (6 1/2 oz)	4
chicken, steamed, 4 (5 3/4 oz)	4
potato, 6 (1" diameter)	2
shrimp, fried, 4 (6 1/2 oz)	4
shrimp, steamed, 4 (5 3/4 oz)	4
vegetarian, fried, 4 (3 1/2" x 2" wide)	3
vegetarian, steamed, 4 (3 1/2" x 2" wide)	3

E

Eclair, 1	9
Edamame	
◆ in pods, 1 cup	1 (5)
◆ shelled, 1/2 cup	2 (5)
Egg curry, 1 cup	2
Egg foo yung	
beef, 1 (3" diameter)	4
chicken, 1 (3" diameter)	4
pork, 1 (3" diameter)	5
shrimp, 1 (3" diameter)	4

◈	POINTS VALUE
Egg roll snacks	
pork or shrimp, store-bought, 3 oz	3
vegetable, store-bought, 3 oz	3
Egg roll wrapper, 1	1
Egg roll	
beef, 1 (4 1/2" long)	5
chicken, 1 (4 1/2" long)	4
chicken, store-bought, 1	3
pork, 1 (4 1/2" long)	5
pork, store-bought, 1 (3 oz)	3
shrimp, 1 (4 1/2" long)	4
shrimp, store-bought, 1 (3 oz)	3
vegetable, store-bought, 1 (3 oz)	3
Egg salad sandwich, 1	11
Egg substitute	
◆ fat-free, 1/4 cup	1 (5)
◆ powder, 1/3 oz	1 (5)
◆ regular, 1/4 cup	2 (5)
Egg white, chicken	
◆ 1	0 (5)
◆ 3	1 (5)
Egg yolk, chicken	
◆ raw, 1	2 (5)
◆ yolk, raw, frozen, 1/2 pound	19 (5)
Egg, whole, chicken	
◆ 1, cooked or raw	2 (5)
deviled, 2 stuffed halves	4

◈	POINTS VALUE
fried, 1 large	2
hard-boiled, 1	2 (5)
poached, 1	2 (5)
scrambled, 2 or 1/2 cup	5
scrambled, fast food, 2	5
Egg, whole, other	
duck, raw, 1	3
goose, raw, 1	7
quail, raw, 1	0
turkey, raw, 1	3
Eggnog	
homemade, with liquor, 1/2 cup	4
reduced-calorie, store-bought (without liquor), 1/2 cup	3
store-bought (without liquor), 1/2 cup	5
Eggplant	
breaded and baked (without oil), 2 slices (3" diameter)	1
breaded and fried, 2 slices (3" diameter)	3
◆ cooked or raw, 1 cup	0
◆ small, medium, or large, 1	0
Eggplant parmesan, frozen, 5 oz	4
Eggplant parmigiana	
with sauce, 3" x 4" with 1/2 cup Italian tomato sauce	13
without sauce, 3" x 4"	11
Eggs Benedict, 2 English muffin halves with 2 eggs and 1/4 cup Hollandaise sauce	16

	POINTS VALUE
Eiderduck, 3 1/2 oz	2
♦ **Elderberries,** 1 cup	1 (2)
♦ **Elk,** cooked or raw, 1 oz	1 (5)
Empanadas, 2 (3" diameter)	5
Emu, cooked, 1 oz	1
Enchilada de camarones, 1 cup	5
Enchilada meal	
beef (2 enchiladas, beans & rice), 1 (11 1/2 oz)	7
cheese (2 enchiladas, beans & rice), 1 (11 1/2 oz)	7
chicken (2 enchiladas, beans & rice), 1 (11 1/2 oz)	7
Enchiladas	
beef, 2 (10 oz)	12
beef, cheese, or chicken, frozen, 1 (4 1/2 oz)	4
cheese, 2 (8 1/2 oz)	10
chicken, 2 (10 1/2 oz)	9
pork, 2 (10 1/2 oz)	12
sour cream, 1 (5 1/2 oz)	8
Endive	
♦ 1 cup	0
♦ head, 1	0
English muffin	
light, any type, 1 (2 oz)	1
regular, any type, 1 (2 oz)	2
Escargots, 6 snails with 2 Tbsp butter	7
♦ **Escarole,** 1 cup	0

	POINTS VALUE
Etouffee	
crawfish, 1 cup	8
crawfish or shrimp, store-bought, 1 cup	8
mix, 2 Tbsp	1
shrimp, 1 cup	9
Extract, any flavor	
1 Tbsp	1
1 tsp	0

F

	POINTS VALUE
Fadge, 1 piece (3 1/4 oz)	2
Fajitas	
beef, 2 (9 oz)	11
beef or chicken, kit, frozen, prepared, 2 (7 1/2 oz)	5
chicken, 2 (8 3/4 oz)	8
pork, 2 (10 1/2 oz)	13
shrimp, 2 (9 oz)	8
vegetarian, 1 (5 1/2 oz)	4
Falafel	
in pita, 1 large pita with 4 falafel patties	10
patties, 4 (2" diameter each)	7
patties, from mix, prepared, 2	4
Fattoush, 2 cups	5
Fennel	
♦ 1 cup	1
♦ bulb, raw, 1 cup	0

	POINTS VALUE
bulb, raw, 1 medium	1
seed, 1 tsp	0
Fettucine Alfredo	
1 cup	16
frozen, 1 cup	7
Fettucine with broccoli and chicken in Alfredo sauce, frozen, 1 cup	9
Fiddlefern (fiddlehead greens), 1 cup	0
Fiddlehead ferns, 1 cup	0
Figs	
canned, water pack, 1 cup	2 (2)
dried, 1	1
fresh, 1 large (2 1/2")	1 (2)
fresh, 2 medium (2 1/4")	1 (2)
Fillo dough, 1 1/2 sheets	2
Fish amandine, 1 fillet (6 oz)	13
Fish	
anchovies, canned in oil, drained, 6 (3/4 oz)	1
arctic char, cooked, 3 oz	4 (5)
arctic char, raw, 3 oz	3 (5)
bass, striped, cooked, 1 fillet (6 oz)	5 (5)
bluefish, cooked, 1 fillet (6 oz)	6 (5)
bluefish, raw, 1 fillet (8 oz)	6 (5)
burbot, cooked, 1 fillet (3 oz)	2 (5)
burbot, raw, 1 fillet (4 oz)	2 (5)
butterfish, cooked or raw, 1 fillet (3/4 oz)	1 (5)
carp, cooked, 1 fillet (6 oz)	7 (5)
carp, raw, 1 fillet (7 oz)	7 (5)

	POINTS VALUE
catfish, cooked, 1 fillet (6 oz)	6 (5)
catfish, raw, 1 fillet (8 oz)	8 (5)
cod, cooked, 1 fillet (6 oz)	4 (5)
cod, raw, 1 fillet (4 oz)	2 (5)
dried, 1 oz	2
eel, cooked, 1 oz	2 (5)
eel, raw, 1 fillet (7 oz)	9 (5)
flounder, cooked, 1 fillet (6 oz)	4 (5)
flounder, raw, 1 fillet (6 oz)	3 (5)
grouper, cooked, 1 fillet (6 oz)	4 (5)
grouper, raw, 1 fillet (8 oz)	4 (5)
haddock, cooked, 1 fillet (6 oz)	4 (5)
haddock, raw, 1 fillet (8 oz)	4 (5)
haddock, smoked, 1 oz (boneless)	1 (5)
halibut, cooked, 1 fillet or steak (6 oz)	5 (5)
halibut, raw, 1/2 fillet (7 oz)	5 (5)
herring, cooked, 1 oz	1 (5)
lox, 1 oz	1 (5)
mackerel, canned in water, 1/2 cup	3 (5)
mackerel, cooked, 1 fillet (6 oz)	8 (5)
mackerel, raw, 1 fillet (8 oz)	9 (5)
mahimahi (dolphinfish), cooked, 1 fillet (6 oz)	4 (5)
mahimahi (dolphinfish), raw, 1 fillet (8 oz)	4 (5)
milkfish, cooked, 3 oz	4 (5)
milkfish, raw, 3 oz	3 (5)
molee, 1 cup	11

Fish (con't)	POINTS VALUE
monkfish, cooked, 3 oz	2 (5)
monkfish, raw, 3 oz	1 (5)
mullet, striped, cooked, 1 fillet (3 oz)	3 (5)
mullet, striped, raw, 1 fillet (4 oz)	3 (5)
orange roughy, cooked, 3 oz	2 (5)
orange roughy, raw, 3 oz	1 (5)
perch, cooked, 1 fillet (6 oz)	4 (5)
perch, raw, 3 oz	2 (5)
pike, cooked, 1 fillet (6 oz)	4 (5)
pike, raw, 1 fillet (7 oz)	4 (5)
pollack, cooked, 1 fillet (6 oz)	4 (5)
pollack, raw, 3 oz	1 (5)
pompano, cooked, 1 fillet (6 oz)	9 (5)
pompano, raw, 3 oz	3 (5)
pout, ocean, cooked, 1/2 fillet (5 oz)	3 (5)
pout, ocean, raw, 1/2 fillet (6 oz)	3 (5)
rockfish, cooked, 1 fillet (6 oz)	4 (5)
rockfish, raw, 1 fillet (8 oz)	5 (5)
roe, cooked, 1 oz	1 (5)
roe, raw, 1 Tbsp	0 (5)
sablefish, cooked, 1/2 fillet (5 oz)	10 (5)
sablefish, raw, 1/2 fillet (7 oz)	10 (5)
sablefish, smoked, 1 oz	2 (5)
salmon, canned, drained, 1/2 cup	4 (5)
salmon, cooked, 1 fillet (6 oz)	9 (5)
salmon, raw, 1 fillet (7 oz)	9 (5)
salmon, smoked, 1 oz	1 (5)

	POINTS VALUE
sardines, canned in oil, drained, 5 (2 oz)	3
sardines, canned in tomato sauce, 1 can (13 oz)	17 (5)
sardines, canned in tomato sauce, 2 oz	3 (5)
sea bass, cooked, 1 fillet (3 1/2 oz)	3 (5)
sea bass, raw, 1 fillet (4 1/2 oz)	3 (5)
shad, cooked, 1 fillet (5 oz)	9 (5)
shad, raw, 1 fillet (6 1/2 oz)	9 (5)
skate, uncooked, 3 1/2 oz	2 (5)
smelt, cooked, 1 oz	1 (5)
smelt, raw, 3 oz	2 (5)
snapper, cooked, 1 fillet (6 oz)	5 (5)
snapper, raw, 1 fillet (7 3/4 oz)	5 (5)
sole, cooked, 1 fillet (6 oz)	4 (5)
sole, raw, 1 fillet (5 3/4 oz)	3 (5)
sturgeon, cooked, 1 piece (4 1/2 x 2 1/8 x 7/8")	5 (5)
sturgeon, raw, 3 oz	2 (5)
sturgeon, smoked, 1 oz	1 (5)
sunfish, pumpkin seed, cooked, 1 fillet (1 1/3 oz)	1 (5)
sunfish, pumpkin seed, raw, 1 fillet (1 3/4 oz)	1 (5)
surimi, 1 oz	1 (5)
swordfish, cooked, 1 fillet or steak (6 oz)	6 (5)
swordfish, raw, 1 fillet or steak (8 oz)	6 (5)
tilapia, cooked, 6 oz	4 (5)
tilapia, raw, 4 oz	2 (5)

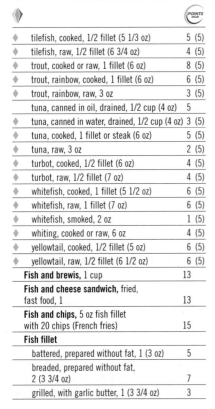

	POINTS VALUE
tilefish, cooked, 1/2 fillet (5 1/3 oz)	5 (5)
tilefish, raw, 1/2 fillet (6 3/4 oz)	4 (5)
trout, cooked or raw, 1 fillet (6 oz)	8 (5)
trout, rainbow, cooked, 1 fillet (6 oz)	6 (5)
trout, rainbow, raw, 3 oz	3 (5)
tuna, canned in oil, drained, 1/2 cup (4 oz)	5
tuna, canned in water, drained, 1/2 cup (4 oz)	3 (5)
tuna, cooked, 1 fillet or steak (6 oz)	5 (5)
tuna, raw, 3 oz	2 (5)
turbot, cooked, 1/2 fillet (6 oz)	4 (5)
turbot, raw, 1/2 fillet (7 oz)	4 (5)
whitefish, cooked, 1 fillet (5 1/2 oz)	6 (5)
whitefish, raw, 1 fillet (7 oz)	6 (5)
whitefish, smoked, 2 oz	1 (5)
whiting, cooked or raw, 6 oz	4 (5)
yellowtail, cooked, 1/2 fillet (5 oz)	6 (5)
yellowtail, raw, 1/2 fillet (6 1/2 oz)	6 (5)
Fish and brewis, 1 cup	13
Fish and cheese sandwich, fried, fast food, 1	13
Fish and chips, 5 oz fish fillet with 20 chips (French fries)	15
Fish fillet	
battered, prepared without fat, 1 (3 oz)	5
breaded, prepared without fat, 2 (3 3/4 oz)	7
grilled, with garlic butter, 1 (3 3/4 oz)	3

	POINTS VALUE
grilled, with lemon pepper, 1 (3 3/4 oz)	3
light, breaded, prepared without fat, 3 3/4 oz	3
Fish portions, from minced fish, breaded or battered, prepared without fat, 3 oz	5
Fish sticks, breaded, frozen, 4 (2 1/2 oz)	5
Fish Veronique, 1 fillet (6 oz)	11
Fish, baked, stuffed, 6 1/2 oz	8
Fish, blackened, 1 fillet (6 oz)	12
Fish, fried	
breaded with flour, 1 fillet (6 oz)	12
fried, without flour, 1 fillet (6 oz)	14
Fish, gefilte, 1 piece (1 1/2 oz)	1
Fish, stuffed, frozen, 1 (5 oz)	5
Fish, whitefish and pike	
large, store-bought, 1	2
small, store-bought, 2	2
Five-spice powder, 1 tsp	0
Flan, 3/4 cup	8
Flanken, 2 slices (4 oz)	8
Flatbreads, 3/4 oz	1
Flauta	
beef, 1 (6" x 1 1/4")	12
chicken, 1 (6" x 1 1/4")	10
pork, 1 (6" x 1 1/4")	11
Flax seed, 1 Tbsp	1

	POINTS VALUE
Flour	
potato, 1 tsp	0
potato, 2 Tbsp	1
soy, 2 Tbsp	1
soy, 1/4 cup	2
wheat, whole-grain, 1 tsp	0
wheat, whole-grain, 2 Tbsp	1
wheat, whole-grain, 1 cup	8
white, 1 tsp	0
white, 2 Tbsp	1
white, 1 cup	9
Focaccia bread, 1 piece (1/4 of 10" diameter)	6
Fondue, cheese, 1/2 cup fondue with 2 oz bread	12
Frankfurter	
on roll, plain, 1 (4 oz)	8
roll or bun, 1 (2 oz)	3
roll or bun, light, 1	1
beef or pork, fat-free, 1 (1 3/4 oz)	1
beef or pork, light, 1 (1 3/4 oz)	2
beef or pork, regular, 1 (2 oz)	5
beef or pork, with cheese, 1 (2 oz)	5
chicken, 1 (2 oz)	4
turkey, 1 (2 oz)	3
turkey, fat-free, 1 (1 1/2 oz)	1
turkey, light, 1 (2 oz)	3
Franks in blankets, frozen, 6 (3 oz)	9

	POINTS VALUE
French fries	
20 (4 1/2" long), 5 1/2 oz	10
fast food, 1 extra large serving	13
fast food, 1 large serving	10
fast food, 1 medium serving	6
frozen (prepared without fat), 15 (3 oz)	3
French toast	
2 slices (4 1/2 oz)	7
frozen, baked, 2 slices (4 oz)	5
French toast sticks	
fast food, 5 pieces	12
frozen, 3 (2 1/2 oz)	6
Fritters	
corn, 3 (2 1/2" x 2" each)	5
vegetable, 1 cup	10
Frog legs, fried, 2 (2 oz)	4
Fromage frais (soft cheese with fruit), 3 1/2 oz	3
Frosting, store-bought, reduced-fat or regular, 2 Tbsp	3
Fructose, high, corn syrup, 1 Tbsp	1
Fruit butter, 1 Tbsp	1
Fruit cocktail, canned, unsweetened, 1/2 cup	1
Fruit compote, 1/2 cup	3
Fruit juice bar, frozen, without sugar, 1	1
Fruit juice cup, frozen, 1 cup	3

	POINTS VALUE
Fruit spread, all spreadable fruit, 1 1/2 Tbsp	1
Fruit, candied, 2 Tbsp	1
Fruit, dried, mixed, 1/4 cup (1 1/2 oz)	1
Fruitcake, 1 slice (2 1/2" x 1 3/4" x 1/2"), or 2 oz	4
Fruit-flavored pieces, 1 package (1 oz)	2
Fruit-flavored roll	
1 large (3/4 oz)	1
1 small (1/2 oz)	1
Fudge, with or without nuts, 1 piece (1" x 2"), or 1 oz	3
Funnel cake, 1/2 (8" diameter)	12

G

	POINTS VALUE
Garam masala, 1/4 tsp	0
Garlic bread	
1 slice (1 1/2 oz)	5
garlic, frozen, 1 piece (1 1/2 oz)	4
Garlic herb seasoning, 2 tsp	0
Garlic powder, 1 tsp	0
Garlic salt, 1 tsp	0
Garlic, fresh	
1 bulb	2
1 clove	0
1 tsp	0

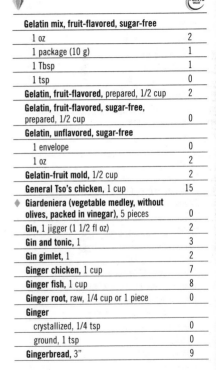

	POINTS VALUE
Gelatin mix, fruit-flavored, sugar-free	
1 oz	2
1 package (10 g)	1
1 Tbsp	1
1 tsp	0
Gelatin, fruit-flavored, prepared, 1/2 cup	2
Gelatin, fruit-flavored, sugar-free, prepared, 1/2 cup	0
Gelatin, unflavored, sugar-free	
1 envelope	0
1 oz	2
Gelatin-fruit mold, 1/2 cup	2
General Tso's chicken, 1 cup	15
♦ **Giardeniera (vegetable medley, without olives, packed in vinegar),** 5 pieces	0
Gin, 1 jigger (1 1/2 fl oz)	2
Gin and tonic, 1	3
Gin gimlet, 1	2
Ginger chicken, 1 cup	7
Ginger fish, 1 cup	8
Ginger root, raw, 1/4 cup or 1 piece	0
Ginger	
crystallized, 1/4 tsp	0
ground, 1 tsp	0
Gingerbread, 3"	9

	POINTS VALUE
Gnocchi	
any type, frozen, 1 cup	7
cheese, 1 cup	11
potato, 1 cup	4
potato, dry, 1 cup	3
potato, refrigerated, 1 cup	5
spinach, 1 cup	12
Goat masala, 1 cup	5
Goat, cooked, 1 oz	1
Gobo (burdock), 1/2 cup (2 oz)	1
Goose	
cooked, with skin, without bone, 2 oz	4
without skin and bone, 2 oz	3
Gooseberries, 1 cup	1 (2)
Gordita, beef, 1 (3" diameter)	10
Gosht shaha korma, 1 cup	14
Gourd, white, flowered, cooked or raw, 1 cup	1
Graham cracker crumbs, 2 Tbsp (1/2 oz)	1
Graham crackers, 2 (2 1/2" square)	1
Granola bar	
chocolate-covered, 1(1 1/4 oz)	4
other than chocolate-covered and reduced-calorie, 1 (1 oz)	3
reduced-calorie, 1 (1 oz)	2
Grape juice, 1/2 cup	2
Grape leaves, 1 cup	0

	POINTS VALUE
Grapefruit	
1 large (approximately 5" diameter)	2 (2)
1 medium (approximately 4" diameter)	1 (2)
1 small (approximately 3 1/2" diameter)	1 (2)
canned, water pack, 1 cup	2 (2)
sections, 1 cup	2 (2)
Grapefruit juice, 1/2 cup	1
Grapes, 1 cup	1 (2)
Gravy	
beef, canned, 1/4 cup	1
brown, 1/4 cup	2
chicken, canned, 1/4 cup	1
cream, 1/4 cup	4
fat-free, canned, 1/2 cup	1
giblet, 1/4 cup	2
sausage, 1/4 cup	4
sausage, canned, 1/4 cup	2
turkey, canned, 1 cup	1
Green bean casserole, 1 cup	5
Green rice, 1 cup	6
Greens, beet, collard, dandelion, kale, mustard, and turnip, cooked or raw, 1 cup	0
Grinder sandwich, 1 (6")	6
Grits, corn, yellow, quick, cooked, 1 cup	3
Guacamole, homemade or store-bought, 1/4 cup	2

	POINTS VALUE
Guava	
◆ 1 cup or 1 medium	1 (2)
◆ strawberry, raw, 1 cup	3 (2)
Guinea hen, cooked, 1 oz	1
Gum, chewing	
sugarless, 1 piece	0
with sugar, 1 piece	0
Gumbo	
base (seasoning mix), 1 1/2 Tbsp	1
chicken, 1 cup	6
seafood, 1 cup	5
seafood, with rice, store-bought, 1 cup	5
with rice mix, 1/4 cup	3
Gyoza, 3	3
Gyro, 1 (6")	15

H

	POINTS VALUE
Halvah	
1 piece (2" x 1 3/4" x 1")	5
store-bought, 1 1/2 oz	6
Ham	
◆ center slice, lean only, 4 oz	5
◆ cooked, lean, 1/2 cup (cubed or shredded) 2 oz	2
◆ cooked, lean, 1 slice (2 oz)	2
cooked, regular, 1 slice or 1/2 cup cubed or shredded (2 oz)	3

	POINTS VALUE
◆ extra lean (approximately 5% fat), roasted, 1 cup	5
glazed with pineapple, 4 oz ham with 1/2 pineapple slice	6
◆ lean only, roasted, 1 cup	5
Ham & cheese sandwich	
1 (4 oz)	9
restaurant-style, grilled, 1	15
Hamantaschen, 1 piece (3" diameter)	3
Hamburger	
large, fast food, 1	13
microwave, 1 small	3
on bun, plain (without mayonnaise, lettuce, and tomato), 1 (3 oz cooked hamburger on 1 1/2 oz bun)	9
roll or bun, 1 (2 oz)	3
roll or bun, light, 1 (1 1/2 oz)	1
small, fast food, 1	6
Hamburger dinner in a box, prepared, 1 cup	7
Haroset, 1/4 cup	1
Hash	
corned beef, canned, 1 cup	10
roast beef, canned, 1 cup	9
Haupia (coconut pudding), 2" square	3
◆ **Hearts of palm (palmetto),** 1 cup (5 oz)	0
Hero sandwich, 1 (6")	6

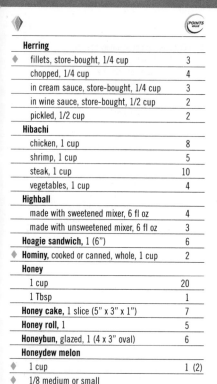

	POINTS VALUE
Herring	
♦ fillets, store-bought, 1/4 cup	3
chopped, 1/4 cup	4
in cream sauce, store-bought, 1/4 cup	3
in wine sauce, store-bought, 1/2 cup	2
pickled, 1/2 cup	2
Hibachi	
chicken, 1 cup	8
shrimp, 1 cup	5
steak, 1 cup	10
vegetables, 1 cup	4
Highball	
made with sweetened mixer, 6 fl oz	4
made with unsweetened mixer, 6 fl oz	3
Hoagie sandwich, 1 (6")	6
♦ **Hominy,** cooked or canned, whole, 1 cup	2
Honey	
1 cup	20
1 Tbsp	1
Honey cake, 1 slice (5" x 3" x 1")	7
Honey roll, 1	5
Honeybun, glazed, 1 (4 x 3" oval)	6
Honeydew melon	
♦ 1 cup	1 (2)
♦ 1/8 medium or small (5 1/4" to 7" diameter)	1 (2)

	POINTS VALUE
Horseradish tree	
♦ leaves, cooked or raw, 1 cup	0
♦ pods, cooked, 1 cup sliced	0
Hot chocolate, homemade	
with whipped topping, 1 cup	7
without whipped topping, 1 cup	6
Hot cross buns, 1	5
Hot dog	
beef or pork, fat-free, 1 (1 3/4 oz)	1
beef or pork, light, 1 (1 3/4 oz)	2
beef or pork, regular, 1 (2 oz)	5
beef or pork, with cheese, 1 (2 oz)	5
chicken, 1 (2 oz)	4
on roll, plain, 1 (4 oz)	8
roll or bun, 1 (2 oz)	3
turkey, 1 (2 oz)	3
turkey, fat-free, 1 (1 1/2 oz)	1
turkey, light, 1 (2 oz)	3
Huevos rancheros, 2 eggs on 2 tortillas	14
Huli huli chicken	
breast (with skin and bone), 1 (7 1/4 oz)	12
drumstick (with skin and bone), 1 (2 oz)	3
thigh (with skin and bone), 1 (3 oz)	5
Hummus	
1/4 cup	3
store-bought, 1/4 cup	2
Hunan beef, 1 cup	9
Hungarian goulash, 1 cup	8

	POINTS VALUE
Hush puppies	
2 (2 1/4 oz)	4
frozen (prepared without fat), 3	2
mix, 1/4 cup	3
I	
Ice cream	
fat-free, sweetened with sugar, 1 scoop or 1/2 cup	2
fat-free, without sugar, 1 scoop or 1/2 cup	2
fried, 1 scoop or 1/2 cup	11
green tea, 1 scoop or 1/2 cup	3
light, sweetened with sugar, 1 scoop or 1/2 cup	3
light, without sugar, 1 scoop or 1/2 cup	2
premium, 1 scoop or 1/2 cup	7
regular, 1 scoop or 1/2 cup	4
Ice cream bar	
chocolate-covered, 1 (3 oz)	5
chocolate-covered with crisp rice, with sugar, 1 (2 oz)	5
Ice cream cone, plain or sugar, 1 small	1
Ice cream soda, 12 fl oz	9
Ice cream sundae	
1 scoop (1/2 cup) ice cream with syrup, nuts, & whipped topping	8
cone, 1 (3 1/2 oz)	8

	POINTS VALUE
Ice cream sandwich	
1 (5" x 1 3/4" x 3/4")	3
reduced-calorie, 1 (3.3 fl oz)	3
Ice pop, fruit-flavored, 1 (1.75 fl oz)	1
Ices	
fruit, 1/2 cup	3
Italian, restaurant-prepared, 1/2 cup	1
water, fruit, reduced calorie, with aspartame, 1 bar	0
Imperial roll, 1 (4 1/2" long)	4
Instant breakfast	
powder, 1 envelope (1 1/4 oz)	3
prepared with 2% milk, 1 (10 fl oz)	5
prepared with fat-free milk, 1 (10 fl oz)	4
prepared with whole milk, 1 (10 fl oz)	6
Irish brown stew, 1 cup	7
Irish coffee, 6 fl oz with 2 Tbsp whipped cream	4
Irish soda bread, 1/12 of 8" round loaf	6
Italian casserole (ground beef, pasta & cheese over rolls)	
1 cup	14
1/8 of a 10" round casserole	16
Italian seasoning, 1 tsp	0
Italian toast snacks, store-bought, 4	3

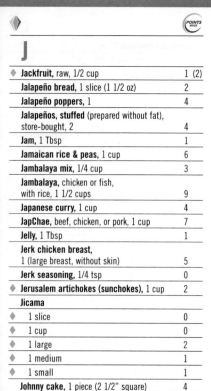

	POINTS VALUE
J	
Jackfruit, raw, 1/2 cup	1 (2)
Jalapeño bread, 1 slice (1 1/2 oz)	2
Jalapeño poppers, 1	4
Jalapeños, stuffed (prepared without fat), store-bought, 2	4
Jam, 1 Tbsp	1
Jamaican rice & peas, 1 cup	6
Jambalaya mix, 1/4 cup	3
Jambalaya, chicken or fish, with rice, 1 1/2 cups	9
Japanese curry, 1 cup	4
JapChae, beef, chicken, or pork, 1 cup	7
Jelly, 1 Tbsp	1
Jerk chicken breast, 1 (large breast, without skin)	5
Jerk seasoning, 1/4 tsp	0
Jerusalem artichokes (sunchokes), 1 cup	2
Jicama	
1 slice	0
1 cup	0
1 large	2
1 medium	1
1 small	1
Johnny cake, 1 piece (2 1/2" square)	4

	POINTS VALUE
Juice	
apple, 1/2 cup	1
carrot, canned, 1/2 cup	1
clam, canned, 1/2 cup	0
clam-tomato, 1 cup	2
coconut, 12 fl oz	3
cranberry cocktail, low-calorie, 1 cup	1
cranberry cocktail, regular, 1/2 cup	1
fruit (combined), 1/2 cup	1
grape, 1/2 cup	2
grapefruit, 1 cup	2
lemon, canned or bottled, 1 Tbsp	0
lemon, canned or bottled, 1 cup	1
lemon, fresh, 1 cup	0
lemon, frozen, unsweetened, single strength, 1 cup	1
lime, canned or bottled, unsweetened, 1 cup	1
lime, fresh, 1 Tbsp	0
lime, fresh, 1 cup	1
orange, 1/2 cup	1
orange-grapefruit, 1/2 cup	1
pineapple, 1/2 cup	1
prune, 1/2 cup	2
tangerine, 1/2 cup	1
tomato, canned, 1/2 cup	0
tomato, canned, 1 cup	1
vegetable, mixed, 1 cup	1

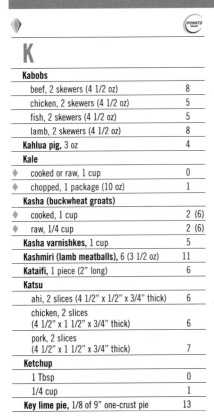

K

	POINTS VALUE
Kabobs	
beef, 2 skewers (4 1/2 oz)	8
chicken, 2 skewers (4 1/2 oz)	5
fish, 2 skewers (4 1/2 oz)	5
lamb, 2 skewers (4 1/2 oz)	8
Kahlua pig, 3 oz	4
Kale	
cooked or raw, 1 cup	0
chopped, 1 package (10 oz)	1
Kasha (buckwheat groats)	
cooked, 1 cup	2 (6)
raw, 1/4 cup	2 (6)
Kasha varnishkes, 1 cup	5
Kashmiri (lamb meatballs), 6 (3 1/2 oz)	11
Kataifi, 1 piece (2" long)	6
Katsu	
ahi, 2 slices (4 1/2" x 1/2" x 3/4" thick)	6
chicken, 2 slices (4 1/2" x 1 1/2" x 3/4" thick)	6
pork, 2 slices (4 1/2" x 1 1/2" x 3/4" thick)	7
Ketchup	
1 Tbsp	0
1/4 cup	1
Key lime pie, 1/8 of 9" one-crust pie	13

	POINTS VALUE
Khal bi, 4 oz	8
Kheer, 1/2 cup	6
Kho-phat (Thai fried rice), 1 cup	8
Kibbe	
baked, 3 pieces (1 1/2" squares)	3
uncooked, 1/2 cup	4
Kielbasa, 1 oz	2
Kim chee, 1/2 cup	0
King ranch chicken casserole, 1 cup	8
Kishke, 1 small piece (3/4 oz)	2
Kiwifruit	
1 cup	1 (2)
1 large (4 oz)	1 (2)
1 medium (2 1/2 oz)	0 (2)
Knish	
potato, 1 (3 1/2" square)	6
potato, store-bought, 1 (4 1/2 oz)	4
Knockwurst, 2 oz	5
Kofta (vegetable balls without sauce), 2	5
Kohlrabi	
cooked, 1 cup	1
raw, 1 cup	0
Kolache	
fruit-filled, 1 (3" diameter)	4
without filling, 1 (3" diameter)	4
Korean barbecue beef, 4 oz	7
Korean barbecue chicken thighs, 1 (5 oz)	12
Korean barbecue short ribs, 4 oz	8

	POINTS VALUE
Korma	
chicken, 1 cup	14
lamb, 1 cup	15
vegetable, 1 cup	11
Kreplach	
boiled, 2 pieces (4" x 3" x 3" each)	6
fried, 2 pieces (4" x 3" x 3" each)	7
Kugel	
lukschen, with fruit, 1 piece (3" x 3 1/4")	7
lukschen, without fruit 1 piece (3 x 3 1/4")	5
noodle, store-bought, 1/2 cup	3
potato, 1 piece (3" x 3 1/4")	4
potato, store-bought, 1/2 cup	4
◆ **Kumquats,** 8 medium (3 oz)	1 (2)
Kung Pao	
beef, 1 cup	10
chicken, 1 cup	8
pork, 1 cup	9
shrimp, 1 cup	9

L

	POINTS VALUE
Ladyfingers, store-bought	
1 large (1/2 oz)	1
2 small (1/2 oz)	1
Lamb	
◆ lean (leg and loin cuts with all visible fat trimmed), cooked, 1 chop, 1/2 cup cubed or shredded, or 1 slice (2 oz)	3 (5)

	POINTS VALUE
◆ heart, cooked, 3 oz	4 (5)
◆ heart, raw, 1 oz	1 (5)
◆ kidneys, cooked, 3 oz	3 (5)
◆ kidneys, raw, 1 oz	1 (5)
leg, cooked, 3 oz	5
leg, cooked, 1 slice (2 oz)	3
leg, cooked, trimmed, 3 oz	5 (5)
leg, trimmed, cooked, 1 slice (2 oz)	3 (5)
leg, trimmed, raw, 3 oz	4 (5)
◆ liver, cooked, 3 oz	4 (5)
◆ liver, raw, 1 oz	1 (5)
loin, cooked, 3 oz	6
loin, cooked, 1 slice (2 oz)	4
loin, cooked, trimmed, 1 slice (2 oz)	4 (5)
loin, cooked, trimmed, 3 oz	6 (5)
loin, trimmed, raw, 3 oz	6 (5)
regular, cooked, 1 chop, 1/2 cup cubed or shredded, or 1 slice (2 oz)	4
rib, cooked, 3 oz	8
shoulder, cooked, 1 slice (2 oz)	5
shoulder, cooked, 3 oz	7
◆ tongue, cooked, 3 oz	6 (5)
◆ tongue, raw, 1 oz	2 (5)
Lamb biryani, 1 cup	14
Lamb masala, 1 cup	6
Lamb stew, 1 cup	5
Lamb, ground	
cooked, 1/2 cup	4
◆ lean, cooked, 3 oz	3 (5)

	POINTS VALUE
Lambsquarters, cooked, 1 cup	1
Lard, 1 Tbsp	3
Lasagna	
cheese, with tomato sauce, 1	8
chicken, 1 cup	5
vegetable, 1 cup	5
vegetarian, with cheese, 10 oz	10
vegetarian, with cheese and spinach, 10 1/2 oz	9
with meat, 4" x 2 1/2" or 1 cup	6
with meat sauce, 1 cup	6
Latte	
made with fat-free milk, 1 small (8 fl oz)	2
made with fat-free milk, 1 tall (12 fl oz)	2
made with fat-free milk, 1 grande (16 fl oz)	3
made with low-fat milk, 1 small (8 fl oz)	3
made with low-fat milk, 1 tall (12 fl oz)	4
made with low-fat milk, 1 grande (16 fl oz)	5
made with whole milk, 1 small (8 fl oz)	3
made with whole milk, 1 tall (12 fl oz)	5
made with whole milk, 1 grande (16 fl oz)	6
Lau lau (pork and fish in taro or spinach leaves), 1	8
Lavash, 1/4 of 10" cracker	5
Lechon asado (roast pork), 3 oz	4
Leeks, cooked or raw, 1 cup	1
Lemon, 1 medium	0 (2)

	POINTS VALUE
Lemon grass (citronella), raw, 1 Tbsp	0
Lemon grass chicken, 1 cup	8
Lemon peel or zest, 1 Tbsp	0
Lemon pepper, 1 tsp	0
Lemonade	
1 cup	2
low calorie, powder, 1 packet (0.42 oz)	1
low calorie, powder, prepared with water, 1 cup	0
Lentils	
cooked, 1/2 cup	2 (5)
dried, 1 cup	13 (5)
sprouted, raw, 1 cup	2 (5)
Lettuce, any type, 1 cup	0
Lettuce wrap	
beef, 2 (each 5" long x 3" wide)	4
chicken, 2 (each 5" long x 3" wide)	3
Licorice	
1 oz	2
1 rope (43" long)	1
Lime peel or zest, 1 Tbsp	0
Lime, 1 medium	0 (2)
Limeade, 1 cup	2
Linguine with red clam sauce, 1 cup linguine with 1/2 cup sauce	6
Linguine with white clam sauce, 1 cup linguine with 1/2 cup sauce	8

41

	POINTS VALUE
Liqueur, any type, 1 jigger (1 1/2 fl oz)	4
Liquor (brandy, gin, rum, scotch, tequila, vodka, whiskey), 1 jigger (1 1/2 fl oz)	2
Litches (lychees)	
dried, 10 nuts	1
raw, 10 medium	1 (2)
Liver paté, 1 slice (4 1/4" x 1 1/2" x 1/2")	3
Liver with bacon, 2 slices (4 oz) with 2 slices bacon	10
Liver with onions, 2 slices (4 oz) with 1/2 cup onions	7
Liver, chopped, 1/4 cup	5
Lo mein	
beef, 1 cup	8
chicken, 1 cup	8
pork, 1 cup	8
shrimp, 1 cup	8
vegetable, 1 cup	7
Lobster bisque, 1 cup	4
Lobster Cantonese, 1 cup	8
Lobster Newburg, 1 cup	14
Lobster roll sandwich, 1	5
Lobster salad sandwich, 1	7
Lobster thermidor, 1 cup	14
Lobster, steamed, 1 1/4 -pound lobster or 4 1/2 oz lobster meat	3 (5)

	POINTS VALUE
Loganberries, 1 cup	1 (2)
Lollipop, 1	2
Lomi lomi salmon, 1/2 cup	1
Long island iced tea, 1 (8 fl oz)	5
Loquats, 10 medium	1 (2)
Lotus root, cooked or raw, 1 cup	1
Lumpia (Filipino spring rolls), 1 (4 1/2" x 1" x 1 1/2")	5
Lumpia wrappers	
1 (12 g)	1
1 oz	2
Luncheon meat	
bologna, beef or pork, 1 slice (1 oz)	2
bologna, turkey, 1 slice (1 oz)	1
bratwurst, 2 oz	5
canned, 2 oz	5
chicken roll, 1 slice (1 oz)	1
fat-free, 2 oz	1
lean (3 g fat or less per oz), 1 slice (1 oz)	1
light, canned, 2 oz	3
liverwurst, 1 oz	3
regular (4 g fat or more per oz), 1 slice (1 oz)	2
salami, beef or pork, 1 slice (1 oz)	2
salami, turkey, 2 slices	3

M

	POINTS VALUE
Macaroni	
cooked, 1 cup	4
dry, 1 cup (elbow)	7
dry, 2 oz	4
dry, 1 pound	32
whole-wheat, cooked, 1 cup (elbow)	3 (6)
whole-wheat, dry, 1 cup	6 (6)
whole-wheat, dry, 2 oz (elbow)	3 (6)
Macaroni and cheese	
1 cup	9
in a cup, 1 (2 oz)	5
frozen, 1 cup	6
package mix, prepared, 1 cup	9
Malai kofta (vegetable balls in cream sauce), 2 kofta with 1/2 cup sauce	9
Malanga	
cooked, 3/4 cup	2
cooked, 1 cup	3
cooked, 1 large	3
uncooked, 1 large	6
Malasadas (Portuguese doughnuts), 1	1
Manapua with char shiu filling, 1	5
Mandarin orange	
1 large (3" diameter)	1 (2)
2 small (2 1/4" diameter)	1 (2)
canned, unsweetened, 1 cup	1 (2)

	POINTS VALUE
Mandelbrot, 1 slice (3" x 2" x 1/2")	5
Mango	
1 cup (8 oz)	2 (2)
1 large	4 (2)
1 small	2 (2)
Mango lassi, 1 cup	3
Manhattan, 1 (2 fl oz)	3
Manicotti	
cheese, with tomato sauce, frozen, 1 (10 oz)	8
cheese, without sauce, frozen, 2 (5 1/2 oz)	6
shells, dry, 2 (1 oz)	2
with meat sauce, 2 shells with 1/2 cup sauce	15
with tomato sauce, 2 shells with 1/2 cup sauce	12
Margarine	
fat-free, 4 Tbsp	1
reduced-calorie, 2 tsp	1
regular, 1 tsp	1
regular, 1 cup	48
Margarita, 1 (4 fl oz)	5
Margarita mix, 1/2 cup	3
Marjoram, dried, 1 tsp	0
Marmalade, 1 Tbsp	1
Marshmallow, 2 medium	1
Marshmallow crème, store-bought, 2 Tbsp (1/2 oz)	1

43

	POINTS VALUE
Martini, 1 (2 1/2 fl oz)	3
Marzipan, 2 Tbsp	4
Masa harina, 1 cup	9
Masala dosa	
with filling, 1 (6" diameter dosa with 1/3 cup potato filling)	11
without filling, 1 (6" diameter)	10
Matzo, 1 board	2
Matzo brie, 1/4 of 10" round or 1 cup	5
Matzo farfel, store-bought, 1/4 cup	1
Matzo meal	
1 tsp	0
3 Tbsp	2
Mayonnaise	
fat-free, 4 Tbsp	1
reduced-calorie, reduced-fat, or light, 2 tsp	1
regular, 1 tsp	1
regular, 1/2 cup	25
Meal replacement/supplement bar for weight loss, 1 (1 oz)	3
Meal replacement/supplement drink	
1 cup	5
for weight loss (prepared from powder using fat-free milk, or canned), 1 cup	3
Meat loaf, 1 slice (5/8" thick)	6
Meat spread, canned, 1/4 cup	3

	POINTS VALUE
Meatballs	
with sauce, 2 meatballs and 1/2 cup Italian tomato sauce	13
without sauce, 2 (1 1/4" diameter each)	10
without sauce, frozen, 6 (3 oz)	6
Melba toast, 6 rounds or 4 slices (3/4 oz)	1
◆ **Melon balls,** 1 cup	1 (2)
Menudo (beef tripe and hominy stew)	
1 cup	6
canned, 1 cup	4
Meringue pie	
1 slice (1/8 of 9" pie)	10
any type, frozen, 1 slice (5 oz)	7
Mexican 7-layer dip, 1/2 cup	3
Mexican coffee, 6 fl oz with 2 Tbsp whipped cream	4
Milk	
buttermilk, dry, 1/4 cup	2
buttermilk, low-fat (1%) or reduced-fat (2%), 1 cup	2
chocolate, low-fat, 1 cup	3
chocolate, reduced-fat, 1 cup	4
chocolate, regular, 1 cup	4
◆ evaporated, fat-free, 1/2 cup	2
evaporated, low-fat, 1/2 cup	2
evaporated, whole, 1/2 cup	4
◆ fat-free, 1 cup	2
goat, 1 cup	4

	POINTS VALUE
♦ instant nonfat dry powder, 1/3 cup	2
♦ instant nonfat dry powder, 1 cup	5
low-fat or light (1/2% or 1%), 1 cup	2
oat, any flavor, 1 cup	2
reduced-fat (2%), 1 cup	3
sweetened condensed, 1/2 cup	11
sweetened condensed, fat-free, 2 Tbsp	2
whole, 1 cup	4
Milk shake	
any flavor, fast food, 1 large	13
any flavor, fast food, 1 medium	10
Millet	
♦ cooked, 1 cup	4
♦ uncooked, 1/4 cup	3
Mimosa, 1 (6 fl oz)	2
Mince pie, frozen, 1 slice (4 1/4 oz)	7
Mincemeat pie	
with meat, 1/8 of 9" two-crust pie	12
without meat, 1/8 of 9" two-crust pie	13
Mincemeat, store-bought, 1/4 cup	3
Mint, chocolate-covered, 1 (2 1/4" diameter)	3
Mirin, 1 fl oz	0
Miso, 1 tsp	0
Mochi	
1 piece (2" square)	2
butter, 1 piece (2" square)	6

	POINTS VALUE
Molasses, 1 Tbsp	1
Molé poblano, 1/4 cup	4
Mongolian beef, 1 cup	8
Monte Cristo sandwich, 1 (3 3/4 oz)	6
Moo goo gai pan, 1 cup	6
Moo shoo	
chicken, 1/2 cup with 2 pancakes	7
pork, 1/2 cup with 2 pancakes	8
tofu, 1/2 cup with 2 pancakes	7
Moose, cooked, 1 oz	1
Moussaka, 1 piece (3" x 4")	12
Mozzarella	
breaded, frozen (prepared without fat), 2 pieces (1 oz)	3
fried, 2 slices (2 3/4" x 1" x 1/2" each)	9
Muffin	
any type, 1 large (3" diameter)	6
any type, 1 mini (1 1/4" diameter)	1
any type, mini, store-bought, 2	6
any type, fast food, 1	9
any type, store-bought, 1 large (4 oz)	10
breakfast (egg and cheese with sausage, ham, or Canadian bacon on English muffin), frozen, 1 (4 1/2 oz)	7
English, any type, 1 (2 oz)	2
fat-free, store-bought, 1 large (4 oz)	4
fat-free, store-bought, 1 small (2 oz)	2
Muffuletta, 1 (6")	20

45

	POINTS VALUE
Mulberries, 1 cup	1 (2)
Mun doo	
fried, 4 (6 1/2 oz)	4
steamed, 4 (5 3/4 oz)	4
Mung beans	
cooked, 1 cup	4
raw, 1 cup	14
sprouted, cooked, 1 cup	0
Mung dal, 1 cup	5
Mushroom gravy and charbroiled beef patty, frozen, 1 patty with gravy (5 3/4 oz)	4
Mushrooms	
breaded (prepared without fat), 7	3
cooked, canned, or raw, 1 cup	0
dried, 4 large or 16 small	1
dried, reconstituted, 1 cup	1
marinated, 1/2 cup	3
shiitake, cooked, 1 cup pieces	1
shiitake, dried, 4	1
stuffed, 4 (2 3/4 oz)	3
Mussaman beef curry, 1 cup	19
Mussels Mariniere, 4 mussels with 3 Tbsp sauce	5
Mustard	
1 Tbsp	0
honey, 1 tsp	0

	POINTS VALUE
Mustard seed, yellow, 1 tsp	0
Mustard spinach, (tendergreen), cooked or raw, 1 cup	0
N	
Naan, 1 piece (7" x 8" diameter)	4
Nachos	
beef, 4 (8 1/2 oz)	13
cheese, 4 (3 oz)	8
cheese and bean, 4 (6 1/2 oz)	9
chicken, 4 (8 1/2 oz)	11
with cheese sauce, 1/2 cup tortilla chips with 1/4 cup cheese sauce	5
Nam prik, 1 Tbsp	1
Napoleon, 1 piece (4 1/2" x 2" x 1 1/2")	14
Nebeyaki udon, 2 cups	5
Nectar, any type, 1/2 cup	1
Nectarine, 1 medium (2 1/2" diameter)	1 (2)
Noodles	
cellophane, cooked, 1 cup	4
cellophone, uncooked, 2 oz	4
chow mein, packaged, 1/2 cup	3
drunken, 1 cup	5
egg, cooked, 1 cup	4
egg, no-yolk, uncooked, 2 oz	4
egg, uncooked, 1 cup	3

	POINTS VALUE
fried, 1 cup	6
Japanese, soba, cooked, 1 cup	2
Japanese, soba, dry, 2 oz	4
lasagna, dry, 2 1/2 noodles	4
Oriental (bean thread), cooked, 1 cup	4
ramen, fresh, 1/2 cup	5
rice, packaged, 1/2 cup	3
soba, with sauce, 1 cup	9
Noodles and sauce mix, prepared, 1/2 cup	3
Nori seaweed, 10 sheets or 2 Tbsp	0
Nuoc cham, 1 Tbsp	0
Nutmeg	
freshly grated, 1 tsp	0
freshly grated, 1 Tbsp	1
ground, 1 tsp	0
Nuts	
Brazil, 8 nuts (1 oz shelled)	5
hazelnuts, 20 nuts (1 oz shelled)	4
macadamia, 12 nuts (1 oz shelled)	5
mixed, 1 oz shelled	4
pecans, 1 cup chopped	21
pecans, 1 cup shelled	20
pecans, 14 halves (1 oz shelled)	5
pignolias (pine nuts), 1 tsp	0
pignolias (pine nuts), 1 Tbsp	1
pignolias (pine nuts), 1 oz	4

	POINTS VALUE
pignolias (pine nuts), 1 cup	20
pistachios, dry roasted, 1 oz shelled	4
pistachios, 1 cup shelled	16
pistachios, 49 (1 oz shelled)	4
wheat-based, 1 oz	5

O

	POINTS VALUE
◆ **Oat bran,** cooked, 1 cup	1
◆ **Oats,** old fashioned, cooked, 1 cup	2
Oats, rolled	
◆ 1/4 cup	1
◆ 1 cup	5
Oil	
canola, 1 tsp	1
flaxseed, 1 tsp	1
olive, 1 tsp	1
safflower, 1 tsp	1
sunflower, 1 tsp	1
vegetable, 1 cup	57
vegetable, 1/4 cup	14
vegetable, 1 tsp	1
whale, 1 Tbsp	4
Okonnmiyaki, without sauce & mayonnaise (Japanese style pizza), 1 (8" diameter)	7

	(POINTS VALUE)
Okra	
breaded, frozen (prepared without fat), 3/4 cup	2
cooked or raw, 1 cup	0
fried, 1 cup	8
Old fashioned, 1 (2 fl oz)	3
Olive spread, store-bought, 1 Tbsp	2
Olives, 6 large or 10 small (1 oz)	1
Omelet	
cheese, 1 (2-egg)	8
ham and cheese, 1 (2-egg)	9
herb or plain, 1 (2-egg)	6
vegetable, 1 (2-egg)	7
Onion powder, 1 tsp	0
Onion rings	
breaded, frozen (prepared without fat), 10 large (3-4" diameter)	7
fast food, 1 serving (8-9 onion rings)	7
fried, 4 (4" diameter each)	6
Onion	
1 large or 1 cup chopped or minced	1
1 small, 1 medium, or 1 cup sliced	0
1 slice (1/8" thick)	0
cooked, 1 cup	1
frozen, chopped, 1 package (10 oz)	1
Onion, blooming, 1/4 (16" diameter onion)	6
Onions, dehydrated flakes, 1/4 cup	1
Opossum, cooked, 1 oz	2

	(POINTS VALUE)
Orange	
1 large (3 1/16" diameter)	1 (2)
1 medium (2 5/8" diameter)	1 (2)
1 small (2 3/8" diameter)	0 (2)
Orange and apricot drink, 1/2 cup	1
Orange chicken, 1 cup	13
Orange juice, 1/2 cup	1
Orange peel or zest, Tbsp	0
Orange sections, 1 cup	1 (2)
Orange-grapefruit juice, 1/2 cup	1
Oregano	
fresh, 1 Tbsp	0
ground, 1 tsp	0
Oriental potato noodles (dang myeon), 2 oz	4
Osso bucco, 6 oz veal with 1/4 cup sauce	12
Ostrich, cooked, 1 oz	1 (5)
Oyster pie, 1 slice (1/8 of 9" pie)	9
Oyster po' boy, 1 (6")	17
Oysters Rockefeller, 4 (2 oz)	3
Oysters, fried, 10 (5 oz)	7

P

Pad Thai (rice noodles with chicken and shrimp), 1 cup	9
Paella, 1 cup	7
Pajun (Korean green onion & shrimp pancake), 1 (6-8" diameter)	8

	POINTS VALUE
Pakora, vegetable, 1 (2" x 3" or 1 3/4 oz)	3
Palak vada (vegetable dumpling)	
fried, 1 (2 1/2" x 1 1/2")	5
steamed, 1 (2 1/2" x 1 1/2")	2
Pan cubano, 1 (6 1/2" x 3")	8
Panang curry	
with beef, 1 cup	13
with chicken, 1 cup	12
with pork, 1 cup	14
Pancake	
any type, from mix, 1 (4" diameter)	1
any type, frozen, 1 (4" diameter)	2
fast food, 1 serving without margarine and syrup (5 1/4 oz)	9
mini, frozen, without syrup, 6 (2 1/4 oz)	3
prepared from scratch, 1 (4" diameter)	3
Chinese, 1	1
Pancake and sausage on a stick, 1 (2 oz)	5
Paneer	
fried, 1 cup	1
fried, 1 oz	2
jalfrezi, 1 cup	5
Panettone, 1/12 of 9" tube or 1 1/2 oz	6
Panini	
chicken, 1 (8 oz)	11
ham & cheese, 1 (7 1/2 oz)	11
vegetable, 1 (13 oz)	10

	POINTS VALUE
Papaya	
◆ fresh, 1 cup	1 (2)
◆ fresh, 1 large (5 3/4" long x 3 1/4" diameter)	2 (2)
◆ fresh, 1 medium (5 1/8" long x 3" diameter)	1 (2)
◆ fresh, 1 small (4 1/2" long x 2 3/4" diameter)	1 (2)
◆ green, 1 cup	1 (2)
Paprika, 1 tsp	0
Paprikash, 1 1/2 cups chicken mixture with 1/2 cup sauce	9
Paratha, 4" triangle	3
Parsley, fresh or dried, 1 cup	0
Parsnips	
◆ cooked, 1 cup	2
◆ raw, 1 medium or 1 cup slices	1
◆ **Passion fruit,** 3 (2 oz)	0 (2)
Passover sponge cake, 1/12 of 9" tube	3
Pasta	
◆ brown rice, 2 oz	4 (6)
cooked, 1 cup	4
spinach, 1 cup cooked or 2 oz uncooked	4
uncooked, 2 oz	4
uncooked, 1 pound	32
◆ whole-wheat, cooked, 1 cup	3 (6)
◆ whole-wheat, uncooked, 2 oz	3 (6)
◆ whole-wheat, uncooked, 1 pound	26 (6)

	POINTS VALUE
Pasta e fagioli, 1 cup	5
Pasta primavera	
with cream sauce, 1 cup pasta and vegetables with 3/4 cup sauce	12
with marinara sauce, 1 cup pasta and vegetables with 3/4 cup sauce	5
Pasta shells, stuffed with ricotta cheese, without sauce, frozen, 1 serving (2-3 pieces)	6
Pasta with garlic and oil, 1 cup	7
Pastitsio, 1 piece (3 1/4" x 3")	13
Pastrami	
beef, 1 slice (1 oz)	3
made from turkey, 1 slice (1 oz)	1
Pâté	
fish, store-bought, 2 oz	3
meat, store-bought, 1/4 cup (2 oz)	5
Paté foie gras, canned, 1 Tbsp	2
Peach	
◆ canned, unsweetened, 1 cup	2 (2)
◆ fresh, 1 large (2 3/4" diameter or 6 oz)	1 (2)
◆ fresh, 1 medium (2 1/2" diameter)	0 (2)
◆ fresh, 1 small (2" diameter)	0 (2)
Peach melba, 1/2 cup ice cream with 2 peach halves and raspberry sauce	7
Peanut brittle	
1 oz	3
store-bought, 4 pieces (1 oz)	3

	POINTS VALUE
Peanut butter	
1 Tbsp	2
reduced-fat, 1 Tbsp	2
Peanut butter and jelly sandwich, 1 (3 1/4 oz)	7
Peanuts	
40 (1 oz shelled)	4
chocolate-covered, 1 oz	3
honey, reduced-fat, 1/4 cup	2
Pear	
◆ 1 large (7 oz)	2 (2)
◆ 1 medium (6 oz)	1 (2)
◆ 1 small (5 oz)	1 (2)
◆ Asian, 1 (2 1/4" high x 2 1/2" diameter)	0 (2)
◆ canned, unsweetened, 1 cup	2 (2)
◆ prickly, 1 (5 oz)	0 (2)
Pear, poached, with 2 Tbsp whipped cream	5
Peas	
◆ split, cooked, 1/2 cup	2 (5)
◆ split, dry, 1/4 cup	3 (5)
Peas and carrots	
◆ canned, 1 cup	1
◆ cooked, 1/2 cup	0
Peas and onions	
◆ canned, solids and liquids, 1 cup	1
◆ cooked, 1 cup	1
Peas, Bahamian style, with rice, 1 cup	7

	POINTS VALUE
Peas, black-eyed	
◆ cooked, 1/2 cup	1 (5)
◆ dry, 1 pound	30 (5)
Peas, chick	
◆ cooked, 1/2 cup	2 (5)
◆ dry, 1 pound	35 (5)
◆ **Peas, green,** cooked or raw, 1 cup	2 (6)
Peas, pigeon	
cooked, 1 cup	3 (5)
dry, 1 cup	14 (5)
◆ **Peas, snow (Chinese pea pods),** 1 cup	1 (6)
◆ **Peas, sugar snap,** 1 cup	1 (6)
Pecan pie	
1/8 of 9" one-crust pie	12
frozen, 1 slice (4 1/2 oz)	10
Pecans	
1 cup halves	20
1 cup chopped	21
14 halves (1 oz)	5
Peking duck, 2 oz duck with 1 piece duck skin and 3 pancakes	10
Penne a la vodka, 1 cup pasta with 1/2 cup sauce	7
Pepper	
◆ any type other than roasted red, cooked or raw, 1 cup	0
◆ roasted red, 1 cup	1
Pepper flakes, red, crushed, 1 tsp	0

	POINTS VALUE
Pepper steak	
6 oz	14
Chinese, 1 cup	5
Pepper, stuffed	
with beef and rice, 1 (8 oz)	8
with beef, in tomato sauce, frozen, 7 oz	4
Peppercorns, ground or whole, any variety, 1 tsp	0
Peppermint, fresh, 2 Tbsp	0
Pepperoni, 1 oz	4
Persimmon	
◆ 1 (2 1/2" diameter, or 6 oz)	2 (2)
Japanese, dried, 1	1
Pesarattu, 1/2 of an 8" diameter	7
Petit fours, 2 (1 3/4" x 1 1/2" x 1" each)	5
Petite marmite, 2 cups	7
Pheasant	
◆ breast, raw, without skin and bone, 1/2 breast	5
cooked, 1 oz	2
◆ leg, raw, without skin and bone, 1 leg	3
Philly cheese steak sandwich, 1 (9 oz)	13
Phyllo dough, frozen, 1 1/2 sheets (1 oz)	2
Picadillo, 1 cup	10
Pickle	
◆ sour, 1 cup	0
sweet, 1 medium or large	1
sweet, 1 midget (2 1/8" long)	0

Pickle (con't)	POINTS VALUE
sweet, 1 oz	1
sweet, 1 small (2 1/2" long)	0
♦ unsweetened, 1 cup or 1 large	0
♦ dill gherkins, 1 cup or 1 medium	0
♦ **Pico de gallo,** 1/2 cup	1
Pie	
any type, frozen, 1 slice (2 1/2" x 1 3/4" x 1/2")	8
fruit, fast food, 1	8
fried, fruit, 1 (5 x 3 3/4")	9
fruit, one-crust, 1 slice (1/8 of 9" pie)	6
fruit, two-crust, 1 slice (1/8 of 9" pie)	9
individual, 1 (5 x 3 3/4")	9
Pie crust	
any type, 1/8 of 9" one-crust pie	5
any type, 1/8 of 9" two-crust pie	7
refrigerated or frozen, 1 slice (1/8 of 9" crust)	2
graham cracker, 1/8 of 9" crust	5
Pie filling	
canned, fruit, 1/3 cup	2
canned, fruit, light, 1/3 cup	1
Pierogies	
cabbage, 2 (3 1/2" each)	7
cheese, 2 (3 1/2" each)	7
meat, 2 (3 1/2" each)	8
potato, 2 (3 1/2" each)	7

	POINTS VALUE
potato and cheese or onion, low-fat, frozen, 3 (4 1/2 oz)	4
potato and cheese, frozen, 3 (4 oz)	4
Pigeon, cooked, 1 oz	1
Pigs' feet, pickled, store-bought, 2 oz	3
Pigs in blankets, 2 (1 oz)	6
Pimiento-cheese spread	
reduced-fat, store-bought, 2 Tbsp	2
regular, store-bought, 2 Tbsp	3
♦ **Pimientos,** canned, 1 cup	0
Piña colada	
1 (6 fl oz)	7
mix, 1/2 cup	4
Pineapple	
♦ canned, unsweetened, 1 cup	2 (2)
♦ fresh, 1/4 medium	1 (2)
♦ fresh, 2 slices (3 1/2" diameter x 1/2" thick), 4 oz, or 1 cup	1 (2)
juice, 1/2 cup	1
Pita	
wheat, 1 small or 1/2 large (1 oz)	1
white, 1 small or 1/2 large (1 oz)	1
Pizza crust dough, refrigerated, frozen or ready-made, 1 oz	2
Pizza pieces, frozen (prepared without fat), 6	5

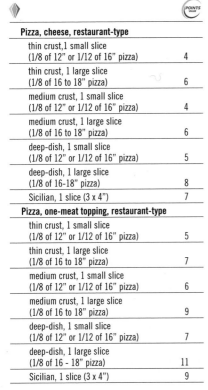

	POINTS VALUE
Pizza, cheese, restaurant-type	
thin crust,1 small slice (1/8 of 12" or 1/12 of 16" pizza)	4
thin crust, 1 large slice (1/8 of 16 to 18" pizza)	6
medium crust, 1 small slice (1/8 of 12" or 1/12 of 16" pizza)	4
medium crust, 1 large slice (1/8 of 16 to 18" pizza)	6
deep-dish, 1 small slice (1/8 of 12" or 1/12 of 16" pizza)	5
deep-dish, 1 large slice (1/8 of 16-18" pizza)	8
Sicilian, 1 slice (3 x 4")	7
Pizza, one-meat topping, restaurant-type	
thin crust, 1 small slice (1/8 of 12" or 1/12 of 16" pizza)	5
thin crust, 1 large slice (1/8 of 16 to 18" pizza)	7
medium crust, 1 small slice (1/8 of 12" or 1/12 of 16" pizza)	6
medium crust, 1 large slice (1/8 of 16 to 18" pizza)	9
deep-dish, 1 small slice (1/8 of 12" or 1/12 of 16" pizza)	7
deep-dish, 1 large slice (1/8 of 16 - 18" pizza)	11
Sicilian, 1 slice (3 x 4")	9

	POINTS VALUE
Pizza, frozen	
Canadian style bacon, 1 slice (5 oz)	7
cheese, frozen, 1 slice (4 1/4 oz)	8
hamburger, 1 slice (5 oz)	7
pepperoni, 1 slice (5 oz)	9
supreme, frozen, 1 slice (5 oz)	9
vegetable, frozen, 1 slice (5 oz)	6
Pizza, frozen, individual pie	
cheese,1 (6 1/2 oz)	13
pepperoni, 1 (6 1/4 oz)	14
sausage, 1 (6 1/4 oz)	14
supreme, 1 (7 1/4 oz)	14
Pizza, fast food	
cheese, thin crust, 1 slice (1/8 of 12" or 1/12 of 16" pizza)	4
cheese, medium crust, 1 slice (1/8 of 12" or 1/12 of 16" pizza)	5
cheese, thick crust, 1 slice (1/8 of 12" or 1/12 of 16" pizza)	7
one meat topping, thin crust, 1 slice (1/8 of 12" or 1/12 of 16" pizza)	5
one meat topping, medium crust, 1 slice (1/8 of 12" or 1/12 of 16" pizza)	6
one meat topping, thick crust, 1 slice (1/8 of 12" or 1/12 of 16" pizza)	7
Pizza, fast food, single serving	
cheese, 1 (6" pizza)	13
one-meat topping, 1 (6" pizza)	15

Food	POINTS VALUE
Pizza bagel, mini, any type, 4 (3 oz)	4
Plantain	
baked or boiled, 1 cup	3
fried, 1 cup	4
raw, 1 cup sliced	3
Plátanos maduros (fried sweet plantains), 1 cup	4
Plums	
1 medium (2 1/8" diameter)	1 (2)
2 small (2" diameter)	1 (2)
canned, purple, juice pack, 1 cup (pitted)	2 (2)
Pocket sandwich, frozen, 1 (4 1/2 oz)	8
Poi, 1/2 cup (4 oz)	3
Poke	
ahi, 1/2 cup	2
tako, 1/2 cup	2
Polenta	
cooked, 1/2 cup	2
dry, 1/4 cup	2
Pomegranate, 1 (3 3/8" diameter)	2 (2)
Pomelo (pummelo), 1	3 (2)
Poor boy sandwich, 1 (6")	6
Popcorn	
buttered, popped, 3 cups	5
butter-flavored, popped, 3 cups	4
caramel-coated, popped, 3 cups	8
cheese-flavored, popped, 3 cups	3
light, butter-flavored, popped, 3 cups	2

Food	POINTS VALUE
light, caramel-coated, popped, 3 cups	6
light, cheese-flavored, popped, 3 cups	3
light, microwave-popped, 3 cups	1
light, plain, popped, 3 cups	2
movie, without butter, 3 cups	3
plain, air-popped, 3 cups	1
plain, microwave-popped, 3 cups	3
plain, oil-popped, 3 cups	3
plain, popped, packaged, 3 cups	4
reduced-fat (94% fat-free), microwave-popped, 5 cups	1
white, air-popped, 1 cup	0
Popcorn cakes	
other than plain or butter-flavored, 1 (1 1/2 oz)	1
plain or butter-flavored, 2 (2/3 oz)	1
mini, 6 (2/3 oz)	1
Popover, 2 (3" diameter, or 1 1/2 oz each)	4
Poppy seeds	
1 Tbsp	1
1 tsp	0
Pork	
barbecue, 1 cup	8
center loin, trimmed, cooked, 3 oz	4 (5)
center loin, trimmed, cooked, 1 slice (2 oz)	2 (5)
heart, cooked, 1 (4 1/2 oz)	4 (5)
heart, raw, 1 oz	1 (5)
kidney, cooked, 1 oz	1 (5)

	POINTS VALUE
kidney, raw, 1 (8 1/4 oz)	5 (5)
lean (leg and loin cuts other than those listed here) trimmed, cooked, 1 chop, 1 slice, or 1/2 cup cubed or shredded (2 oz)	2 (5)
lean boneless pork chop, cooked, 3 oz	4
leg, cooked, 3 oz	6
leg, cooked, 1 slice (2 oz)	4
leg, trimmed, cooked, 2 oz	3 (5)
liver, cooked, 3 oz	3 (5)
liver, raw, 1 oz	1 (5)
loin, trimmed, cooked, 2 oz	2 (5)
regular, cooked, 1 chop, 1 slice, or 1/2 cup cubed or shredded (2 oz)	5
shoulder, trimmed, cooked, 1 slice (2 oz)	3
sirloin, trimmed, cooked, 2 oz	3 (5)
sirloin, trimmed, raw, 3 oz	3 (5)
tenderloin, trimmed, cooked, 1 cup	4 (5)
tenderloin, trimmed, cooked, 3 oz	3 (5)
tenderloin, trimmed, cooked, 1 slice (2 oz)	2 (5)
tenderloin, trimmed, raw, 1 oz	1 (5)
tongue, cooked, 3 oz	6 (5)
tongue, raw, 1 oz	2 (5)
top loin, trimmed, cooked, 3 oz	3 (5)
top loin, trimmed, cooked, 1 slice (2 oz)	2 (5)
top loin, trimmed, raw, 3 oz	3 (5)
Pork and beans, canned, 1/2 cup	2
Pork and broccoli, 1 cup	3
Pork hash, 4	6
Pork in barbecue sauce, frozen, 1/4 cup	2

	POINTS VALUE
Pork with cashews, 1 cup	10
Pork rinds, 1 oz	4
Pork stir-fry with garlic or black bean sauce, 1 cup	8
Pork, Chinese roast, 1 cup	5
Pork, sweet and sour, 1 cup	12
Portuguese sweet bread, 1/8 loaf	5
Pot pie	
any type, fast food, 1	19
beef, chicken, or turkey, frozen, 1 (7 oz)	11
chicken, homemade, 8 1/2 oz	10
Pot sticker (filled wontons)	
pork or vegetable, frozen, 1 large or 2 small (1 1/2 oz)	2
vegetarian, fried or steamed, 4 (3 1/2" x 2" each)	3
Potato chips	
baked, 11 (1 oz)	2
fat-free (made with fat substitute), 1 oz	1
reduced-calorie, 14 (1 oz)	3
regular, 14 (1 oz)	4
Potato flakes, dry, 1/3 cup	1
Potato latkes, 2 (3 1/2" diameter)	6
Potato leaves, sweet, cooked or raw, 1 cup	0
Potato mix, flavored, prepared, 1/2 cup	3
Potato pancake	
mix, 3 Tbsp	1
frozen, 1 (2 oz)	1
1 (3 1/4 oz)	2

	POINTS VALUE
Potato puffs (appetizer pastry), frozen, 2	4
Potato skins	
frozen, 2 (4 oz)	5
with cheese, bacon & sour cream, 2 (7 oz)	9
Potato tots, frozen (prepared without fat), 9 (3 oz)	4
Potatoes	
baked, plain, 1 large (7 oz)	3 (6)
baked, plain, 1 small (3 oz)	1 (6)
boiled, 1 (2 1/2" diameter)	2 (6)
raw, 1/2 cup diced	1 (6)
raw, 1 large (9 oz)	3 (6)
raw, 1 small (4 oz)	1 (6)
Potatoes au gratin, 1 cup	13
Potatoes O'Brien	
frozen (prepared without fat), 1 cup	1 (6)
home-prepared, 1 cup	3
Potatoes, baby	
cooked, 1 (2 oz)	1 (6)
raw, 1 (2 1/2 oz)	1 (6)
Potatoes, baked	
with cheese sauce and bacon, fast food, 1	11
with sour cream and chives, fast food, 1	10
with vegetables and cheese, fast food, 1	10

	POINTS VALUE
Potatoes, baked, stuffed	
with bacon & cheese, 1 (9 1/2 oz)	11
with vegetables and cheese, 1 (13 1/2 oz)	9
Potatoes, bliss	
cooked, 1 (2 oz)	1 (6)
uncooked, 1 (2 1/2 oz)	1 (6)
Potatoes, garlic mashed, 1/2 cup	4
Potatoes, hash brown	
1 cup	7
fast food, 1/2 cup	4
hash brown patty, frozen (prepared without fat), 1	1
patty, frozen (prepared without fat), 1 cup	8
Potatoes, home fried, 1 cup	5
Potatoes, mashed	
1/2 cup	2
in a cup, 1	3
Potatoes, new	
cooked, 1 (2 oz)	1 (6)
uncooked, 1/2 cup diced	1 (6)
uncooked, 1 small (1 3/4 to 2 1/4" diameter)	1 (6)
Potatoes, scalloped, 1/2 cup	4
Potatoes, shoestring, canned, 1 cup	6
Potatoes, stuffed	
with cheese, 1 (5 1/2 oz)	4
with sour cream and chives, 1 (5 1/2 oz)	4

	POINTS VALUE
Potatoes, sweet	
baked, 1 medium (2" diameter, 5" long)	2 (6)
canned, mashed, 1 cup	4
cooked, 1 cup (7 oz)	3 (6)
cooked, 1 large (5") or 7 oz	3 (6)
cooked, 1 medium (4 1/2 oz)	2 (6)
cooked, 1 small (3 oz)	1 (6)
frozen, cooked, 1 cup cubes	3 (6)
raw, 1 cup cubes	2 (6)
raw, 1 large (8 oz)	4 (6)
raw, 1 medium (7 oz)	3 (6)
raw, 1 small (4 1/2 oz)	2 (6)
Potatoes, white or red	
canned, drained solids, 1 cup	1 (6)
cooked, 1 cup	2 (6)
cooked, 1 large (5") or 7 oz	3 (6)
cooked, 1 small (2" diameter) or 3 oz	1 (6)
Potatoes, Yukon gold	
uncooked, 1/2 cup diced	1 (6)
uncooked, 1 medium or large (2 1/4" or larger)	2 (6)
uncooked, 1 small (1 3/4 to 2 1/4" diameter)	1 (6)
Poultry seasoning, 1 tsp	0
Pound cake, store-bought, 1 slice (2 1/2 oz)	6
Poutine, 20 French fries with 2 oz cheese and 1/2 cup sauce	17
Pozole, 1 cup	4

	POINTS VALUE
Praline, 1 (2 1/2" diameter, or 1 1/2 oz)	5
Preserves, 1 Tbsp	1
Pretzels	
regular twists, 2 (3/4 oz)	2
small twists, 15 (3/4 oz)	2
Bavarian or hard, 1 (3/4 oz)	2
soft, 1 (2 1/2 oz)	3
soft, Philadelphia, 1 (4 1/2 x 4")	3
rods, 2 (3/4 oz)	2
sticks, 45 (3/4 oz)	2
yogurt-covered, 7 (1 oz)	3
Prickly pear (cactus pear), 1 (5 oz)	0
Profiterole, 1 oz	3
Prune juice, 1/2 cup	2
Prunes, 2 (3/4 oz)	1
Ptarmigan, muscle, raw, 3 1/2 oz	3
Pudding	
any flavor, 1/2 cup	3
any flavor, 1 cup	7
banana, 1 cup	7
banana, instant, fat-free, sugar free, with pie filling mix, 1 oz	1
bread, 1 cup	13
butterscotch, instant, fat-free, sugar free, with pie filling mix, 1 oz	1
chocolate, instant, fat-free, sugar free, with pie filling mix, 1 oz	1

◆ *Pudding (con't)*

	POINTS VALUE
from fat-free, sugar-free mix, made with fat-free milk, 1 cup	3
from regular mix, made with fat-free milk, 1 cup	6
Indian, 1 cup	7
plum, 1/2 cup with 1 Tbsp sauce	9
ready-made, 1/2 cup	3
ready-made, reduced-calorie, 1/2 cup	2
rice, 1 cup	8
tapioca, 1 cup	5
Thai tapioca, 1/2 cup	4
◆ vanilla, instant, fat-free, sugar free, with pie filling mix, 1 oz	1
Puff pastry, frozen, baked, 1 oz	4
Pumpkin	
◆ canned, 1 cup	1
◆ fresh, cooked or raw, 1 cup	0
Pumpkin bread, 1 slice (3/4" thick)	7
Pumpkin pie	
1/8 of 9" one-crust pie	9
frozen, 1 slice (5 oz)	6
Pumpkin pie spice, 1 tsp	0
Pumpkin seeds	
1 Tbsp	2
1 tsp	1
Puris, 4" diameter	2

Q

	POINTS VALUE
Quail	
breast, meat only, raw, 1 breast (2 oz)	2
cooked, 1 oz	2
meat only, raw, 1 (3 1/4 oz)	3
Quenelles, 8 (2 1/2" x 1 1/2" x 3/4")	12
Quesadilla	
beef, 1/2 of 6" diameter	7
cheese, 1/2 of 6" diameter	5
chicken, 1/2 of 6" diameter	6
vegetable, 1/2 of 6" diameter	6
Quiche	
appetizer, frozen, any type, 2 (1 1/2 oz)	3
crab, frozen, 5 oz	11
vegetable, 1/8 of 9" pie	8
vegetable, frozen, 5 oz	9
Quiche Lorraine	
1/8 of 9" pie	10
frozen, 5 1/2 oz	10
◆ **Quince,** 1 (3 1/4 oz)	1 (2)
Quinoa	
◆ cooked, 1 cup	4 (6)
◆ uncooked, 2 Tbsp	1 (6)

R

Food	POINTS VALUE
Rabbit, cooked, 1 oz	1
Raccoon, cooked, 1 oz	2
Radicchio, raw, 1 cup shredded	0
Radish seeds, sprouted, raw, 1 cup	1
Radishes, 1 cup	0
Raisins	
1/4 cup (1 1/2 oz)	2
chocolate-covered, 1 oz	2
yogurt-covered, 2 oz	3
Raita, 1/2 cup	1
Rajmah, 1 cup	6
Raspberries, 1 1/2 cups	1 (2)
Ratatouille, 1 cup	4
Ravioli	
beef or chicken, without sauce, frozen, 1 cup	4
beef, breaded, frozen, 6 (4 oz)	5
beef, in meat sauce, canned, 1 cup	5
cheese, breaded, frozen, 6 (4 oz)	7
cheese, with tomato sauce, 8 pieces or 1 cup with 1/2 cup sauce	16
cheese, without sauce, 8 pieces or 1 cup	13
cheese, without sauce, frozen, 1 cup	6
meat, with tomato sauce, 8 pieces or 1 cup with 1/2 cup sauce	14
meat, without sauce, 8 pieces or 1 cup	12

Food	POINTS VALUE
Red snapper Veracruz, 6 oz, cooked fillet with 3/4 cup sauce	11
Relish, any type, 1 tsp	0
Reuben sandwich, 1 (8 oz)	17
Rhubarb	
cooked, with sugar, 1 cup	5
cooked or raw, 1 cup	0 (2)
Rhubarb pie, 1/8 of 9" two-crust pie	11
Rice cakes	
any type other than plain, 1 (1/2 oz)	1
plain, mini, 6 (3/4 oz)	1
plain, regular, 2 (3/4 oz)	1
Rice crackers, 8 (1/2 oz)	1
Rice drink	
any type other than those listed here, 1 cup	3
chocolate, 1 cup	4
fat-free, 1 cup	2
Rice mix, flavored, any type, prepared, 1/2 cup	3
Rice pilaf, 1 cup	5
Rice, brown	
cooked, 1 cup	4 (6)
instant, 1/2 cup	3 (6)
quick cooking, 1/2 cup	3 (6)
uncooked, 1/4 cup	3 (6)
uncooked, 1 cup	13 (6)
Rice, crisp, and marshmallow treat, store-bought, 1 small (3/4 oz)	2

	POINTS VALUE
Rice, Cuban, 1 cup	4
Rice, dirty	
1 cup	9
mix (prepared without fat), 1 cup	3
Rice, fried	
plain, 1 cup	8
with beef, 1 cup	8
with chicken, 1 cup	8
with chicken or pork, frozen, 1/2 cup	2
with pork, 1 cup	8
with shrimp, 1 cup	8
Rice, Spanish	
1 cup	5
canned, 1 cup	3
Rice, sushi, cooked, 1/2 cup	2
Rice, white	
cooked, 1 cup	4
uncooked, 1/4 cup	3
uncooked, 1 cup	13
Rice, wild	
♦ cooked, 1 cup	3 (6)
♦ uncooked, 1 cup	11 (6)
Rice, with pigeon peas (arroz con gandules), 1 cup	8
Risotto, 1/2 cup	5
Roast beef sandwich, 1 (7 1/2 oz)	9
Rocky mountain oysters, 2 slices (1 oz each)	10

	POINTS VALUE
Rogan josh, 1 cup	10
Roll	
crescent dinner, store-bought, 1 (1 oz)	2
dinner, 1 (2 oz)	3
hard, 1 (2 oz)	3
high fiber (3 grams or more dietary fiber per roll), 1 (2 oz)	1
light, 1 (2 oz)	1
Ropa vieja, 1 cup	9
Rosemary, fresh or dried, 1 Tbsp	0
Roux, store-bought, 2 Tbsp	5
Rugalach, 1 piece (2 1/2" x 1 1/4")	3
Rum, 1 jigger (1 1/2 fl oz)	2
Runza, 1 (5 1/2 oz)	8
♦ **Rutabaga,** cooked or raw, 1 cup	1

S

	POINTS VALUE
Saag gosht, 1 cup	6
Saag paneer, 1 cup	6
Saccharin, 1 packet or tablet	0
Sachertorte, 1/16 of 9" cake	7
Saffron, 1 tsp	0
Saganaki, 1 piece (1" x 2" x 1/2" thick)	6
Sage, fresh or dried, 1 Tbsp	0
Saimin, 1 cup	2
Sake, 1/2 cup	3

Salad	POINTS
Caesar, 3 cups	7
carrot and raisin, 1/2 cup	7
chef's, fast food, 1	5
chef's, with dressing, 4 cups	8
chef's, without dressing, 4 cups	6
chicken macaroni, 1 cup	6
chicken, 1/2 cup	6
chicken, Oriental, 2 cups	7
chicken, store-bought, 1/2 cup	5
cobb, without dressing, 3 cups	10
conch, 1 cup	2
egg, 1/2 cup	8
fruit, 1 cup	2
Greek, with dressing, 3 cups	9
Greek, without dressing, 3 cups	2
green papaya, with pork and shrimp, 1 cup	3
green papaya, without meat, 1 cup	1
grilled chicken, without dressing, fast food, 1	4
herring, store-bought, 1/4 cup	3
lobster, 1/2 cup	4
◆ mixed greens, 1 cup	0
macaroni, 1/2 cup	6
macaroni, store-bought, 1/2 cup	5
Niçoise, with dressing, 4 cups	18
◆ Niçoise, without dressing, 4 cups	8

	POINTS
pasta mix, packaged (prepared according to directions), 1/2 cup	4
pasta, 1/2 cup	3
pasta, store-bought, 1/2 cup	3
potato macaroni, 1/2 cup	10
potato, 1/2 cup	7
potato, German, 1/2 cup	2
potato, hot, with ham, 1 cup	6
potato, store-bought, 1/2 cup	4
salmon, kippered (with mayonnaise), store-bought, 2 oz	5
seafood, store-bought, 1/2 cup	6
seaweed, 1/2 cup	1
shrimp, 1/2 cup	3
side, without dressing, fast food, 1	0
spinach, with dressing, 2 cups	7
taco, with shell, without dressing, fast food, 1	16
taco, without shell and dressing, fast food, 1	9
Thai beef, 1 cup	14
Thai chicken, 1 cup	11
Thai seafood, 2 cups	10
three-bean, 1/2 cup	4
◆ three-bean, canned, without oil, 1/2 cup	1
tomato and mozzarella, without dressing, 2 large tomato slices with 2 oz cheese	4
◆ tossed, without dressing, 2 cups	0
tuna macaroni, 1 cup	5

COMPLETE A-Z FOOD LIST

Salad (con't)	POINTS VALUE
tuna, 1/2 cup	7
tuna, store-bought, 1/2 cup	5
turkey macaroni, 1 cup	5
Waldorf, 1/2 cup	4
whitefish, store-bought, 1 1/2 oz	5
yogurt and cucumber, 1/2 cup	1
Salami	
beef or pork, 1 slice (1 oz)	2
dry or hard, pork, 1 slice (3 1/8" diameter x 1/16" thick)	1
turkey, 2 slices (2 oz)	3
Salisbury steak, with gravy, frozen, 1 steak with gravy	4
Salmon, grilled, frozen, 3 oz	2
Salsa	
black bean & corn, 1/2 cup	1
con queso, store-bought, 2 Tbsp	2
fat-free, 2 Tbsp	0
fat-free, 1/2 cup	0
Salsify (oyster plant), cooked or raw, 1 cup	1
Salt	
kosher, 1 tsp	0
sea, 1 tsp	1
table, 1 tsp	0
Samosa, 1 (2 1/2" x 2 1/2" x 3" triangle)	3

	POINTS VALUE
Sandwich	
barbecue beef, frozen, microwave, 1	9
cheese, grilled, restaurant-type, 1 (4 oz)	13
chicken, fried, fast food, 1	11
Cuban, 1/2 (6 1/2" x 3" x 4")	11
egg and cheese, fast food, 1	8
fish and cheese, fried, fast food, 1	13
fish fillet, 1 (4 1/2 oz)	8
grilled chicken, fast food, 1	7
grilled chicken, frozen, 1 (4 1/2 oz)	6
roast beef, fast food, 1	9
steak, frozen, 1 (2 oz)	5
turkey, 1 (4 oz)	6
Sandwich spread, pork or beef, 2 Tbsp	2
Sangria, 4 fl oz	2
Sashimi	
except mackerel or mackerel, 4 pieces (2 oz)	1 (5)
mackerel, 4 pieces (2 oz)	3 (5)
salmon, 4 pieces (2 oz)	2 (5)
Satay	
beef, with peanut sauce, 2 skewers with 1/4 cup sauce	11
beef, without peanut sauce, 2 skewers (3 oz)	5
chicken, with peanut sauce, 2 skewers with 1/4 cup sauce	11
chicken, without peanut sauce, 2 skewers (3 oz)	3

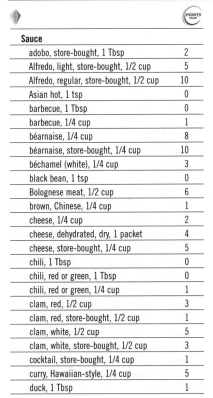

	POINTS VALUE
Sauce	
adobo, store-bought, 1 Tbsp	2
Alfredo, light, store-bought, 1/2 cup	5
Alfredo, regular, store-bought, 1/2 cup	10
Asian hot, 1 tsp	0
barbecue, 1 Tbsp	0
barbecue, 1/4 cup	1
béarnaise, 1/4 cup	8
béarnaise, store-bought, 1/4 cup	10
béchamel (white), 1/4 cup	3
black bean, 1 tsp	0
Bolognese meat, 1/2 cup	6
brown, Chinese, 1/4 cup	1
cheese, 1/4 cup	2
cheese, dehydrated, dry, 1 packet	4
cheese, store-bought, 1/4 cup	5
chili, 1 Tbsp	0
chili, red or green, 1 Tbsp	0
chili, red or green, 1/4 cup	1
clam, red, 1/2 cup	3
clam, red, store-bought, 1/2 cup	1
clam, white, 1/2 cup	5
clam, white, store-bought, 1/2 cup	3
cocktail, store-bought, 1/4 cup	1
curry, Hawaiian-style, 1/4 cup	5
duck, 1 Tbsp	1

	POINTS VALUE
enchilada, canned, 1/2 cup	1
fish, ready-to-serve, 1 Tbsp	0
hoisin, 1 tsp	0
hollandaise, 1/4 cup	8
hollandaise, store-bought, 1/4 cup	4
horseradish, 1 Tbsp	0
horseradish, store-bought, 2 Tbsp	3
hot, 1 tsp	0
kung pao, 2 Tbsp	1
marinara, 1/2 cup	3
marinara, store-bought, 1/2 cup	2
meat, 1/2 cup	5
mole, store-bought, brown, 2 Tbsp	5
mole, store-bought, green, 2 Tbsp	4
mornay, 1/4 cup	3
oyster, 1 tsp	0
pasta, bottled, any type, 1/2 cup	2
pasta, bottled, any type, reduced-fat, 1/2 cup	1
peanut, spicy, 2 Tbsp	4
peanut, Thai, canned, 2 Tbsp	2
pepper, 1 tsp	0
pesto, 2 Tbsp	4
pesto, store-bought, 2 Tbsp	3
pizza, store-bought, 1/4 cup	1
plum, 1 Tbsp	1

Sauce (con't)	POINTS VALUE
puttanesca, 1/2 cup	11
remoulade, 2 Tbsp	4
Sloppy Joe, store-bought, 1/4 cup	1
sofrito, 1/2 cup	6
soy (shoyu),1 Tbsp	0
soy (shoyu), low sodium, 1 Tbsp	0
spaghetti, bottled, any type, 1/2 cup	2
spaghetti, bottled, any type, reduced-fat, 1/2 cup	1
spaghetti, dehydrated, dry, 1 packet	2
Spanish, 1/2 cup	2
steak, 1 Tbsp	0
sweet and sour, 2 Tbsp	1
sweet and sour, dehydrated, dry, 2 Tbsp	1
taco 1 Tbsp	0
tahini, 2 Tbsp	5
tamari, 1 Tbsp	0
teriyaki, 1 Tbsp	1
teriyaki, dehydrated, dry, 1 packet	3
tartar, 1 Tbsp	2
tartar, fat-free, 1/4 cup	1
♦ tomato, canned, 1/2 cup	0
tomato, canned, Spanish style, 1 cup	1
tomato, Italian, 1/2 cup	3
♦ tomato, with onions, canned, 1 cup	1
♦ tomato, with onions, green peppers, and celery, canned, 1 cup	1

	POINTS VALUE
♦ tomato, with tomato tidbits, canned, 1 cup	1
tzatziki, 1/2 cup	1
Vietnamese spring roll dipping, 2 Tbsp	0
white, medium, 1/4 cup	2
white, thin, 1/4 cup	2
wine, 1/4 cup	2
Worcestershire, 1 Tbsp	0
Sauerbraten, 3 oz beef with 2 Tbsp gravy	6
♦ **Sauerkraut,** 1 cup	0
Sausage	
beef or pork, cooked, 1 link or patty (1 oz)	3
chicken, cooked, 1 1/2 oz	2
chicken, raw, 2 oz	2
chorizo, 1 link (5 1/2" long)	12
low-fat (1 g fat or less per oz), 2 oz	2
mini, 6 (2 oz)	5
turkey, raw, 3 oz	4
Sausage biscuit	
fast food, 1	12
frozen, 1 large (2 oz)	7
frozen, 2 small (2 oz)	7
Sausage in brioche, 1 slice (2" thick)	15
Sausage on a roll, plain, 1 (5 1/4 oz)	12
Savory, ground, 1 tsp	0
Scallion pancake, 1 (5" diameter)	6
♦ **Scallions,** 1 cup	0
Scallops, fried, 20 small (3 1/2 oz)	5

	POINTS VALUE
Schaum torte	
with whipped cream, 1/10 10" pan	8
without whipped cream, 1/10 10" pan	3
Schav, canned, 1 cup	0
Schmaltz, 1 Tbsp	3
Schnapps, any flavor, 1 jigger (1 1/2 fl oz)	4
Scone	
1 regular (2 1/2 oz)	6
1 small (1 1/2 oz)	3
Scotch, 1 jigger (1 1/2 fl oz)	2
Scrapple, 1 slice (4 1/2" x 3/4" x 3/8" thick, or 2 oz)	3
Screwdriver, 1 (6 fl oz)	3
Seafood cakes (Haw Mok Thalay), 3/4 cup	8
Seaweed, 2 Tbsp	0
Sechuan pork hotpot, 1 cup	5
Seitan	
dry mix, prepared, 2 oz	2
slices, 2 slices (2 oz)	1
Seltzer, plain or flavored, unsweetened, 1 can or bottle (12 fl oz)	0
Sesame candy, 1 piece (2" x 1")	2
Sesame noodles, 1 cup	5
Sesame seeds	
1 tsp	0
1 Tbsp	1
Sesame sticks, store-bought, 1/3 cup (1 oz)	4

	POINTS VALUE
Shabu shabu, 4 oz beef, 2 oz tofu, and 1 1/2 cups vegetables	9
Shallots	
freeze-dried, 1/4 cup	0
raw, 1 medium	0
Shark, cooked, 1 steak (6 oz)	5
Sharon fruit, 3 oz	0
Shawarma, chicken	
1/2 cup	6
1 thigh (without skin and bone) 2 oz	5
Shellfish	
abalone, cooked or raw, 3 oz	2 (5)
clam, cooked, 1/2 cup (2 oz)	2 (5)
clam, raw, 1 pound (with shell)	1 (5)
clams, fried, frozen (prepared without fat), 3 oz	6
clams, stuffed, frozen (prepared without fat), 3 oz	2
conch, cracked, 1 (6" long x 3")	9
conch, fritters, 2 (1 3/4 oz)	2
crab, cooked or canned, 1/2 cup (2 oz)	1 (5)
crab, cooked or canned, 1 cup	3 (5)
crab, cooked or raw, 3 oz	2 (5)
crab, imitation, 1/2 cup (3 oz)	2 (5)
crab, stuffed, frozen, 1 (3 oz)	3
crabmeat, canned, 1 cup	3 (5)
crabmeat, canned, 1/2 cup	1 (5)

Shellfish (con't)

		POINTS VALUE
◆	crayfish, cooked, 16 (2 oz)	1 (5)
◆	crayfish, raw, 8 (1 oz)	0 (5)
◆	crayfish, wild, cooked, 3 oz	1 (5)
◆	lobster, cooked, 1/2 cup (2 oz)	1 (5)
◆	lobster, raw, 1 (5 1/2 oz)	3 (5)
◆	lobster, spiny, cooked or raw, 1 (7 1/2 oz)	5 (5)
◆	mussel, blue, raw (without shell), 1 cup	3 (5)
◆	mussel, cooked, 1/2 cup (2 oz)	2 (5)
◆	mussels, raw, in shell, 3 medium (20 mussels per pound)	1 (5)
◆	mussels, raw, in shell, 4 small (25 mussels per pound)	1 (5)
◆	mussels, raw, in shell, 1 pound	6 (5)
◆	octopus, cooked, 3 oz	3 (5)
◆	oyster, canned or cooked, 1/2 cup	2 (5)
◆	oyster, cooked, 6 medium (2 oz)	1 (5)
◆	oyster, raw, 6 medium (3 oz)	1 (5)
◆	scallops, cooked, 10 small or 4 large (2 oz)	1 (5)
◆	scallops, imitation, 3 oz	2 (5)
◆	scallops, raw, 3 oz	2 (5)
	scallops, fried, frozen (prepared without fat), 3 1/4 oz	5
	shrimp, butterfly, breaded, frozen (prepared without fat), 3 1/2 oz	6
◆	shrimp, canned, 1/2 cup	2 (5)
◆	shrimp, cooked, 1/2 cup (2 oz)	1 (5)
◆	shrimp, imitation, 3 oz	2 (5)
◆	shrimp, raw, 1 oz	1 (5)

		POINTS VALUE
	squid, fried, 3 oz	4
◆	squid, cooked, 3 oz	2 (5)
◆	squid, raw, 1 oz	1 (5)
Shells, stuffed with cheese, no sauce, frozen, 2 (4 1/2 oz)		6
Shepherd's pie, 1 cup		9
Sherbet, 1/2 cup		2
Sherry, dry or sweet, 1/2 cup		3
Shish kabob (lamb), 2 small skewers (4 1/2 oz)		8
Shortcakes, store-bought, 2 (1 oz each)		4
Shortening, 1 cup		53
Shoyu chicken, 1 thigh (3 1/4 oz)		6
Shrimp		
	barbecued, 4 large shrimp with 1/4 cup sauce	11
	broiled, stuffed, 6 large (6 oz)	18
	fried, 10 (5 oz)	8
	fried, stuffed, 6 large (9 1/2 oz)	9
	popcorn, breaded, frozen (prepared without fat), 1 cup	5
	stir-fry, with garlic or black bean sauce, 1 cup	7
	sweet and sour, 1 cup	10
Shrimp and broccoli, 1 cup		2
Shrimp Cantonese, 1 cup		8
Shrimp po' boy, 1 (6")		18
Shrimp puffs, 6 (1 1/2" rounds)		5

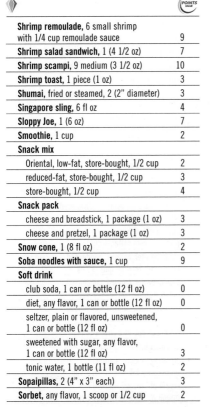

	POINTS VALUE
Shrimp remoulade, 6 small shrimp with 1/4 cup remoulade sauce	9
Shrimp salad sandwich, 1 (4 1/2 oz)	7
Shrimp scampi, 9 medium (3 1/2 oz)	10
Shrimp toast, 1 piece (1 oz)	3
Shumai, fried or steamed, 2 (2" diameter)	3
Singapore sling, 6 fl oz	4
Sloppy Joe, 1 (6 oz)	7
Smoothie, 1 cup	2
Snack mix	
Oriental, low-fat, store-bought, 1/2 cup	2
reduced-fat, store-bought, 1/2 cup	3
store-bought, 1/2 cup	4
Snack pack	
cheese and breadstick, 1 package (1 oz)	3
cheese and pretzel, 1 package (1 oz)	3
Snow cone, 1 (8 fl oz)	2
Soba noodles with sauce, 1 cup	9
Soft drink	
club soda, 1 can or bottle (12 fl oz)	0
diet, any flavor, 1 can or bottle (12 fl oz)	0
seltzer, plain or flavored, unsweetened, 1 can or bottle (12 fl oz)	0
sweetened with sugar, any flavor, 1 can or bottle (12 fl oz)	3
tonic water, 1 bottle (11 fl oz)	2
Sopaipillas, 2 (4" x 3" each)	3
Sorbet, any flavor, 1 scoop or 1/2 cup	2

	POINTS VALUE
Soufflé	
cheese, 1 cup	5
fruit, 1/2 cup	4
Soup	
asparagus crab, 1 cup	2
avgolemono, 1 cup	4
bean and bacon, canned (made with water), 1 cup	3
bean and ham, canned (made with water), 1 cup	3
beef broth bouillon and consomme, canned, condensed, 1 can (10.5 oz)	1
beef broth, cubed, dry, 1 cube (6 fl oz prepared)	0
beef noodle mix in a cup, 1 (2 oz)	4
beef vegetable, canned (made with water), 1 cup	1
beef, canned (made with water), 1 cup	2
beef, canned, chunky, ready-to-serve, 1 cup	4
black bean, 1 cup	2
black bean in cup, 1 (2 oz)	3
black bean, canned (made with water), 1 cup	1
bouillon, any type, 1 cup	0
broccoli cheese, 1 cup	7
broccoli cheese, canned (made with fat-free milk), 1 cup	3

Soup (con't)	POINTS VALUE
broccoli cheese, canned (made with low-fat milk), 1 cup	4
broccoli cheese, canned (made with whole milk), 1 cup	4
broccoli cheese, low-fat, canned (made with fat-free or low-fat milk), 1 cup	2
broth, any type, 1 cup	0
cabbage, 1 cup	1
cauliflower, dehydrated, prepared with water, 1 cup (8 fl oz)	2
cheddar cheese, 1 cup	9
cheddar cheese, canned (made with fat-free milk), 1 cup	4
cheddar cheese, canned (made with low-fat milk), 1 cup	4
cheddar cheese, canned (made with whole milk), 1 cup	5
cherry, 1 cup	7
chicken and stars, canned (made with water), 1 cup	1
chicken enchilada, 1 cup	5
chicken noodle, 1 cup	3
chicken noodle mix, prepared, 1 cup	1
chicken noodle mix, prepared, 1 cup	1
chicken noodle, canned (made with water), 1 cup	2
chicken noodle, in a cup, 1 (2 oz)	2
chicken vegetable, canned, chunky, ready-to-serve, 1 cup	4

	POINTS VALUE
chicken vegetable, canned, condensed, 1 can (10.5 oz)	4
chicken vegetable, dehydrated, dry, 1	1
chicken vegetable, in cup, 1 (2 oz)	2
chicken with rice, canned (made with water), 1 cup	2
chicken, canned, chunky, ready-to-serve, 1 cup (8 fl oz)	4
chicken, with matzo balls, 1 cup soup with 2 (1 1/2") matzo balls	3
chicken, with tortilla strips and shredded cheese, 1 cup	4
chicken, without matzo balls (broth only), 1 cup	0
consomme with gelatin, dehydrated, dry, 1 packet (2 oz)	2
consomme, dehydrated, prepared with water, 1 cup	0
corn chowder, canned, condensed, made with fat-free milk, 1 cup	4
corn chowder, canned, condensed, made with low-fat milk, 1 cup	4
corn chowder, canned, condensed, made with whole milk, 1 cup	5
corn chowder, in a cup, 1 (2 oz)	3
cream of broccoli, 1 cup	6
cream of broccoli, canned (made with fat-free milk), 1 cup	3
cream of broccoli, canned (made with low-fat milk), 1 cup	3

	POINTS VALUE
cream of broccoli, canned (made with whole milk), 1 cup	4
cream of broccoli, low-fat, canned (made with fat-free milk), 1 cup	3
cream of broccoli, low-fat, canned (made with low-fat milk), 1 cup	3
cream of celery, canned (made with fat-free milk), 1 cup	3
cream of celery, canned (made with low-fat milk), 1 cup	3
cream of celery, canned (made with whole milk), 1 cup	4
cream of celery, canned, condensed, 1 can (10.75 oz)	5
cream of celery, low-fat, canned (made with fat-free milk), 1 cup	2
cream of celery, low-fat, canned (made with low-fat milk), 1 cup	3
cream of chicken, canned (made with fat-free milk), 1 cup	4
cream of chicken, canned (made with low-fat milk), 1 cup	4
cream of chicken, canned (made with whole milk), 1 cup	5
cream of chicken, canned, condensed, 1 can (10.75 oz)	7
cream of chicken, dehydrated, dry, 1 packet (2/3 oz)	2
cream of chicken, low-fat, canned (made with fat-free milk), 1 cup	3

	POINTS VALUE
cream of chicken, low-fat, canned (made with low-fat milk), 1 cup	3
cream of mushroom, 1 cup	9
cream of mushroom, canned (made with fat-free milk), 1 cup	3
cream of mushroom, canned (made with low-fat milk), 1 cup	4
cream of mushroom, canned (made with whole milk), 1 cup	4
cream of mushroom, canned, condensed, 1 can (10.75 oz)	8
cream of mushroom, low-fat, canned (made with fat-free milk), 1 cup	2
cream of mushroom, low-fat, canned (made with low-fat milk), 1 cup	3
cream of potato, 1 cup	2
cream of potato, canned (made with fat-free milk), 1 cup	3
cream of potato, canned (made with low-fat milk), 1 cup	4
cream of potato, canned (made with whole milk), 1 cup	4
cream of tomato, 1 cup	4
egg drop, 1 cup	1
◆ escarole, canned, ready-to-serve, 1 cup	1
French onion au gratin, 1 cup	7
gazpacho, 1 cup	3
◆ gazpacho, canned (made with water), 1 cup	1
◆ gazpacho, canned, ready-to-serve, 1 cup	1

Soup (con't)	POINTS VALUE
hot and sour, 1 cup	2
hot and spicy chicken, 1 cup	3
Italian wedding, 1 cup	5
leek, dehydrated, dry, 1 packet (2 3/4 oz)	6
lentil, 1 cup	3
lentil with ham, canned, ready-to-serve, 1 cup	3
lentil with ham, canned, ready-to-serve, 1 cup	3
lentil, in a cup, 1 (2 oz)	3
lobster bisque, canned (made with fat-free milk), 1 cup	2
lobster bisque, canned (made with low-fat milk), 1 cup	3
lobster bisque, canned (made with whole milk), 1 cup	3
Manhattan clam chowder, 1 cup	4
Manhattan clam chowder, canned (made with water), 1 cup	1
matzo ball, canned (ready-to-serve), 1 cup	2
minestrone, 1 cup	4
minestrone in a cup, 1 (2 oz)	2
minestrone, low-fat, canned (made with water), 1 cup	1
miso, 1 cup	2
mulligatawny, 1 cup	6
mushroom barley, 1 cup	3

	POINTS VALUE
mushroom barley, canned, condensed, 1 can (10.75 oz)	4
mushroom with beef stock, canned, condensed, 1 can (10.75 oz)	5
mushroom, dehydrated, prepared with water, 1 cup	2
New England clam chowder, 1 cup	4
New England clam chowder, canned (made with fat-free milk), 1 cup	3
New England clam chowder, canned (made with low-fat milk), 1 cup	3
New England clam chowder, canned (made with whole milk), 1 cup	4
New England clam chowder, low-fat, canned (made with fat-free milk), 1 cup	2
New England clam chowder, low-fat, canned (made with low-fat milk), 1 cup	3
onion mix, 1 cup prepared or 1/4 envelope	0
onion, canned, condensed, 1 can (10.5 oz)	3
onion, dehydrated, prepared with water, 1 cup	0
Oriental, mix in a cup, 1 (2 oz)	2
oxtail, 1 cup	1
oxtail, dehydrated, dry, 1 packet (2 2/3 oz)	6
oxtail, dehydrated, prepared with water, 1 cup	1
oxtail soup, Hawaiian-style, 1 cup	7
oyster stew, canned (made with fat-free milk), 1 cup	3

	POINTS VALUE
oyster stew, canned (made with low-fat milk), 1 cup	4
oyster stew, canned (made with whole milk), 1 cup	4
pasta with vegetables, canned (made with water), 1 cup	2
◆ pea, green, mix, dehydrated, dry form, 1 packet (1 oz)	2
◆ pea, green, mix, dehydrated, prepared with water, 1 cup	2
◆ pea, split with ham, canned, chunky, ready-to-serve, 1 cup	3
Persian noodle, store-bought, 1 cup	3
Persian pomegranate, store-bought, 1 cup	4
Pigeon pea and dumpling soup, 1 1/2 cups	7
Portuguese bean, 1 cup	5
potato leek, in a cup, 1 (2 oz)	2
potato, frozen, 1 (7 1/2 oz)	1
pozole (pork and hominy), canned (ready-to-serve), 1 cup	3
ramen noodle mix, 1 (3 oz)	8
ramen noodle mix, low-fat, 1 (3 oz)	6
ramen in a cup, low-fat, 1 (2 oz)	3
red beans and rice in a cup, 1 (2 oz)	3
Scotch broth, 1 cup	5
◆ Scotch broth, canned, condensed, 1 can (10.5 oz)	4

	POINTS VALUE
shark fin, 1 cup	2
◆ split pea, 1 cup	3
◆ split pea with ham, canned (made with water), 1 cup	4
◆ split pea, frozen, 1 package (7 1/2 oz)	2
◆ split pea in a cup, 1 (2 oz)	3
◆ stock, fish, home-prepared, 1 cup	1
◆ stockpot, canned, condensed, 1 can (11 oz)	6
Thai chicken coconut, 1 cup	8
Thai coconut ginger, canned (ready-to-serve), 1 cup	3
tomato, 1 cup	2
◆ tomato vegetable mix, dehydrated, dry form, 1 packet (1 1/3 oz)	2
◆ tomato vegetable, dehydrated, prepared with water, 1 cup	1
◆ tomato, canned (made with fat-free milk), 1 cup	2
tomato, canned (made with low-fat milk), 1 cup	3
◆ tomato, canned (made with water), 1 cup	2
tomato, canned (made with whole milk), 1 cup	3
◆ tomato, dehydrated, dry, 1 packet (3/4 oz)	2
◆ tomato, dehydrated, prepared with water, 1 cup	2
tortilla, 1 cup	6

COMPLETE A-Z FOOD LIST

Soup (con't)	POINTS VALUE
turkey noodle, canned (made with water), 1 cup	1
turkey vegetable, canned, condensed, 1 can (10.5 oz)	4
turtle, 1 cup	2
vichyssoise, 1 cup	2
vegetable, 1 cup	2
vegetable beef, canned (made with water), 1 cup	1
vegetable beef, dehydrated, dry, 1 packet (2 2/3 oz)	5
vegetable mix, prepared, 1 cup	1
vegetable with beef broth, canned, condensed, 1 can (10.5 oz)	4
vegetable, canned (made with water), 1 cup	3
vegetable, canned, chunky, ready-to-serve, 1 cup	3
vegetable, mix, 1 packet (1 2/3 oz)	3
vegetable, mix, 2 Tbsp	1
vegetarian vegetable in a cup, 1 (2 oz)	3
Vietnamese beef noodle, 1 cup	2
wonton, 1 cup with 4 wontons	4
yogurt and cucumber, 1 cup	2
Sour apple martini, 3 fl oz	5
Soursop (guanabana), 1/2 cup pulp	1 (2)
Souvlaki	
chicken, 1 large or 2 small skewers (4 1/2 oz)	5

	POINTS VALUE
chicken, in pita bread, 1 (6 1/2 oz)	7
lamb, 1 large or 2 small skewers (4 3/4 oz)	8
lamb, in pita bread, 1 (6 1/2 oz)	8
Soy beverage drink	
1 cup	3
reduced-fat, 1 cup	3
Soy burger, 1 (2 1/2 oz)	2 (5)
Soy cheese	
fat-free, 1 oz	1
fat-free, 1 slice (3/4 oz)	1
regular, 1 oz	2
regular, 1 slice (3/4 oz)	1
Soy crumbles, meatless, 1/2 cup	1 (5)
Soy milk, calcium-fortified, flavored or unflavored, 1 cup	2
Soy sour cream, 1 oz	1
Soy yogurt	
flavored, 3/4 cup (6 oz)	3
plain, 3/4 cup (6 oz)	3
Soybean nuts, 1/4 cup (1 oz)	3
Soybeans	
cooked, 1/2 cup	3 (5)
dry, 1 pound	45 (5)
green, cooked, 1 cup	5
green, raw, 1 cup	8
roasted, 1 cup	19

	POINTS VALUE
Spaetzle, 1/2 cup	5
Spaghetti	
cooked, 1 cup	4
uncooked, 2 oz	4
♦ whole wheat, cooked, 1 cup	3 (6)
♦ whole-wheat, uncooked, 2 oz	3 (6)
Spaghetti bolognese, 1 cup spaghetti with 1/2 cup sauce	10
Spaghetti carbonara, 1 cup	11
Spaghetti with marinara sauce, 1 cup spaghetti with 1/2 cup sauce	6
Spaghetti with meat sauce, 1 cup spaghetti with 1/2 cup sauce	9
Spaghetti with tomato sauce and meatballs, 1 cup spaghetti, 1/2 cup sauce and 2 meatballs	16
Spaghetti, in tomato sauce, with cheese, canned, 1 cup	3
Spaghetti, in tomato sauce, with meatballs, canned, 1 cup	5
Spanakopita	
1 (3" square) or 1 cup	8
frozen, 2 pieces (1 oz each)	4
Spareribs	
barbecued, 4 small (4" long each)	8
barbecued, 6 (6 1/4 oz)	12
Chinese, barbecued, 2 (4" long each)	4
♦ **Spinach,** cooked or raw, 1 cup	0

	POINTS VALUE
Spinach soufflé, home-prepared, 1 cup	6
Sponge cake, 1/12 of 9" tube	3
Spoon bread, 1/2 cup	4
Sports drink, 1 cup	1
Spread, hazelnut and chocolate, 1 Tbsp	2
Spring roll	
beef or pork, 1 (4 1/2" long)	5
chicken, 1 (4 1/2" long)	4
fresh, Vietnamese, 1 (1 3/4 oz)	2
fried, Vietnamese, 1 (4" long)	4
shrimp, 1 (4 1/2" long)	4
Thai, 1 (4" long)	4
Sprinkles, any type, 1 Tbsp	1
Sprouts	
♦ alfalfa, 1 cup	0
♦ bean, 1 cup	0
Spumoni, 1/2 cup	7
Squab, (pigeon)	
breast, without skin and bone, raw, 1 breast	3
meat only, raw, 1 (6 oz)	6
without skin and bone, cooked, 1 oz	1
Squash	
♦ spaghetti, 1 medium (8 oz)	1
♦ spaghetti, cooked or raw, 1 cup	0
♦ summer, all varieties, cooked or raw, 1 cup	0

Squash (con't)	POINTS VALUE
winter, acorn, 1 medium (4" diameter)	3
winter, all varieties except butternut and hubbard, cooked, 1 cup	1
winter, all varieties, raw, 1 cup	1
winter, butternut or hubbard, cooked, 1 cup	2
Squash leaves, 1 cup	0
Squirrel, cooked, 1 oz	1
Star anise, 1 tsp	0
Starfruit (carambola), 2 large (4 1/2" long)	1 (2)
Steak au poivre, 6 oz steak with 1 Tbsp sauce	14
Steak, blackened, 6 oz	17
Steak, chicken fried	
without gravy, 6 oz	13
with cream gravy, 6 oz with 1/4 cup cream gravy	17
Steak, Salisbury, 6 oz	11
Sticky rice with mango, 1 cup sliced mangoes with 1/2 cup sticky rice	9
Stir-fried beef with garlic or black bean sauce, 1 cup	8
Stir-fried chicken with garlic or black bean sauce, 1 cup	7
Stir-fried pork with garlic or black bean sauce, 1 cup	8
Stir-fried shrimp with garlic or black bean sauce, 1 cup	7

	POINTS VALUE
Stir-fried vegetables	
1 cup	3
with beef, 1 cup	4
with chicken, 1 cup	2
with pork, 1 cup	3
without sauce, frozen, 1 cup	0
Strawberries	
fresh, 1 1/2 cups whole or sliced	1 (2)
frozen, unsweetened, 1 cup thawed	1 (2)
Strawberry shortcake, 1/12 of 9" cake or 1 filled individual shortcake	7
Stromboli, 1 slice (1" thick) or 2 oz	4
Strudel, any type, 1 piece (5 1/2" x 2")	9
Stuffing	
1/2 cup	4
bread, from mix, prepared, 1/2 cup	4
Submarine sandwich, 1 (6")	6
Succotash, (corn and limas)	
cooked, 1 cup	4
frozen, cooked, 1 cup	2
canned, with cream style or whole kernel corn, 1 cup	3
Sucralose, 1 tsp	0
Sugar apple	
1/3 cup	1 (2)
1/2 (2 3/4 oz)	1 (2)
Sugar substitute, 1 tsp	0

	POINTS VALUE
Sugar, brown	
1 Tbsp unpacked	1
1 cup packed	17
Sugar, white	
1 Tbsp	1
1 cup	15
Suimono, 1 cup	1
Sukiyaki with sauce, 2 cups with 1/4 cup sauce	12
Summer squash casserole, 1 cup	9
Sunflower seeds	
1 tsp	0
1 Tbsp	1
Sunomono, 1/2 cup	0
Sushi, Alaskan roll, 2 pieces (1" high x 1 3/4" diameter)	3
Sushi, California roll, 4 large pieces (1" high X 1 3/4" diameter) or 1 oz each	3
Sushi, cone, 1	2
Sushi, inari, 1	2
Sushi, kappa maki (cucumber roll)	
6 small pieces (1" diameter, 1" thick)	2
4 medium (1 1/2" diameter, 3/4" thick)	2
Sushi, maki (vegetables and rice rolled with seaweed)	
6 small pieces (1" diameter, 1" thick)	2
4 medium pieces (1 1/2" diameter, 3/4" thick)	2

	POINTS VALUE
Sushi, nigiri (sliced raw fish over rice)	
albacore (white tuna),amaebi (sweet shrimp), conch, ebi (cooked shrimp), hamachi (yellow tail), hirame (fluke), hokigai (surf clam), ika (squid), ikura (salmon roe), kani (crab), maguro (tuna), masago (smelt roe), saba (mackerel), sake (fresh salmon), smoked salmon, suzuki (sea bass), suzume, tai (red snapper), tairagai (scallops), tako (octopus), todiko (flying fish roe), unagi (fresh water eel), uni (sea urchin), 4 pieces (2" long, 3/4" wide)	2
Sushi, nori maki (raw fish and rice rolled with seaweed), 4 medium (1 1/2" diameter, 3/4" thick) or 6 small (1"diameter, 1" thick)	2
Sushi, Philadelphia roll, 2 large pieces (1" high x 1 3/4" diameter)	3
Sushi, rainbow roll, 6 small (1" diameter, 1" thick) or 4 medium (1 1/2" diameter, 3/4" thick)	2
Sushi, shrimp tempura roll, 6 pieces (1 1/2" diameter x 1" thick)	8
Sushi, spider roll, 6 pieces (2" diameter x 1" thick)	9
Sushi, tamago-yaki (omelet roll), 2 pieces (3/4" wide)	3
Sushi, tuna roll, 6 small (1" diameter, 1" thick) or 4 medium (1 1/2" diameter, 3/4" thick)	2
Sushi, tuna roll, spicy, 6 pieces (2" diameter x 1" thick)	5

	POINTS VALUE
Sushi, unagi maki, 6 small (1" diameter, 1" thick) or 4 medium (1 1/2" diameter, 3/4" thick)	2
Sushi, uni maki, 6 small (1" diameter, 1" thick) or 4 medium (1 1/2" diameter, 3/4" thick)	2
Sushi, yellow tail roll, 6 small (1" diameter, 1" thick) or 4 medium (1 1/2" diameter, 3/4" thick)	2
◆ **Swamp cabbage, (skunk cabbage),** cooked or raw, 1 cup	0
Swedish meatballs	
6 (1" diameter)	9
with noodles, frozen, 1 cup	7
Sweet and sour	
beef, 1 cup	12
chicken, 1 cup	10
pork, 1 cup	12
shrimp, 1 cup	10
◆ **Sweet potato leaves,** cooked, 1 cup	0
Sweet potato pie, 1/8 of 9" pie	9
Sweet potatoes, candied, 1/2 cup	4
Sweet roll	
1 large (4 oz)	5
pecan-swirl, store-bought, 2 (2 oz)	5
store-bought, 1 (2 3/4" square)	5
◆ **Sweetbreads,** cooked, 1 oz	1 (5)

	POINTS VALUE
Sweetsop (sugar apple)	
◆ 1/3 cup	1 (2)
◆ 1/2 (2 7/8" diameter)	1 (2)
Syrup	
chocolate, 1 Tbsp	1
maple, 1 Tbsp	1
maple, 1 cup	17
pancake, low-calorie, 2 Tbsp	1
pancake, regular, 1 Tbsp	1
Szechuan chicken, frozen, 1 cup	5

T

	POINTS VALUE
Tabouli, 1/2 cup	4
Taco	
beef, 1 (3 1/2 oz)	5
breakfast, 1 (3 3/4 oz)	5
chicken, 1 (3 1/2 oz)	4
fish, 1 (4 1/4 oz)	4
hard, dinner kit in a box, prepared, 2 (5 1/2 oz)	7
hard, fast food, 1	3
pork, 1 (3 1/2 oz)	4
soft, fast food, 1	3
soft, kit in a box, prepared, 2 (5 1/2 oz)	9

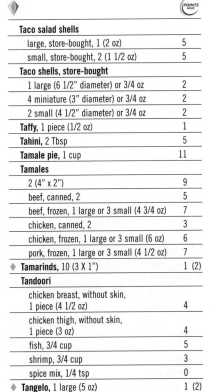

	POINTS VALUE
Taco salad shells	
large, store-bought, 1 (2 oz)	5
small, store-bought, 2 (1 1/2 oz)	5
Taco shells, store-bought	
1 large (6 1/2" diameter) or 3/4 oz	2
4 miniature (3" diameter) or 3/4 oz	2
2 small (4 1/2" diameter) or 3/4 oz	2
Taffy, 1 piece (1/2 oz)	1
Tahini, 2 Tbsp	5
Tamale pie, 1 cup	11
Tamales	
2 (4" x 2")	9
beef, canned, 2	5
beef, frozen, 1 large or 3 small (4 3/4 oz)	7
chicken, canned, 2	3
chicken, frozen, 1 large or 3 small (6 oz)	6
pork, frozen, 1 large or 3 small (4 1/2 oz)	7
◆ **Tamarinds,** 10 (3 X 1")	1 (2)
Tandoori	
chicken breast, without skin, 1 piece (4 1/2 oz)	4
chicken thigh, without skin, 1 piece (3 oz)	4
fish, 3/4 cup	5
shrimp, 3/4 cup	3
spice mix, 1/4 tsp	0
◆ **Tangelo,** 1 large (5 oz)	1 (2)

	POINTS VALUE
Tangerine	
◆ 1 large (3" diameter)	1 (2)
◆ 2 medium (2 3/8" diameter)	1 (2)
◆ 2 small (2 1/4" diameter)	1 (2)
Tapioca, uncooked, 1 tsp	0
Taquitos	
beef, 1 (5 1/2" x 1 1/2")	4
chicken, 1 (5 1/2" x 1 1/2")	2
frozen, 2 (2 oz)	3
Taro	
◆ cooked, 1 cup	3
◆ raw, 1 cup	2
◆ **Tahitian,** cooked or raw, 1 cup	1
◆ **Taro leaves,** cooked or raw, 1 cup	0
Taro shoots	
◆ cooked, 1 cup	1
◆ raw, 1/2 cup	0
Tarragon, fresh or dried, 1 tsp	0
Tart shell, 1 (4" diameter)	6
Tarte aux fruits	
1/8 of 9" tart	8
individual, 1 (4")	11
Tea	
black, decaffeinated or regular, without sugar, 1 cup	0
decaffeinated or regular, sweetened, 1 cup	2

Tea (con't)	POINTS VALUE
instant, unsweetened, powder, 1 tsp	0
instant, unsweetened, powder, prepared, 1 cup	0
sweetened, 1 Tbsp	2
◆ Tempeh (fermented soybean cake), 1/4 cup (1 1/2 oz)	2
Tempura	
batter mix, 1/4 cup	2
shrimp, 4 jumbo	12
vegetable, 1 cup	8
Teppan yaki (mixed grill of beef, chicken, shrimp and vegetables), 1 1/2 cups	12
Tequila, 1 jigger (1 1/2 fl oz)	2
Teriyaki	
beef, 2 slices (4 oz)	7
chicken, 2 slices (4 oz)	6
fish other than salmon, 4 oz	5
salmon, 4 oz	7
tofu, 1 cup	4
Texas trash (cereal and nut mix), 1 cup	8
Textured vegetable protein	
◆ 1/3 cup (3/4 oz dry)	1 (5)
◆ 1 oz	2 (5)
Thai chicken with basil, 1 breast (without skin and bone), 3 oz	5
Thai coffee or tea, 1 cup	7
Thai crisp noodles, 1 cup	8

	POINTS VALUE
Thai curry paste, 1 Tbsp	1
Thai grilled beef (Nuea nam tok), 1/2 cup on lettuce leaves	5
Thai paste, 2 Tbsp	2
Thyme, fresh or dried, 1 tsp	0
Tirami-su, 2 1/4" square	10
Toasted cheese sandwich, 1 (3 3/4 oz)	8
Toaster pastry	
low-fat, 1 (1 3/4 oz)	4
regular, any type, 1 (1 3/4 oz)	5
Tofu	
◆ extra firm, 3 oz	2 (5)
◆ firm, lite, 3 oz	1 (5)
◆ firm, regular, 1/5 block, 1/3 cup, or 3 oz	2 (5)
◆ low-fat, 1/5 block, 1/3 cup, or 3 oz	1 (5)
◆ silken, 3 oz	1 (5)
◆ silken, lite, 3 oz	0 (5)
◆ soft, regular, 1/5 block, 1/3 cup, or 3 oz	1 (5)
◆ **Tofu, okara,** 1 cup	2 (5)
Tofu, frozen, 1/2 cup	5
Tom Collins, 6 fl oz	2
Tom yum kung, 1 cup	2
◆ **Tomatillos,** 1 small, medium or large or 1/2 cup	0
Tomato or mixed vegetable juice, 1 cup	1
Tomato paste	
◆ canned, 2 Tbsp	0
◆ canned, 1/2 cup	1

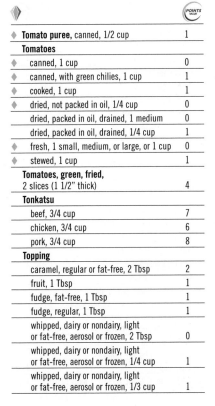

	POINTS VALUE
Tomato puree, canned, 1/2 cup	1
Tomatoes	
canned, 1 cup	0
canned, with green chilies, 1 cup	1
cooked, 1 cup	1
dried, not packed in oil, 1/4 cup	0
dried, packed in oil, drained, 1 medium	0
dried, packed in oil, drained, 1/4 cup	1
fresh, 1 small, medium, or large, or 1 cup	0
stewed, 1 cup	1
Tomatoes, green, fried, 2 slices (1 1/2" thick)	4
Tonkatsu	
beef, 3/4 cup	7
chicken, 3/4 cup	6
pork, 3/4 cup	8
Topping	
caramel, regular or fat-free, 2 Tbsp	2
fruit, 1 Tbsp	1
fudge, fat-free, 1 Tbsp	1
fudge, regular, 1 Tbsp	1
whipped, dairy or nondairy, light or fat-free, aerosol or frozen, 2 Tbsp	0
whipped, dairy or nondairy, light or fat-free, aerosol or frozen, 1/4 cup	1
whipped, dairy or nondairy, light or fat-free, aerosol or frozen, 1/3 cup	1

	POINTS VALUE
Tortellini	
beef, chicken, or pork, without sauce, frozen, 1 cup	5
cheese, without sauce, 10 (2/3 cup)	3
cheese, without sauce, frozen, 1 cup	6
meat, without sauce, 10 (2/3 cup)	3
mushroom, without sauce, frozen, 1 cup	6
sausage, without sauce, frozen, 1 cup	7
Tortiere (Canadian meat pie), 1/8 of 9" pie	9
Tortilla chips	
12 (1 oz)	3
baked, low-fat, 12 (1 oz)	2
reduced-fat, 12 (1 oz)	2
Tortilla, corn	
2 (4" diameter), 1 oz	1
1 (6" diameter), 1 oz	1
1/2 (10" diameter), 1 oz	1
Tortilla, flour	
2 (4" diameter), 1 oz	2
1 (6" diameter), 1 oz	2
1 (8" diameter), 1 1/2 oz	3
1/2 (10" diameter), 1 oz	2
fat-free, 2 (4" diameter), 1 oz	1
fat-free, 1 (6" diameter), 1 oz	1
fat-free, 1 (10" diameter), 2 oz	2
Tortilla, whole wheat, 1 medium (7")	1
Tortoni, 2 1/2 oz	7

	POINTS VALUE
Tostada	
beef, 1 (8 1/4 oz)	10
chicken, 1 (8 1/4 oz)	8
with beans and cheese, fast food, 1	5
Tostada shells, store-bought, 2 (1 oz)	2
Trail mix	
1/4 cup	4
tropical, 1/4 cup	3
with chocolate chips, 1/4 cup	5
Trifle, 1 cup	5
Tripe, beef, cooked, 1 oz	1 (5)
Tropical fruit, canned, in passion fruit juice, 1/2 cup	1
Tuna dinner in a box, prepared, 1 cup	7
Tuna melt sandwich, 1 (5 3/4 oz)	9
Tuna noodle casserole, 1 cup	9
Tuna salad sandwich, 1 (6 1/4 oz)	10
Tuna, grilled, frozen, 3 oz	2 (5)
Turkey breast	
cooked, with skin, 1 slice (2 oz)	2
cooked, without skin, 1 slice, 2 oz or 1/2 cup cubed or shredded	2 (5)
without skin or bone, raw, 1/2 breast (13 3/4 oz)	9 (5)
without skin or bone, raw, 4 oz	3 (5)
Turkey burger, frozen (prepared), 1 (3 oz)	5

	POINTS VALUE
Turkey croquette, breaded, with gravy, frozen, 1 (3 1/2 oz)	3
Turkey roll, 1 slice (1 oz)	1
Turkey tetrazzini, 1 1/2 cups	14
Turkey giblets, cooked, 1 cup (chopped or diced)	5 (5)
Turkey gizzard, cooked, 1 cup (chopped or diced)	5 (5)
Turkey heart, cooked, 1 cup chopped or diced	6 (5)
Turkey leg (thigh and drumstick with skin), cooked 1 (1 1/4 pounds)	27
Turkey liver, cooked, 1 cup chopped or diced	5 (5)
Turkey neck, cooked, 1 (bone and skin removed), 5 1/2 oz	6 (5)
Turkey thigh, cooked, with skin, 1 slice (2 oz)	3
Turkey, canned, 1/2 cup	4 (5)
Turkey, dark meat	
cooked, without skin, 1 slice, 2 oz or 1/2 cup cubed or shredded	2 (5)
cooked, meat and skin, 1 cup chopped or diced	8
Turkey, ground	
93% lean/7% fat, cooked, 1/2 cup or 2 oz	3 (5)
93% lean/7% fat, cooked, 1 patty (3 oz)	4 (5)

	POINTS VALUE
93% lean/7% fat, cooked, 12 oz (1 pound raw)	16 (5)
93% lean/7% fat, raw, 4 oz	3 (5)
breast, ground, raw, 4 oz	3 (5)
regular, cooked, 1/2 cup or 2 oz	3 (5)
regular, cooked, 1 patty (3 oz)	5 (5)
regular, cooked, 12 oz (1 pound raw)	20 (5)
regular, raw, 4 oz	5 (5)
Turkey, light meat, cooked, without skin, 1 slice, 2 oz or 1/2 cup cubed or shredded	2 (5)
Turkey, meat only, roasted, 1 cup chopped or diced	5
Turkey, with gravy, frozen, 1 cup	4
Turmeric, ground, 1 tsp	0
Turnips, cooked or raw, 1 cup	0
Turnover, fruit, any type	
1 (3" x 1 1/2")	5
fast food, 1	7
Twice-cooked pork, 1 cup	10
Tyropitas, frozen, 2 (2 oz)	4
Tzimmes, vegetable, 3/4 cup	2

U

Urad dal, 1 cup	4

V

Veal	
brain, cooked, 3 oz	3 (5)
brain, raw, 1 oz	1 (5)
breast, cooked, 3 oz	6
breast, lean only, cooked, 3 oz	4 (5)
breast, trimmed, cooked, 3 oz	5 (5)
cubed, lean only, cooked, 3 oz	4 (5)
cubed, lean only, raw, 1 oz	1 (5)
heart, cooked, 3 oz	4 (5)
heart, raw, 1 oz	1 (5)
kidneys, cooked, 3 oz	3 (5)
kidneys, raw, 1 oz	1 (5)
lean (leg and loin cuts with all visible fat trimmed), cooked, 1 slice or 1/2 cup cubed or shredded (2 oz)	3 (5)
lean (leg and loin cuts with all visible fat trimmed), raw, 1 oz	1 (5)
leg, cooked, 3 oz	4
leg, trimmed, cooked, 3 oz	4 (5)
leg, trimmed, raw, 1 oz	1 (5)
liver, cooked, 3 oz	3 (5)
liver, raw, 1 oz	1 (5)
loin, cooked, 3 oz	6
loin, trimmed, cooked, 3 oz	4 (5)
loin, trimmed, raw, 1 oz	1 (5)

Veal (con't)

	POINTS VALUE
regular, cooked, 1 slice or 1/2 cup cubed or shredded (2 oz)	3
rib, cooked, 3 oz	5
rib, trimmed, cooked, 3 oz	4
shank, cooked, 3 oz	4
◆ shank, lean only, cooked, 3 oz	3 (5)
◆ shank, lean only, raw, 1 oz	1 (5)
shoulder, cooked, 3 oz	5
◆ shoulder, trimmed, cooked, 3 oz	4 (5)
◆ shoulder, trimmed, raw, 1 oz	1 (5)
sirloin, cooked, 3 oz	5
sirloin, lean and fat, cooked, 3 oz	5
◆ sirloin, trimmed, cooked, 3 oz	4 (5)
◆ sirloin, trimmed, raw, 1 oz	1 (5)
◆ tongue, cooked, 3 oz	4 (5)
◆ tongue, raw, 1 oz	1 (5)
Veal cutlet, breaded, fried, 4 oz	8
Veal marsala, 4 oz veal with sauce	13
Veal parmigiana	
without sauce, 5 1/2 oz	10
with sauce, 5 oz with 1/2 cup tomato sauce	12
Veal piccata, 2 slices (4 oz)	10
Veal scaloppine, 2 pieces (4 1/2 oz)	8
Veal with peppers, 5 oz	11
Vegetable juice, mixed	
1/2 cup	0
1 cup	1

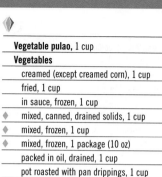

	POINTS VALUE
Vegetable pulao, 1 cup	3
Vegetables	
creamed (except creamed corn), 1 cup	2
fried, 1 cup	4
in sauce, frozen, 1 cup	2
◆ mixed, canned, drained solids, 1 cup	1
◆ mixed, frozen, 1 cup	1
◆ mixed, frozen, 1 package (10 oz)	3
packed in oil, drained, 1 cup	3
pot roasted with pan drippings, 1 cup	2
sautéed, 1 cup	6
◆ stir-fry, without sauce, 1 cup	0
Vegetables, Chinese, prepared without oil, 1 cup	2
Vegetarian breakfast link (sausage-type), 2 (1 1/2 oz)	3
Vegetarian breakfast patty (sausage-type), 1 (1 1/3 oz)	1
Vegetarian breakfast strips, 4 (1 oz)	3
◆ **Vegetarian burger, black bean,** frozen, 1 (1 1/2 oz)	2 (5)
◆ **Vegetarian burger, fat-free,** frozen, 1 (2 3/4 oz)	1 (5)
◆ **Vegetarian burger,** frozen, 1 (2 3/4 oz)	2 (5)
Vegetarian chicken patty, frozen, 1 (3 oz)	2
Vegetarian chicken pieces (nugget-style), frozen, 4 (2 3/4 oz)	2
Vegetarian deli slices, frozen, 3 (2 3/4 oz)	1

	POINTS VALUE
Vegetarian frankfurter, fat-free, frozen, 1/2 large (2 1/2 oz)	1
Vegetarian frankfurter, fat-free, frozen, 1 small (2 1/2 oz)	1
Vegetarian frankfurter, regular, frozen, 1/2 large (3 oz)	1
Vegetarian frankfurter, regular, frozen, 1 small (3 oz)	1
Vegetarian ground "meat", frozen, 1/2 cup	1 (5)
Vegetarian sausage, frozen, 1 1/2 oz	2
Vegetarian topping (made with soy), 2 Tbsp	1
Venison	
cooked, 1 oz	1 (5)
raw, 4 oz	4 (5)
Vienna sausage	
canned, beef and pork, 3 (2" long each)	4
chicken, canned, 3 (2" long each)	3
Vietnamese beef balls (Thit bo vien), 6 (1 1/2 oz)	2
Vietnamese chicken curry, 1 cup	7
Vindaloo	
chicken, 1 cup	8
lamb, 1 cup	16
pork, 1 cup	9
Vinegar, 1 Tbsp	0
Vitello tonnato, 2 slices veal (4 oz) with 1/2 cup sauce	16
Vodka, 1 jigger (1 1/2 fl oz)	2
Vodka gimlet, 2 1/2 fl oz	2

W

	POINTS VALUE
Waffle	
any type other than those listed here, 1 (7" square)	5
any type, frozen, 1 (4" round or square), or 1 1/4 oz	2
any type, made from mix, 1 (4" round or square)	2
Belgian, frozen, 1 (1 oz)	2
low-fat, any type, frozen, 2 (4" round or square)	3
mini, frozen, 4 (1 3/4 oz)	2
sticks, frozen, 1 large or 2 small (2 oz)	3
Walnuts	
1 cup chopped, pieces, or chips	21
1 cup ground	14
14 halves (1 oz)	5
1 Tbsp	1
Wasabi	
powder, 1 tsp	0
root, raw, 1 cup sliced	2
Water chestnuts	
1/2 cup	1
canned, 1 cup	1
Chinese, (matai), raw, 1/2 cup slices	1
Water or mineral water, 1 cup	0

83

	POINTS VALUE
Watercress, 1 cup	0
Watermelon, 1 cup or 1 slice (2")	1 (2)
Wax gourd (Chinese winter melon), cooked or raw, 1 cup	0
Wheat germ	
2 Tbsp	1
3 Tbsp	1
Whiskey, 1 jigger (1 1/2 fl oz)	2
Whiskey sour, 3 fl oz	2
Wiener schnitzel, 1 slice (3 oz)	9
Wine	
1 small glass (4 fl oz)	2
dessert, dry, 2 fl oz	1
dessert, sweet, 2 fl oz	2
light, 1 small glass (4 fl oz)	1
non-alcoholic, 1/2 cup	1
Wine cooler, 8 fl oz	2
Wine spritzer, 8 fl oz	2
Wonton skins (wrappers), 5 (3 1/2" squares)	2
Wontons	
boiled, 6 (6 oz)	5
fried, 6 (4 oz)	11

Y

	POINTS VALUE
Yaki-soba	
beef, 1 cup (1/2 cup noodles with 1/2 cup mixed vegetables)	4
chicken, 1 cup (1/2 cup noodles with 1/2 cup chicken & vegetables)	4
pork, 1 cup (1/2 cup noodles with 1/2 cup pork & vegetables)	4
Yakitori, 1 skewer (7 1/2 oz)	5
Yam	
cooked, 3/4 cup	2 (6)
cooked, 1 cup	3 (6)
cooked, 1 large (5"), or 7 oz	3 (6)
sweet, canned, in syrup, 1 cup	3
uncooked, 1 cup cubes	3 (6)
uncooked, 1 large (8 oz)	4 (6)
Yam patty, frozen, 1 (4 oz)	1 (6)
Yeast, 1 tsp	0
Yogurt	
fat-free, flavored (vanilla, lemon, coffee), sweetened with sugar, 1 cup	3
fat-free, fruit-flavored, sweetened with sugar, 1 cup	4
fat-free, plain, 1 cup	2
light (artificially sweetened), 1 cup	2

	POINTS VALUE
low-fat, flavored (vanilla, lemon, coffee), sweetened with sugar, 1 cup	4
low-fat, plain, 1 cup	3
low-fat, fruit-flavored, sweetened with sugar, 1 cup	5
plain, whole milk, 1 cup	4
Yogurt, frozen	
fat-free, no sugar added, 1 scoop or 1/2 cup	2
frozen, fat-free, sweetened with sugar, 1 scoop or 1/2 cup	2
frozen, low-fat, 1 scoop or 1/2 cup	3
Yogurt bar, chocolate-covered, frozen, 1 (2.8 fl oz)	5
Yogurt drink, 1 cup	5
Yorkshire pudding, 1 piece (4" square)	6
Yosenabe, 2 cups	4
Yuca, raw, 1 cup	6

Z

	POINTS VALUE
Zabaglione, 1/2 cup	4
Zeppole, 1 (4" diameter)	6
Ziti, baked	
with meat, 1 cup	9
without meat, 1 cup	6
Zucchini	
breaded, prepared without fat, 6 pieces (4 oz)	4
cooked or raw, 1 cup	0
Zucchini, Italian style, canned, 1 cup	2
Zucchini bread, 1 slice (3/4" thick)	5
Zuppa di pesce, 2 cups	11
Zuppa Inglese, 1/16 of 10" cake	8
Zwieback, 4	2

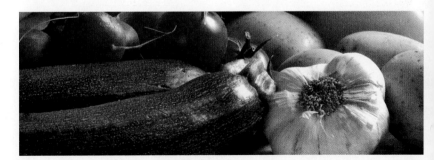

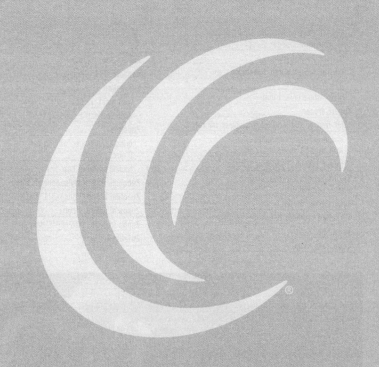

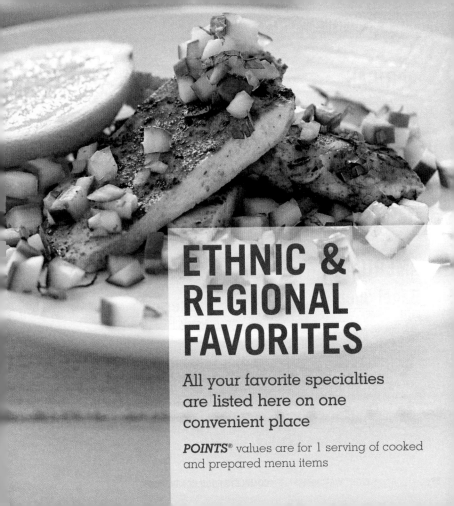

ETHNIC & REGIONAL FAVORITES

All your favorite specialties
are listed here on one
convenient place

***POINTS*®** values are for 1 serving of cooked
and prepared menu items

AFRICAN

	POINTS VALUE
Chutney, any type, 2 Tbsp	1
Couscous, cooked, 1 cup	3
Curry	
African, fish, 1/2 cup	6
African, shrimp, 1/2 cup	6
Doro wat, 1 cup	7
Fish, fried, breaded with flour, 1 fillet (6 oz)	12
Ostrich, cooked, 3 oz	3 (5)
Fritters, vegetable, 1 cup	10
Rice, white, cooked, 1 cup	4

AMERICAN

Bagel Shop

	POINTS VALUE
Bagel	
any type, 1/2 large (4 1/2" diameter or 2 oz)	3
any type, 1 large (4 oz)	6
any type, 1 mini (2 1/2" diameter)	1
any type, 1 small (3" diameter or 2 oz)	3
Bagel, with cream cheese and lox, 1 large (6 1/2 oz)	12
Butter, regular, 1 tsp	1

	POINTS VALUE
Cheese, cream	
light, 1 Tbsp	1
regular, 1 Tbsp	1
Egg, whole, chicken, fried, 1 large	2
Hummus, 1/4 cup	3
Muffin, any type, 1 large (3" diameter)	6
Peanut butter, 1 Tbsp	2
Salad	
chicken, 1/2 cup	6
tuna, 1/2 cup	7
Soup	
chicken, with matzo balls, 1 cup soup with 2 (1 1/2") matzo balls	3
chicken, without matzo balls (broth only), 1 cup	0
minestrone, 1 cup	4

Bakery

	POINTS VALUE
Brownie, 1 (2" square)	5
Cake	
angel food, 1 slice (1/16 of 10" tube)	2
carrot, with cream cheese icing, 1/12 of 9" layer cake, or 3" square	16
coffee, 3" square, or 1/12 of 9" tube	8
pineapple upside-down, 2 1/2" square	5
pineapple upside-down, 1/8 of 10" skillet cake	10

	POINTS VALUE
pound, 1 slice (5" x 3" x 1")	8
with icing, 1/12 of 9" layer cake or 3" square	12
Cheesecake, with or without fruit topping, 1/16 of 10" cake	10
Cinnamon bun	
1 large	6
any type, 1 cup	10
Cobbler, fruit, any type, 1 cup	10
Muffin, any type, 1 large (3" diameter)	6
Pie	
chiffon, 1/8 of 9" one-crust pie	9
coconut custard pie, 1/8 of 9" one-crust pie	9
custard pie, 1/8 of 9" one-crust pie	8
fruit, one-crust, 1/8 of 9" pie	6
fruit, two-crust, 1/8 of 9" pie	9
key lime pie, 1/8 of 9" one-crust pie	13
rhubarb pie, 1/8 of 9" two-crust pie	11
meringue, 1/8 of 9" pie	10
mincemeat, with meat, 1/8 of 9" two-crust pie	12
mincemeat, without meat, 1/8 of 9" two-crust pie	13
pecan, 1/8 of 9" one-crust pie	12
pumpkin, 1/8 of 9" one-crust pie	9

	POINTS VALUE
Bar/Pub	
Beer	
light, 1 can or bottle (12 fl oz)	2
regular, 1 can or bottle (12 fl oz)	3
Buffalo wings, 3 (4 1/2 oz)	9
Carrot sticks, 1 cup	0
Celery sticks, 1 cup	0
Cheeseburger on bun, plain (without mayonnaise, lettuce, and tomato), 1	11
Chili dog on roll, 1	10
Dressing, salad, creamy, regular, 2 Tbsp	4
Fish, fried, breaded with flour, 1 fillet (6 oz)	12
French fries, 20 (4 1/2" long), 5 1/2 oz	10
Hamburger on bun, plain (without mayonnaise, lettuce, and tomato), 1 (3 oz cooked hamburger on 1 1/2 oz bun)	9
Hot dog, on roll, plain, 1 (4 oz)	8
Hummus, 1/4 cup	3
Liquor (brandy, gin, rum, scotch, tequila, vodka, whiskey), 1 jigger (1 1/2 fl oz)	2
Nachos	
beef, 4 (8 1/2 oz)	13
cheese, 4 (3 oz)	8
cheese and bean, 4 (6 1/2 oz)	9
chicken, 4 (8 1/2 oz)	11
with cheese sauce, 1/2 cup tortilla chips with 1/4 cup cheese sauce	5

	POINTS VALUE
Peanuts, 40 (1 oz shelled)	4
Philly cheese steak sandwich, 1 (9 oz)	13
Pita, 1 small or 1/2 large (1 oz)	1
Pretzels	
7 regular (3/4 oz)	2
15 small (3/4 oz)	2
45 sticks (3/4 oz)	2
Salsa, fat-free, 2 Tbsp	0
Sloppy Joe, 1 (6 oz)	7
Tortilla chips, 12 (1 oz)	3
Wine	
1 small glass (4 fl oz)	2
light, 1 small glass (4 fl oz)	1
Wine spritzer, 8 fl oz	2

Barbecue

	POINTS VALUE
Beans	
baked, 1/2 cup	5
green, cooked, 1 cup	0
Sauce	
barbecue, 1 Tbsp	0
barbecue, 1/4 cup	1
hot, 1 tsp	0
Beef	
brisket, cooked, 3 oz	9
shortribs, cooked, 3 oz	11

	POINTS VALUE
Chicken breast	
barbecued, with skin and bone, 1 (4 1/2 oz)	6
cooked, without skin and bone, 1 (3 oz)	3 (5)
Chicken drumstick, barbecued, with skin and bone, 1 (1 1/2 oz)	2
Chicken thigh, barbecued, with skin and bone, 1 (1 oz)	5
Cobbler, fruit, any type, 1 cup	10
Collards, cooked or raw, 1 cup	0
Corn on the cob	
1 large (8")	2 (6)
1 medium (7")	1 (6)
1 small (5 1/2")	1 (6)
Cornbread, 1 piece (2" square)	3
French fries, 20 (4 1/2" long), 5 1/2 oz	10
Ketchup	
1 Tbsp	0
1/4 cup	1
Lemonade, 1 cup	2
Pecan pie, 1/8 of 9" one-crust pie	12
Pickle, unsweetened, 1 cup or 1 large	0
Pork, barbecued, 1 cup	8
Potatoes, baked, plain, 1 large (7 oz)	3 (6)
Shrimp, barbecued, 4 large shrimp with 1/4 cup sauce	11
Spareribs	
barbecued, 4 small (4" long each)	8
barbecued, 6 (6 1/4 oz)	18

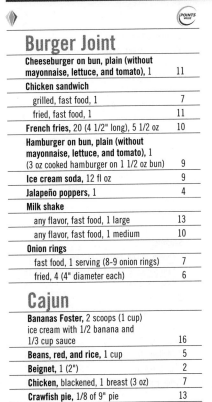

POINTS VALUE

Burger Joint

Cheeseburger on bun, plain (without mayonnaise, lettuce, and tomato), 1 — 11

Chicken sandwich
- grilled, fast food, 1 — 7
- fried, fast food, 1 — 11

French fries, 20 (4 1/2" long), 5 1/2 oz — 10

Hamburger on bun, plain (without mayonnaise, lettuce, and tomato), 1 (3 oz cooked hamburger on 1 1/2 oz bun) — 9

Ice cream soda, 12 fl oz — 9

Jalapeño poppers, 1 — 4

Milk shake
- any flavor, fast food, 1 large — 13
- any flavor, fast food, 1 medium — 10

Onion rings
- fast food, 1 serving (8-9 onion rings) — 7
- fried, 4 (4" diameter each) — 6

Cajun

Bananas Foster, 2 scoops (1 cup) ice cream with 1/2 banana and 1/3 cup sauce — 16

Beans, red, and rice, 1 cup — 5

Beignet, 1 (2") — 2

Chicken, blackened, 1 breast (3 oz) — 7

Crawfish pie, 1/8 of 9" pie — 13

POINTS VALUE

Creole
- chicken, without rice, 1 cup — 6
- shrimp, without rice, 1 cup — 4

Etouffee
- crawfish, 1 cup — 8
- shrimp, 1 cup — 9

Fish, blackened, 1 fillet (6 oz) — 12

Green rice, 1 cup — 6

Gumbo
- chicken, 1 cup — 6
- seafood, 1 cup — 5

Jambalaya, chicken or fish, with rice, 1 1/2 cups — 9

Muffuletta, 1 (6") — 20

Oyster pie, 1 slice (1/8 of 9" pie) — 9

Oyster po' boy, 1 (6") — 17

Praline, 1 (2 1/2" diameter, or 1 1/2 oz) — 5

Sauce, remoulade, 2 Tbsp — 4

Rice, dirty, 1 cup — 9

Soup, turtle, 1 cup — 2

Steak, blackened, 6 oz — 17

Diner

Bacon, lettuce, and tomato sandwich, 1 — 12

Butter, regular, 1 tsp — 1

Cantaloupe, 1/4 large (6 1/2" diameter) — 1 (2)

91

	POINTS VALUE
Egg, whole, chicken	
poached, 1	2 (5)
scrambled, 2 or 1/2 cup	5
English muffin, any type, 1 (2 oz)	2
Fish	
cod, cooked, 1 fillet (6 oz)	4 (5)
grouper, cooked, 1 fillet (6 oz)	4 (5)
haddock, cooked, 1 fillet (6 oz)	4 (5)
tuna, canned in water, drained, 1/2 cup	3 (5)
French fries, 20 (4 1/2" long), 5 1/2 oz	10
Hamburger on bun, plain (without mayonnaise, lettuce, and tomato), 1 (3 oz cooked hamburger on 1 1/2 oz bun)	9
Honey, 1 Tbsp	1
Muffin, any type, 1 large (3" diameter)	6
Omelet	
cheese, 1 (2-egg)	8
ham and cheese, 1 (2-egg)	9
herb or plain, 1 (2-egg)	6
vegetable, 1 (2-egg)	7
Pancake, prepared from scratch, 1 (4" diameter)	3
Peanut butter, 1 Tbsp	2
Pie	
fruit, one-crust, 1/8 of 9" pie	6
fruit, two-crust, 1/8 of 9" pie	9
Potatoes, baked, plain, 1 large (7 oz)	3 (6)

	POINTS VALUE
Potatoes, hash brown, 1 cup	7
Potatoes, sweet, baked, 1 medium (2" diameter, 5" long)	2 (6)
Preserves, 1 Tbsp	1
Pudding	
any flavor, 1/2 cup	3
any flavor, 1 cup	7
rice, 1 cup	8
tapioca, 1 cup	5
Salad	
chef's, with dressing, 4 cups	8
chef's, without dressing, 4 cups	6
fruit, 1 cup	2
Greek, with dressing, 3 cups	9
Greek, without dressing, 3 cups	2
Sandwich	
cheese, grilled, restaurant-type, 1 (4 oz)	13
ham & cheese, grilled, restaurant-type, 1	15
turkey, 1 (4 oz)	6
Soup	
black bean, 1 cup	2
chicken noodle, 1 cup	3
Salad	
chicken, 1/2 cup	6
tuna, 1/2 cup	7
Syrup, pancake, regular, 1 Tbsp	1

Ice Cream Shop

	POINTS VALUE
Banana split, 3 scoops (1 1/2 cups) ice cream, 1 banana, 3 Tbsp syrup, and 1/2 cup whipped cream	19
Ice cream	
premium, 1 scoop or 1/2 cup	7
regular, 1 scoop or 1/2 cup	4
Ice cream cone, plain or sugar, 1 small	1
Ice cream soda, 12 fl oz	9
Ice cream sundae	
1 scoop (1/2 cup) ice cream with syrup, nuts, & whipped topping	8
cone, 1 (3 1/2 oz)	8
Soft drink	
diet, any flavor, 1 can or bottle (12 fl oz)	0
sweetened with sugar, any flavor, 1 can or bottle (12 fl oz)	3
Sprinkles, any type, 1 Tbsp	1

Salad Bar

	POINTS VALUE
Bacon bits, imitation, 1 tsp	0
Beans, garbanzo, cooked, 1/2 cup	2 (5)
Beets	
cooked, 1 cup	1
pickled, 1/2 cup	1
Carrots, raw, 1 cup	0
Cheese, cottage, regular (4%), 1 cup	5

	POINTS VALUE
Cheese, hard or semisoft, regular, 3 Tbsp grated or 4 Tbsp shredded (1 oz)	3
Corn, kernels, cooked, 1 cup	2 (6)
Croutons, packaged, regular, 1/2 cup	3
Cucumber, 1 cup	0
Dressing, salad, creamy	
fat-free, 2 Tbsp	1
reduced-calorie, reduced-fat, or light, 2 Tbsp	2
regular, 2 Tbsp	4
Dressing, salad, Italian-type (not creamy)	
fat-free, 2 Tbsp	0
reduced-calorie, reduced-fat, or light, 2 Tbsp	1
regular, 2 Tbsp	4
Egg, whole, chicken, hard-boiled, 1	2 (5)
Gelatin, fruit-flavored, prepared, 1/2 cup	2
Ham, cooked, regular, 1/2 cup cubed or shredded (2 oz)	3
Lettuce, any type, 1 cup	0
Olives, 6 large or 10 small (1 oz)	1
Onion, 1 cup chopped or minced	1
Pepper	
any type other than roasted red, cooked or raw, 1 cup	0
roasted red, 1 cup	1
Pineapple, fresh, 1 cup	1 (2)
Radishes, 1 cup	0

	POINTS VALUE
Salad	
Caesar, 3 cups	7
chicken, 1/2 cup	6
tuna, 1/2 cup	7
pasta, 1/2 cup	3
Sprouts	
alfalfa, 1 cup	0
bean, 1 cup	0
Sunflower seeds	
1 tsp	0
1 Tbsp	1
Tomatoes, fresh, 1 cup	0
Yogurt	
low-fat, flavored (vanilla, lemon, coffee), sweetened with sugar, 1 cup	4
low-fat, fruit-flavored, sweetened with sugar, 1 cup	5

Seafood

	POINTS VALUE
Butter, regular, 1 tsp	1
Crab cakes, 2 (2 1/4 oz each, or 3" round)	4
Cream, sour, regular, 1 Tbsp	1
Fish	
bass, striped, cooked, 1 fillet (6 oz)	5 (5)
cod, cooked, 1 fillet (6 oz)	4 (5)
haddock, cooked, 1 fillet (6 oz)	4 (5)
halibut, cooked, 1 fillet or steak (6 oz)	5 (5)

	POINTS VALUE
mahimahi (dolphinfish), cooked, 1 fillet (6 oz)	4 (5)
salmon, cooked, 1 fillet (6 oz)	9 (5)
snapper, cooked, 1 fillet (6 oz)	5 (5)
swordfish, cooked, 1 fillet or steak (6 oz)	6 (5)
tuna, cooked, 1 fillet or steak (6 oz)	5 (5)
Fish, baked, stuffed, 6 1/2 oz	8
Fish, blackened, 1 fillet (6 oz)	12
Fish, fried, breaded with flour, 1 fillet (6 oz)	12
Lemon, 1 medium	0 (2)
Lobster Newburg, 1 cup	14
Lobster thermidor, 1 cup	14
Potatoes, baked, plain, 1 large (7 oz)	3 (6)
Sauce	
cocktail, 1/4 cup	1
tartar, 1 Tbsp	2
Shellfish	
crab, cooked or canned, 1 cup	3 (5)
lobster, cooked, 1/2 cup (2 oz)	1 (5)
lobster, steamed, 1 1/4-pound lobster or 4 1/2 oz lobster meat	3 (5)
scallops, cooked, 2 oz	1 (5)
scallops, fried, 20 small (3 1/2 oz)	5
shrimp, cooked, 1/2 cup (2 oz)	1 (5)
shrimp, broiled, stuffed, 6 large (6 oz)	18
shrimp, fried, 10 (5 oz)	8
shrimp, fried, stuffed, 6 large (9 1/2 oz)	9

Soup

	POINTS VALUE
Manhattan clam chowder, 1 cup	4
New England clam chowder, 1 cup	4

Southern/Soul Food

Apple brown Betty, 1 cup	5
◆ **Beans, green,** cooked, 1 cup	0
Biscuit, 1 small (2" diameter)	3
Pudding, bread, 1 cup	13
Pot pie, chicken, 8 1/2 oz	10
Chicken thigh, fried, with skin and bone, 1 (3 oz)	7
Cobbler, fruit, any type, 1 cup	10
Corn on the cob	
◆ 1 large (8")	2 (6)
◆ 1 medium (7")	1 (6)
◆ 1 small (5 1/2")	1 (6)
Cornbread, 1 piece (2" square)	3
Fish, fried, breaded with flour, 1 fillet (6 oz)	12
Gravy	
brown, 1/4 cup	2
cream, 1/4 cup	4
◆ **Greens, beet, collard, dandelion, kale, mustard, and turnip,** cooked or raw, 1 cup	0
◆ **Grits, corn, yellow, quick,** cooked, 1 cup	3

Gumbo

	POINTS VALUE
chicken, 1 cup	6
seafood, 1 cup	5
Ham, cooked, regular, 1 slice or 1/2 cup cubed or shredded (2 oz)	3
Hush puppies, 2 (2 1/4 oz)	4
Macaroni and cheese, 1 cup	9
Okra	
◆ cooked or raw, 1 cup	0
fried, 1 cup	8
Pie	
pecan, 1/8 of 9" one-crust pie	12
sweet potato, 1/8 of 9" pie	9
Pork, regular, cooked, 1 chop or 1 slice (2 oz)	5
Potatoes	
au gratin, 1 cup	13
mashed, 1/2 cup	2
Salad, potato, 1/2 cup	7
◆ **Soup, split pea,** 1 cup	3
Stuffing, 1/2 cup	4

Steakhouse

Bread, any type (white, wheat, rye, Italian, French, pumpernickel), 1 slice (1 oz)	2
Butter, regular, 1 tsp	1
◆ **Chicken breast, cooked, without skin and bone,** 1 (3 oz)	3 (5)

	POINTS VALUE
Cream, sour, regular, 1 Tbsp	1
French fries, 20 (4 1/2" long), 5 1/2 oz	10
Onion rings, fried, 4 (4" diameter each)	6
Onion, blooming, 1/4 (16" diameter onion)	6
Oysters, cooked, 6 medium (2 oz)	1 (5)
Mushrooms, cooked, 1 cup	0
Potatoes	
baked, plain, 1 large (7 oz)	3 (6)
garlic mashed, 1/2 cup	4
mashed, 1/2 cup	2
Salad, cobb, without dressing, 3 cups	10
Sauce	
barbecue, 1 Tbsp	0
barbecue, 1/4 cup	1
cocktail, 1/4 cup	1
steak, 1 Tbsp	0
Shrimp, cooked, 1/2 cup (2 oz)	1 (5)
Spareribs	
barbecued, 4 small (4" long each)	8
barbecued, 6 (6 1/4 oz)	18
Spinach, cooked or raw, 1 cup	0
Steak	
blackened, 6 oz	17
filet mignon, trimmed, cooked, 1 small (4 oz)	6 (5)
KC strip, cooked, 1 small (4 oz)	7
KC strip, trimmed, cooked, 1 small (4 oz)	5 (5)

	POINTS VALUE
lean, cooked (round or loin cuts with all visible fat trimmed), 2 oz	3 (5)
New York steak, cooked, 1 small (4 oz)	8
New York steak, trimmed, cooked, 1 small (4 oz)	6 (5)
strip sirloin, cooked, 1 small (4 oz)	7
strip sirloin, trimmed, cooked, 1 small (4 oz)	5 (5)
T-bone steak, cooked, 1 small (4 oz)	9
T-bone steak, trimmed, cooked, 1 small (4 oz)	7 (5)

CANADIAN

	POINTS VALUE
Bacon, Canadian-style, cooked, 1 slice	1 (5)
Caribou, cooked, 1 oz	1
Corn, cream-style, 1 cup	3
Donair, 4 oz meat with onion, tomato and 2 Tbsp sauce	14
Donair sauce, 2 Tbsp	2
Fiddlefern (fiddlehead greens), 1 cup	0
Fish and brewis, 1 cup	13
Poutine, 20 French fries with 2 oz cheese and 1/2 cup sauce	17
Rabbit, cooked, 1 oz	1
Rice, wild, cooked, 1 cup	3 (6)
Soup, split pea, 1 cup	3
Tortiere (Canadian meat pie), 1/8 of 9" pie	9
Venison, cooked, 1 oz	1 (5)

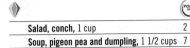

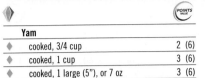

POINTS VALUE

Yam

cooked, 3/4 cup	2 (6)
cooked, 1 cup	3 (6)
cooked, 1 large (5"), or 7 oz	3 (6)

CARIBBEAN

Bahamian macaroni and cheese, 1 cup	9
Bahamian style peas and rice, 1 cup	7
Beans, black, and rice, 1 cup	4
Bistec de palomilla (Cuban fried steak), 1 steak	10
Carne guisado (Cuban beef stew), 1 cup	5
Chicken asopao, 1 cup with 1 piece chicken	8
Chicken breast, jerk, 1 (large breast, without skin)	5
Chuleta, 1 pork chop	10
Conch, cracked, 1 (6" long x 3")	9
Cuban sandwich, 1/2 (6 1/2" x 3" x 4")	11
Curry goat, 4 oz	5
Jamaican rice & peas, 1 cup	6
Lechon asado (roast pork), 3 oz	4
Pan Cubano, 1 (6 1/2" x 3")	8
Plantain	
baked or boiled, 1 cup	3
fried, 1 cup	4
Plátanos maduros (fried sweet plantains), 1 cup	4
Rice, Cuban, 1 cup	4

POINTS VALUE

Salad, conch, 1 cup	2
Soup, pigeon pea and dumpling, 1 1/2 cups	7

CHINESE

Beef and broccoli, 1 cup	4
Beef stir-fry, with garlic or black bean sauce, 1 cup	8
Beef, orange-ginger, 1 cup	11
Broccoli stir fry, 1 cup	3
Char shiu bao (roast pork bun), 1 (2 oz)	4
Chicken and broccoli, 1 cup	2
Chicken breast, five spice, with skin and bone, 1 (4 1/2 oz)	7
Chicken leg, five spice, 1 leg (thigh and drumstick, with skin and bone)	9
Chicken stir-fry with garlic or black bean sauce, 1 cup	7
Chicken subgum chow mein, 1 cup	4
Chicken with cashews, 1 cup	9
Chinese pepper steak, 1 cup	5
Chinese vegetables	
with beef, 1 cup	6
with chicken, 1 cup	5
with pork, 1 cup	7
with shrimp, 1 cup	4
with tofu, 1 cup	4
prepared without oil, 1 cup	2
Chicken, sesame, 1 cup	9

	POINTS VALUE
Chicken, sweet and sour, 1 cup	10
Chop suey	
beef, 1 cup	5
chicken, 1 cup	4
pork, 1 cup	4
vegetable, 1 cup	4
Chow fun	
beef, 1 cup	7
chicken, 1 cup	7
pork, 1 cup	7
shrimp, 1 cup	7
Chow mein	
beef, 1 cup	5
beef, chicken, or pork, canned, 1 cup	1
chicken, 1 cup	4
pork, 1 cup	5
Cookies, Chinese almond, 2 (1 oz)	3
Crab Rangoon, 1 large (4 1/2") or 5 mini	5
Dim sum	
bean curd roll with shrimp and vegetables, 1 (5" long x 2" wide)	2
bean curd roll with vegetables, 1 (5" long x 1.5" wide)	2
sesame seed balls, 1 (3" x 3")	5
Dumplings	
beef or pork, fried, 4 (6 1/2 oz)	6
beef or pork, steamed, 4 (5 3/4 oz)	6

	POINTS VALUE
chicken, fried, 4 (6 1/2 oz)	4
chicken, steamed, 4 (5 3/4 oz)	4
shrimp, fried, 4 (6 1/2 oz)	4
shrimp, steamed, 4 (5 3/4 oz)	4
vegetarian, fried, 4 (3 1/2" x 2" wide)	3
vegetarian, steamed, 4 (3 1/2" x 2" wide)	3
Egg foo yung	
beef, 1 (3" diameter)	4
chicken, 1 (3" diameter)	4
pork, 1 (3" diameter)	5
shrimp, 1 (3" diameter)	4
Egg roll	
beef, 1 (4 1/2" long)	5
chicken, 1 (4 1/2" long)	4
pork, 1 (4 1/2" long)	5
shrimp, 1 (4 1/2" long)	4
General Tso's chicken, 1 cup	15
Ginger chicken, 1 cup	7
Ginger fish, 1 cup	8
Kung Pao	
beef, 1 cup	10
chicken, 1 cup	8
pork, 1 cup	9
shrimp, 1 cup	9
Lobster Cantonese, 1 cup	8

	POINTS VALUE
Lo mein	
beef, 1 cup	8
chicken, 1 cup	8
pork, 1 cup	8
shrimp, 1 cup	8
vegetable, 1 cup	7
Mongolian beef, 1 cup	8
Moo goo gai pan, 1 cup	6
Moo shoo	
chicken, 1/2 cup with 2 pancakes	7
pork, 1/2 cup with 2 pancakes	8
tofu, 1/2 cup with 2 pancakes	7
Noodles, fried, 1 cup	6
Orange chicken, 1 cup	13
Pancake, Chinese, 1	1
Peking duck, 2 oz duck with 1 piece duck skin and 3 pancakes	10
Pork and broccoli, 1 cup	3
Pork stir-fry with garlic or black bean sauce, 1 cup	8
Pork with cashews, 1 cup	10
Pork, Chinese roast, 1 cup	5
♦ **Rice, brown,** cooked, 1 cup	4 (6)
Rice, fried	
plain, 1 cup	8
with beef, 1 cup	8
with chicken, 1 cup	8
with pork, 1 cup	8
with shrimp, 1 cup	8

	POINTS VALUE
Sauce	
black bean, 1 tsp	0
brown, Chinese, 1/4 cup	1
hoisin, 1 tsp	0
kung pao, 2 Tbsp	1
oyster, 1 tsp	0
plum, 1 Tbsp	1
soy (shoyu),1 Tbsp	0
soy (shoyu), low sodium, 1 Tbsp	0
sweet and sour, 2 Tbsp	1
Scallion pancake, 1 (5" diameter)	6
Sesame noodles, 1 cup	5
Shrimp	
Cantonese, 1 cup	8
stir-fry, with garlic or black bean sauce, 1 cup	7
sweet and sour, 1 cup	10
Shrimp and broccoli, 1 cup	2
Shrimp toast, 1 piece (1 oz)	3
Soup	
egg drop, 1 cup	1
hot and sour, 1 cup	2
wonton, 1 cup with 4 wontons	4
Spareribs, Chinese, barbecued, 2 (4" long each)	4
Spring roll	
beef or pork, 1 (4 1/2" long)	5
chicken, 1 (4 1/2" long)	4
shrimp, 1 (4 1/2" long)	4

	POINTS VALUE
Stir-fried beef with garlic or black bean sauce, 1 cup	8
Stir-fried chicken with garlic or black bean sauce, 1 cup	7
Stir-fried pork with garlic or black bean sauce, 1 cup	8
Stir-fried shrimp with garlic or black bean sauce, 1 cup	7
Stir-fried vegetables	
1 cup	3
with beef, 1 cup	4
with chicken, 1 cup	2
with pork, 1 cup	3
Sweet and sour	
beef, 1 cup	12
chicken, 1 cup	10
pork, 1 cup	12
shrimp, 1 cup	10
Twice-cooked pork, 1 cup	10
Wontons	
boiled, 6 (6 oz)	5
fried, 6 (4 oz)	11

EASTERN EUROPEAN

	POINTS VALUE
Beef Stroganoff with noodles, 1 cup stroganoff with 1 cup noodles	15
Borscht, 1 cup with 2 Tbsp sour cream	4

	POINTS VALUE
Chicken Kiev, 1 (4 x 8")	18
Chruscik, 1	1
Hungarian goulash, 1 cup	8
Kolache	
fruit-filled, 1 (3" diameter)	4
without filling, 1 (3" diameter)	4
Pierogies	
cabbage, 2 (3 1/2" each)	7
cheese, 2 (3 1/2" each)	7
meat, 2 (3 1/2" each)	8
potato, 2 (3 1/2" each)	7
potato and cheese, frozen, 3 (4 oz)	4
Rice pilaf, 1 cup	5

ENGLISH/IRISH

	POINTS VALUE
Beans, baked, 1/2 cup	5
Beef Wellington, 1 slice (3 1/2 x 2 1/2 x 1 1/2")	12
Bubble & squeak, 1 cup	3
Cabbage, all varieties, cooked or raw, 1 cup	0
Carrots and parsnips, 1 cup	4
Colcannon, 1 cup	7
Cornish hen	
cooked, with skin, 1/2 (4 1/2 oz)	9
cooked, without skin, 1/2 (3 3/4 oz)	3 (5)

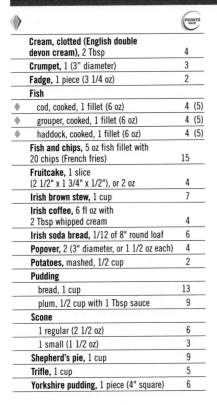

	POINTS VALUE
Cream, clotted (English double devon cream), 2 Tbsp	4
Crumpet, 1 (3" diameter)	3
Fadge, 1 piece (3 1/4 oz)	2
Fish	
cod, cooked, 1 fillet (6 oz)	4 (5)
grouper, cooked, 1 fillet (6 oz)	4 (5)
haddock, cooked, 1 fillet (6 oz)	4 (5)
Fish and chips, 5 oz fish fillet with 20 chips (French fries)	15
Fruitcake, 1 slice (2 1/2" x 1 3/4" x 1/2"), or 2 oz	4
Irish brown stew, 1 cup	7
Irish coffee, 6 fl oz with 2 Tbsp whipped cream	4
Irish soda bread, 1/12 of 8" round loaf	6
Popover, 2 (3" diameter, or 1 1/2 oz each)	4
Potatoes, mashed, 1/2 cup	2
Pudding	
bread, 1 cup	13
plum, 1/2 cup with 1 Tbsp sauce	9
Scone	
1 regular (2 1/2 oz)	6
1 small (1 1/2 oz)	3
Shepherd's pie, 1 cup	9
Trifle, 1 cup	5
Yorkshire pudding, 1 piece (4" square)	6

	POINTS VALUE
# FRENCH	
Baba au rhum, 1 (3 1/4 oz)	8
Beef Bourguignon, 1 1/2 cups	20
Blanquette of veal, 2 cups	13
Bouillabaisse, 2 cups	7
Brioche, 1 slice (1 oz)	3
Cassoulet, 1 cup	11
Chicken cordon bleu, 1 piece (5 1/2 oz)	13
Chocolate mousse, 1 cup	12
Coq au vin, 2 cups	13
Coquilles St. Jacques, 2 shells (13 2/3 oz)	8
Cream puff, 1 (2 oz)	7
Creme brulee, 3/4 cup	11
Creme caramel, 1 cup	7
Creme fraiche, 2 Tbsp	3
Crepes	
1 (6" diameter)	2
chicken, 2 (10 1/2 oz)	12
seafood, 2 (11 oz)	11
Suzette, 2 (4 3/4 oz)	10
Croissant	
chocolate filled, 1 (5" long)	6
plain, 1 (5" long)	5
Croque monsieur, 1 (6 1/2 oz)	11
Croquettes	
beef, 2 (2-1/2 oz each)	10
chicken, 2 (2 1/2 oz each)	9

	POINTS VALUE
Duck a l'orange, 1/4 duck with 2 Tbsp sauce	13
Eclair, 1	9
Escargots, 6 snails with 2 Tbsp butter	7
Fish amandine, 1 fillet (6 oz)	13
Fish Veronique, 1 fillet (6 oz)	11
Fondue, cheese, 1/2 cup fondue with 2 oz bread	12
Frog legs, fried, 2 (2 oz)	4
Fromage frais (soft cheese with fruit), 3 1/2 oz	3
Liver paté, 1 slice (4 1/4" x 1 1/2" x 1/2")	3
Mussels Mariniere, 4 mussels with 3 Tbsp sauce	5
Napoleon, 1 piece (4 1/2" x 2" x 1 1/2")	14
Oysters Rockefeller, 4 (2 oz)	3
Peach melba, 1/2 cup ice cream with 2 peach halves and raspberry sauce	7
Petit fours, 2 (1 3/4" x 1 1/2" x 1" each)	5
Petite marmite, 2 cups	7
Potatoes au gratin, 1 cup	13
Profiterole, 1 oz	3
Quenelles, 8 (2 1/2" x 1 1/2" x 3/4")	12
Quiche Lorraine, 1/8 of 9" pie	10
Quiche, vegetable, 1/8 of 9" pie	8
Ratatouille, 1 cup	4
Salad	
Niçoise, with dressing, 4 cups	18
◆ Niçoise, without dressing, 4 cups	8

	POINTS VALUE
Sauce	
béarnaise, 1/4 cup	8
hollandaise, 1/4 cup	8
mornay, 1/4 cup	3
Soup	
French onion au gratin, 1 cup	7
vichyssoise, 1 cup	2
Sausage in brioche, 1 slice (2" thick)	15
Sorbet, any flavor, 1/2 cup	2
Soufflé	
cheese, 1 cup	5
fruit, 1/2 cup	4
Steak au poivre, 6 oz steak with 1 Tbsp sauce	14
Tarte aux fruits	
1/8 of 9" tart	8
individual, 1 (4")	11

GERMAN

	POINTS VALUE
◆ **Applesauce, unsweetened,** 1 cup	2 (2)
Beef Stroganoff with noodles, 1 cup stroganoff with 1 cup noodles	15
Beer, regular, 1 can or bottle (12 fl oz)	3
Bratwurst, 2 oz	5
Cream, sour, regular, 1 Tbsp	1
Dumplings, potato, 6 (1" diameter)	2
Herring, pickled, 1/2 cup	2

	POINTS VALUE
Potato pancake, 1 (3 1/4 oz)	2
Salad, potato, German, 1/2 cup	2
Sachertorte, 1/16 of 9" cake	7
◆ **Salmon,** cooked, 1 fillet (6 oz)	9 (5)
Sauerbraten, 3 oz beef with 2 Tbsp gravy	6
◆ **Sauerkraut,** 1 cup	0
Spaetzle, 1/2 cup	5
Strudel, any type, 1 piece (5 1/2" x 2")	9
Wine, 1 small glass (4 fl oz)	2
Wiener schnitzel, 1 slice (3 oz)	9

GREEK

	POINTS VALUE
Baba ganosh, 1/4 cup	3
Baklava, 1 piece (2" square)	4
Cheese, feta, 1/4 cup (crumbled)	3
Dolma, 4 (3 1/2 oz)	4
Falafel	
in pita, 1 large pita with 4 falafel patties	10
patties, 4 (2" diameter each)	7
Gyro, 1 (6")	15
Halvah, 1 piece (2" x 1 3/4" x 1")	5
Hummus, 1/4 cup	3
Kataifi, 1 piece (2" long)	6
Moussaka, 1 piece (3" x 4")	12
◆ **Olives,** 6 large or 10 small (1 oz)	1 (2)
Pastitsio, 1 piece (3 1/4" x 3")	13

	POINTS VALUE
Pita, 1 small or 1/2 large (1 oz)	1
Saganaki, 1 piece (1" x 2" x 1/2" thick)	6
Salad	
Greek, with dressing, 3 cups	9
Greek, without dressing, 3 cups	2
yogurt and cucumber, 1/2 cup	1
Shish kabob (lamb), 2 small skewers (4 1/2 oz)	8
Soup, avgolemono, 1 cup	4
Souvlaki	
chicken, 1 large or 2 small skewers (4 1/2 oz)	5
chicken, in pita bread, 1 (6 1/2 oz)	7
lamb, 1 large or 2 small skewers (4 3/4 oz)	8
lamb, in pita bread, 1 (6 1/2 oz)	8
Spanakopita, 1 (3" square) or 1 cup	8

HAWAIIAN

	POINTS VALUE
◆ **Lomi lomi salmon,** 1/2 cup	1
◆ **Mahimahi (dolphinfish),** cooked, 1 fillet (6 oz)	4 (5)
Manapua with char shiu filling, 1	5
Mun doo	
fried, 4 (6 1/2 oz)	4
steamed, 4 (5 3/4 oz)	4
Nuts, macadamia, 12 nuts (1 oz shelled)	5
◆ **Poi,** 1/2 cup (4 oz)	3

	POINTS VALUE
Poke	
◆ ahi, 1/2 cup	2
◆ tako, 1/2 cup	2
Saimin, 1 cup	2

INDIAN

	POINTS VALUE
Aloo palak, 1 cup	3
Bean and lentil stew (Dal maharani), 1 cup	6
Biryani, chicken, 1 cup	9
Chana dal, 1 cup	4
Chapati, 1 piece (5" diameter)	2
Chicken tikka, 4 oz	5
Chili fish (Macher jhol), 1 fillet (6 oz)	12
Coconut rice, Indian, 1 cup	5
Curry	
beef, 1 cup	10
Bengali fish, 1 fillet (4 1/2 oz) and 1 cup vegetables	10
chicken, 1 cup	10
lamb, 1 cup	10
Dhansak, 1 cup	6
Fritters, vegetable, 1 cup	10
◆ **Garam masala,** 1/4 tsp	0
Gosht shaha korma, 1 cup	14
Kashmiri (lamb meatballs), 6 (3 1/2 oz)	11

	POINTS VALUE
Kheer, 1/2 cup	6
Korma	
chicken, 1 cup	14
lamb, 1 cup	15
vegetable, 1 cup	11
Lamb biryani, 1 cup	14
Lamb masala, 1 cup	6
Mango lassi, 1 cup	3
Masala dosa	
with filling, 1 (6" diameter dosa with 1/3 cup potato filling)	11
without filling, 1 (6" diameter)	10
Mung dal, 1 cup	5
Naan, 1 piece (7" x 8" diameter)	4
Pakora, vegetable, 1 (2" x 3" or 1 3/4 oz)	3
Palak vada (vegetable dumpling)	
fried, 1 (2 1/2" x 1 1/2")	5
steamed, 1 (2 1/2" x 1 1/2")	2
Paratha, 4" triangle	3
Puris, 4" diameter	2
Raita, 1/2 cup	1
Saag gosht, 1 cup	6
Saag paneer, 1 cup	6
Samosa, 1 (2 1/2" x 2 1/2" x 3" triangle)	3
Soup, mulligatawny, 1 cup	6
Tandoori	
chicken breast, without skin, 1 piece (4 1/2 oz)	4

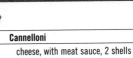

	POINTS VALUE
chicken thigh, without skin, 1 piece (3 oz)	4
fish, 3/4 cup	5
shrimp, 3/4 cup	3
Urad dal, 1 cup	4
Vindaloo	
chicken, 1 cup	8
lamb, 1 cup	16
pork, 1 cup	9

ITALIAN
Italian Restaurant

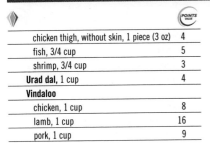

	POINTS VALUE
Artichokes	
marinated, 1/2 cup	3
stuffed, 1	14
Biscotti	
chocolate, 1 regular, 2 small, or 8 mini (1 oz)	3
fat-free, 1 regular, 2 small, or 8 mini (1 oz)	2
plain, 1 regular, 2 small, or 8 mini (1 oz)	3
Bruschetta, 1 slice (3 oz)	3
Calamari	
fried, 1/2 cup	11
◆ grilled, 1/2 cup	1 (5)
Calzone, ham and cheese, 1 (5 1/4 x 6")	12

	POINTS VALUE
Cannelloni	
cheese, with meat sauce, 2 shells with 1/2 cup sauce	15
cheese, with tomato sauce, 2 shells with 1/2 cup sauce	12
meat, with cream sauce, 2 shells with 1/2 cup sauce	17
meat, with tomato sauce, 2 shells with 1/2 cup sauce	14
spinach and cheese, with cream sauce, 2 shells with 1/2 cup sauce	15
spinach and cheese, with tomato sauce, 2 shells with 1/2 cup sauce	12
Cannoli, 1 (3 1/2" long)	9
Caponata (eggplant appetizer), 1/4 cup	1
Cappuccino	
◆ made with fat-free milk, 1 small (8 fl oz)	1
◆ made with fat-free milk, 1 tall (12 fl oz)	2
◆ made with fat-free milk, 1 grande (16 fl oz)	2
made with low-fat milk, 1 small (8 fl oz)	2
made with low-fat milk, 1 tall (12 fl oz)	3
made with low-fat milk, 1 grande (16 fl oz)	3
made with whole milk, 1 small (8 fl oz)	2
made with whole milk, 1 tall (12 fl oz)	3
made with whole milk, 1 grande (16 fl oz)	4
ready-made, from machine, any flavor, 1 cup	2

	POINTS VALUE
Cheese, Parmesan	
2 Tbsp grated	1
1 oz	3
Chicken cacciatore, 1/2 breast or 1 thigh and leg (6 1/2 oz)	10
Chicken marsala, 4 oz chicken without bone, with sauce	15
Chicken parmigiana	
without sauce, 5 1/2 oz	8
with sauce, 5 oz with 1/2 cup sauce	10
Chicken tetrazzini, 1 1/2 cups	14
Cioppino, 2 cups	13
Clams, baked, 6	7
Clams, fried, 1 cup	11
Cookies	
amaretti, 1 (1" diameter)	2
sesame seed, 2 (2" long)	3
Eggplant parmigiana	
with sauce, 3" x 4" with 1/2 cup Italian tomato sauce	13
without sauce, 3" x 4"	11
Eggplant	
breaded and baked (without oil), 2 slices (3" diameter)	1
breaded and fried, 2 slices (3" diameter)	3
Fettucine Alfredo, 1 cup	16
Focaccia bread, 1 piece (1/4 of 10" diameter)	6

	POINTS VALUE
Garlic bread, 1 slice (1 1/2 oz)	5
Gnocchi	
cheese, 1 cup	11
potato, 1 cup	4
spinach, 1 cup	12
Ices, Italian, restaurant-prepared, 1/2 cup	1
Italian casserole (ground beef, pasta & cheese over rolls)	
1 cup	14
1/8 of a 10" round casserole	16
Italian toast snacks, store-bought, 4	3
Lasagna	
cheese, with tomato sauce, 1	8
chicken, 1 cup	5
vegetable, 1 cup	5
vegetarian, with cheese, 10 oz	10
vegetarian, with cheese and spinach, 10 1/2 oz	9
with meat, 4" x 2 1/2" or 1 cup	6
with meat sauce, 1 cup	6
Latte	
made with fat-free milk, 1 small (8 fl oz)	2
made with fat-free milk, 1 tall (12 fl oz)	2
made with fat-free milk, 1 grande (16 fl oz)	3
made with low-fat milk, 1 small (8 fl oz)	3
made with low-fat milk, 1 tall (12 fl oz)	4
made with low-fat milk, 1 grande (16 fl oz)	5

	POINTS VALUE
made with whole milk, 1 small (8 fl oz)	3
made with whole milk, 1 tall (12 fl oz)	5
made with whole milk, 1 grande (16 fl oz)	6
Linguine with red clam sauce, 1 cup linguine with 1/2 cup sauce	6
Linguine with white clam sauce, 1 cup linguine with 1/2 cup sauce	8
Manicotti	
with meat sauce, 2 shells with 1/2 cup sauce	15
with tomato sauce, 2 shells with 1/2 cup sauce	12
Meatballs	
with sauce, 2 meatballs and 1/2 cup Italian tomato sauce	13
without sauce, 2 (1 1/4" diameter each)	10
Mozzarella, fried, 2 slices (2 3/4" x 1" x 1/2" each)	9
Mushrooms, marinated, 1/2 cup	3
Osso bucco, 6 oz veal with 1/4 cup sauce	12
Panettone, 1/12 of 9" tube or 1 1/2 oz	6
Panini	
chicken, 1 (8 oz)	11
ham & cheese, 1 (7 1/2 oz)	11
vegetable, 1 (13 oz)	10
Pasta e fagioli, 1 cup	5
Pasta primavera	
with cream sauce, 1 cup pasta and vegetables with 3/4 cup sauce	12

	POINTS VALUE
with marinara sauce, 1 cup pasta and vegetables with 3/4 cup sauce	5
Pasta with garlic and oil, 1 cup	7
Pasta, cooked, 1 cup	4
Penne a la vodka, 1 cup pasta with 1/2 cup sauce	7
Ravioli	
cheese, with tomato sauce, 8 pieces or 1 cup with 1/2 cup sauce	16
cheese, without sauce, 8 pieces or 1 cup	13
meat, with tomato sauce, 8 pieces or 1 cup with 1/2 cup sauce	14
meat, without sauce, 8 pieces or 1 cup	12
Risotto, 1/2 cup	5
Salad	
Caesar, 3 cups	7
tomato and mozzarella, without dressing, 2 large tomato slices with 2 oz cheese	4
Sauce	
Bolognese meat, 1/2 cup	6
clam, red, 1/2 cup	3
clam, white, 1/2 cup	5
marinara, 1/2 cup	3
meat, 1/2 cup	5
pesto, 2 Tbsp	4
tomato, Italian, 1/2 cup	3
Shrimp scampi, 9 medium (3 1/2 oz)	10

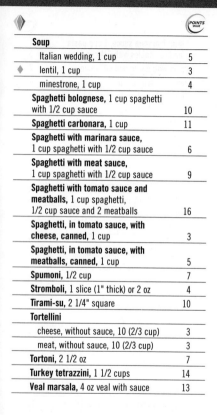

	POINTS VALUE
Soup	
Italian wedding, 1 cup	5
♦ lentil, 1 cup	3
minestrone, 1 cup	4
Spaghetti bolognese, 1 cup spaghetti with 1/2 cup sauce	10
Spaghetti carbonara, 1 cup	11
Spaghetti with marinara sauce, 1 cup spaghetti with 1/2 cup sauce	6
Spaghetti with meat sauce, 1 cup spaghetti with 1/2 cup sauce	9
Spaghetti with tomato sauce and meatballs, 1 cup spaghetti, 1/2 cup sauce and 2 meatballs	16
Spaghetti, in tomato sauce, with cheese, canned, 1 cup	3
Spaghetti, in tomato sauce, with meatballs, canned, 1 cup	5
Spumoni, 1/2 cup	7
Stromboli, 1 slice (1" thick) or 2 oz	4
Tirami-su, 2 1/4" square	10
Tortellini	
cheese, without sauce, 10 (2/3 cup)	3
meat, without sauce, 10 (2/3 cup)	3
Tortoni, 2 1/2 oz	7
Turkey tetrazzini, 1 1/2 cups	14
Veal marsala, 4 oz veal with sauce	13

	POINTS VALUE
Veal parmigiana	
without sauce, 5 1/2 oz	10
with sauce, 5 oz with 1/2 cup tomato sauce	12
Veal piccata, 2 slices (4 oz)	10
Veal scaloppine, 2 pieces (4 1/2 oz)	8
Veal with peppers, 5 oz	11
Vitello tonnato, 2 slices veal (4 oz) with 1/2 cup sauce	16
Wine, 1 small glass (4 fl oz)	2
Zabaglione, 1/2 cup	4
Zeppole, 1 (4" diameter)	6
Ziti, baked	
with meat, 1 cup	9
without meat, 1 cup	6
Zuppa di pesce, 2 cups	11
Zuppa Inglese, 1/16 of 10" cake	8

Pizzeria

	POINTS VALUE
Basil, fresh or dried, 1 tsp	0
Beer	
light, 1 can or bottle (12 fl oz)	2
regular, 1 can or bottle (12 fl oz)	3
Cheese, Parmesan, 2 Tbsp grated	1
Garlic bread, 1 slice (1 1/2 oz)	5
Garlic powder, 1 tsp	0
Garlic, fresh, 1 tsp	0

◆	POINTS VALUE
Oregano	
fresh, 1 Tbsp	0
ground, 1 tsp	0
Pizza, cheese, restaurant-type	
thin crust, 1 small slice (1/8 of 12" or 1/12 of 16" pizza)	4
thin crust, 1 large slice (1/8 of 16 to 18" pizza)	6
medium crust, 1 small slice (1/8 of 12" or 1/12 of 16" pizza)	4
medium crust, 1 large slice (1/8 of 16 to 18" pizza)	6
deep-dish 1 small slice (1/8 of 12" or 1/12 of 16" pizza)	5
deep-dish, 1 large slice (1/8 of 16-18" pizza)	8
Sicilian, 1 slice (3 x 4")	7
Pizza, one-meat topping, restaurant-type	
thin crust, 1 small slice (1/8 of 12" or 1/12 of 16" pizza)	5
thin crust, 1 large slice (1/8 of 16 to 18" pizza)	7
medium crust, 1 small slice (1/8 of 12" or 1/12 of 16" pizza)	6
medium crust, 1 large slice (1/8 of 16 to 18" pizza)	9
deep-dish, 1 small slice (1/8 of 12" or 1/12 of 16" pizza)	7
deep-dish, 1 large slice (1/8 of 16-18" pizza)	11
Sicilian, 1 slice (3 x 4")	9

◆	POINTS VALUE
Pizza, fast food	
cheese, thin crust, 1 slice (1/8 of 12" or 1/12 of 16" pizza)	4
cheese, medium crust, 1 slice (1/8 of 12" or 1/12 of 16" pizza)	5
cheese, thick crust, 1 slice (1/8 of 12" or 1/12 of 16" pizza)	7
one meat topping, thin crust, 1 slice (1/8 of 12" or 1/12 of 16" pizza)	5
one meat topping, medium crust, 1 slice (1/8 of 12" or 1/12 of 16" pizza)	6
one meat topping, thick crust, 1 slice (1/8 of 12" or 1/12 of 16" pizza)	7
Pizza, fast food, single serving	
cheese, 1 (6" pizza)	13
one-meat topping, 1 (6" pizza)	15
Sauce, tomato, Italian, 1/2 cup	3

JAPANESE

	POINTS VALUE
Dressing, salad, ginger, 2 Tbsp	2
Edamame	
◆ in pods, 1 cup	1 (5)
◆ shelled, 1/2 cup	2 (5)
Gyoza, 3	3
Hibachi	
chicken, 1 cup	8
shrimp, 1 cup	5
steak, 1 cup	10
vegetables, 1 cup	4

ETHNIC & REGIONAL FAVORITES

	POINTS VALUE
Ice cream, green tea, 1 scoop or 1/2 cup	3
Nebeyaki udon, 2 cups	5
Noodles	
ramen, fresh, 1/2 cup	5
soba, with sauce, 1 cup	9
Salad, seaweed, 1/2 cup	1
Sashimi	
except mackerel or mackerel, 4 pieces (2 oz)	1 (5)
mackerel, 4 pieces (2 oz)	3 (5)
salmon, 4 pieces (2 oz)	2 (5)
Shabu shabu, 4 oz beef, 2 oz tofu, and 1 1/2 cups vegetables	9
Shumai, fried or steamed, 2 (2" diameter)	3
Soup, miso, 1 cup	2
Suimono, 1 cup	1
Sukiyaki with sauce, 2 cups with 1/4 cup sauce	12
Sunomono, 1/2 cup	0
Sushi, Alaskan roll, 2 pieces (1" high x 1 3/4" diameter)	3
Sushi, California roll, 4 large pieces (1" high x 1 3/4" diameter) or 1 oz each	3
Sushi, cone, 1	2
Sushi, inari, 1	2
Sushi, kappa maki (cucumber roll)	
6 small pieces (1" diameter, 1" thick)	2
4 medium (1 1/2" diameter, 3/4" thick)	2

	POINTS VALUE
Sushi, maki (vegetables and rice rolled with seaweed)	
6 small pieces (1" diameter, 1" thick)	2
4 medium pieces (1 1/2" diameter, 3/4" thick)	2
Sushi, nigiri (sliced raw fish over rice)	
albacore (white tuna), amaebi (sweet shrimp), conch, ebi (cooked shrimp), hamachi (yellow tail), hirame (fluke), hokigai (surf clam), ika (squid), ikura (salmon roe), kani (crab), maguro (tuna), masago (smelt roe), saba (mackerel), sake (fresh salmon), smoked salmon, suzuki (sea bass), suzume, tai (red snapper), tairagai (scallops), tako (octopus), todiko (flying fish roe), unagi (fresh water eel), uni (sea urchin), 4 pieces (2" long, 3/4" wide)	2
Sushi, nori maki (raw fish and rice rolled with seaweed), 4 medium (1 1/2" diameter, 3/4" thick) or 6 small (1" diameter, 1" thick)	2
Sushi, Philadelphia roll, 2 large pieces (1" high x 1 3/4" diameter)	3
Sushi, rainbow roll, 6 small (1" diameter, 1" thick) or 4 medium (1 1/2" diameter, 3/4" thick)	2
Sushi, shrimp tempura roll, 6 pieces (1 1/2" diameter x 1" thick)	8
Sushi, spider roll, 6 pieces (2" diameter x 1" thick)	9
Sushi, tamago-yaki (omelet roll), 2 pieces (3/4" wide)	3

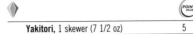

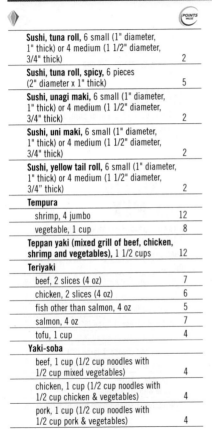

	POINTS VALUE
Sushi, tuna roll, 6 small (1" diameter, 1" thick) or 4 medium (1 1/2" diameter, 3/4" thick)	2
Sushi, tuna roll, spicy, 6 pieces (2" diameter x 1" thick)	5
Sushi, unagi maki, 6 small (1" diameter, 1" thick) or 4 medium (1 1/2" diameter, 3/4" thick)	2
Sushi, uni maki, 6 small (1" diameter, 1" thick) or 4 medium (1 1/2" diameter, 3/4" thick)	2
Sushi, yellow tail roll, 6 small (1" diameter, 1" thick) or 4 medium (1 1/2" diameter, 3/4" thick)	2
Tempura	
shrimp, 4 jumbo	12
vegetable, 1 cup	8
Teppan yaki (mixed grill of beef, chicken, shrimp and vegetables), 1 1/2 cups	12
Teriyaki	
beef, 2 slices (4 oz)	7
chicken, 2 slices (4 oz)	6
fish other than salmon, 4 oz	5
salmon, 4 oz	7
tofu, 1 cup	4
Yaki-soba	
beef, 1 cup (1/2 cup noodles with 1/2 cup mixed vegetables)	4
chicken, 1 cup (1/2 cup noodles with 1/2 cup chicken & vegetables)	4
pork, 1 cup (1/2 cup noodles with 1/2 cup pork & vegetables)	4

	POINTS VALUE
Yakitori, 1 skewer (7 1/2 oz)	5
Yosenabe, 2 cups	4

JEWISH

	POINTS VALUE
Bagel	
any type, 1/2 large (4 1/2" diameter or 2 oz)	3
any type, 1 large (4 oz)	6
any type, 1 mini (2 1/2" diameter)	1
any type, 1 small (3" diameter or 2 oz)	3
Bagel, with cream cheese and lox, 1 large (6 1/2 oz)	12
Beets, pickled, 1/2 cup	1
Bialy, 1 (3 oz)	5
Blintz, cheese, 1 (4 3/4 oz)	5
Borscht, 1 cup with 2 Tbsp sour cream	4
Cabbage, stuffed, 2 (2 x 2 1/2")	6
Challah bread, 1 slice (5" x 3" x 3/4")	2
Cheesecake, with or without fruit topping, 1/16 of 10" cake	10
Chicken and meatball fricassee, 2 cups	9
Chicken in the pot, without skin, 2 cups	10
Cholent, 1 cup	4
Fruit compote, 1/2 cup	3
Hamantaschen, 1 piece (3" diameter)	3
Haroset, 1/4 cup	1
Honey cake, 1 slice (5" x 3" x 1")	7

	POINTS VALUE
Herring	
chopped, 1/4 cup	4
pickled, 1/2 cup	2
Kasha varnishkes, 1 cup	5
Knish, potato, 1 (3 1/2" square)	6
Kreplach	
boiled, 2 pieces (4" x 3" x 3" each)	6
fried, 2 pieces (4" x 3" x 3" each)	7
Kugel	
lukschen, with fruit, 1 piece (3" x 3 1/4")	7
lukschen, without fruit 1 piece (3" x 3 1/4")	5
potato, 1 piece (3" x 3 1/4")	4
Liver, chopped, 1/4 cup	5
Mandelbrot, 1 slice (3" x 2" x 1/2")	5
Matzo, 1 board	2
Matzo brie, 1/4 of 10" round or 1 cup	5
Passover sponge cake, 1/12 of 9" tube	3
Pastrami, beef, 1 slice (1 oz)	3
Potato latkes, 2 (3 1/2" diameter)	6
Rugalach, 1 piece (2 1/2" x 1 1/4")	3
Soup	
cabbage, 1 cup	1
chicken, with matzo balls, 1 cup soup with 2 (1 1/2") matzo balls	3
chicken, without matzo balls (broth only), 1 cup	0
mushroom barley, 1 cup	3

	POINTS VALUE
Turkey, light meat, cooked, without skin, 1 slice (2 oz)	2 (5)
Tzimmes, vegetable, 3/4 cup	2

KOREAN

JapChae, beef, chicken, or pork, 1 cup	7
Khal bi, 4 oz	8
Kim chee, 1/2 cup	0

MEXICAN/ TEX-MEX

Arroz con pollo, 3 oz chicken with 1 1/2 cup rice	13
Beans, refried, 1/2 cup	3
Burrito	
bean, 1 large (8")	8
bean, 1 small (6")	5
bean, fast food, 1	7
beef and cheese, 1 large (8")	8
beef and cheese, 1 small (6")	5
chicken and cheese, 1 large (8")	7
chicken and cheese, 1 small (6")	5
vegetable, 1 large (made with 10" tortilla)	10
vegetable, 1 small (made with 6" tortilla)	5

	POINTS VALUE
Carne asada, 4 oz	10
Carnitas, 1 cup	9
Chalupa (pork & bean dish), 1 cup	6
Cheese, hard or semisoft, regular, 1 cube (1"), 3 Tbsp grated, or 4 Tbsp shredded (1 oz)	3
Cheese, Mexican	
queso anejo, 1 cup (crumbled)	13
queso asadero, 1 cup (shredded)	11
queso chihuahua, 1 cup (shredded)	11
Chicken adobo, 1 thigh (4 oz)	6
Chicken mole, 1 cup	8
Chili con carne	
with beans, 1 cup	8
without beans, 1 cup	8
Chili con queso	
1/4 cup	5
canned, 1/4 cup	2
frozen, 1/4 cup	5
Chili rellenos, beef and cheese, without sauce, 2	18
Sauce, chili, red or green, 1 Tbsp	0
Chimichanga	
beef, 1 (3 x 3 1/2")	11
chicken, 1 (3 x 3 1/2")	9
Cookies, Mexican wedding, 2 (each 1 1/2" wide)	2
Corn cake, sweet, 1/2 cup	8

	POINTS VALUE
Cornbread, Mexican, 1 piece (1/12 of 10" round or 3 1/3 oz)	7
Empanadas, 2 (3" diameter)	5
Enchilada de camarones, 1 cup	5
Enchiladas	
beef, 2 (10 oz)	12
cheese, 2 (8 1/2 oz)	10
chicken, 2 (10 1/2 oz)	9
pork, 2 (10 1/2 oz)	12
sour cream, 1 (5 1/2 oz)	8
Fajitas	
beef, 2 (9 oz)	11
chicken, 2 (8 3/4 oz)	8
pork, 2 (10 1/2 oz)	13
shrimp, 2 (9 oz)	8
vegetarian, 1 (5 1/2 oz)	4
Flauta	
beef, 1 (6" x 1 1/4")	12
chicken, 1 (6" x 1 1/4")	10
pork, 1 (6" x 1 1/4")	11
Gordita, beef, 1 (3" diameter)	10
Guacamole, 1/4 cup	2
Huevos rancheros, 2 eggs on 2 tortillas	14
Ice cream, fried, 1 scoop or 1/2 cup	11
Jalapeño poppers, 1	4
Margarita, 1 (4 fl oz)	5
Menudo (beef tripe and hominy stew), 1 cup	6

	POINTS VALUE
Mexican 7-layer dip, 1/2 cup	3
Mexican coffee, 6 fl oz with 2 Tbsp whipped cream	4
Molé poblano, 1/4 cup	4
Nachos	
beef, 4 (8 1/2 oz)	13
cheese, 4 (3 oz)	8
cheese and bean, 4 (6 1/2 oz)	9
chicken, 4 (8 1/2 oz)	11
with cheese sauce, 1/2 cup tortilla chips with 1/4 cup cheese sauce	5
Picadillo, 1 cup	10
Pico de gallo, 1/2 cup	1
Pozole, 1 cup	4
Quesadilla	
beef, 1/2 of 6" diameter	7
cheese, 1/2 of 6" diameter	5
chicken, 1/2 of 6" diameter	6
vegetable, 1/2 of 6" diameter	6
Rice, Spanish, 1 cup	5
Salad	
taco, with shell, without dressing, fast food, 1	16
taco, without shell and dressing, fast food, 1	9

	POINTS VALUE
Salsa	
black bean & corn, 1/2 cup	1
fat-free, 2 Tbsp	0
fat-free, 1/2 cup	0
Sangria, 4 fl oz	2
Sauce	
sofrito, 1/2 cup	6
taco, 1 Tbsp	0
Sausage, chorizo, 1 link (5 1/2" long)	12
Sopaipillas, 2 (4" x 3" each)	3
Soup	
black bean, 1 cup	2
chicken enchilada, 1 cup	5
chicken, with tortilla strips and shredded cheese, 1 cup	4
gazpacho, 1 cup	3
tortilla, 1 cup	6
Taco	
beef, 1 (3 1/2 oz)	5
breakfast, 1 (3 3/4 oz)	5
chicken, 1 (3 1/2 oz)	4
fish, 1 (4 1/4 oz)	4
hard, fast food, 1	3
pork, 1 (3 1/2 oz)	4
soft, fast food, 1	3
Tamale pie, 1 cup	11

	POINTS VALUE
Tamales, 2 (4" x 2")	9
Taquitos	
beef, 1 (5 1/2" x 1 1/2")	4
chicken, 1 (5 1/2" x 1 1/2")	2
Tortilla chips, 12 (1 oz)	3
Tortilla, corn	
2 (4" diameter), 1 oz	1
1 (6" diameter), 1 oz	1
1/2 (10" diameter), 1 oz	1
Tortilla, flour	
2 (4" diameter), 1 oz	2
1 (6" diameter), 1 oz	2
1 (8" diameter), 1 1/2 oz	3
1/2 (10" diameter), 1 oz	2
Tostada	
beef, 1 (8 1/4 oz)	10
chicken, 1 (8 1/4 oz)	8
with beans and cheese, fast food, 1	5

MIDDLE EASTERN

	POINTS VALUE
Baba ganosh, 1/4 cup	3
Baklava, 1 piece (2" square)	4
Couscous (semolina), cooked, 1 cup	3
Dolma, 4 (3 1/2 oz)	4
Falafel	
in pita, 1 large pita with 4 falafel patties	10
patties, 4 (2" diameter each)	7

	POINTS VALUE
Hummus, 1/4 cup	3
Kibbe	
baked, 3 pieces (1 1/2" squares)	3
uncooked, 1/2 cup	4
Lavash, 1/4 of 10" cracker	5
Rice pilaf, 1 cup	5
Sauce, tzatziki, 1/2 cup	1
Sesame candy, 1 piece (2" x 1")	2
Shawarma, chicken	
1/2 cup	6
1 thigh (without skin and bone) 2 oz	5
Shish kabob (lamb), 2 small skewers (4 1/2 oz)	8
Soup, yogurt and cucumber, 1 cup	2
Souvlaki	
chicken, 1 large or 2 small skewers (4 1/2 oz)	5
chicken, in pita bread, 1 (6 1/2 oz)	7
lamb, 1 large or 2 small skewers (4 3/4 oz)	8
lamb, in pita bread, 1 (6 1/2 oz)	8

SPANISH

	POINTS VALUE
Calamari, fried, 1/2 cup	11
Ceviche, 1/2 cup	2
Flan, 3/4 cup	8
Paella, 1 cup	7

	POINTS VALUE
Red snapper Veracruz, 6 oz cooked fillet with 3/4 cup sauce	11
Rice, Spanish, 1 cup	5
Sangria, 4 fl oz	2
Sausage, chorizo, 1 link (5 1/2" long)	12
Sauce, Spanish, 1/2 cup	2
◆ Soup, black bean, 1 cup	2

THAI

	POINTS VALUE
Coconut rice, Thai, 1 cup	8
Curry paste	
green, 1/4 cup	1
panang, 1/4 cup	1
red, 1/4 cup	1
Curry, green chicken (Gaeng Kheow Wan Gai), 1 cup	7
Ginger chicken, 1 cup	7
Kho-phat (Thai fried rice), 1 cup	8
Mussaman beef curry, 1 cup	19
Nam prik, 1 Tbsp	1
Pad Thai (rice noodles with chicken and shrimp), 1 cup	9
Pudding, Thai tapioca, 1/2 cup	4
Rice, white, cooked, 1 cup	4
Sauce, peanut, spicy, 2 Tbsp	4

	POINTS VALUE
Salad	
Thai beef, 1 cup	14
Thai chicken, 1 cup	11
Thai seafood, 2 cups	10
Satay	
beef, with peanut sauce, 2 skewers with 1/4 cup sauce	11
beef, without peanut sauce, 2 skewers (3 oz)	5
chicken, with peanut sauce, 2 skewers with 1/4 cup sauce	11
chicken, without peanut sauce, 2 skewers (3 oz)	3
Seafood cakes (Haw Mok Thalay), 3/4 cup	8
Soup	
hot and spicy chicken, 1 cup	3
Thai chicken coconut, 1 cup	8
Spring roll, Thai, 1 (4" long)	4
Thai chicken with basil, 1 breast (without skin and bone), 3 oz	5
Thai coffee or tea, 1 cup	7
Thai crisp noodles, 1 cup	8
Thai curry paste, 1 Tbsp	1
Thai grilled beef (Nuea nam tok), 1/2 cup on lettuce leaves	5
Thai paste, 2 Tbsp	2
Tom yum kung, 1 cup	2

POINTS
VALUE

VIETNAMESE

Imperial roll, 1 (4 1/2" long)	4
Lemon grass chicken, 1 cup	8
Nuoc cham, 1 Tbsp	0
Sauce	
Vietnamese spring roll dipping, 2 Tbsp	0
Soup	
asparagus crab, 1 cup	2
Vietnamese beef noodle, 1 cup	2
Spring roll	
fresh, Vietnamese, 1 (1 3/4 oz)	2
fried, Vietnamese, 1 (4" long)	4
Vietnamese beef balls (Thit bo vien), 6 (1 1/2 oz)	2
Vietnamese chicken curry, 1 cup	7

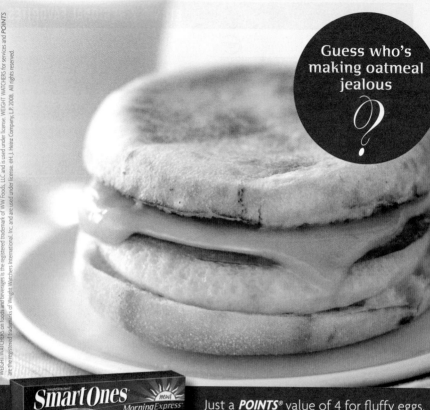

Guess who's making oatmeal jealous ?

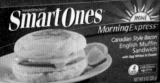

Smart Ones
new!
Morning Express
Canadian Style Bacon
English Muffin
Sandwich
with Egg Whites & Cheese

COOK THOROUGHLY
2 INDIVIDUALLY WRAPPED SANDWICHES

Just a **POINTS**® value of 4 for fluffy eggs, Canadian style bacon and gooey cheese a hot, toasty muffin.

Special savings at eatyourbest.cc

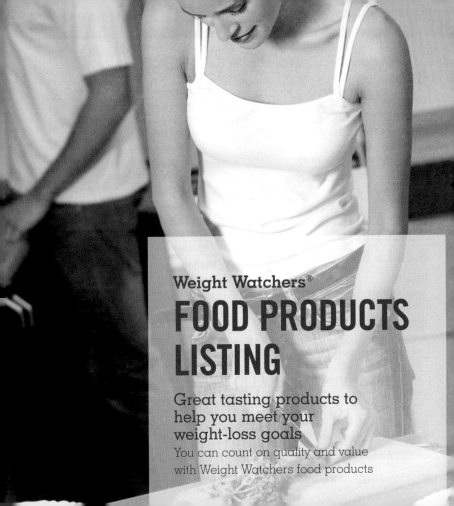

Weight Watchers®

FOOD PRODUCTS LISTING

Great tasting products to
help you meet your
weight-loss goals

You can count on quality and value
with Weight Watchers food products

WEIGHT WATCHERS® FOOD PRODUCTS LISTING

Beverages

Lemonade
Weight Watchers Mix-Ins
Lemonade, 1/2 packet	0

Smoothies
Weight Watchers Smoothie Drink Mix
♦ Creamy chocolate, 1 packet	1
♦ French vanilla, 1 packet	1

Tea/Iced Tea
Weight Watchers Mix-Ins
Peach iced tea, 1/2 packet	0

Bread & Baked Goods

Bagels
Weight Watchers
Hearth baked bagel, 1	2

Bread
Weight Watchers
100% whole wheat bread, 2 slices	1
Fork split English muffin, 1	1
Lite seedless rye bread, 2 slices	1
Multi-grain, 2 slices	1
Wheat English muffin, 1	1

Brownies
Weight Watchers Smart Ones
Brownie a la mode, 1 serving (89 g)	4

Cakes
Weight Watchers
Caramel cake with caramel icing, 1 cake	1
Carrot cake with cream cheese icing, 1 cake	1
Chocolate cake with chocolate icing, 1 cake	1
Golden sponge cake with creamy filling, 1 cake	1
Lemon cake with lemon icing, 1 cake	1
Weight Watchers Smart Ones
Double fudge cake, 1 serving (77 g)	4
Strawberry shortcake, 1 serving (94 g)	4

Flatbread/Pita
Weight Watchers
Whole wheat pita, 1	1

Muffins
Weight Watchers
Berries and crème muffins, 1 muffin	3
Blueberry muffin, 1muffin	3
Caramel apple muffin, 1 muffin	3
Double chocolate muffin, 1 muffin	3

Pastries
Weight Watchers Smart Ones
Chocolate eclair, 1 serving (59 g)	3

Rolls
Weight Watchers
Wheat sandwich rolls, 1	2

Breakfast, Cereals & Cereal Bars

Cereal Bars
Weight Watchers Snack Bars

	POINTS VALUE
Blueberry crumbcake, 1 bar	2
Chocolate caramel, 1 bar	2
Lemon dream, 1 bar	2
Double chocolate delight, 1 bar	2
Mint cookie crisp, 1 bar	2
Sweet & salty, 1 bar	2

Weight Watchers Mini Bars

Chewy oatmeal raisin, 1 bar	1
Chocolate caramel, 1 bar	1
Dark chocolate raspberry, 1 bar	1
Peanut butter bliss, 1 bar	1

Oatmeal
Weight Watchers

Maple brown sugar oatmeal, 1 serving (39 g)	2

Candy, Cookies & Desserts

Candy, non-chocolate
Weight Watchers Fruities

Blackberry, 3 pieces	0
Cherry, 3 pieces	0
Strawberry, 3 pieces	0

Chocolate Candy
Weight Watchers by Whitman's

	POINTS VALUE
Almond nougat, 1 piece	1
Caramel drops, 7 pieces	3
Caramel medallions, 1 piece	1
Coconut, 1 piece	1
Crispy butter cream caramel, 1 piece	1
Double chocolate mousse, 1 piece	1
English toffee squares, 1 piece	1
Mint patties, 1 piece	1
Nougienuttychew, 1 piece	1
Peanut butter cups, 1 piece	2
Peanut butter crunch, 1 piece	1
Pecan crowns, 1 piece	1

Cookies
Weight Watchers

Chocolate chip soft cookies, 1	1
Oatmeal raisin soft cookies, 1	1

Ice Cream
Weight Watchers

Chocolate chip cookie dough, 1 cup	2
Chocolate fudge brownie, 1 cup	2
Chocolate mousse bar, 1	1
Chocolate round ice cream sandwiches, 1	2
English toffee crunch bar, 1 bar	2
Giant chocolate cookies & cream bar, 1 bar	2
Giant chocolate fudge sundae cone, 1 cone	2

	POINTS VALUE
Giant cookies & cream bar, 1 bar	2
Giant fudge bar, 1 bar	1
Giant latte bars, 1 bar	1
Giant orange sorbet & ice cream bar, 1 bar	2
Giant vanilla fudge sundae cone, 1 cone	2
Giant wildberry sorbet & ice cream bar, 1 bar	2
Key lime sherbet & ice cream bar, 1 bar	1
Mint chocolate chip, 1 cup	2
Passion fruit sherbet & ice cream bar, 1 bar	1
Strawberry sherbet & ice cream bar, 1 bar	1
Turtle sundae, 1 cup	3
Vanilla ice cream sandwich, 1	2
Vanilla round ice cream sandwiches, 1	2

Weight Watchers Smart Ones

Chocolate chip cookie dough sundae, 1 serving (75 g)	3
Mint chocolate chip sundae, 1 serving (69 g)	3
Mocha fudge sundae, 1 serving (69 g)	3
Peanut butter cup sundae, 1 serving (65 g)	3

Mousses

Weight Watchers Smart Ones

Chocolate mousse, 1 serving (77 g)	3

Pies

Weight Watchers Smart Ones

Key lime pie, 1 serving (79 g)	4

	POINTS VALUE

Dairy & Eggs

Cheese
Weight Watchers

Light string cheese, 1 piece	1
Reduced fat cheddar cheese snacks, 1 piece	1
Reduced fat cream cheese spread, 1 container	1
Reduced fat shredded 4 cheese Mexican style blend, 1/3 cup	2
Reduced fat shredded cheddar cheese, 1 pouch	2
Reduced fat shredded mozzarella cheese, 1/3 cup	2
Reduced fat whipped cream cheese, 2 Tbsp	1
Singles, 1 slice	1

Yogurt and Yogurt Drinks
Weight Watchers

Amaretto cheesecake nonfat yogurt, 6 oz	1
Berries 'n cream nonfat yogurt, 6 oz	1
Black cherry fat free yogurt, 4 oz	1
Black cherry nonfat yogurt, 6 oz	1
Boston crème pie nonfat yogurt, 6 oz	1
Cherry cheesecake nonfat yogurt, 6 oz	1
Key lime pie nonfat yogurt, 6 oz	1
Lemon cream pie fat free yogurt, 4 oz	1
Lemon cream pie nonfat yogurt, 6 oz	1

	POINTS VALUE
Peach nonfat yogurt, 4 oz	1
Peach nonfat yogurt, 6 oz	1
Raspberry nonfat yogurt, 6 oz	1
Smooth & creamy strawberry shortcake fat free yogurt, 4 oz	1
Smooth & creamy white chocolate cheesecake fat free yogurt, 4 oz	1
Strawberry banana nonfat yogurt, 6 oz	1
Strawberry nonfat yogurt, 6 oz	1
Strawberry nonfat yogurt, 4 oz	1
Vanilla fat free yogurt, 4 oz	1
Vanilla nonfat yogurt, 6 oz	1
White chocolate raspberry nonfat yogurt, 6 oz	1

Prepared Foods, Salads & Sides

Ethnic Entrees
Weight Watchers Smart Ones

	POINTS VALUE
Chicken enchilada suiza, 1 package	6
Chicken oriental, 1 package	4
Szechuan style vegetables & chicken, 1 package	4
Traditional lasagna with meat sauce, 1 package	6

Weight Watchers Smart Ones Anytime Selections

	POINTS VALUE
Calzone Italiano, 1 serving (283 g)	6
Chicken and cheese quesadilla, 1 serving (226 g)	4

Weight Watchers Smart Ones Bistro Selections

Chicken carbonara, 1 package	5
Chicken enchiladas monterey, 1 package	6
Chicken fettucini, 1 package	7
Chicken santa fe, 1 package	2
Dragon shrimp lo mein, 1 package	5
Fajita chicken supreme, 1 package	5
Picante chicken and pasta, 1 package	5
Sweet & sour chicken, 1 package	3
Teriyaki chicken and vegetables, 1 package	4
Thai style chicken & rice noodles, 1 package	5

Fish and Seafood Entrees
Weight Watchers Smart Ones

Shrimp marinara with linguini, 1 package	3
Tuna noodle gratin, 1 package	5

Meat and Poultry Entrees
Weight Watchers Smart Ones

Chicken mirabella, 1 package	4
Honey dijon chicken, 1 package	4

Prepared Foods, Salads & Sides, Weight Watchers Smart Ones Bistro Selections (con't)

	POINTS VALUE
Lemon herb chicken piccata, 1 package	4
Roast turkey medallions, 1 package	4
Salisbury steak with macaroni & cheese, 1 package	5
Santa fe style rice & beans, 1 package	6
Swedish meatballs, 1 package	5

Weight Watchers Smart Ones Bistro Selections

Beef pot roast, 1 package	3
Chicken marsala with broccoli, 1 package	4
Chicken parmesan, 1 package	5
Creamy parmesan chicken with garden vegetables, 1 package	4
Meatloaf with mashed potatoes, 1 package	5
Pepper steak, 1 package	5
Roast beef with gravy, 1 package	5
Roast beef with portabello gravy, 1 package	4
Roasted chicken with sour cream & chive mashed potatoes, 1 package	4
Salisbury steak and asparagus, 1 package	4
Sirloin beef and Asian style vegetables, 1 package	3
Slow-roasted turkey breast, 1 package	4
Stuffed turkey breast, 1 package	6
Teriyaki chicken & vegetables, 1 package	4
Turkey medallions with mushroom gravy and green beans, 1 package	4

Weight Watchers Smart Ones Fruit Inspirations

	POINTS VALUE
Cranbury turkey medallions, 1 serving (255 g)	7
Honey mango barbeque chicken, 1 serving (255 g)	5
Orange sesame chicken, 1 serving (255 g)	7
Pineapple beef teriyaki, 1 serving (255 g)	6

Pasta Entrees

Weight Watchers Smart Ones

Angel hair marinara, 1 package	3
Creamy rigatoni with broccoli & chicken, 1 package	6
Fettucini alfredo, 1 package	6
Lasagna Bolognese, 1 package	5
Lasagna florentine, 1 package	6
Macaroni & cheese, 1 package	5
Pasta Primavera, 1 package	5
Ravioli florentine, 1 package	5
Spaghetti bolognese, 1 package	6
Three cheese macaroni, 1 package	6
Three cheese ziti marinara, 1 package	6

Weight Watchers Smart Ones Bistro Selections

Penne pollo, 1 package	6

Pizza
Weight Watchers Smart Ones Bistro Selections

Four cheese pizza, 1 pizza	8
Pepperoni pizza, 1 pizza	8

Potato, Rice and Grain Sides
Weight Watchers Smart Ones

Broccoli & cheddar roasted potatoes, 1 package	4

Sandwiches
Weight Watchers Smart Ones Morning Express

Breakfast quesadilla, 1 serving (113 g)	4
English muffin sandwich, 1 serving (113 g)	4
English muffin sandwich with Canadian bacon, 1 serving (113 g)	4
Stuffed breakfast sandwich, 1 serving (113 g)	5

Weight Watchers Smart Ones Bistro Selections

Smartwich, pepperoni pizza, 1 serving (127 g)	6

Snacks

Cheese Snacks
Weight Watchers

Cheddar twists, 1 pouch	2

Pretzels
Weight Watchers

Sourdough pretzel thins, 1 pouch	2

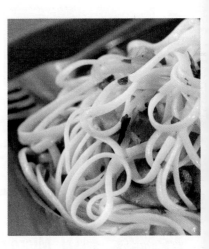

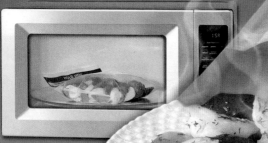

Ziploc® BRAND BAGS · Zip'n Steam™

CAUTION: Hot steam. Open carefully away from body.

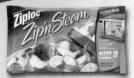

Microwave healthy meals in minutes!
Great for cooking vegetables, seafood, chicken & beef

SC Johnson
A FAMILY COMPANY

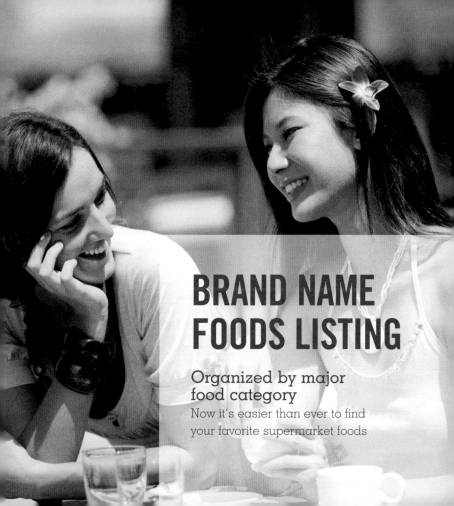

BRAND NAME FOODS LISTING

Organized by major food category

Now it's easier than ever to find your favorite supermarket foods

Baking Powders
Calumet

	POINTS VALUE
Baking powder, 1/8 tsp	0

Gaylord Hauser

Brewer's yeast, 2 Tbsp (rounded)	2

Bread, Biscuit and Popover Mixes and Doughs
Athens

Fillo twin pack, 5 sheets	4
Mini fillo shells, 2	1

Betty Crocker

Banana mix, prepared, 1 slice (1/12 loaf)	4
Banana, no cholesterol/low-fat recipe, prepared, 1 slice	3
Cinnamon streusel mix, prepared, 1 slice (1/14 loaf)	4
Cinnamon streusel, no cholesterol/reduced fat recipe, prepared, 1 slice	4
Cranberry orange mix, prepared, 1 slice (1/12 loaf)	4
Cranberry orange, no cholesterol/low-fat recipe, prepared, 1 slice	3

Bisquick

Heart smart baking mix, 1/3 cup	3
Original all purpose baking mix, 1/3 cup	3

Hodgson Mill

Multi purpose baking mix, 1/4 cup	2
Whole wheat insta-bake mix, 1/3 cup	2

Tony Chachere's

	POINTS VALUE
Shredded coconut batter mix, 1/4 cup	3

Schwan's LiveSmart

Frozen bread dough, white or honey wheat, 1 serving (1/9 loaf)	2

Brownie Mixes
Arrowhead Mills

Brownie mix, 1 serving (1/20 package)	2
Brownie mix, 1 serving (41 g)	3
Gluten free brownie mix, 1 serving (1/20 package)	2
Gluten free brownie mix, prepared, 1 serving (41 g)	4

Betty Crocker

Fudge brownie mix (pouch), prepared, 1 piece (1/9 pan)	4

Betty Crocker Supreme Brownie Mixes

Chocolate chunk supreme, prepared, 1 piece (1/20 pan)	4
Dark chocolate (with Hershey's syrup pouch), prepared, 1 piece (1/20 pan)	4
Dark chocolate fudge, prepared, 1 piece (1/20 pan)	4
Frosted brownie supreme, prepared, 1 piece (1/20 pan)	5
Fudge traditional chewy (family size), prepared, 1 piece (1/20 pan)	4
Hershey's triple chocolate chunk, prepared, 1	4

◆	POINTS VALUE
Hershey's ultimate fudge, prepared, 1 piece (1/20 pan)	4
Low fat fudge, mix, 1 serving (1/18 package)	3
Original fudge with syrup pouch, prepared, 1 piece (1/20 pan)	4
Peanut butter, 1 piece (1/20 pan)	4
Triple chunk, 1 piece (1/20 pan)	4
Turtle, prepared, 1 piece (1/20 pan)	4
Walnut chocolate chunk supreme, 1 piece (1/20 pan)	4
Walnut supreme, prepared, 1 piece (1/20 pan)	4
Betty Crocker Warm Delights Dessert Bowl	
Hot fudge brownie mix, 1 package	8
Peanut butter flavored brownie mix, 1 package	9
Cherrybrook Kitchen	
Fudge brownie mix, 1 serving (mix for 1 brownie)	3
Gluten free fudge brownie mix, 1	3
Dr. Oetker	
Frosted brownie mix, 1 serving (1/9 package)	4
Eagle Brand Premium Dessert Kits	
Decadent fudge, 1 piece (1" x 1")	5
Hodgson Mill	
Brownie mix made with whole wheat flour & milled flaxseed, 3 Tbsp	2

◆	POINTS VALUE
No Pudge!	
Fat free fudge brownie mix - cappuccino, prepared, 1 square (1/16 pan)	2
Fat free fudge brownie mix - mint, prepared, 1 square (1/16 pan)	2
Fat free fudge brownie mix - original, prepared, 1 square (1/16 pan)	2
Fat free fudge brownie mix - raspberry, prepared, 1 square (1/16 pan)	2

Cake Mixes
Aunt Jemima

Easy mix coffee cake, 1/8 package	4
Betty Crocker Classic Cake Mixes	
Gingerbread mix, prepared, 1 slice (1/8 cake)	5
Pineapple upside down cake mix & topping, prepared, 1 slice (1/6 cake)	9
Pound cake, prepared, 1 slice (1/8 cake)	6
Betty Crocker Complete Desserts	
Triple chocolate hot fudge cake mix, prepared, 1 serving (1/6 package)	9
Betty Crocker Supreme Dessert Bar Mixes	
Cake lovers cake & frosting kit, prepared, 1 serving (1/12 cake & 2 Tbsp frosting)	9
Betty Crocker Warm Delights Dessert Bowl	
Cinnamon swirl cake mix, 1 package	8
Lemon swirl cake mix, 1 package	8
Molten caramel cake mix, 1 package	7
Molten chocolate cake mix, 1 package	8

BAKING MIXES, INGREDIENTS & DOUGHS

Cake Mixes (con't)	POINTS VALUE
Cherrybrook Kitchen	
Chocolate cake mix, 1 serving (1/12 of cake mix)	3
Wheat free/gluten free chocolate cake mix, 1 serving (1/8 of cake mix)	3
Yellow cake mix, 1 serving (1/12 of cake mix)	3
Chi-Chi's	
Sweet corn cake mix, 1/2 cup	2
Dromedary	
Pound cake mix, prepared, 1 serving (1/8 cake)	6
Manischewitz	
Angel food cake mix, 3 Tbsp	2
Sponge cake mix, 2 Tbsp	3
SuperMoist	
Butter pecan mix, prepared, 1 slice (1/12 cake)	6
Butter recipe chocolate mix, prepared, 1 slice (1/12 cake)	6
Butter recipe white mix, whole egg recipe, prepared, 1 slice (1/12 cake)	6
Butter recipe yellow mix, prepared, 1 slice (1/12 cake)	6
Carrot cake mix, prepared, 1 slice (1/10 cake)	8
Cherry chip mix, prepared, 1 slice (1/10 cake)	7
Chocolate fudge mix, prepared, 1 slice (1/12 cake)	6

	POINTS VALUE
Cinnamon swirl mix, prepared, 1 slice (1/12 cake)	7
Confetti angel food cake mix, prepared, 1 slice (1/12 cake)	3
Dark chocolate mix, prepared, 1 slice (1/12 cake)	7
Devils food mix, prepared, 1 slice (1/12 cake)	6
French vanilla mix, prepared, 1 slice (1/12 cake)	6
German chocolate mix, prepared, 1 slice (1/12 cake)	6
Golden vanilla mix, prepared, 1 slice (1/12 cake)	6
Lemon mix, prepared, 1 slice (1/12 cake)	6
Milk chocolate mix, prepared, 1 slice (1/12 cake)	6
Party rainbow chip mix, prepared, 1 slice (1/10 cake)	7
Spice mix, prepared, 1 slice (1/12 cake)	6
Strawberry mix, prepared, 1 slice (1/12 cake)	6
Triple chocolate fudge mix, prepared, 1 slice (1/12 cake)	6
White angel food mix, prepared, 1 slice (1/12 cake)	3
White mix, prepared, 1 slice (1/12 cake)	5
White mix, whole egg recipe, prepared, 1 slice (1/12 cake)	6
Yellow mix, prepared, 1 slice (1/12 cake)	6

	POINTS VALUE
Sweet 'N Low	
Banana snack cake mix, 1 serving (1/5 package)	3
Chocolate snack cake mix, 1 serving (1/5 package)	3
Gingerbread snack cake mix, 1 serving (1/5 package)	3
Lemon snack cake mix, 1 serving (1/5 package)	3
White snack cake mix, 1 serving (1/5 package)	3
Yellow snack cake mix, 1 serving (1/5 package)	3

Candy, non-chocolate
Hershey's

Heath baking bits - English toffee, 1 Tbsp	4

Tree of Life

Malt sweetened carob chips, 50	2

Chocolate
Baker's

225th anniversary bittersweet chocolate bar, 2 squares	1
Bittersweet chocolate bar, 1/2 square	2
Chocolate melts, 6 wafers	2
German's sweet chocolate bar, 1 serving (13 g)	1
Milk dipping chocolate, 6 wafers	2

	POINTS VALUE
Semi sweet (dark) dipping chocolate, 6 wafers	2
Semi-sweet chocolate bar, 1/2 square	2
Semi-sweet chocolate shavings, 1 tsp	0
Unsweetened bar, 1/2 square	2
White chocolate bar, 1/2 square	2
Hershey's	
Cocoa, 1 Tbsp	0
M&M's	
Milk chocolate mini baking bits, 1/2 oz (about 1 Tbsp)	2
Semisweet chocolate mini baking bits, 1/2 oz (about 1 Tbsp)	1
Nestle	
Choco bake, 1/2 oz	2
Cocoa for baking, 1 Tbsp	0

Coconut
A Taste of Thai

Coconut milk, 1/3 cup	4
Lite coconut milk, 1/3 cup	1

Dole

Coconut, 1 cup	7

Port Arthur

Coconut milk, 1/4 cup	2
Lite coconut milk, 1/4 cup	1

Tropical Nut & Fruit

Angel flake coconut, 2 Tbsp	2

	POINTS VALUE
Cookie Mixes and Doughs	
Betty Crocker	
Rainbow chocolate candy cookie mix, prepared, 2	4
Walnut chocolate chip cookie mix, prepared, 2	4
Betty Crocker Cookie Mixes (Pouch)	
Chocolate chip cookie mix, prepared, 2	4
Chocolate chip snack size, prepared, 2	4
Chocolate peanut butter chip cookie mix, prepared, 2	4
Double chocolate chunk cookie mix, prepared, 2	4
Hershey's kisses peanut butter, prepared, 1	3
Oatmeal chocolate chip cookie mix, prepared, 2	4
Oatmeal cookie mix, prepared, 2	4
Peanut butter cookie mix, prepared, 2	4
Peanut butter snack size, prepared, 2	3
Betty Crocker Pouch Dessert Mixes	
Sugar cookie mix, prepared, 2	4
Betty Crocker Warm Delights Dessert Bowl	
Fudgy chocolate chip mix, 1 package	7
Cherrybrook Kitchen	
Chocolate chip cookie mix, 1 serving (mix for 1 cookie)	2
Sugar cookie mix, 1 serving (mix for 1 cookie)	1

	POINTS VALUE
Wheat free/gluten free chocolate chip cookie mix, 1 serving (mix for 1 cookie)	2
Wheat free/gluten free sugar cookies mix, 1 serving (mix for 1 cookie)	1
Eagle Brand Premium Dessert Kits	
Magic cookie bar, 1 piece (1 1/2" x 1 1/2")	3
Pillsbury	
Holiday shapes (sugar), 2	3
Sugar cookie dough sheets, 1 serving (1/12 package)	4
Pillsbury Create 'N Bake	
Chocolate chip cookies, 1 ball	3
Chocolate chip walnut cookies, 1 ball	3
Double chocolate chip & chip cookies, 1 ball	3
Oatmeal chocolate chip cookies, 1 ball	3
Peanut butter cookies, 1 ball	3
Sugar cookies, 1 slice	3
Pillsbury Ready To Bake!	
Chocolate candy cookies, 1	2
Chocolate chip, 1	2
Chocolate chip mini bites, 4	3
Chocolate chip with walnuts, 1	2
Chocolate chunk & chip, 1	2
Oatmeal chocolate chip cookies, 1	2
Peanut butter blossom cookies, 1	3
Reeses pieces, 1	2
S'mores, 1	2
Sugar, 1	2
Sugar free chocolate chip, 1	2

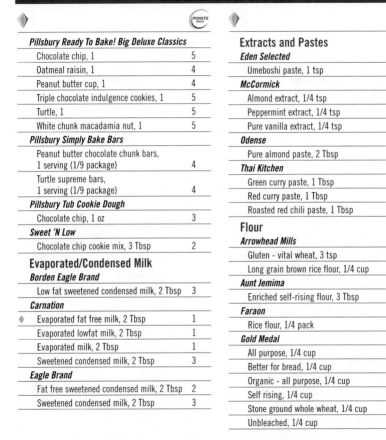

	POINTS VALUE
Pillsbury Ready To Bake! Big Deluxe Classics	
Chocolate chip, 1	5
Oatmeal raisin, 1	4
Peanut butter cup, 1	4
Triple chocolate indulgence cookies, 1	5
Turtle, 1	5
White chunk macadamia nut, 1	5
Pillsbury Simply Bake Bars	
Peanut butter chocolate chunk bars, 1 serving (1/9 package)	4
Turtle supreme bars, 1 serving (1/9 package)	4
Pillsbury Tub Cookie Dough	
Chocolate chip, 1 oz	3
Sweet 'N Low	
Chocolate chip cookie mix, 3 Tbsp	2

Evaporated/Condensed Milk
Borden Eagle Brand

Low fat sweetened condensed milk, 2 Tbsp	3

Carnation

Evaporated fat free milk, 2 Tbsp	1
Evaporated lowfat milk, 2 Tbsp	1
Evaporated milk, 2 Tbsp	1
Sweetened condensed milk, 2 Tbsp	3

Eagle Brand

Fat free sweetened condensed milk, 2 Tbsp	2
Sweetened condensed milk, 2 Tbsp	3

Extracts and Pastes
Eden Selected

	POINTS VALUE
Umeboshi paste, 1 tsp	0

McCormick

Almond extract, 1/4 tsp	0
Peppermint extract, 1/4 tsp	0
Pure vanilla extract, 1/4 tsp	0

Odense

Pure almond paste, 2 Tbsp	4

Thai Kitchen

Green curry paste, 1 Tbsp	0
Red curry paste, 1 Tbsp	0
Roasted red chili paste, 1 Tbsp	1

Flour
Arrowhead Mills

Gluten - vital wheat, 3 tsp	1
Long grain brown rice flour, 1/4 cup	2

Aunt Jemima

Enriched self-rising flour, 3 Tbsp	2

Faraon

Rice flour, 1/4 pack	3

Gold Medal

All purpose, 1/4 cup	2
Better for bread, 1/4 cup	2
Organic - all purpose, 1/4 cup	2
Self rising, 1/4 cup	2
Stone ground whole wheat, 1/4 cup	1
Unbleached, 1/4 cup	2

Flour (con't)

  POINTS VALUE

Hodgson Mill

100% whole grain stone ground whole wheat flour, 1/4 cup	1
100% whole wheat stone ground pastry flour, 1/4 cup	1
Brown rice flour, 1/4 cup	2
Buckwheat flour, 1/4 cup	1
Oat bran flour, 1/4 cup	2
Oat bran flour blend, 1/4 cup	2
Organic rye flour, 1/4 cup	1
Organic soy flour, 1/4 cup	2
Organic spelt flour, 1/4 cup	1
Organic whole wheat graham flour, 1/4 cup	1
Organic whole wheat pastry flour, 1/4 cup	1
Semolina pasta flour, 1/4 cup	2
Soy flour, 1/4 cup	1
White whole wheat flour, 1/4 cup	1
Whole grain rye flour, 1/4 cup	1

Manischewitz

Cake meal, 1/4 cup	3
Potato starch, 1 Tbsp	1

Wondra

Flour, 1/4 cup	2

Frosting/Icing

Betty Crocker Homestyle Frosting

Fluffy white, mix (box), 3 Tbsp	2

 POINTS VALUE

Betty Crocker Ready-To-Spread Rich & Creamy

Coconut pecan, 2 Tbsp	3

Betty Crocker Rich & Creamy

Butter cream, 2 Tbsp	3
Caramel (dulce de leche), 2 Tbsp	3
Cherry, 2 Tbsp	3
Chocolate, 2 Tbsp	3
Cream cheese, 2 Tbsp	3
Creamy white, 2 Tbsp	3
Dark chocolate, 2 Tbsp	3
Lemon, 2 Tbsp	3
Milk chocolate, 2 Tbsp	3
Rainbow chip, 2 Tbsp	3
Sour cream chocolate, 2 Tbsp	3
Triple chocolate fudge chip, 2 Tbsp	3
Vanilla creamy white, 2 Tbsp	3

Betty Crocker Whipped

Butter cream, 2 Tbsp	3
Chocolate, 2 Tbsp	2
Cream cheese, 2 Tbsp	3
Fluffy white, 2 Tbsp	3
Milk chocolate, 2 Tbsp	2
Strawberry mist, 2 Tbsp	3
Vanilla, 2 Tbsp	3
Whipped cream, 2 Tbsp	2

	POINTS VALUE
Cherrybrook Kitchen	
Chocolate frosting mix, 1 Tbsp	1
Vanilla frosting mix, 1 Tbsp	1
Litehouse	
Blueberry glaze, 3 Tbsp	1
Peach glaze, 3 Tbsp	1
Strawberry glaze, 3 Tbsp	1
Sugar free strawberry glaze, 3 Tbsp	1
Naturally Fresh	
Strawberry glaze, 1 serving (1 oz)	1
Sweet 'N Low	
Chocolate flavor whipped frosting & fudge topping mix, 4 Tbsp	1
White whipped frosting mix, 2 Tbsp	1
T. Marzetti	
Glaze for blueberries, 3 Tbsp	1
Glaze for peaches, 3 Tbsp	1
Glaze for strawberries, 3 Tbsp	1

Fruit Crisps
Betty Crocker Complete Desserts

Old fashion apple crisp mix, 1 serving (1/6 package)	6

T. Marzetti

Apple crisp mix, 1 serving (1/8 package)	2

	POINTS VALUE
## Gelatins	
Certo	
Fruit pectin, 2 pouches	0
Sure Jell	
Fruit pectin for homemade jams & jellies, 1 serving (0.5 g)	0
Fruit pectin for lower sugar recipes, 1 serving (0.5 g)	0
Jam pectin no cook, 1 serving (0.5 g)	0

Honey, Syrups and Molasses
Aunt Jemima

Butter lite syrup, 1/4 cup	2
Butter rich syrup, 1/4 cup	4
Country rich syrup, 1/4 cup	4
Original syrup, 1/4 cup	4

Brer Rabbit

Molasses, blackstrap, 1 Tbsp	1
Molasses, full flavored, 1 Tbsp	1
Molasses, mild flavored, 1 Tbsp	1

DaVinci Gourmet

Sugar free caramel syrup, 2 Tbsp	0
Sugar free hazelnut syrup, 2 Tbsp	0
Sugar free kahlua coffee liqueur flavored syrup, 2 Tbsp	0
Sugar free raspberry syrup, 2 Tbsp	0
Sugar free vanilla syrup, 2 Tbsp	0

Honey, Syrups & Molasses (con't)

	POINTS VALUE
Eden Organic	
Barley malt syrup, 1 Tbsp	1
Grandma's	
Original molasses, 1 Tbsp	1
Hershey's	
Sugar free strawberry syrup, 2 Tbsp	0
Syrup, 2 Tbsp	2
Joseph's	
Original sugar free maple flavor syrup, 1 oz	1
Kellogg's Eggo	
Butter pecan flavored syrup, 1/4 cup	5
Syrup buttery, 1/4 cup	3
Syrup lite, 1/4 cup	2
Syrup original, 1/4 cup	5
Syrup, cinnamon French toast flavored, 1/4 cup	3
Log Cabin	
100% pure maple syrup, 1/4 cup	4
Lite syrup, 1/4 cup	2
Original syrup, 1/4 cup	4
Sugar free syrup, 1/4 cup	1
Manischewitz	
Clover honey, 1 Tbsp	1
Golden honey, 1 Tbsp	1
Orange blossom honey, 1 Tbsp	1
Wild flower honey, 1 Tbsp	1

	POINTS VALUE
Maple Grove	
Sugar free butter flavor syrup, 1/4 cup	1
Sugar free maple flavor syrup, 1/4 cup	1
Vermont sugar free pancake syrup, 1/4 cup	0
Mrs. Butterworth's	
Lite syrup, 1/4 cup	2
Original syrup, 1/4 cup	4
Sugar free syrup, 1/4 cup	1
Muirhead	
Pomegranate syrup, 1 Tbsp	1
Naturally Fresh	
Maple mountain sugar free syrup, 2 Tbsp	0
Nesquik	
Chocolate syrup, 2 Tbsp	2
Strawberry syrup, 2 Tbsp	2
Smucker's	
Sugar free breakfast syrup, 1/4 cup	1
Tree of Life	
Blackstrap molasses, unsulphered, 1 Tbsp	1
Honey, 1 Tbsp	1
Maple syrup, 1/4 cup	4
Vermont Maid	
Lite syrup, 1/4 cup	2
Sugar free butter lite, 1/4 cup	1
Sugar free syrup, 1/4 cup	1
Syrup, 1/4 cup	4

	POINTS VALUE
Walden Farms	
Blueberry syrup, 1/4 cup	0
Chocolate syrup, 2 Tbsp	0
Pancake syrup, 1/4 cup	0
Strawberry syrup, 2 Tbsp	0

Mincemeat
Muirhead
Green tomato mincemeat, 1 Tbsp	1

Muffin Mixes
Betty Crocker
Apple cinnamon mix (pouch), 1 serving (1/5 pouch)	3
Apple streusel mix (box), no-cholesterol/low fat recipe, prepared, 1	4
Apple streusel mix (box), prepared, 1	5
Authentic corn bread mix (pouch), prepared, 1	4
Banana nut mix (box), no-cholesterol/low fat recipe, prepared, 1	3
Banana nut mix (box), prepared, 1	5
Banana nut mix (pouch), 1 serving (1/6 pouch)	3
Blueberry mix (pouch), 1 serving (1/6 pouch)	3
Chocolate chip mix (box), no cholesterol/reduced fat recipe, prepared, 1	4
Chocolate chip mix (pouch), 1 serving (1/5 pouch)	3

	POINTS VALUE
Chocolate chip muffin & quick bread mix (box), prepared, 1	5
Chocolate chip muffin & quick bread mix (box), reduced fat, no cholesterol recipe, prepared, 1	4
Cinnabon cinnamon streusel jumbo muffin mix (box), prepared, 1	14
Cinnamon streusel mix (box), prepared, 1	5
Cinnamon streusel mix (box), prepared, no-cholesterol/reduced fat recipe, 1	3
Double chocolate mix (box), no-cholesterol recipe, prepared, 1	4
Double chocolate mix (box), prepared, 1	5
Lemon poppyseed mix (pouch), 1 serving (1/6 pouch)	3
Sunkist lemon poppyseed mix (box), no-cholesterol/low fat recipe, prepared, 1	3
Sunkist lemon poppyseed mix (box), prepared, 1	5
Triple berry mix, 1 serving (1/6 pouch)	3
Twice the blueberries mix (box), no-cholesterol/low fat recipe, prepared, 1	3
Twice the blueberries mix (box), prepared, 1	4
Wild blueberry mix (box), no-cholesterol/low fat recipe, prepared, 1	3
Wild blueberry mix (box), prepared, 1	4
Cherrybrook Kitchen	
Chocolate chip muffin mix, 1	3

BAKING MIXES, INGREDIENTS & DOUGHS

 Muffin Mixes (con't)

Hodgson Mill

	POINTS VALUE
Apple cinnamon muffin mix, 1/4 cup	2
Bran muffin mix, 1/4 cup	2
Cornbread & muffin mix, 1/4 cup	2
Jalapeno (Mexican style) cornbread mix, 1/4 cup (dry)	2
Whole wheat muffin mix, 1/4 cup	2
Whole wheat wild blueberry muffin mix, 1/4 cup	2

Pancake Syrup
Aunt Jemima

	POINTS VALUE
Butter lite syrup, 1/4 cup	2
Butter rich syrup, 1/4 cup	4
Country rich syrup, 1/4 cup	4
Original syrup, 1/4 cup	4

Kellogg's Eggo

	POINTS VALUE
Butter pecan flavored syrup, 1/4 cup	5
Syrup buttery, 1/4 cup	3
Syrup lite, 1/4 cup	2
Syrup original, 1/4 cup	5
Syrup, cinnamon French toast flavored, 1/4 cup	3

Log Cabin

	POINTS VALUE
100% pure maple syrup, 1/4 cup	4
Lite syrup, 1/4 cup	2
Original syrup, 1/4 cup	4
Sugar free syrup, 1/4 cup	1

Maple Grove

	POINTS VALUE
Vermont sugar free pancake syrup, 1/4 cup	0

Mrs. Butterworth's

	POINTS VALUE
Lite syrup, 1/4 cup	2
Original syrup, 1/4 cup	4
Sugar free syrup, 1/4 cup	1

Walden Farms

	POINTS VALUE
Calorie free pancake syrup, 1/4 cup	0

Pie Filling and Mixes
Betty Crocker Supreme Dessert Bar Mixes

	POINTS VALUE
7 layer bar kit, prepared, 1 bar	5
Almond joy dessert bar mix, prepared, 1 bar	5
Heath dessert bar mix, prepared, 1 bar	4
Reese's dessert bar mix, prepared, 1 bar	4
Sunkist lemon bar, prepared, 1 piece	3

Comstock

	POINTS VALUE
Lite cherry, 1/3 cup	1
More fruit apple, 1/3 cup	1
More fruit blueberry, 1/3 cup	2
More fruit cherry, 1/3 cup	2
More fruit cinnamon 'n spice apple, 1/3 cup	2
More fruit lite cherry, 1/3 cup	1
More fruit peach, 1/3 cup	2
No sugar added apple, 1/3 cup	1
No sugar added cherry, 1/3 cup	1
Original country cherry, 1/3 cup	2
Premium apricot, 1/3 cup	2

	POINTS VALUE
Premium blackberry, 1/3 cup	2
Premium dark sweet cherry, 1/3 cup	2
Premium pineapple, 1/3 cup	2
Premium raspberry, 1/3 cup	1
Premium strawberry, 1/3 cup	2
Quick & easy lemon, 1/3 cup	3
Durkee	
Lemon pie filling, 1 Tbsp	1
Jell-O Instant	
Chocolate dirt cup kit mix, 1 serving (1/6 box)	3
Chocolate dirt cup kit, prepared, 1/2 cup	5
Easy Southern banana pudding dessert kit, 1 serving (1/12 package)	2
Easy southern banana pudding dessert kit, 1/2 cup	3
Jell-O No Bake	
Cherry cheesecake mix, 1 serving (1/8 cake)	4
Cherry cheesecake, prepared, 1 serving (1/9 package)	6
Chips ahoy, as packaged, 1 serving (60 g)	6
Chips ahoy, prepared, 1 serving (1/6 package)	8
Double chocolate pie mix, 1 serving (1/6 package)	4
Double chocolate pie, prepared, 1 serving (1/6 package)	7
Homestyle cheesecake mix, 1 serving (1/8 cake)	5

	POINTS VALUE
Homestyle cheesecake, prepared, 1 serving (1/6 package)	8
Oreos and creme mix, 1 serving (62 g)	6
Oreos and crème, prepared, 1 serving (1/6 package)	8
Peanut butter cup mix, 1 serving (1/8 dessert)	7
Peanut butter cup, prepared, 1/8 package	9
Pumpkin style pie mix, 1 serving (34 g)	3
Pumpkin style pie, prepared, 1 serving (1/6 package)	6
Real cheesecake mix, 1 serving (1/8 cake)	5
Real cheesecake, prepared, 1 serving (1/6 package)	8
Strawberry cheesecake mix, 1 serving (1/8 cake)	4
Strawberry cheesecake, prepared, 1 serving (1/9 package)	6
Lucky Leaf	
Apple pie filling, 1/3 cup	2
Apple pie filling, no sugar added, 1/3 cup	0
Blueberry pie filling, 1/3 cup	2
Cherry pie filling, 1/3 cup	2
Cherry pie filling, no sugar added, 1/3 cup	1
Lemon pie filling, 1/3 cup	2
Peach pie filling, 1/3 cup	2
Strawberry pie filling, 1/3 cup	1
Payaso	
Flan dessert mix, 1/4 pack	1

Pie Filling and Mixes (con't) | POINTS VALUE

Philadelphia

Ready to eat cheesecake filling, as packaged, 1/8 package	7
Ready to eat cheesecake filling, prepared, 1/8 package	9

Pie/Pastry Dough and Crusts

Betty Crocker

Pie crust mix (box), 1 serving (1/8 of 9" crust)	3
Pizza crust mix (pouch), 1 serving (1/4 crust)	3

Keebler

Graham cracker crumbs, 3 Tbsp	1

Mrs. Smith's

9" pie crust, deep dish, 1 serving (1/8 pie crust)	3
9" pie crust, regular, 1 serving (1/8 pie crust)	3

Nabisco

Nilla pie crust, 1 serving (1/8 pie crust)	3
Nilla wafers crumbs, 2 1/2 Tbsp	2
Oreo basecake - crumbs, 1/4 cup	3
Oreo pie crust, 1/6 crust (19 g)	2
Oreo pie crust, 1/6 crust (28 g)	3

Nabisco Honey Maid

Graham pie crust, 1 serving (1/8 pie crust)	3

Oronoque Orchards

9" pie crust, deep dish, ready to bake, 1 serving (1/8 pie crust)	3
9" pie crust, regular, ready to bake, 1 serving (1/8 pie crust)	2

Pillsbury

All ready pie crust, refrigerated, rolled, 1/8	3
Pie crusts - frozen 9", 1 serving (1/8 of pie crust)	3

Pillsbury Pet-Ritz

Deep dish 9", frozen, 1/8	2
Deep dish, frozen, vegetable oil, 1/8	2
Large 9 5/8", frozen, 1/8	3
Regular 9", frozen, 1/8	2

Ready Crust

Chocolate pie crust (6 oz), 1/8	2
Graham cracker pie crust (10"), 1 serving (1/10 crust)	3
Graham cracker pie crust (6 oz), 1/8	2
Reduced fat graham cracker pie crust (6 oz), 1/8	2
Shortbread pie crust (6 oz), 1/8	3
Tart graham cracker crusts (4 oz), 1 crust	2

Shortening/Lard

Earth Balance

Natural shortening stick, 1 Tbsp	4

Smart Balance

Vegetable shortening, 1 Tbsp	3

	POINTS VALUE
Spectrum Naturals	
Organic shortening, 1 Tbsp	3
Spices	
Durkee	
Basil leaf, 1 serving (4 g)	0
Bay leaf, whole, 1 serving (4 g)	0
Chili powder, mild, 1/4 tsp	0
Cinnamon, ground, 1/4 tsp	0
Cumin seed, ground, 1/4 tsp	0
Garlic powder, 1/4 tsp	0
Lemon pepper, 1/4 tsp	0
Nutmeg, ground, 1/4 tsp	0
Pepper, black ground, 1/4 tsp	0
McCormick	
Alum, 1/4 tsp	0
Caraway seed, 1/4 tsp	0
Celery flakes, 1/4 tsp	0
Celery seed, 1/4 tsp	0
Chives, 1/4 tsp	0
Cilantro leaves, 1/4 tsp	0
Cream of tartar, 1/4 tsp	0
Cumin seeds, 1/4 tsp	0
Curry powder, 1/4 tsp	0
Dill seed, 1/4 tsp	0
Dill weed, 1/4 tsp	0
Fennel seed, 1/4 tsp	0
Garlic powder, 1/4 tsp	0

	POINTS VALUE
Ground allspice, 1/4 tsp	0
Ground black pepper, 1/4 tsp	0
Ground cinnamon, 1/4 tsp	0
Ground cloves, 1/4 tsp	0
Ground cumin, 1/4 tsp	0
Ground ginger, 1/4 tsp	0
Ground mace, 1/4 tsp	0
Ground marjoram, 1/4 tsp	0
Ground mustard, 1/4 tsp	0
Ground nutmeg, 1/4 tsp	0
Ground oregano, 1/4 tsp	0
Ground red pepper, 1/4 tsp	0
Ground sage, 1/4 tsp	0
Ground thyme, 1/4 tsp	0
Ground turmeric, 1/4 tsp	0
Ground white pepper, 1/4 tsp	0
Italian seasoning, 1/4 tsp	0
Marjoram leaves, 1/4 tsp	0
Mustard seeds, 1/4 tsp	0
Onion powder, 1/4 tsp	0
Oregano leaves, 1/4 tsp	0
Paprika, 1/4 tsp	0
Parsley flakes, 1/4 tsp	0
Pickling spice, 1/4 tsp	0
Poppy seeds, 1/4 tsp	0
Pumpkin pie spice, 1/4 tsp	0
Rosemary leaves, 1/4 tsp	0

BAKING MIXES, INGREDIENTS & DOUGHS

Spices, McCormick (con't)	POINTS VALUE
Rubbed sage, 1/4 tsp	0
Sesame seeds, 1/4 tsp	0
Tarragon leaves, 1/4 tsp	0
Thyme leaves, 1/4 tsp	0
Whole allspice, 1/4 tsp	0
Whole basil leaves, 1/4 tsp	0
Whole bay leaves, 1/4 tsp	0
Whole cloves, 1/4 tsp	0
Nu-Salt	
Salt substitute, 1 packet	0
Salt substitute, 1 serving (1/6 tsp)	0
Spice Islands	
Basil leaf, 1 serving	0
Cayenne pepper, 1 serving	0
Curry powder, 1/4 tsp	0
Dill weed, 1 serving	0
Tree of Life	
Bee pollen, 1 tsp	1
Crystallized ginger, 7 pieces	3
Sesame seeds, 1/4 cup	5
Turmeric in brine, 1 Tbsp	0

Sugar/Sugar Substitutes
Equal

	POINTS VALUE
Sweetener, 1 packet	0
Sweetener, 1 tsp	0

	POINTS VALUE
Estee	
Fructose natural sweetener, 1 packet	0
Fructose natural sweetener, 1 tsp	0
Joseph's	
Maltitol sweetener, 1 serving (1 oz)	1
McNeil Nutritionals	
SPLENDA brown sugar blend, 1/2 tsp	0
SPLENDA No calorie sweetener, 1 packet	0
SPLENDA No calorie sweetener, 1 tsp (granulated)	0
SPLENDA sugar blend for baking, 1/2 tsp	0
NatraTaste	
Sugar substitute, 1 packet	0
Sans Sucre	
Cinnamon sugar, 1/2 tsp	0
Splenda	
Café sticks, 1 stick	0
No calorie sweetener, flavor accents, lemon, 1 packet	0
No calorie sweetener, flavor accents, raspberry, 1 packet	0
Quick pack no-calorie sweetener pouches, 1/8 package	0
Sugar in the Raw	
Turbinado sugar from natural cane, 1 packet	0
Turbinado sugar from natural cane, 1 tsp	0

POINTS VALUE

Sugar Twin	
Calorie free sweetener, 1 packet	0
Calorie free sweetener, white, 1 tsp	0
Spoonable brown, 1 tsp	0
Sweet & Slender	
Natural sweetener packets, 1/2 packet	0
Natural sweetener shaker jar, 1/8 tsp	0
Sweet 'N Low	
Brown zero calories sweetener, 1 serving (1/10 tsp)	0
Low calorie sweetener tablets, 1 tablet	0
Zero calorie sweetener, 1 serving (1/10 tsp)	0
Zero calorie sweetener, 1 packet	0
Zero-calorie liquid sweetener, 10 drops	0
Sweet One	
Granulated sugar substitute, 1 packet	0
SweetLeaf	
Stevia extract powder, 1 serving (1/40 tsp)	0
Steviaclear liquid stevia extract, 2 drops	0
Steviaplus fiber, 1/2 packet	0
Steviatabs, 1 tablet	0
Tree of Life	
Fructose, 1 tsp	0
Turbinado sugar, 1 tsp	0

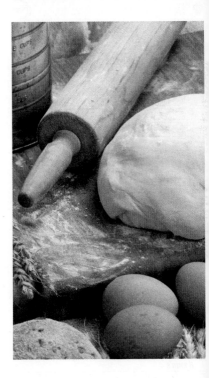

Beer

Budweiser

Bud dry, 1 can or bottle	3
Bud ice, 1 can or bottle	3
Bud ice light, 1 can or bottle	2
Bud light, 1 can or bottle	2
Budweiser, 1 can or bottle	3
Budweiser select, 1 can or bottle	2

Busch

Busch, 1 can or bottle	3
Busch ice, 1 can or bottle	3
Busch light, 1 can or bottle	2
Busch non-alcoholic beer, 1 can or bottle	1

Cerveza

Cerveza aquila, 1 can or bottle	2
Cerveza cristal, 1 can or bottle	3

Cusquena

Cusquena, 1 can or bottle	3

Fosters

Fosters, 1 can or bottle	3
Fosters special bitter, 1 can or bottle	3

Frederick Miller

Frederick miller classic chocolate lager, 1 can or bottle	4

Hamm's

Golden draft, 12 fl oz	3
Hamm's, 1 can or bottle	3
Special light, 12 fl oz	2

Henry Weinhard's

Henry Weinhard's blue boar, 1 can or bottle	3
Henry Weinhard's classic dark lager, 1 can or bottle	3
Henry Weinhard's northwest trail blond lager, 1 can or bottle	3
Henry Weinhard's summer wheat, 1 can or bottle	3
Private reserve dark, 12 fl oz	3

Leinenkugel's

Leinenkugel's amber light, 1 can or bottle	2
Leinenkugel's apple spice, 1 can or bottle	4
Leinenkugel's berry weiss, 1 can or bottle	4
Leinenkugel's big butt, 1 can or bottle	4
Leinenkugel's creamy dark, 1 can or bottle	3
Leinenkugel's honey weiss, 1 can or bottle	3
Leinenkugel's light, 1 can or bottle	2
Leinenkugel's northwoods lager, 1 can or bottle	3
Leinenkugel's oktoberfest, 1 can or bottle	3
Leinenkugel's original lager, 1 can or bottle	3
Leinenkugel's red lager, 1 can or bottle	3
Leinenkugel's sunset wheat, 1 can or bottle	3

Magnum

Malt liquor, 1 can or bottle	3

Michelob

Michelob, 1 can or bottle	3
Michelob amberbock, 1 can or bottle	3

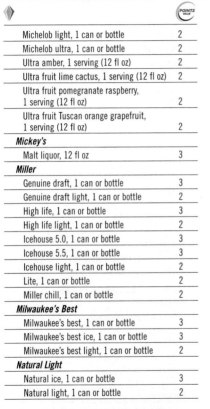

	POINTS VALUE
Michelob light, 1 can or bottle	2
Michelob ultra, 1 can or bottle	2
Ultra amber, 1 serving (12 fl oz)	2
Ultra fruit lime cactus, 1 serving (12 fl oz)	2
Ultra fruit pomegranate raspberry, 1 serving (12 fl oz)	2
Ultra fruit Tuscan orange grapefruit, 1 serving (12 fl oz)	2
Mickey's	
Malt liquor, 12 fl oz	3
Miller	
Genuine draft, 1 can or bottle	3
Genuine draft light, 1 can or bottle	2
High life, 1 can or bottle	3
High life light, 1 can or bottle	2
Icehouse 5.0, 1 can or bottle	3
Icehouse 5.5, 1 can or bottle	3
Icehouse light, 1 can or bottle	2
Lite, 1 can or bottle	2
Miller chill, 1 can or bottle	2
Milwaukee's Best	
Milwaukee's best, 1 can or bottle	3
Milwaukee's best ice, 1 can or bottle	3
Milwaukee's best light, 1 can or bottle	2
Natural Light	
Natural ice, 1 can or bottle	3
Natural light, 1 can or bottle	2

	POINTS VALUE
O'Doul's	
O'Doul's amber non-alcoholic beer, 1 can or bottle	2
O'Doul's non-alcoholic beer, 1 can or bottle	1
Olde English 800	
Olde English 800, 12 fl oz	3
Olde English 800 7.5, 1 can or bottle	4
Olde English high gravity 800, 1 can or bottle	4
Peroni Nastro Azzurro	
Peroni nastro azzurro, 1 can or bottle	3
Pilsner Urquell	
Pilsner urquell, 1 can or bottle	3
Red Dog	
Red dog, 1 can or bottle	3
Sharp's	
Sharp's, 1 can or bottle	1
Sheaf Stout	
Sheaf stout, 1 can or bottle	4
Southpaw	
Southpaw light, 1 can or bottle	2
Sparks	
Sparks, 1 can or bottle	5
Sparks light, 1 can or bottle	3
Sparks plus 6%, 1 can or bottle	5
Sparks plus 7%, 1 can or bottle	6

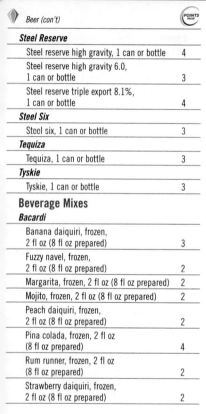

Beer (con't)

	POINTS VALUE
Steel Reserve	
Steel reserve high gravity, 1 can or bottle	4
Steel reserve high gravity 6.0, 1 can or bottle	3
Steel reserve triple export 8.1%, 1 can or bottle	4
Steel Six	
Steel six, 1 can or bottle	3
Tequiza	
Tequiza, 1 can or bottle	3
Tyskie	
Tyskie, 1 can or bottle	3

Beverage Mixes
Bacardi

	POINTS VALUE
Banana daiquiri, frozen, 2 fl oz (8 fl oz prepared)	3
Fuzzy navel, frozen, 2 fl oz (8 fl oz prepared)	2
Margarita, frozen, 2 fl oz (8 fl oz prepared)	2
Mojito, frozen, 2 fl oz (8 fl oz prepared)	2
Peach daiquiri, frozen, 2 fl oz (8 fl oz prepared)	2
Pina colada, frozen, 2 fl oz (8 fl oz prepared)	4
Rum runner, frozen, 2 fl oz (8 fl oz prepared)	2
Strawberry daiquiri, frozen, 2 fl oz (8 fl oz prepared)	2

	POINTS VALUE
Chincoteague	
Bloody Mary mix, 5 fl oz	1
Del Monte	
Snap-E-Tom from concentrate, 1 cup	1
Snap-E-Tom from concentrate, 1 small can	1
Seagram's	
Black cherry seltzer naturals, 8 fl oz	0
Club soda, 8 fl oz	0
Diet tonic water, 8 fl oz	0
Lemon lime seltzer naturals, 8 fl oz	0
Orange seltzer naturals, 8 fl oz	0
Original seltzer, 8 fl oz	0
Raspberry seltzer naturals, 8 fl oz	0
Tonic water, 8 fl oz	2
Tonic water with a twist of lime, 8 fl oz	2
Tree of Life	
Pomegranate concentrate, 8 tsp	2
Wild blueberry concentrate, 8 tsp	2

Cocoa and Chocolate Drinks
CocoaVia

	POINTS VALUE
Rich chocolate indulgence beverage, 1 bottle	3
Flavia	
Hot chocolate beverage, choco, 1 sachet	1
Hot chocolate beverage, milky way swirl, 1 sachet	1
Hershey's	
1% no sugar added chocolate milk, 1 cup	2

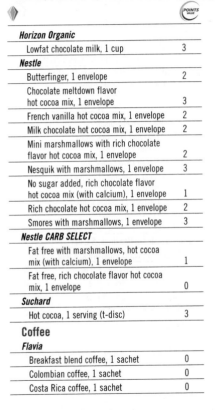

	POINTS VALUE
Horizon Organic	
Lowfat chocolate milk, 1 cup	3
Nestle	
Butterfinger, 1 envelope	2
Chocolate meltdown flavor hot cocoa mix, 1 envelope	3
French vanilla hot cocoa mix, 1 envelope	2
Milk chocolate hot cocoa mix, 1 envelope	2
Mini marshmallows with rich chocolate flavor hot cocoa mix, 1 envelope	2
Nesquik with marshmallows, 1 envelope	3
No sugar added, rich chocolate flavor hot cocoa mix (with calcium), 1 envelope	1
Rich chocolate hot cocoa mix, 1 envelope	2
Smores with marshmallows, 1 envelope	3
Nestle CARB SELECT	
Fat free with marshmallows, hot cocoa mix (with calcium), 1 envelope	1
Fat free, rich chocolate flavor hot cocoa mix, 1 envelope	0
Suchard	
Hot cocoa, 1 serving (t-disc)	3
Coffee	
Flavia	
Breakfast blend coffee, 1 sachet	0
Colombian coffee, 1 sachet	0
Costa Rica coffee, 1 sachet	0

	POINTS VALUE
Espresso roast coffee, 1 sachet	0
French roast coffee, 1 sachet	0
French roast decaf coffee, 1 sachet	0
French vanilla coffee, 1 sachet	0
Hazelnut coffee, 1 sachet	0
Hazelnut decaf coffee, 1 sachet	0
House blend coffee, 1 sachet	0
House blend decaf coffee, 1 sachet	0
Intense dark roast coffee, 1 sachet	0
Irish crème coffee, 1 sachet	0
Italian roast coffee, 1 sachet	0
Kenyan dawn coffee, 1 sachet	0
Sidamo gold coffee, 1 sachet	0
Sumatra coffee, 1 sachet	0
General Foods	
Vanilla crème drink mix, 1 1/3 Tbsp	1
Vanilla crème sugar free drink mix, 1 1/3 Tbsp	1
General Foods International Coffee	
Café francais, prepared, 8 fl oz	1
Café Vienna, prepared, 1 serving (16 g)	2
Cappuccino café mocha decaffeinated single serve coffee mix, 1 envelope	2
Cappuccino café mocha single serve coffee mix, 1 envelope	2
Cappuccino coolers French vanilla, 1 serving (8 oz)	3

Coffee, General Foods International
Coffee (con't)

	POINTS VALUE
Cappuccino coolers hazelnut, 1 serving (8 oz)	3
Cappuccino French vanilla decaffeinated single serve coffee mix, 1 envelope	2
Cappuccino French vanilla single serve coffee mix, 1 envelope	2
Crème caramel mix, 1 serving (15 g)	1
French vanilla cafe decaffeinated, prepared, 1 serving (14 g)	1
French vanilla cafe, prepared, 1 serving (14 g)	1
French vanilla nut coffee mix, 1 1/3 Tbsp	1
Hazelnut Belgian cafe, prepared, 8 fl oz	2
Italian cappuccino, prepared, 8 fl oz	1
Orange cappuccino, prepared, 1 serving (13 g)	1
Pumpkin spice coffee mix, 1 1/3 Tbsp	2
Sugar free café Vienna, 1 Tbsp	1
Sugar free decaffeinated French vanilla café, 1 Tbsp	1
Sugar free French vanilla café, 1 Tbsp	1
Sugar free Suisse mocha, 1 Tbsp	1
Sugar free Suisse mocha decaffeinated, 1 Tbsp	1
Suisse mocha, prepared, 1 serving (13 g)	1
Swiss white chocolate, 1 serving (16 g)	2
Viennese chocolate café, 1 serving (13 g)	1

	POINTS VALUE
Gevalia	
Decaffeinated cappuccino, 1 serving (1 coffee t-disc & 1 milk creamer t-disc)	1
Decaffeinated latte, 1 serving (1 coffee t-disc & 1 milk creamer t-disc)	2
Gevalia Café Collection	
Cappuccino, 1 serving (1 coffee t-disc & 1 milk creamer t-disc)	1
Latte, 1 serving (1 coffee t-disc & 1 milk creamer t-disc)	2
Maxwell House Café Collection	
Cappuccino, 1 serving (1 coffee t-disc & 1 milk creamer t-disc)	1
Latte, 1 serving (1 coffee t-disc & 1 milk creamer t-disc)	2
Starbucks	
Double shot coffee drink, 8 fl oz	4
Double shot light coffee drink, 8 fl oz	2
Frappuccino - caramel, 8 fl oz	4
Frappuccino - coffee, 8 fl oz	4
Frappuccino - mocha, 8 fl oz	3
Frappuccino - mocha lite, 8 fl oz	2
Frappuccino - vanilla, 8 fl oz	4
Iced coffee, 8 fl oz	1
Iced coffee light, 8 fl oz	1

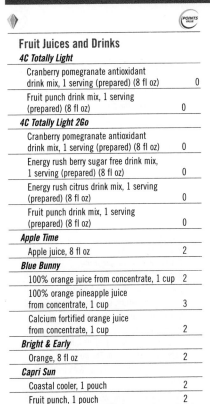

Fruit Juices and Drinks

4C Totally Light

	POINTS VALUE
Cranberry pomegranate antioxidant drink mix, 1 serving (prepared) (8 fl oz)	0
Fruit punch drink mix, 1 serving (prepared) (8 fl oz)	0

4C Totally Light 2Go

Cranberry pomegranate antioxidant drink mix, 1 serving (prepared) (8 fl oz)	0
Energy rush berry sugar free drink mix, 1 serving (prepared) (8 fl oz)	0
Energy rush citrus drink mix, 1 serving (prepared) (8 fl oz)	0
Fruit punch drink mix, 1 serving (prepared) (8 fl oz)	0

Apple Time

Apple juice, 8 fl oz	2

Blue Bunny

100% orange juice from concentrate, 1 cup	2
100% orange pineapple juice from concentrate, 1 cup	3
Calcium fortified orange juice from concentrate, 1 cup	2

Bright & Early

Orange, 8 fl oz	2

Capri Sun

Coastal cooler, 1 pouch	2
Fruit punch, 1 pouch	2
Grape, 1 pouch	2
Mountain cooler, 1 pouch	2
Orange, 1 pouch	2
Pacific cooler, 1 pouch	2
Red berry, 1 pouch	2
Splash cooler, 1 pouch	2
Strawberry, 1 pouch	2
Strawberry-kiwi, 1 pouch	2
Surfer cooler, 1 pouch	2
Tropical punch, 1 pouch	2
Wild cherry, 1 pouch	2

Capri Sun On the Go

Sport lightspeed lemon lime, prepared, 1 serving (8.45 fl oz)	1
Sport thunder punch, prepared, 1 serving (8.45 fl oz)	1

Cascadian Farm

Orange juice frozen concentrate, 2 fl oz	2
Organic apple juice from concentrate, 60 ml	2
Organic cranberry cocktail concentrate, 60 ml	2
Organic grape juice from concentrate, 60 ml	3
Organic raspberry juice from concentrate, 60 ml	3

Fruit Juices and Drinks (con't)

Ceres 100% Pure Fruit Juice Blend

Apricot juice, 8 fl oz	2
Cranberry & kiwi juice, 8 fl oz	2
Guava juice, 8 fl oz	2
Litchi juice, 8 fl oz	2
Mango juice, 8 fl oz	2
Medley of fruits, 8 fl oz	2
Papaya juice, 8 fl oz	2
Passion fruit juice, 8 fl oz	2
Peach juice, 8 fl oz	2
Pear juice, 8 fl oz	2
Pineapple juice, 8 fl oz	2
Secrets of the valley, 8 fl oz	2
Strawberry juice, 8 fl oz	2
White grape juice, 8 fl oz	3
Youngberry juice, 8 fl oz	2

Crystal Light

Energy wild strawberry, sugar free, 8 fl oz	0
Fruit punch, sugar free, prepared, 8 fl oz	0
Immunity berry pomegranate, sugar free, 8 fl oz	0
Pineapple-orange mix, sugar free, prepared, 8 fl oz	0
Ruby red grapefruit mix, sugar free, prepared, 1 serving (8 fl oz)	0
Strawberry-kiwi, sugar free, prepared, 8 fl oz	0
Strawberry-orange-banana mix, sugar free, prepared, 8 fl oz	0

Tangerine strawberry, sugar free, prepared, 8 fl oz	0

Crystal Light Calcium

Raspberry peach mix, sugar free, prepared, 8 fl oz	0

Crystal Light On the Go

Cherry pomegranate, prepared, 1 serving (8.45 fl oz)	0
Fruit punch, prepared, 1 serving (8.45 fl oz)	0
Hydration berry splash, prepared, 1 serving (8.45 fl oz)	0
Hydration lightly lemon, prepared, 1 serving (8.45 fl oz)	0
Raspberry ice mix, 1 serving (8.45 fl oz)	0
Wild strawberry, prepared, 1 serving (8.45 fl oz)	0

Crystal Light Sunrise

Classic orange mix, sugar free, prepared, 8 fl oz	0
Classic orange on the go, 1 packet	0
Ruby red grapefruit, sugar free, 8 fl oz	0
Strawberry-kiwi mix, sugar free, 1 serving (2 g)	0
Tangerine strawberry, prepared, 8 fl oz	0

Crystal Light Sunrise On The Go

Orange, prepared, 1 serving (8.45 fl oz)	0

Del Monte

Pineapple juice from concentrate, 1 cup	3
Pineapple juice from concentrate, 5 1/2 fl oz	2

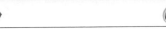

	POINTS VALUE
Dole	
Apple juice, 8 fl oz	2
Apple juice, 1 can (11.5 fl oz)	3
Cranberry grape, 1 serving (8 fl oz)	3
Cranberry grape, 1 can (11.5 fl oz)	5
Cranberry juice cocktail, 1 can (11.5 fl oz)	3
Grape raspberry, 1 serving (8 fl oz)	3
Grape raspberry, 1 can (11.5 fl oz)	4
Grape raspberry cocktail, frozen concentrate, 1/4 cup	3
Orange (no pulp & w/pulp), 8 fl oz	2
Orange (no pulp & w/pulp), 1 can (11.5 fl oz)	3
Orange guava, 8 fl oz	2
Orange Pacific passion, 1 can (8.4 oz)	3
Orange peach mango, 8 fl oz	2
Orange peach mango, frozen concentrate, 1/4 cup	2
Orange strawberry banana, 11 1/2 fl oz	5
Orange strawberry banana, 8 fl oz	3
Orange strawberry banana, frozen concentrate, 1/4 cup	3
Orange tropical, 8 fl oz	2
Orange tropical, frozen concentrate, 1/4 cup	3
Orange with calcium, 8 fl oz	2
Orange with double vitamin C, 8 fl oz	2
Orchard peach, 1 bottle (10 fl oz)	3
Paradise blend, 1 can (11.5 fl oz)	3

	POINTS VALUE
Paradise blend, 1 serving (8 fl oz)	2
Pineapple citrus, 1 serving (8 fl oz)	2
Pineapple citrus, 1 can (11.5 fl oz)	3
Pineapple juice, canned, 8 fl oz	2
Pineapple juice, reconstituted, 8 fl oz	2
Pineapple juice, reconstituted, 1 can (177 ml)	2
Pineapple juice, refrigerated, 8 fl oz	3
Pineapple orange, 8 fl oz	2
Pineapple orange banana, 8 fl oz	3
Pineapple orange banana, frozen concentrate, 1/4 cup	3
Pineapple orange strawberry, 8 fl oz	2
Pineapple orange strawberry, frozen concentrate, 1/4 cup	3
Pineapple orange, frozen concentrate, 1/4 cup	2
Pineapple passionfruit mango, 8 fl oz	3
Pineapple, frozen concentrate, 1/4 cup	2
Pine-grapefruit juice, 1 can (177 ml)	2
Pine-orange juice, 1 can (177 ml)	2
Pine-orange-banana juice, 1 can (177 ml)	2
Pink pine grapefruit drink, 8 fl oz	3
Pink pine grapefruit drink, 1 can (177 ml)	2
Raspberry kiwi, 8 fl oz	2
Ruby red grapefruit juice, 1 bottle (10 fl oz)	4
Ruby red grapefruit juice, 1 can (11.5 fl oz)	4
Sparklers - orange tangerine, 8 fl oz	1

BEVERAGES

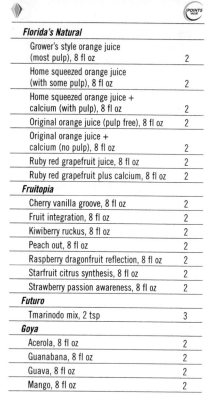

Fruit Juices and Drinks, Dole (con't)	
Sparklers - pink grapefruit, 8 fl oz	1
Sparklers - pomegranate blueberry, 8 fl oz	1
Sparklers, cranberry raspberry, 8 fl oz	1
Strawberry kiwi, 1 serving (8 fl oz)	4
Strawberry splash, 1 can (250 ml)	3
Dole 100% Juice	
Apple juice, 8 fl oz	2
Cranberry juice, 8 fl oz	3
Orange, 8 fl oz	2
Pineapple peach mango juice, 8 fl oz	3
Ruby red grapefruit juice, 8 fl oz	3
Strawberry kiwi juice, 8 fl oz	3
Dole Plus	
Apple, 8 fl oz	2
Fruit punch, 8 fl oz	2
Mixed berry, 8 fl oz	2
Orange, 8 fl oz	2
Eden Organic	
Apple juice, 8 oz	2
Apple juice concentrate, 2 Tbsp	2
Cherry concentrate, 2 Tbsp	2
Cherry juice (Montmorency tart cherries), 1 serving (8 oz)	3
Five Alive	
Citrus, 8 fl oz	2
Citrus, frozen, 2 fl oz (8 fl oz prepared)	2

Florida's Natural	
Grower's style orange juice (most pulp), 8 fl oz	2
Home squeezed orange juice (with some pulp), 8 fl oz	2
Home squeezed orange juice + calcium (with pulp), 8 fl oz	2
Original orange juice (pulp free), 8 fl oz	2
Original orange juice + calcium (no pulp), 8 fl oz	2
Ruby red grapefruit juice, 8 fl oz	2
Ruby red grapefruit plus calcium, 8 fl oz	2
Fruitopia	
Cherry vanilla groove, 8 fl oz	2
Fruit integration, 8 fl oz	2
Kiwiberry ruckus, 8 fl oz	2
Peach out, 8 fl oz	2
Raspberry dragonfruit reflection, 8 fl oz	2
Starfruit citrus synthesis, 8 fl oz	2
Strawberry passion awareness, 8 fl oz	2
Futuro	
Tmarinodo mix, 2 tsp	3
Goya	
Acerola, 8 fl oz	2
Guanabana, 8 fl oz	2
Guava, 8 fl oz	2
Mango, 8 fl oz	2

	POINTS VALUE
Papaya, 8 fl oz	2
Passion & papaya, 8 fl oz	2
Passion fruit, 8 fl oz	2
Tamarind, 8 fl oz	2
Herdez	
Tropical fruit juice, 1 can	3
Hi-C	
Blast orange supernova, 1 bottle	3
Blazin' blueberry, 1 box	2
Boppin' strawberry, 1 box	2
Crazy citrus cooler, 1 box	2
Flashin' fruit punch, 1 box	2
Frightening fruit punch, 1 box	2
Grabbin' grape, 1 box	2
Kids + minis apple juice, 1 box	1
Kids + minis fruit punch, 1 box	1
Kids + minis grape, 1 box	1
Kids + orange juice, 1 box	2
Orange lavaburst, 1 box	2
Smashin' wild berry, 1 box	2
Strawberry kiwi kraze, 1 box	2
Torrential tropical punch, 1 box	2
Wild cherry, 1 box	2
Hi-C Blast	
Berry blue, 8 fl oz	3
Blue watermelon, 1 pouch	2

	POINTS VALUE
Fruit punch, 8 fl oz	2
Fruit punch, 1 pouch	2
Orange, 8 fl oz	2
Orange, 1 pouch	2
Raspberry kiwi, 1 pouch	2
Strawberry, 1 pouch	2
Strawberry kiwi, 8 fl oz	3
Wild berry, 8 fl oz	2
Wild berry, 1 pouch	2
Hi-C Sour Blast	
Green apple, 1 pouch	2
Indian Summer	
Apple juice, 8 fl oz	2
Apple juice with vitamin c added, 8 fl oz	2
Cherry pomegranate juice, 8 fl oz	3
Natural apple juice, 8 fl oz	2
Red tart cherry juice, 8 fl oz	3
Juicy Juice	
Apple-banana, 8 fl oz	2
Apple-raspberry, 8 fl oz	2
Kool-Aid	
Cherry sugar-free mix, prepared, 8 fl oz	0
Cherry sugar-sweetened mix, prepared, 8 fl oz	1
Grape mix, unsweetened, 1 packet	0
Grape sugar-free mix, prepared, 8 fl oz	0

Fruit Juices and Drinks, Kool-Aid (con't)

	POINTS VALUE
Ice kool arctic green apple mix, sugar sweetened, 1 serving (17 g)	1
Ice kool arctic green apple mix, unsweetened, 1 packet	0
Ice kool lemon ice mix, sugar sweetened, 1 serving (17 g)	1
Ice kool lemon ice mix, unsweetened, 1 packet	0
Orange mix, unsweetened, 1 packet	0
Tropical punch mix, unsweetened, 1 packet	0
Tropical punch sugar free-mix, prepared, 8 fl oz	0
Tropical punch sugar-sweetened mix, prepared, 8 fl oz	1
Kool-Aid Bursts	
Berry blue, 1 bottle	2
Cherry, 1 bottle	2
Grape, 1 bottle	2
Lime, 1 bottle	2
Strawberry-kiwi, 1 bottle	2
Tropical punch, 1 bottle	2
Kool-Aid Jammers	
Blue raspberry, 1 pouch	2
Cherry, 1 pouch	1
Grape, 1 pouch	2
Green apple, 1 pouch	2
Kiwi strawberry, 1 pouch	2
Orange, 1 pouch	2
Tropical punch, 1 pouch	2

	POINTS VALUE
Kool-Aid Jammers 10	
Cherry, 1 pouch	0
Kiwi strawberry, 1 pouch	0
Tropical punch, 1 pouch	0
Kool-Aid Magic Twists	
Grape illusion mix, sugar sweetened, 1 serving (17 g)	1
Kool-Aid On The Go	
Tropical punch, sugar free, prepared, 1 serving (250 ml)	0
Kool-Aid Singles	
Cherry, prepared, 1 packet	1
Grape, prepared, 1 packet	1
Orange, prepared, 1 packet	1
Tropical punch, prepared, 1 serving (8 fl oz)	1
Libby's Juicy Juice	
Apple, 1 box	2
Apple, 1 small box	1
Apple, 1 cup	2
Apple concentrate, 1 serving (2 fl oz)	2
Apple-grape, 1 cup	2
Berry, 1 cup	2
Berry, 1 small box	1
Berry, 1 box	2
Berry concentrate, 1 serving (2 fl oz)	3
Cherry, 1 cup	2
Cherry, 1 small box	1
Cherry, 1 box	2

	POINTS VALUE
Cherry concentrate, 1 serving	3
Cranberry apple, 1 cup	2
Cranberry apple concentrate, 1 serving (2 fl oz)	3
Grape, 1 cup	2
Grape, 1 small box	1
Grape, 1 box	2
Grape concentrate, 1 serving (2 fl oz)	3
Kiwi strawberry, 1 box	2
Kiwi strawberry, 1 small box	1
Kiwi strawberry, 1 cup	2
Kiwi strawberry concentrate, 1 serving (2 fl oz)	2
Mango, 1 serving (8 fl oz)	2
Orange tangerine, 1 cup	3
Orange tangerine, 1 box	2
Orange tangerine, 1 small box	1
Peach, 1 serving (8 fl oz)	2
Punch, 1 small box	1
Punch, 1 cup	2
Punch, 1 box	2
Punch concentrate, 1 serving (2 fl oz)	2
Tropical, 1 cup	2
Watermelon, 1 serving (8 fl oz)	2
White grape, 1 cup	3
White grape concentrate, 1 serving (2 fl oz)	3

	POINTS VALUE
Lucky Leaf	
Apple juice, 8 fl oz	2
Premium apple juice, 8 fl oz	2
Premium apple juice with calcium and vitamin c, 8 fl oz	2
Sparkling cider, 8 fl oz	3
Manischewitz	
Apple juice, 8 fl oz	2
Apple juice, 1 box	2
Grape juice, 8 fl oz	3
White grape juice, 8 fl oz	3
Market Day	
Tropicana orange juice singles, 1 carton	2
Minute Maid	
Apple juice, 1 box	2
Apple juice, frozen concentrate, 2 fl oz (8 fl oz prepared)	2
Apple strawberry juice, 1 box	2
Berry kiwi, 12 fl oz	3
Berry kiwi, 8 fl oz	2
Berry punch, 8 fl oz	2
Berry punch, frozen concentrate, 2 fl oz (8 fl oz prepared)	2
Breakfast blends, berry, 8 fl oz	3
Breakfast blends, citrus, 8 fl oz	3
Breakfast blends, tropical, 8 fl oz	3
Cherry limeade, 8 fl oz	3

Fruit Juices and Drinks, Minute Maid (con't)	POINTS VALUE
Citrus punch, 8 fl oz	2
Citrus punch, frozen concentrate, 2 fl oz (8 fl oz prepared)	2
Country style orange juice, 8 fl oz	2
Country style orange juice, frozen concentrate, 2 fl oz (8 fl oz prepared)	2
Enhanced juice/active, orange juice, 8 fl oz	3
Enhanced juice/heart wise, orange juice, 8 fl oz	2
Enhanced juice/multi-vitamin, orange juice, 8 fl oz	3
Fruit medley, 8 fl oz	2
Fruit punch, 1 box	2
Fruit punch, 8 fl oz	2
Fruit punch, 1 can (8 fl oz)	2
Fruit punch, 1 can (12 fl oz)	4
Fruit punch, frozen concentrate, 2 fl oz (8 fl oz prepared)	2
Grape, 1 box	2
Grape juice cocktail, frozen concentrate, 2 fl oz (8 fl oz prepared)	3
Grape punch, 8 fl oz	2
Grapefruit juice, frozen concentrate, 2 fl oz (8 fl oz prepared)	2
Home squeezed style orange juice, 8 fl oz	2
Home squeezed style orange juice with calcium & vitamin D, 8 fl oz	2
Kids + orange juice, 8 fl oz	2

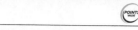

	POINTS VALUE
Lemon juice, frozen single strength, 1 serving (5 ml)	0
Lime juice, 1 serving (5 ml)	0
Limeade, 8 fl oz	2
Limeade, 1 can	4
Low acid orange juice, 8 fl oz	2
Low acid orange juice, frozen concentrate, 2 fl oz (8 fl oz prepared)	2
Mixed berry, 1 box	2
Orange juice, 8 fl oz	2
Orange juice with C, E & zinc, 8 fl oz	2
Orange juice with C, E & zinc, frozen concentrate, 2 fl oz (8 fl oz prepared)	2
Orange juice with calcium, frozen concentrate, 2 fl oz	3
Orange juice, frozen concentrate, 2 fl oz	2
Orange passion, 8 fl oz	3
Orange passion, frozen concentrate, 2 fl oz (8 fl oz prepared)	3
Orange tangerine, 8 fl oz	2
Orange tangerine, frozen concentrate, 2 fl oz (8 fl oz prepared)	2
Orange tropical, 8 fl oz	3
Orangeade, 1 can (12 oz)	3
Orangeade, 12 fl oz	5
Orangeade, 1 bottle (16.9 fl oz)	5
Orangeade, 8 fl oz	2
Original orange juice, 8 fl oz	2

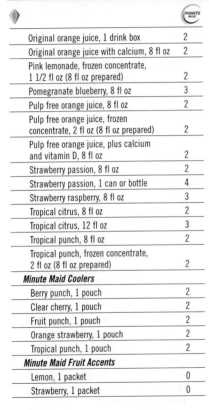

	POINTS VALUE
Original orange juice, 1 drink box	2
Original orange juice with calcium, 8 fl oz	2
Pink lemonade, frozen concentrate, 1 1/2 fl oz (8 fl oz prepared)	2
Pomegranate blueberry, 8 fl oz	3
Pulp free orange juice, 8 fl oz	2
Pulp free orange juice, frozen concentrate, 2 fl oz (8 fl oz prepared)	2
Pulp free orange juice, plus calcium and vitamin D, 8 fl oz	2
Strawberry passion, 8 fl oz	2
Strawberry passion, 1 can or bottle	4
Strawberry raspberry, 8 fl oz	3
Tropical citrus, 8 fl oz	2
Tropical citrus, 12 fl oz	3
Tropical punch, 8 fl oz	2
Tropical punch, frozen concentrate, 2 fl oz (8 fl oz prepared)	2
Minute Maid Coolers	
Berry punch, 1 pouch	2
Clear cherry, 1 pouch	2
Fruit punch, 1 pouch	2
Orange strawberry, 1 pouch	2
Tropical punch, 1 pouch	2
Minute Maid Fruit Accents	
Lemon, 1 packet	0
Strawberry, 1 packet	0

	POINTS VALUE
Minute Maid Juices To Go	
Apple juice, 8 fl oz	2
Cranberry apple cocktail, 1 can	4
Cranberry apple raspberry, 8 fl oz	2
Cranberry grape, 8 fl oz	3
Fruit medley, 8 fl oz	3
Fruit punch, 1 bottle	3
Grape, 1 bottle	3
Grape, 1 can	4
Mixed berry, 1 bottle	3
Mixed berry, 1 can	4
Orange juice with calcium, 8 fl oz	2
Orange juice with calcium & vitamin D, 8 fl oz	2
Orange tropical, 1 can	4
Ruby red grapefruit, 8 fl oz	3
Ruby red grapefruit, 8 fl oz	3
Strawberry raspberry, 8 fl oz	2
Minute Maid Light	
Cherry limeade, 1 can (12 oz)	0
Limeade, 8 fl oz	1
Mango tropical, 1 can (12 oz)	0
Orange juice beverage, 8 fl oz	1
Orange tangerine, 8 fl oz	1
Orangeade, 8 fl oz	0
Orangeade, 1 can (12 oz)	0
Raspberry passion, 8 fl oz	0
Raspberry passion, 1 can (12 oz)	0

BEVERAGES

	POINTS VALUE
Minute Maid Simply	
Grapefruit juice, 8 fl oz	2
Limeade, 8 fl oz	2
Limeade, 1 bottle	4
Original pasteurized orange juice - pulp free, 8 fl oz	2
Pure pressed apple juice, 8 fl oz	3
Musselman's	
Apple juice, 8 fl oz	2
Premium apple juice, 8 fl oz	2
Premium apple juice with calcium and vitamin c, 8 fl oz	2
Sparkling cider, 8 fl oz	3
Ocean Spray	
100% grapefruit juice, 8 fl oz	2
100% juice blend, cranberry & pomegranate, 1 serving (250 ml)	3
100% juice cranberry & blueberry, 8 fl oz	3
100% juice cranberry and concord grape, 8 fl oz	3
100% juice cranberry and Pacific raspberry, 8 fl oz	3
100% juice cranberry blend, 8 fl oz	3
100% juice no sugar added, cranberry, 1 cup	3
100% juice pink grapefruit blend, 8 fl oz	2
100% juice ruby red grapefruit with calcium, 8 fl oz	3
100% juice white cranberry, 8 fl oz	3
100% juice white grapefruit, 8 fl oz	2
Cran-apple cranberry juice drink, 8 fl oz	3
Cran-cherry cranberry juice drink, 8 fl oz	3
Cran-grape cranberry juice drink, 8 fl oz	3
Cran-raspberry cranberry juice drink, 8 fl oz	2
Cran-strawberry cranberry strawberry juice drink, 8 fl oz	2
Cran-tangerine cranberry juice drink, 8 fl oz	3
Cranberry cocktail, 8 fl oz	3
Cranberry grape cocktail, 8 fl oz	3
Cranberry juice cocktail with calcium, 8 fl oz	3
Diet cranberry spray, 8 fl oz	0
Diet cran-grape juice, 8 fl oz	0
Light - cran apple, 1 cup	1
Light cranberry cocktail, 8 fl oz	1
Light cran-grape cocktail, 1 serving (250 ml)	1
Light cran-raspberry cocktail, 1 serving (250 ml)	1
Light ruby red grapefruit juice, 8 fl oz	1
Organic 100% cranberry blend, 8 fl oz	3
Pure cranberry 100% unsweetened cranberry juice, 8 fl oz	1
Refreshers cranberry, 8 fl oz	2
Ruby grapefruit juice, 1 serving (250 ml)	3
Ruby red grapefruit juice drink, 8 fl oz	2
Ruby tangerine grapefruit juice drink, 8 fl oz	2

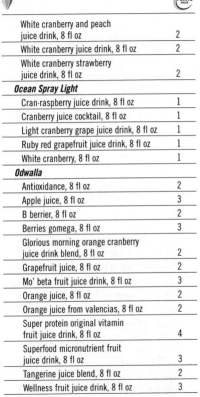

	POINTS VALUE
White cranberry and peach juice drink, 8 fl oz	2
White cranberry juice drink, 8 fl oz	2
White cranberry strawberry juice drink, 8 fl oz	2
Ocean Spray Light	
Cran-raspberry juice drink, 8 fl oz	1
Cranberry juice cocktail, 8 fl oz	1
Light cranberry grape juice drink, 8 fl oz	1
Ruby red grapefruit juice drink, 8 fl oz	1
White cranberry, 8 fl oz	1
Odwalla	
Antioxidance, 8 fl oz	2
Apple juice, 8 fl oz	3
B berrier, 8 fl oz	2
Berries gomega, 8 fl oz	3
Glorious morning orange cranberry juice drink blend, 8 fl oz	2
Grapefruit juice, 8 fl oz	2
Mo' beta fruit juice drink, 8 fl oz	3
Orange juice, 8 fl oz	2
Orange juice from valencias, 8 fl oz	2
Super protein original vitamin fruit juice drink, 8 fl oz	4
Superfood micronutrient fruit juice drink, 8 fl oz	3
Tangerine juice blend, 8 fl oz	2
Wellness fruit juice drink, 8 fl oz	3

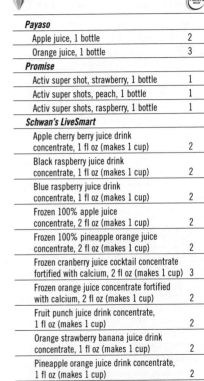

	POINTS VALUE
Payaso	
Apple juice, 1 bottle	2
Orange juice, 1 bottle	3
Promise	
Activ super shot, strawberry, 1 bottle	1
Activ super shots, peach, 1 bottle	1
Activ super shots, raspberry, 1 bottle	1
Schwan's LiveSmart	
Apple cherry berry juice drink concentrate, 1 fl oz (makes 1 cup)	2
Black raspberry juice drink concentrate, 1 fl oz (makes 1 cup)	2
Blue raspberry juice drink concentrate, 1 fl oz (makes 1 cup)	2
Frozen 100% apple juice concentrate, 2 fl oz (makes 1 cup)	2
Frozen 100% pineapple orange juice concentrate, 2 fl oz (makes 1 cup)	2
Frozen cranberry juice cocktail concentrate fortified with calcium, 2 fl oz (makes 1 cup)	3
Frozen orange juice concentrate fortified with calcium, 2 fl oz (makes 1 cup)	2
Fruit punch juice drink concentrate, 1 fl oz (makes 1 cup)	2
Orange strawberry banana juice drink concentrate, 1 fl oz (makes 1 cup)	2
Pineapple orange juice drink concentrate, 1 fl oz (makes 1 cup)	2
Tropical punch juice drink concentrate, 1 fl oz (makes 1 cup)	2

Fruit Juices and Drinks, Schwan's LiveSmart (con't)   (POINTS VALUE)

Wild cherry juice drink concentrate, 1 fl oz (makes 1 cup)	2

SoBe

Adrenaline rush, 1 serving (8 fl oz)	3
Elixir 3C - cranberry grapefruit, 8 fl oz	2
Elixir 3C - orange carrot, 8 fl oz	2
Elixir 3C - pomegranate cranberry, 8 fl oz	2
Elixir 3C-concord-white grape, 8 fl oz	2
No fear, 8 fl oz	3
No fear gold, 8 fl oz	3
Sugar free adrenaline rush, 1 serving (8 fl oz)	0
Sugar free no fear, 8 fl oz	0
Synergy - fruit punch, 8 fl oz	1
Synergy - grape, 8 fl oz	1
Synergy - kiwi strawberry, 8 fl oz	1
Synergy - mango orange, 8 fl oz	1

Sun-Rype

Blue label apple juice, 1 serving (100 ml)	1
Calcium enriched orange juice from concentrate, 1 serving (250 ml)	2
Pure unsweetened fruit juice combo from concentrate, 1 serving (250 ml)	1
Pure unsweetened orange juice from concentrate, 1 serving (250 ml)	1

Sunsweet

Plumsmart plum juice, 8 fl oz	3
Prune juice, 8 fl oz	3

 (POINTS VALUE)

Tang

Orange (with fruitrition), prepared, 8 fl oz	1
Tangerine strawberry (with fruitrition), prepared, 8 fl oz	1
Wild berry (with fruitrition), prepared, 8 fl oz	1

Tree of Life

Apple juice, east coast, 8 fl oz	3
Black cherry concentrate, 8 tsp	2
Concord grape concentrate, 9 tsp	3
Noni juice, 2 Tbsp	0

Tropicana

Antioxidant advantage, orange juice with C, E & selenium, 8 fl oz	2
Apple, 8 fl oz	2
Apple, 1 carton	2
Apple cranberry, 1 can	4
Berry punch, 8 fl oz	3
Cranberry, 1 container	5
Cranberry, 8 fl oz	3
Fruit punch, 1 can (11.5 oz)	6
Fruit punch, 8 fl oz	4
Grape, 1 container	5
Grape, 1 fl oz	3
Grape, 1 can	4
Grape punch, 8 fl oz	2
Healthy kids orange juice with A, C, E & D & calcium, 8 fl oz	2

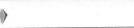

	POINTS VALUE
Heart healthy orange juice with omega 3, 8 fl oz	2
Low acid orange juice, 8 fl oz	2
Orange cranberry frozen concentrate, 1 serving (60 ml)	3
Orange juice with fiber, 8 fl oz	2
Orange peach frozen concentrate, 1 serving (1/4 cup)	2
Orange pulp free & with pulp frozen concentrate, 1 serving	2
Orange strawberry banana frozen concentrate, 1 serving (1/4 cup)	3
Orangeade, 8 fl oz	3
Orchard berry, 8 fl oz	2
Organic orange juice, 8 fl oz	2
Organic orchard medley, 8 fl oz	2
Peach orchard punch, 8 fl oz	3
Peach papaya, 8 fl oz	2
Strawberry melon, 8 fl oz	2
Strawberry splash punch, 8 fl oz	2
Sugar free orangeade, 8 fl oz	0
Tropical orange, 8 fl oz	2
Tropical orange pineapple, 8 fl oz	2
Tropical punch, 8 fl oz	2
Tropicana fruit punch, 8 fl oz	2
Tropicana Light 'N Healthy	
Orange juice beverage with calcium, 8 fl oz	1
Orange juice beverage with pulp, 8 fl oz	1

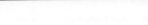

	POINTS VALUE
Tropicana Pure	
Indian river grapefruit juice, 8 fl oz	2
Peach papaya mango juice, 8 fl oz	3
Pomegranate blueberry, 8 fl oz	3
Raspberry acai, 8 fl oz	3
Valencia juice with pulp, 8 fl oz	2
Valencia mango, 8 fl oz	3
Valenia orange, 8 fl oz	2
Tropicana Pure Premium	
Golden grapefruit, 8 fl oz	2
Orange juice, 8 fl oz	2
Orange juice, 1 carton (177 ml)	2
Orange juice, 1 large container (414 ml)	4
Orange juice, 1 container (296 ml)	3
Orange juice, 1 carton (250 ml)	2
Orange juice - lots of pulp, 8 fl oz	2
Orange juice - original, some pulp, 8 fl oz	2
Orange juice - original, some pulp, 1 container	4
Orange juice + calcium & vitamin D- lots of pulp, 8 fl oz	2
Orange pineapple, 8 fl oz	3
Orange strawberry banana, 8 fl oz	3
Orange tangerine, 8 fl oz	2
Orange with calcium & vitamin D, 8 fl oz	2
Ruby red grapefruit, 8 fl oz	2
Sweet grapefruit, 8 fl oz	3
Triple berry, 8 fl oz	2
Tropical orange, 8 fl oz	2

Fruit Juices and Drinks (con't) (POINTS VALUE)

Tropicana Pure Tropics

Orange peach mango, 8 fl oz	2
Orange pineapple, 8 fl oz	2
Orange, strawberry, banana, 8 fl oz	2

Tropicana Seasons Best

Apple, 8 fl oz	2
Apple, 1 carton	2
Apple + calcium and vit C, 10 fl oz	3
Apple juice, 1 can	3
Apple juice, 1 bottle	3
Cranberry cocktail, 10 fl oz	3
Cranberry cocktail, 8 fl oz	2
Cranberry grape, 8 fl oz	3
Fruit punch + calcium & vits. A, C, E, 10 fl oz	3
Grape juice, 8 fl oz	3
Orange pineapple, 8 fl oz	2
Ruby red grapefruit, 8 small fl oz	2
Ruby red grapefruit, 10 large fl oz	3

Tropicana Season's Best

Apple juice, 1 bottle	3
Grapefruit + vit C, 8 fl oz	2
Grapefruit juice, 1 small bottle	1
Grapefruit juice, 1 bottle	2
Grapefruit juice, 8 fl oz	2
Grapefruit juice, 1 cup	2
Grapefruit juice, 1 bottle (10 fl oz)	2

Orange + vit. C, 8 fl oz	2
Orange juice, 1 bottle	2
Orange juice, 1 can	3
Orange juice, pulp free & with pulp, 8 fl oz	2
Pineapple orange banana + calcium & vits. A, C, E, 10 fl oz	3

Tropicana Twister

Grape, 8 fl oz	2
Orange, 8 fl oz	3
Strawberry, 8 fl oz	2

Very Fine

Apple cranberry juice cocktail, 8 fl oz	3
Apple juice, 8 fl oz	2
Apple strawberry, 8 fl oz	3
Apricot nectar, 10 fl oz	4
Cranberry juice cocktail, 8 fl oz	3
Fruit punch, 8 fl oz	2
Fruit punch 100% vitamin c & 10% calcium, 8 fl oz	3
Grape juice, 8 fl oz	3
Guava nectar, 10 fl oz	4
Orange juice, 8 fl oz	2
Orange tangerine, 8 fl oz	2
Peach nectar, 10 fl oz	3
Pear nectar, 10 fl oz	3
Tropical fusion, 8 fl oz	3

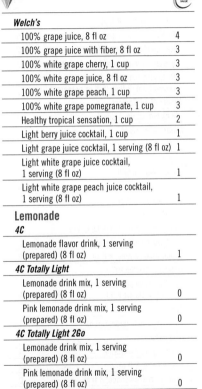

Welch's	POINTS VALUE
100% grape juice, 8 fl oz	4
100% grape juice with fiber, 8 fl oz	3
100% white grape cherry, 1 cup	3
100% white grape juice, 8 fl oz	3
100% white grape peach, 1 cup	3
100% white grape pomegranate, 1 cup	3
Healthy tropical sensation, 1 cup	2
Light berry juice cocktail, 1 cup	1
Light grape juice cocktail, 1 serving (8 fl oz)	1
Light white grape juice cocktail, 1 serving (8 fl oz)	1
Light white grape peach juice cocktail, 1 serving (8 fl oz)	1

Lemonade

4C	
Lemonade flavor drink, 1 serving (prepared) (8 fl oz)	1

4C Totally Light	
Lemonade drink mix, 1 serving (prepared) (8 fl oz)	0
Pink lemonade drink mix, 1 serving (prepared) (8 fl oz)	0

4C Totally Light 2Go	
Lemonade drink mix, 1 serving (prepared) (8 fl oz)	0
Pink lemonade drink mix, 1 serving (prepared) (8 fl oz)	0

Blue Bunny	POINTS VALUE
Natural lemonade, 1 cup	2

Capri Sun	
Lemonade, 1 pouch	2

Cascadian Farm	
Lemonade frozen concentrate, 1 serving (1.6 fl oz)	2

Country Time	
Lemonade large ready to drink pouches, 1 pouch	4
Lemonade, prepared, 8 fl oz	1
Lite lemonade, prepared, 8 fl oz	1
Lite pink lemonade, prepared, 8 fl oz	1
Pink lemonade, prepared, 8 fl oz	1
Raspberry lemonade, prepared, 8 fl oz	2
Strawberry lemonade, prepared, 8 fl oz	2

Country Time On the Go	
Lemonade yellow, prepared, 1 serving (8.45 fl oz)	1

Crystal Light	
Hydration pink lemonade, sugar free, 8 fl oz	0
Lemonade mix, sugar free, prepared, 8 fl oz	0
Lemonade, sugar free, 8 fl oz	0
Pink lemonade mix, sugar free, prepared, 8 fl oz	0
Pink lemonade, sugar free, 8 fl oz	0
Raspberry lemonade, sugar free, prepared, 8 fl oz	0

Lemonade (con't)

POINTS VALUE

	POINTS VALUE
Crystal Light On the Go	
Lemonade mix, 1 packet	0
Raspberry lemonade, prepared, 1 serving (8.45 fl oz)	0
Goya	
Lemonade, 8 fl oz	2
Hi-C	
Poppin' lemonade, 1 box	2
Kellogg's	
Special K20 protein water mix, pink lemonade, 1 packet	0
Kool-Aid	
Lemonade mix, unsweetened, 1 packet	0
Lemonade sugar-free mix, prepared, 8 fl oz	0
Soarin' strawberry lemonade sugar-free mix, prepared, 8 fl oz	0
Kool-Aid Jammers	
Lemonade, 1 pouch	2
Minute Maid	
Country style lemonade, frozen concentrate, 1 1/2 fl oz (8 fl oz prepared)	2
Frozen lemonade, frozen concentrate, 1 1/2 fl oz (8 fl oz prepared)	2
Lemonade, 1 box	2
Lemonade, 8 fl oz	2
Lemonade, 1 can	3
Lemonade, 1 can (squat can)	2
Pink lemonade, 1 can	2

	POINTS VALUE
Pink lemonade, 8 fl oz	2
Pink lemonade, 1 bottle (16.9 fl oz)	5
Raspberry lemonade, 8 fl oz	2
Raspberry lemonade, 1 can or bottle	3
Raspberry lemonade, frozen concentrate, 2 fl oz (8 fl oz prepared)	2
Minute Maid Coolers	
Pink lemonade, 1 pouch	2
Minute Maid Light	
Lemonade, 8 fl oz	0
Lemonade, 1 can	0
Minute Maid Simply	
Lemonade, 1 bottle	4
Lemonade, 8 fl oz	2
Odwalla	
Pure squeezed lemonade, 8 fl oz	2
Strawberry lemonade, 8 fl oz	2
Summertime lime, 8 fl oz	2
Schwan's LiveSmart	
Frozen lemonade concentrate, 2 fl oz (makes 1 cup)	3
SoBe	
Synergy - lemonade, 8 fl oz	1
Tropicana	
Lemonade, 1 container	4
Lemonade, 8 fl oz	2
Sugar free lemonade, 8 fl oz	0

Weight Watchers Mix-Ins

	POINTS VALUE
Lemonade, 1/2 packet	0

Meal Replacement Drinks

Balanced

Chocolate, 1 can	4
Vanilla, 1 can	4

Gatorade

Nutrition shake, chocolate, 1 can	8
Nutrition shake, vanilla, 1 can	8

Kashi GOLEAN

Chocolate shake mix, 2 scoops	4
Vanilla shake mix, 2 scoops	4

Nestle Carnation

Instant breakfast mix, chocolate malt, no sugar added, 1 packet	1
Instant breakfast mix, classic chocolate malt, 1 packet	2
Instant breakfast mix, classic French vanilla, 1 packet	3
Instant breakfast mix, classic French vanilla, no sugar added, 1 packet	1
Instant breakfast mix, dark chocolate powder, 1 packet	2
Instant breakfast mix, rich milk chocolate, 1 packet	2
Instant breakfast mix, rich milk chocolate, no sugar added, 1 packet	1
Instant breakfast mix, strawberry sensation, 1 packet	3
Instant breakfast mix, strawberry sensation, no sugar added, 1 packet	1
Instant breakfast, creamy milk chocolate, 1 can	5
Instant breakfast, creamy milk chocolate, no sugar added, 1 can	3
Instant breakfast, French vanilla, 1 can	5
Instant breakfast, French vanilla, no sugar added, 1 can	3
Instant breakfast, strawberry crème, 1 can	5

Milk and Milk Based Drinks

Alba

Chocolate, prepared, 8 fl oz	1
Double fudge, prepared, 8 fl oz	1
Nonfat dry milk, prepared, 8 fl oz	2
Strawberry, prepared, 8 fl oz	1
Vanilla, prepared, 8 fl oz	1

Starbucks

Frappuccino - strawberries & crème, 8 fl oz	4

Smoothies

8th Continent

Chocolate strawberry banana soymilk smoothie, 8 fl oz	2

Fruitfull

Berry berry best, 1 serving (4 fl oz)	3
Make mine mango, 1 serving (4 fl oz)	3
Strawberry and banana, 1 serving (4 fl oz)	2

Smoothies (con't)   POINTS VALUE POINTS VALUE

Horizon Organic Fat Free Yogurt Smoothies

Strawberry banana splash, 1 container	2
Tropical fruit punch, 1 container	2
Wild berry blast, 1 container	2

Jell-O Smoothie Snacks

Mixed berry, 1 container	2
Strawberry banana, 1 container	2

Lightfull Satiety Smoothie

Cafe latte, 1 container	1
Chocolate satisfaction, 1 container	1
Mango oasis, 1 container	1
Peachy cream, 1 container	1
Strawberry bliss, 1 container	1

Odwalla

Blackberry fruit shake fruit smoothie blend, 8 fl oz	3
Blueberry b monster vitamin b fruit smoothie blend, 8 fl oz	3
Citrus c monster vitamin c fruit smoothie blend, 8 fl oz	3
Mango tango fruit smoothie blend, 8 fl oz	3
Raspberry cha cha fruit smoothie blend, 8 fl oz	2
Strawberry banana fruit smoothie blend, 8 fl oz	3
Strawberry c monster vitamin c fruit smoothie blend, 8 fl oz	3
Tropical calci-yum monster calcium fruit smoothie blend, 8 fl oz	4

Silk Live!

Cultured soy - peach, 1 container	4
Cultured soy - raspberry, 1 container	4
Cultured soy - strawberry, 1 container	4

Tropicana

Mixed berry fruit smoothie, 11 fl oz	4
Strawberry banana fruit smoothie, 11 fl oz	4
Tropical fruit - fruit smoothie, 11 fl oz	4

Weight Watchers Smoothie Drink Mix

Creamy chocolate, 1 packet	1
French vanilla, 1 packet	1

Yoplait Go-Gurt Smoothies

Punch, 1 container	2
Strawberry, 1 container	2
Strawberry banana, 1 container	2
Wild berry, 1 container	2

Yoplait Light

Peach, 1 bottle	1

Yoplait Light Smoothies

Strawberry, 1 container	1
Strawberry banana, 1 container	1

Yoplait Nouriche Super Smoothie

Mixed berry, 1 container	4
Peach, 1 container	4
Raspberry, 1 container	4
Strawberry, 1 container	4
Strawberry banana, 1 container	4

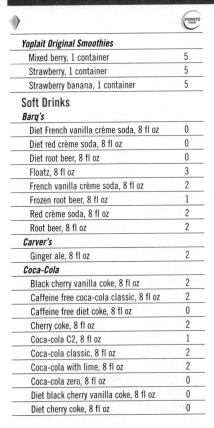

Yoplait Original Smoothies

	POINTS VALUE
Mixed berry, 1 container	5
Strawberry, 1 container	5
Strawberry banana, 1 container	5

Soft Drinks

Barq's

Diet French vanilla crème soda, 8 fl oz	0
Diet red crème soda, 8 fl oz	0
Diet root beer, 8 fl oz	0
Floatz, 8 fl oz	3
French vanilla crème soda, 8 fl oz	2
Frozen root beer, 8 fl oz	1
Red crème soda, 8 fl oz	2
Root beer, 8 fl oz	2

Carver's

Ginger ale, 8 fl oz	2

Coca-Cola

Black cherry vanilla coke, 8 fl oz	2
Caffeine free coca-cola classic, 8 fl oz	2
Caffeine free diet coke, 8 fl oz	0
Cherry coke, 8 fl oz	2
Coca-cola C2, 8 fl oz	1
Coca-cola classic, 8 fl oz	2
Coca-cola with lime, 8 fl oz	2
Coca-cola zero, 8 fl oz	0
Diet black cherry vanilla coke, 8 fl oz	0
Diet cherry coke, 8 fl oz	0

	POINTS VALUE
Diet coke, 8 fl oz	0
Diet coke sweetened with splenda, 8 fl oz	0
Diet coke with lime, 8 fl oz	0
Diet inca kola, 8 fl oz	0
Diet vanilla coke, 8 fl oz	0
Frozen classic, 8 fl oz	1
Frozen vanilla coke, 8 fl oz	2
Inca kola, 8 fl oz	2
Manzana mia, 8 fl oz	2
Vanilla coke, 8 fl oz	2

Crystal Light

Raspberry ice, sugar free, 8 fl oz	0

Crystal Light Sunrise

Classic orange, 8 fl oz	0

Diet Steaz Sparkling Green Tea

Black cherry, 1 cup	1
Cola, 1 cup	1
Lemon lime, 1 cup	1

Fanta

Apple, 8 fl oz	2
Berry, 8 fl oz	2
Black cherry, 8 fl oz	2
Citrus, 8 fl oz	2
Grape, 8 fl oz	2
Lemon, 8 fl oz	2
Orange, 8 fl oz	2
Peach, 8 fl oz	2
Pineapple, 8 fl oz	2

BEVERAGES

Soft Drinks, Fanta (con't)	POINTS VALUE		*Fresca*	POINTS VALUE
Pink grapefruit, 8 fl oz	2		*Fresca*	
Red tangerine, 8 fl oz	3		Fresca, 8 fl oz	0
Strawberry, 8 fl oz	2		Fresca black cherry, 8 fl oz	0
Zero orange, 8 fl oz	0		Fresca peach, 8 fl oz	0
Fanta Frozen			*Master*	
Banana, 8 fl oz	1		Frozen chill strawberry crème, 8 fl oz	1
Blue raspberry, 8 fl oz	2		*Mello Yello*	
Grape, 8 fl oz	1		Cherry, 8 fl oz	2
Green lemon lime, 8 fl oz	2		Diet mello yello, 8 fl oz	0
Kiwi strawberry, 8 fl oz	1		Frozen mello yello, 8 fl oz	1
Master chill cherry limeade, 8 fl oz	1		Mello yello, 8 fl oz	2
Orange, 8 fl oz	1		Melon, 8 fl oz	2
Orange crème, 8 fl oz	1		*Minute Maid*	
Peach, 8 fl oz	1		Frozen blueberry, 8 fl oz	1
Pina colada, 8 fl oz	1		Grape, 8 fl oz	2
Pineapple, 8 fl oz	1		Strawberry, 8 fl oz	2
Purple berry cherry, 8 fl oz	2		*Miranda*	
Strawberry, 8 fl oz	2		Orange, 8 fl oz	3
Strawberry banana, 8 fl oz	1		Pink grapefruit, 8 fl oz	2
Super sour apple, 8 fl oz	1		Strawberry, 8 fl oz	2
Super sour cherry, 8 fl oz	1		*Mountain Dew*	
Super sour watermelon, 8 fl oz	2		Caffeine free, 8 fl oz	2
Watermelon, 8 oz	1		Code red, 8 fl oz	2
White cherry, 8 fl oz	1		Diet, 8 fl oz	0
Wild cherry, 8 fl oz	2		Diet caffeine free, 8 fl oz	0
			Diet code red, 8 fl oz	0
			MDX, 8 fl oz	3

	POINTS VALUE		POINTS VALUE
Mountain dew code red freeze, 8 fl oz	1	Jazz - strawberries & cream, 8 fl oz	0
Mountain dew freeze, 8 fl oz	1	Pepsi freeze, 8 fl oz	1
Regular, 8 fl oz	2	Pepsi lime, 8 fl oz	2
Mr. Pibb		Pepsi one, 8 fl oz	0
Diet Mr. Pibb, 8 fl oz	0	Regular, 8 fl oz	2
Pibb xtra, 8 fl oz	2	Wild cherry, 8 fl oz	2
Pibb zero, 8 fl oz	0	Wild cherry pepsi freeze, 8 fl oz	1
Mug		***Red Flash***	
Cream soda, 8 fl oz	2	Red Flash, 8 fl oz	2
Diet cream soda, 8 fl oz	0	***Seagram's***	
Diet root beer, 8 fl oz	0	Diet ginger ale, 8 fl oz	0
Root beer, 8 fl oz	2	Diet raspberry ginger ale, 8 fl oz	0
Northern Neck		Ginger ale, 8 fl oz	2
Diet ginger ale, 8 fl oz	0	Raspberry ginger ale, 8 fl oz	2
Ginger ale, 8 fl oz	2	***Sierra Mist***	
Payaso		Sierra Mist, 8 fl oz	2
Horchata drink mix, 3 tsp	3	Sierra mist free, 8 fl oz	0
Pepsi		***Sprite***	
Caffeine free, 8 fl oz	2	Diet sprite zero, 8 fl oz	0
Diet, 8 fl oz	0	Frozen sprite, 8 fl oz	1
Diet caffeine free, 8 fl oz	0	Sprite, 8 fl oz	2
Diet pepsi freeze, 8 fl oz	0	Sprite remix Aruba jam, 8 fl oz	2
Diet pepsi lime, 8 fl oz	0	***Steaz Green Tea Soda***	
Diet pepsi max, 8 fl oz	0	Cola, 8 fl oz	2
Diet vanilla, 8 fl oz	0	Ginger ale, 8 fl oz	2
Diet wild cherry, 8 fl oz	0	Grape, 8 fl oz	2
Jazz - caramel cream, 8 fl oz	0	Key lime, 8 fl oz	2

BEVERAGES

Soft Drinks, Steaz Green Tea Soda (con't)	POINTS VALUE
Lemon dew, 8 fl oz	2
Orange, 8 fl oz	2
Raspberry, 8 fl oz	2
Root beer, 8 fl oz	2
Tab	
Tab, 8 fl oz	0
Tropicana Twister	
Diet orange, 8 fl oz	0
Waist Watcher	
Diet black cherry, 1 can	0
Diet black raspberry soda, 8 oz	0
Diet caffeine free cola, 1 can	0
Diet chocolate soda, 8 oz	0
Diet chocolate soda, 1 can	0
Diet citrus frost, 1 can	0
Diet ginger ale, 1 can	0
Diet lemon up, 1 can	0
Diet orange, 1 can	0
Diet raspberry ginger ale, 1 can	0
Diet root beer, 1 can	0
Diet tonic water, 8 oz	0
Diet vanilla cream, 1 can	0

Soy, Rice and Chai Drinks
8th Continent

	POINTS VALUE
Chocolate soy milk, 8 fl oz	3
◆ Fat free original soy milk, 8 fl oz	1
Fat free vanilla soy milk, 8 fl oz	1
Light chocolate soy milk, 8 fl oz	2

	POINTS VALUE
◆ Light original soy milk, 8 fl oz	1
Light vanilla soy milk, 8 fl oz	1
Original soy milk, 8 fl oz	2
Vanilla soy milk, 8 fl oz	2
Better Than Milk	
Rice original, powder, 1 serving (19 g)	2
Rice vanilla, powder, 1 serving (19 g)	1
Soy chocolate, powder, 1 serving (30 g)	2
Soy light, powder, 1 serving (19 g)	2
Soy original, powder, 1 serving (23 g)	2
Soy vanilla, powder, 1 serving (20 g)	2
Eden Organic	
Edenblend, 8 fl oz	2
Edensoy chocolate, 8 oz	4
◆ Edensoy extra original, 8 oz	2
Edensoy extra vanilla, 8 oz	3
◆ Edensoy light original, 8 oz	2
Edensoy light vanilla, 8 oz	3
◆ Edensoy original, 8 oz	3
◆ Edensoy unsweetened, 8 oz	3
Edensoy vanilla, 8 oz	3
Fearn	
Chocolate, 8 fl oz	2
Original, 8 fl oz	2
Soyness, chocolate, 8 fl oz	2
Soyness, original, 8 fl oz	2
Soyness, vanilla, 8 fl oz	2
Vanilla, 8 fl oz	2

	POINTS VALUE
General Foods International Coffee	
Sugar free chai latte, 1 Tbsp	1
House Foods Soy Time	
Banana, 8 fl oz	2
Original, 8 fl oz	2
Vanilla, 8 fl oz	2
Oregon Chai	
Sugar free original chai tea latte, 1/2 cup	0
Pacific Chai	
Caffeine free spice liquid concentrate, 4 fl oz	2
Decaf vanilla, 2 Tbsp	2
Decaffeinated spice, 2 Tbsp	2
Green tea, 2 Tbsp	2
Mocha chai latte, 2 Tbsp	2
Spice chai latte, 2 Tbsp	2
Spice liquid concentrate, 4 fl oz	2
Vanilla, 2 Tbsp	2
Vanilla liquid concentrate, 4 fl oz	2
Rice Dream	
Classic carob, 8 oz	3
Classic original, 8 oz	3
Classic vanilla, 8 oz	3
Enriched chocolate, 8 oz	3
Enriched original, 8 oz	3
Enriched vanilla, 8 oz	3
Heartwise original, 8 oz	2
Heartwise vanilla, 8 oz	2
Horchata original, 8 oz	3

	POINTS VALUE
Silk	
Chai, 1 cup	3
Chocolate, 1 cup	3
Coffee, 1 cup	3
Coffee soylatte, 11 fl oz	5
Coffee soylatte, 1 cup	3
Cultured soy - banana-strawberry, 1 container	3
Cultured soy - black cherry, 1 container	3
Cultured soy - blueberry, 1 container	3
Cultured soy - key lime, 1 container	3
Cultured soy - plain, 8 oz	3
Cultured soy - vanilla (6 oz), 1 container	3
Enhanced, 1 cup	2
Light chocolate, 1 cup	2
Mocha, 1 cup	3
Nog, 1/2 cup	2
Organic plain, 1 cup	3
Organic plain, 11 oz	4
Organic unsweetened, 1 cup	2
Organic vanilla, 1 cup	2
Plain light, 1 cup	1
Plus dha omega-3, 1 cup	2
Plus fiber, 1 cup	1
Pumpkin spice, 1 cup	3
Spice soylatte, 11 fl oz	4
Vanilla light, 1 cup	2
Very vanilla, 1 cup	3

BEVERAGES

	POINTS VALUE
Soy Dream	
Classic original, 8 oz	3
Classic vanilla, 8 oz	3
Enriched chocolate, 8 oz	3
Enriched original, 8 oz	2
Enriched vanilla, 8 oz	2
Vitasoy	
Chocolate banana soymilk, 8 fl oz	3
Classic original soymilk, shelf, 8 fl oz	3
Creamy original soymilk, shelf, 8 fl oz	3
Green tea soy drink, 1 serving	3
Holly nog, 8 fl oz	3
Light chocolate drink, shelf, 8 fl oz	2
Light original, shelf, 8 fl oz	1
Light vanilla, shelf, 8 fl oz	2
Organic holly nog, 8 fl oz	3
Organic peppermint chocolate, 8 fl oz	3
Peppermint chocolate, 8 fl oz	3
Rich chocolate soy milk, shelf stable, 8 fl oz	3
Smooth vanilla soymilk, 8 fl oz	3
Strawberry banana soymilk, 8 fl oz	3
Unsweetened original soymilk, shelf, 8 fl oz	2
Vanilla delight, shelf, 8 fl oz	3
WestSoy	
Lite plain soymilk, 8 oz	2
Lite vanilla soymilk, 8 oz	2
Low fat soy drink plain, 8 oz	2

	POINTS VALUE
Low fat soy drink vanilla, 8 oz	2
Lowfat soymilk, plain, 1 cup	2
Lowfat soymilk, vanilla, 1 cup	2
Non fat plain soymilk, 1 cup	1
Non fat soymilk, plain, 1 cup	1
Non fat soymilk, vanilla, 1 cup	1
Non fat vanilla soymilk, 1 cup	1
Organic original soymilk, 1 cup	2
Plus soymilk, plain, 1 cup	2
Plus vanilla soymilk, 1 cup	2
Rice plain, 8 oz	2
Rice vanilla, 8 oz	2
Shake chocolate, 8 oz	3
Shake vanilla, 8 oz	3
Unsweetened, 1 cup	1
Unsweetened almond soymilk, 1 cup	1
Unsweetened chocolate soymilk, 1 cup	2
Unsweetened original soymilk, 1 cup	1
Unsweetened vanilla soymilk, 1 cup	2
Unsweetened, almond, 1 cup	1
Unsweetened, chocolate, 1 cup	2
WestSoy drink plain, 1 cup	2
WestSoy lite plain, 1 cup	2
WestSoy lite vanilla, 1 cup	2
WestSoy Soy Slender	
Cappuccino, 8 oz	1
Chocolate, 8 oz	1

	POINTS VALUE
Sugar free soymilk, cappuccino, 1 cup	1
Sugar free soymilk, chocolate, 1 cup	1
Sugar free soymilk, vanilla, 1 cup	1
Vanilla, 8 oz	1

Sports Drinks

AMP Energy

	POINTS VALUE
Amp energy, 8 fl oz	2
Amp energy, overdrive, 8 fl oz	2

Fearn

Liquid lecithin, 1 Tbsp	4
Natural mint flavor liquid lecithin, 1 Tbsp	4

Gatorade

All flavors, 8 small fl oz	1
Powder, all flavors, 1 serving (makes 8 fl oz)	1

Gatorade All Stars

Berry, 8 fl oz	1
Fruit punch, 8 fl oz	1
Grape, 8 fl oz	1
Ice punch, 8 fl oz	1
Lemon-lime, 8 fl oz	1
Orange, 8 fl oz	1
Strawberry, 8 fl oz	1

Market Day

Gatorade kid size variety pack, 1 bottle	2

Powerade

	POINTS VALUE
Arctic shatter, 8 fl oz	1
Black cherry lime, 8 fl oz	1
Citrus blend, 8 fl oz	1
Flava 23 sourberry, 8 fl oz	1
Flava 23 sourmelon, 8 fl oz	1
Fruit punch, 8 fl oz	1
Green squall, 8 fl oz	1
Jagged ice, 8 fl oz	1
Lemon-lime, 8 fl oz	1
Mango, 8 fl oz	1
Mountain blast, 8 fl oz	1
NHRA, 8 fl oz	2
Olympic (citrus), 8 fl oz	1
Option black cherry, 8 fl oz	0
Option lemon, 8 fl oz	0
Option strawberry, 8 fl oz	0
Orange, 8 fl oz	1
Strawberry melon, 8 fl oz	1

SoBe

Essential energy, berry, 8 fl oz	3
Essential energy, orange, 8 fl oz	3

Steaz Energy

Organic fuel, 8 fl oz	2

Tea/Iced Tea

4C

	POINTS VALUE
Decaffeinated iced tea mix with sugar and natural lemon flavor, 1 serving(8 fl oz) (prepared)	2
Green antioxidant with honey & lemon, 1 serving (prepared) (8 fl oz)	2
Green tea with sugar, honey and natural lemon flavor, 1 serving (prepared) (8 fl oz)	2
Iced tea mix with sugar and natural lemon flavor, 1 serving (prepared) (8 fl oz)	1
Peach iced tea mix with sugar and natural peach flavor, 1 serving (prepared) (8 fl oz)	2

4C Light

Decaffeinated low calorie iced tea mix with natural lemon flavor, 1 serving (prepared) (8 fl oz)	0
Low calorie green tea with honey and lemon, 1 serving (prepared) (8 fl oz)	0
Low calorie iced tea mix with natural lemon flavor, 1 serving (prepared) (8 fl oz)	0

4C Totally Light

Iced tea mix antioxidant green tea, 1 serving (prepared) (8 fl oz)	0
Iced tea mix, antioxidant green tea, 1 serving (prepared) (8 fl oz)	0
Iced tea mix, natural decaffeinated natural lemon flavor, 1 serving (prepared) (8 fl oz)	0
Iced tea mix, natural lemon flavor, 1 serving (prepared) (8 fl oz)	0

4C Totally Light Tea 2Go

Iced tea mix, green antioxidant with honey and natural lemon flavor, 1 serving (8 fl oz)	0

4C Totally Light Tea2Go

Iced tea mix naturally decaffeinated natural lemon flavor, 1 serving (prepared) (8 fl oz)	0
Iced tea mix variety pack, decaffeinated, 1 serving (prepared) (8 fl oz)	0
Iced tea mix variety pack, green tea, 1 serving (prepared) (8 fl oz)	0
Iced tea mix variety pack, lemon, 1 serving (prepared) (8 fl oz)	0
Iced tea mix variety pack, raspberry, 1 serving (prepared) (8 fl oz)	0
Iced tea mix, lemon, 1 serving (prepared) (8 fl oz)	0

Country Time

Lemonade iced tea classic mix, 1 serving (23 g)	2
Lemonade iced tea peach mix, 1 serving (23 g)	2
Lemonade iced tea raspberry mix, 1 serving (23 g)	2

Crystal Light

Green tea raspberry, sugar free, prepared, 8 fl oz	0
Iced tea decaffeinated mix, sugar free, prepared, 8 fl oz	0
Iced tea mix, sugar free, prepared, 8 fl oz	0

	POINTS VALUE
Lemon tea, sugar free, 8 fl oz	0
Peach iced tea mix, sugar free, prepared, 8 fl oz	0
Raspberry iced tea mix, sugar free, prepared, 8 fl oz	0

Crystal Light On the Go

Green tea honey lemon, sugar free, prepared, 1 serving (8.45 fl oz)	0
Iced tea mix, sugar free, 1 packet	0
Peach tea mix, sugar free, 1 packet	0
White tea blueberry, 1 serving (8.45 fl oz)	0

Eden Organic

Lotus root tea, 1 tsp	0
Organic matcha tea, 1 serving (1 g)	0

Flavia

Decaffeinated English breakfast tea, 1 sachet	0
Earl grey tea, 1 sachet	0
English breakfast tea, 1 sachet	0
Exotic chai tea, 1 sachet	0
Green tea with jasmine, 1 sachet	0
Japanese green tea, 1 sachet	0
White tea and orange, 1 sachet	0

General Foods

Instant chai latte flavored tea mix, 1 1/3 Tbsp	2

Kellogg's

Special K20 protein water mix, iced tea, 1 packet	0

Lipton

	POINTS VALUE
Diet green tea with citrus, 8 fl oz	0
Diet green tea with citrus, 8 fl oz	0
Diet green tea with mixed berry, 8 fl oz	0
Diet iced tea with lemon, 8 fl oz	0
Diet iced tea with peach, 8 fl oz	0
Diet white tea with raspberry, 8 fl oz	0
Green tea with citrus, 8 fl oz	2
Iced tea with lemon, 8 fl oz	1
Iced tea with peach, 8 fl oz	2
Original - diet lemon, 8 fl oz	0
White tea with raspberry, 8 fl oz	1

Lipton Brisk

Diet iced tea with lemon, 8 fl oz	0
Green tea, 8 fl oz	2
Iced tea with lemon, 8 fl oz	2
Raspberry iced tea, 8 fl oz	2

Lipton PureLeaf

Diet sweet tea, 8 fl oz	0
Diet sweet tea with lemon, 8 fl oz	0
Extra sweet tea, 8 fl oz	2
Green tea with honey, 8 fl oz	1
Green tea with passion fruit, 8 fl oz	1
Lemon tea, 8 fl oz	1
Peach tea, 8 fl oz	1
Raspberry tea, 8 fl oz	1
Sweetened tea, 8 fl oz	1

Tea/Iced Tea, Lipton PureLeaf (con't)	POINTS VALUE
Unsweetened tea, 8 fl oz	0
White tea with tangerine, 8 fl oz	1
Lipton To Go	
Apple cranberry white iced tea, 1/2 packet	0
Cherry green iced tea, 1/2 packet	0
Citrus green iced tea, 1/2 packet	0
Lemon black iced tea, 1/2 packet	0
Mandarin mango green iced tea, 1/2 packet	0
Peach black iced tea, 1/2 packet	0
Raspberry white iced tea, 1/2 packet	0
Minute Maid	
Lemonade iced tea, 8 fl oz	2
Nestea	
100% decaf tea iced tea mix, 2 tsp	0
100% tea iced tea mix, 2 tsp	0
Brewed unsweetened, 8 fl oz	0
Cool, 8 fl oz	2
Cool lemonade tea, 8 fl oz	2
Cool peach frrreezer, 8 fl oz	2
Cool raspbrrry cooler, 8 fl oz	2
Decaffeinated sweetened tea, 8 fl oz	1
Diet green, 8 fl oz	0
Diet lemon, 8 fl oz	0
Diet Nestea sweetened with splenda, 8 fl oz	0
Green, 8 fl oz	2
Green tea concentrate, 1 fl oz	2
Herb tea lemon bliss iced tea mix, 1 Tbsp	0

	POINTS VALUE
Honey lemon green tea, 8 fl oz	2
Lemon, 8 fl oz	2
Lemon & sugar iced tea mix, 1 1/3 Tbsp	1
Lemon concentrate, 1 fl oz	2
Lemon iced tea mix, 2 tsp	0
Lemon sweet, 8 fl oz	2
Lemonade tea iced tea mix, 1 1/3 Tbsp	1
Nestea ice lemon green tea, 8 fl oz	2
Nestea ice lime iced tea, 8 fl oz	2
Peach concentrate, 2 Tbsp	2
Peach iced tea, 8 fl oz	2
Raspberry, 8 fl oz	2
Raspberry concentrate, 1 fl oz	2
Sugar free decaf iced tea mix, 2 tsp	0
Sugar free iced tea mix, 2 tsp	0
Sweetened, 8 fl oz	2
Unsweetened, 8 fl oz	0
Unsweetened concentrate, 2 Tbsp	0
SoBe	
Black tea, 8 fl oz	2
Green tea, 8 fl oz	2
Lean diet green tea, 8 fl oz	0
Lean diet peach tea, 8 fl oz	0
Oolong tea, 8 fl oz	2
Zen tea, 8 fl oz	2
Steaz Green Tea Soda	
Diet black cherry, 8 fl oz	1
Diet blueberry pomegranate, 8 fl oz	1

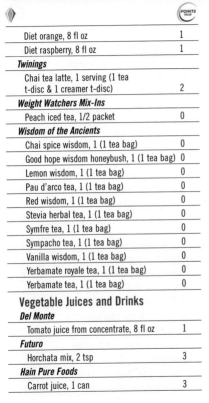

	POINTS VALUE
Diet orange, 8 fl oz	1
Diet raspberry, 8 fl oz	1
Twinings	
Chai tea latte, 1 serving (1 tea t-disc & 1 creamer t-disc)	2
Weight Watchers Mix-Ins	
Peach iced tea, 1/2 packet	0
Wisdom of the Ancients	
Chai spice wisdom, 1 (1 tea bag)	0
Good hope wisdom honeybush, 1 (1 tea bag)	0
Lemon wisdom, 1 (1 tea bag)	0
Pau d'arco tea, 1 (1 tea bag)	0
Red wisdom, 1 (1 tea bag)	0
Stevia herbal tea, 1 (1 tea bag)	0
Symfre tea, 1 (1 tea bag)	0
Sympacho tea, 1 (1 tea bag)	0
Vanilla wisdom, 1 (1 tea bag)	0
Yerbamate royale tea, 1 (1 tea bag)	0
Yerbamate tea, 1 (1 tea bag)	0

Vegetable Juices and Drinks
Del Monte
Tomato juice from concentrate, 8 fl oz	1

Futuro
Horchata mix, 2 tsp	3

Hain Pure Foods
Carrot juice, 1 can	3

Herdez
Original vegetable juice, 1 can	1
Picante limon vegetable juice, 1 can	1

Odwalla
Carrot juice, 8 fl oz	1

Water
Aquafina
Aquafina, 8 fl oz	0
Aquafina alive - berry pomegranate, 8 fl oz	0
Aquafina alive - orange lime, 8 fl oz	0
Aquafina alive - peach mango, 8 fl oz	0
Aquafina sparkling - citrus twist, 8 fl oz	0

Aquafina Essentials FlavorSplash
Citrus blend, 8 fl oz	0
Wild berry, 8 fl oz	0

Aquafina FlavorSplash
Raspberry, 8 fl oz	0

Aquafina Sparkling
Berry burst, 8 fl oz	0

Dasani
Dasani, 8 fl oz	0
Dasani with lemon, 8 fl oz	0
Dasani with raspberry, 8 fl oz	0
Dasani with strawberry, 8 fl oz	0

Fruit 2 O
Energy raspberry, 8 fl oz	0
Hydration strawberry tangerine, 8 fl oz	0

BEVERAGES

	POINTS VALUE
Immunity berry pomegranate, 8 fl oz	0
Natural cherry, 8 fl oz	0
Natural grape, 8 fl oz	0
Natural lemon, 8 fl oz	0
Natural lime, 8 fl oz	0
Natural orange, 8 fl oz	0
Natural peach, 6 fl oz	0
Natural raspberry, 8 fl oz	0
Natural strawberry, 8 fl oz	0
Relax tropical fruit, 8 fl oz	0
Tropical fruit, 8 fl oz	0
Fruit 2 0 Plus 10	
Natural apple, 8 fl oz	0
Natural berry, 8 fl oz	0
Watermelon kiwi, 8 fl oz	0
Kellogg's	
Special K20 protein strawberry kiwi, 1 bottle	0
Special K20 protein water lemon, 1 bottle	0
Special K20 protein water mix, strawberry kiwi, 1 packet	0
Special K20 protein water tropical blend, 1 bottle	0
Special K20 protein water, mixed berry, 1 bottle	0
Minute Maid	
Just 10 - fruit punch, 1 pouch	0

	POINTS VALUE
Minute Maid Fruit Falls	
Berry water beverage, 1 pouch	0
Tropical water beverage, 1 pouch	0
Naturally Fresh	
Mountain spring water, 2 Tbsp	0
Propel	
Berry, 8 fl oz	0
Black cherry, 8 fl oz	0
Grape, 8 fl oz	0
Kiwi strawberry, 8 fl oz	0
Lemon, 8 fl oz	0
Mandarin orange with calcium, 8 fl oz	0
Mango with calcium, 8 fl oz	0
Mixed berry with calcium, 8 fl oz	0
SoBe	
Lifewater - blackberry grape, 8 fl oz	1
Lifewater - orange tangerine, 8 fl oz	1
Lifewater - passionfruit citrus, 8 fl oz	1
Lifewater - pomegranate cherry, 8 fl oz	1
Lifewater - strawberry kiwi, 8 fl oz	1

Wine and Wine Coolers
Eden

	POINTS VALUE
Mirin (rice cooking wine), 1 Tbsp	1
Fanci Food	
Cooking wine, burgundy, 2 Tbsp	1
Cooking wine, sherry, 2 Tbsp	1

Little Boomey

	POINTS VALUE
Cabernet merlot, 1/2 cup	2
Cabernet sauvignon, 1/2 cup	2
Chardonnay, 1/2 cup	2
Merlot, 1/2 cup	2
Shiraz, 1/2 cup	2
Shiraz cabernet, 1/2 cup	2

Ola

Cooking wine, 1 tsp	0

Regina

Cooking wine, burgundy, 2 Tbsp	1
Cooking wine, sauterne, 2 Tbsp	0
Cooking wine, sherry, 2 Tbsp	1

Regina Select

Cabernet sauvignon cooking wine, 2 Tbsp	0
Chardonnay cooking wine, 2 Tbsp	0
Marsala cooking wine, 2 Tbsp	1

Sutter Home

Cabernet sauvignon, 1/2 cup	2
Chardonnay, 1/2 cup	2
Johannisberg riesling, 1/2 cup	2
Merlot, 1/2 cup	2
Pinot grigio, 1/2 cup	2
Pinot noir, 1/2 cup	2
Shiraz, 1/2 cup	2
White merlot, 1/2 cup	2
White zinfandel, 1/2 cup	2
Zinfandel, 1/2 cup	2

Sutter Home Fre

	POINTS VALUE
Dealcoholized chardonnay, 1/2 cup	1
Dealcoholized merlot, 1/2 cup	1
Dealcoholized sparkling brut, 1/2 cup	1
Dealcoholized white zinfandel, 1/2 cup	1

Trinity Oaks

Cabernet sauvignon, 1/2 cup	2
Chardonnay, 1/2 cup	2
Merlot, 1/2 cup	2
Pinot grigio, 1/2 cup	2
White merlot, 1/2 cup	2
Zinfandel, 1/2 cup	2

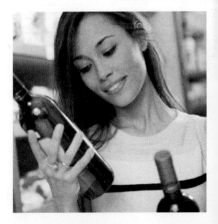

	POINTS VALUE
Bagels	
Alvarado	
Sprouted spelt bagel, 1	4
Sprouted wheat bagel, 1	4
Sprouted wheat cinnamon raisin bagel, 1	5
Sprouted wheat granola crunch bagel, 1	5
Sprouted wheat onion poppyseed bagel, 1	6
Sprouted wheat sesame seed bagels, 1	6
Cobblestone Mill	
Cinnamon raisin bagels, 1	5
Multigrain bagels, 1	5
Plain bagels, 1	5
French Meadow Bakery	
Healthy hemp, 1	7
Sourdough bagel, 1	5
Spelt bagel (alternative grain), 1	5
Sprouted bagels with Ezekiel 4:9 grains, 1	5
Sprouted wheat raisin & cinnamon, 1	5
Healthy Life Original	
100% whole wheat light bagels, 1	2
Market Day	
Cinnamon brown sugar bagel-ers, 1	4
Original plain bagel-ers, 1	4
Otis Spunkmeyer	
Blueberry, 1 (113 g)	5
Blueberry, 1 (85 g)	4
Cinnamon raisin, 1 (113 g)	5

	POINTS VALUE
Cinnamon raisin, 1 (85 g)	4
Onion, 1 (113 g)	5
Onion, 1 (85 g)	4
Plain, 1 (85 g)	4
Pepperidge Farm	
Plain bagels, 1	5
Thomas'	
100% whole wheat mini bagels, 1	2
Brown sugar cinnamon mini bagel, 1	3
Cinnamon raisin swirl bagel, 1	5
Cinnamon raisin swirl mini bagel, 1	2
Cinnamon raisin toaster bagel, 1	4
Cinnamon swirl bagel, 1	5
Egg toaster bagel, 1	4
Everything bagel, 1	6
Everything square bagel, 1	6
Hearty grains 100% whole wheat bagel, 1	5
New York style plain bagel, 1	5
Onion bagel, 1	5
Plain mini bagel, 1	2
Plain square bagel, 1	6
Plain toaster bagel, 1	4
Sesame seed bagel, 1	6
Weight Watchers	
Hearth baked bagel, 1	2
Western Bagel	
New York style bialy, 1	4

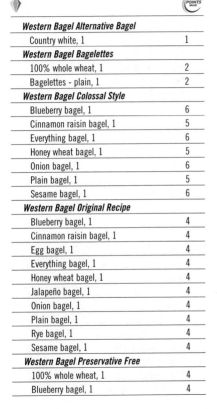

	POINTS VALUE
Western Bagel Alternative Bagel	
Country white, 1	1
Western Bagel Bagelettes	
100% whole wheat, 1	2
Bagelettes - plain, 1	2
Western Bagel Colossal Style	
Blueberry bagel, 1	6
Cinnamon raisin bagel, 1	5
Everything bagel, 1	6
Honey wheat bagel, 1	5
Onion bagel, 1	6
Plain bagel, 1	5
Sesame bagel, 1	6
Western Bagel Original Recipe	
Blueberry bagel, 1	4
Cinnamon raisin bagel, 1	4
Egg bagel, 1	4
Everything bagel, 1	4
Honey wheat bagel, 1	4
Jalapeño bagel, 1	4
Onion bagel, 1	4
Plain bagel, 1	4
Rye bagel, 1	4
Sesame bagel, 1	4
Western Bagel Preservative Free	
100% whole wheat, 1	4
Blueberry bagel, 1	4

	POINTS VALUE
Cinnamon raisin bagel, 1	4
Everything bagel, 1	4
Onion bagel, 1	4
Plain bagel, 1	4
Sesame bagel, 1	5
Western Bagel Preservative Free	
Cinnamon spice, 1	1
Sweet wheat, 1	1
Western Bagel Preservative Free Bagelettes	
100% whole wheat, 1	2
Plain, 1	2
Western Bagel The Alternative Bagel	
Cinnamon spice, 1	1
Roasted onion bagel, 1	1
Sweet wheat, 1	1
Very blueberry, 1	1
Western Bagel The Perfect 10 Bagel	
Healthy grain, 1	2

Biscuits

Alexia

Biscuits, 1	4

Bisquick Complete Biscuit Mixes

Buttermilk, 1/3 cup	3
Cheese garlic, 1/3 cup	4
Honey butter, 1/3 cup	3
Three cheese, 1/3 cup	4

Biscuits (con't) POINTS VALUE

Market Day	
Homestyle biscuit dough, 1 piece	5
Pillsbury	
Buttermilk, 3	3
Cheddar flaky layers, 1	5
Country biscuits, 3	3
Flaky layer buttermilk, 3	3
Reduced fat biscuits - flaky layers, 1	4
Pillsbury Golden Layers	
Butter tastin flaky, 1	2
Buttermilk flaky, 1	3
Honey butter, 1	3
Original flaky, 1	3
Pillsbury Grands!	
Homestyle shortcake biscuits, 1	4
Pillsbury Grands! Flaky	
Butter tastin', 1	4
Buttermilk, 1	4
Original, 1	4
Pillsbury Grands! Homestyle	
Butter tastin', 1	4
Buttermilk, 1	4
Buttermilk, reduced fat, 1	4
Extra rich, 1	5
Original, 1	4
Southern style, 1	4
Wheat, reduced fat, 1	4

  POINTS VALUE

Pillsbury Homestyle	
Butter tastin' fluffy, 1	2
Buttermilk fluffy, 1	2
Pillsbury Oven Baked	
Butter tastin', 1	4
Buttermilk, 1	4
Cheddar garlic, 1	4
Extra-large easy split, 1	6
Flaky layers, 1	4
Southern style, 1	4
Pillsbury Perfect Portions	
Butter tastin', 1	4
Buttermilk, 1	4
Buttermilk reduced fat, 1	4
Flaky layers, 1	4

Bread

Alexia	
Garlic baguette, 2 pieces	3
Alvarado	
100% whole wheat 7-grain bread, 1 slice	1
100% whole wheat bread, 1 slice	1
100% whole wheat oatmeal bread, 1 slice	1
California style complete protein bread, 1 slice	1
Diabetic lifestyle bread, 1 slice	1
Essential flax seed bread, 2 slices	2

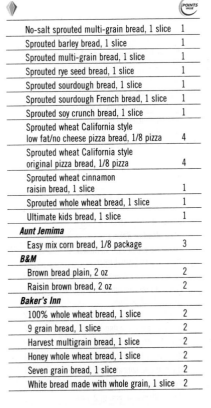

	POINTS VALUE
No-salt sprouted multi-grain bread, 1 slice	1
Sprouted barley bread, 1 slice	1
Sprouted multi-grain bread, 1 slice	1
Sprouted rye seed bread, 1 slice	1
Sprouted sourdough bread, 1 slice	1
Sprouted sourdough French bread, 1 slice	1
Sprouted soy crunch bread, 1 slice	1
Sprouted wheat California style low fat/no cheese pizza bread, 1/8 pizza	4
Sprouted wheat California style original pizza bread, 1/8 pizza	4
Sprouted wheat cinnamon raisin bread, 1 slice	1
Sprouted whole wheat bread, 1 slice	1
Ultimate kids bread, 1 slice	1
Aunt Jemima	
Easy mix corn bread, 1/8 package	3
B&M	
Brown bread plain, 2 oz	2
Raisin brown bread, 2 oz	2
Baker's Inn	
100% whole wheat bread, 1 slice	2
9 grain bread, 1 slice	2
Harvest multigrain bread, 1 slice	2
Honey whole wheat bread, 1 slice	2
Seven grain bread, 1 slice	2
White bread made with whole grain, 1 slice	2

	POINTS VALUE
Be Happy & Healthy	
Almond cherry, 1/2 slice	6
Apple spice, 1/2 slice	5
Banana, 1/2 slice	4
Cappuccino-chocolate chip, 1/2 slice	6
Carrot, 1/2 slice	5
Chocolate, 1/2 slice	3
Old fashion pound cake, 1/2 slice	6
Orange cranberry, 1/2 slice	3
Pumpkin, 1/2 slice	3
Sweet potato, 1/2 slice	4
Zucchini, 1/2 slice	5
Beefsteak	
Hearty rye bread, 1 slice	1
Light soft rye bread, 2 slices	1
Soft rye bread, 1 slice	1
Butternut	
Honey wheat bread, 2 slices	2
White bread, 1 slice	1
Cobblestone Mill	
Cinnamon raisin swirl breakfast bread, 1 slice	2
Cinnamon swirl breakfast bread, 1 slice	2
Crunchy oat meal bread, 1 slice	2
Jewish rye specialty bread, 1 slice	1
Pumpernickel specialty bread, 1 slice	1
Sour dough specialty bread, 1 slice	1

BREAD & BAKED GOODS

Bread (con't)	POINTS VALUE
DiGiorno Microwave Thin Crust	
Grilled chicken & vegetable (dual serve), 1/2 small	6
Grilled chicken & vegetable (dual serve), 1	12
Dromedary	
Gingerbread cake & cookie mix, prepared, 2 oz	4
Hot roll mix, prepared, 1 roll	2
Flatout	
Carbdown Italian herb, 1	1
Garden spinach, 1	2
Harvest wheat, 1	2
Italian herb, 1	2
Multi-grain, 1	1
No crust & soft kidz original, 1	0
Southwest chipotle, 1	2
Sundried tomato, 1	2
Sundried tomato light, 1	1
The original, 1	2
The original carbdown, 1	1
Whole grain white, 1	2
Flatout Mini	
Harvest wheat, 1	1
Food for Life	
7-sprouted grains, 1/2	1
7-sprouted grains, 1 slice	1
Cinnamon raisin 7-sprouted grains, 1 slice	1
Ezekiel 4:9 sprouted grain, 1/2	1

	POINTS VALUE
Ezekiel 4:9 sprouted grain cinnamon raisin, 1/2	1
Ezekiel 4:9 sprouted grains, 1 slice	1
Genesis 1:29 sprouted grain, 1/2	1
Organic bran for life bread, 1 slice	1
Organic Ezekiel 4:9 cinnamon raisin sprouted grains, 1 slice	1
Organic Ezekiel 4:9 low sodium sprouted grain bread, 1 slice	1
Organic Ezekiel 4:9 sprouted with sesame, 1 slice	1
Organic Genesis 1:29 sprouted grains bread, 1 slice	1
Organic low sodium 7-sprouted grains bread, 1 slice	1
Sprouted whole wheat, 1 slice	1
French Meadow Bakery	
100% rye bread with sunflower seed, 1 slice (wheat free)	1
Brown rice with whole wheat, 2 slice	3
European sour dough rye (wheat-free), 1 slice	1
Flax & sunflower (round), 1 slice	2
Healthy hemp sprouted bread, 1 slice	2
Kamut (alternative grain), 2 slice	3
Rye flaxseed (wheat-free), 1 slice	1
Rye salt free (wheat-free), 1 slice	1
Rye whole grain (wheat-free), 1 slice	1
Spelt (alternative grain), 2 slice	2

	POINTS VALUE
Spelt cinnamon raisin (alternative grain), 2 slice	3
Sprouted health seed spelt, 2 oz	3
Sprouted men's bread with soy isoflavones, 1 slice	2
Sprouted woman's bread with soy isoflavones, 1 slice	1
Summer (round), 1 slice	2
White spelt bread, 21 slice	3
Healthy Life 100% Natural	
Farmer's 12 grain bread, 1 slice	1
Whole grain 100% whole wheat bread, 1 slice	1
Whole grain flaxseed bread, 1 slice	1
Healthy Life Original	
100% whole grain sugar free rye bread made with caraway seeds, 2 slices	1
100% whole grain sugar free rye bread no seeds, 2 slices	1
100% whole grain sugar free wheat bread, 2 slices	1
100% whole wheat whole grain bread, 2 slices	1
100% whole wheat whole grain flaxseed bread, 2 slices	1
Italian bread, 2 slices	1
Light English muffins, 1	1
Sourdough bread, 2 slices	1
White bread, 2 slices	1

	POINTS VALUE
Healthy Life Southern Country Style	
100% whole wheat, 2 slices	2
100% whole wheat bread, 1 slice	1
Oatmeal, 2 slices	3
Whole grain white, 2 slices	2
Hodgson Mill	
Barley bread mix with soy, 1/4 cup	2
Caraway rye bread mix with soy, 1/4 cup	2
Honey whole wheat bread mix with soy, 1/4 cup	2
Nine grain bread mix with soy, 1/4 cup	2
Whole wheat gingerbread mix, 1/4 cup	2
Home Pride Butter Top	
Wheat bread, 1 slice	1
White bread, 1 slice	1
Market Day	
Cherry braided bread, 1 serving (1/10 loaf)	3
Cream cheese braided bread, 1 slice	3
Stuffed appetizer bread, 1/4 loaf	10
Merita	
Autumn grain bread, 1 slice	1
Calcium fortified old fashioned white bread, 1 slice	1
Millbrook	
Cracked wheat bread, 1 slice	2
Wheat bread, 2 slices	2

Bread (con't)

Nature's Own

100% whole wheat bread made with organic flour, specialty bread, all-natural, 1 slice	2
100% whole wheat bread/100% whole grain bread, 1 slice	1
100% whole wheat specialty bread, all-natural, 1 slice	2
12 grain bread, 1 slice	1
9 grain specialty bread, all-natural, 1 slice	2
All natural 12 grain specialty bread, 1 slice	1
All natural 7 cereal grains specialty bread, 1 slice	2
All natural double fiber wheat specialty bread, 1 slice	1
All natural honey white made with whole grain specialty bread, 1 slice	2
Butterbread, 1 slice	1
Double fiber wheat bread, 1 slice	0
Honey 7 grain/with whole grain nutrition bread, 1 slice	1
Honey wheat, 1 slice	1
Honey wheat bread made with organic flour, specialty bread, all-natural, 1 slice	1
Light honey wheat bread, 2 slices	1
Light wheat, 2 slices	1
Light white, 2 slices	1
Wheat n' fiber/9-grams carb per slice bread, 1 slice	1
Whitewheat loaf bread, 1 slice	0

Nature's Path

Carrot raisin manna bread, 1 slice	2
Cinnamon date manna bread, 1 slice	2
Fruit and nut manna bread, 1 slice	2
Millet rice manna bread, 1 slice	2
Multigrain manna bread, 1 slice	2
Sun seed manna bread, 1 slice	3
Whole rye manna bread, 1 slice	2
Whole wheat manna bread, 1 slice	2

Otis Spunkmeyer

Apple spice mini loaf, 1	8
Banana walnut mini loaf, 1	11
Chocolate fudge pecan mini loaf, 1	10

Otis Spunkmeyer Café Collection

Chocolate marble bread slices, 1 slice	11
Vanilla pound cake, 1 slice	11
Yogurt lemon poppy, 1 slice	10

Paraclete

Bread, 1 slice	0
Wheat bread, 1 slice	0

Pepperidge Farm

100% natural whole grain 100% whole wheat bread, 1 slice	2
100% whole wheat English muffins, 1	2
Carb style 7 grain bread, 1 slice	1
Carb style whole wheat bread, 1 slice	1
Cinnamon swirl, 1 slice	2
Farmhouse 12 grain bread, 1 slice	2

	POINTS VALUE
Light style seven grain bread, 3 slices	2
Light style whole grain white bread, 3 slices	2
Original English muffins, 1	3
Original white thin sliced enriched bread, 1 slice	1
Raisin cinnamon swirl bread, 1 slice	2
Pepperidge Farm Farmhouse	
Country white bread, 1 slice	2
Harvest 7 grain bread, 1 slice	2
Hearty white bread, 1 slice	2
Pepperidge Farm Light Style	
Oatmeal bread, 3 slices	2
Soft wheat bread, 3 slices	2
Pepperidge Farm Natural Whole Grain	
9 grain bread, 1 slice	2
Pillsbury	
Cinnamon mini bites, 3 pieces	4
Crusty French loaf, 1 slice (1/5 loaf)	2
Roman Meal	
100% whole wheat, 1 slice	1
12 grain bread, 1 slice	2
Healthy white bread, 2 slices	2
High fiber 100% whole grain bread, 1 slice	1
Honey & oat bran with fiber bread, 1 slice	2
Honey wheatberry bread, 1 slice	2
Round top bread, 2 slices	2
Sandwich bread, 1 slice	1
Superseed bread, 1 slice	2

	POINTS VALUE
Rudi's Organic Bakery	
100% whole wheat bun, 1	3
14 grain, 1 slice	1
7 grain with flax, 1 slice	1
Apple 'n spice, 1 slice	2
Cinnamon raisin, 1 slice	3
Colorado cracked wheat, 1 slice	2
Country French, 1 slice	2
Country morning white, 1 slice	2
European multigrain, 1 slice	2
Honey sweet whole wheat, 1 slice	2
Jewish light rye, 1 slice	2
Multi-grain oat, 1 slice	2
Multigrain with flax English muffin, 1	2
Rocky mountain sourdough, 1 slice	2
Rosemary olive oil, 1 slice	2
Spelt ancient grain bread, 1 slice	2
Spelt bread, 1 slice	2
Spelt English muffins, 1	2
Tuscan roasted garlic, 1 slice	2
Wheat and oat, 1 slice	1
Whole grain wheat English muffin, 1	2
Rudi's Organic Bakery Right Choice	
Low-carb bread, 1 slice	0
Schwan's LiveSmart	
French baguette bread, 1/4 loaf	2
Multi grain loaf, 1/2 loaf	2

187

Bread (con't)

	POINTS VALUE
Thomas'	
100% whole wheat cinnamon raisin swirl toasting bread, 1 slice	2
Cinnamon raisin English muffin, 1	2
Cinnamon swirl toasting bread, 1 slice	3
Corn toasting bread, 1 slice	2
Cranberry English muffin, 1	3
Date nut loaf, 2 oz (approximately 1" slice)	4
English muffin toasting bread, 1 slice	2
Hearty grains 100% whole wheat English muffin, 1	2
Hearty grains 12 grain English muffin, 1	2
Hearty grains honey wheat English muffin, 1	2
Hearty grains multi-grain English muffin, 1	3
Hearty grains oat bran English muffin, 1	2
Light multi-grain English muffin, 1	1
Oatmeal raisin swirl toasting bread, 1 slice (approx. 1" slice)	2
Original English muffin, 1	2
Raisin cinnamon swirl toasting bread, 1 slice	2
Sourdough English muffin, 1	2
Super size original English muffin, 1	4
Weight Watchers	
100% whole wheat bread, 2 slices	1
Fork split English muffin, 1	1
Lite seedless rye bread, 2 slices	1

	POINTS VALUE
Multi-grain, 2 slices	1
Wheat English muffin, 1	1
Western Bagel English Muffins	
Cinnamon raisin, 1	3
Original, 1	3
Sourdough, 1	3
Western Bagel The Alternative English	
Plain English muffin, 1	1
Wonder	
100% whole grain bread, 1 slice	1
Cinnamon swirl bread, 1 slice	2
Kid's white bread, 1 slice	1
Made with whole grain honey wheat bread, 2 slices	3
Made with whole grain wheat bread, 2 slices	2
White bread, 1 slice	1
White made with whole grain bread, 2 slices	2
Wonder English Muffins	
Cinnamon raisin English muffin, 1	3
Original English muffin, 1	2
Sourdough English muffin, 1	2
Wonder Light	
Italian bread, 2 slices	1
Sourdough bread, 2 slices	1
Wheat bread, 2 slices	1
White bread, 2 slices	1

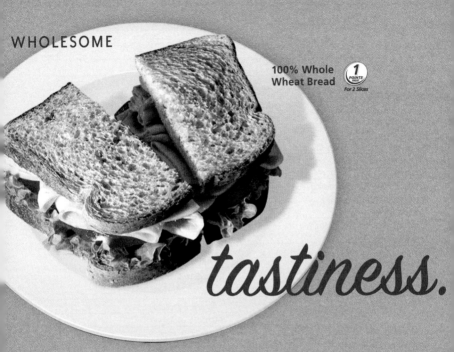

WHOLESOME

100% Whole
Wheat Bread

1 POINTS VALUE
For 2 Slices

tastiness.

With eight scrumptious varieties, it's easier than
ever to make smart choices that taste great.

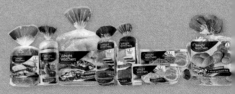

WeightWatchers®

Go to WeightWatchers.com/bread
to learn more about all of our delicious breads.

◆ | (POINTS VALUE) | ◆ | (POINTS VALUE)

Bread crumbs

4C

Carb careful plain crumbs, 1 serving (30 g)	1
Carb careful seasoned crumbs, 1 serving (30 g)	1
Plain bread crumbs, 1 serving (30 g)	2
Plain kosher bread crumbs, 1 serving (30 g)	2
Seasoned bread crumbs, 1 serving (30 g)	2
Seasoned kosher bread crumbs, 1 serving (30 g)	2
Seasoned salt free bread crumbs, 1 serving (30 g)	2

Contadina

Roasted garlic and savory spices bread crumbs, 1/4 cup	2
Three cheese bread crumbs, 1/4 cup	2
Unseasoned bread crumbs, 1/4 cup	2

Ian's

Italian breadcrumb, 1 Tbsp	1
Original breadcrumb, 1 Tbsp	1
Original panko breadcrumb, 1 Tbsp	1
Whole wheat breadcrumb, 1 Tbsp	1

Kellogg's

Corn flake crumbs, 6 Tbsp	2

Lance

Cracker meal, 1/4 cup	2

Nabisco

Cracker meal, 1 serving (26 g)	2

Old London

Bread crumbs, lemon pepper, 1/4 cup	2
Bread crumbs, plain, 1/4 cup	2
Bread crumbs, roasted garlic, 1/4 cup	2
Bread crumbs, seasoned, 1/4 cup	2

Progresso

Garlic & herb, 1/4 cup	2
Italian style, 1/4 cup	2
Panko crispy bread crumbs - Italian style, 1/4 cup	3
Panko crispy bread crumbs - plain, 1/4 cup	2
Parmesan, 1/4 cup	2
Plain, 1/4 cup	2

Breadsticks

Lance

Cheese, 2 packages	1
Garlic, 2 packages	1
Plain, 2 packages	1
Sesame, 2 packages	1

Market Day

Bosco breadsticks, 1 piece	5
French breadsticks, 1	2

Pillsbury

Cornbread twists, 1	3
Garlic flavored, 2	4

	POINTS VALUE
Italian garlic with herb, 2	4
Italian parmesan with garlic, 2	4
Original, soft, 2	3
Stella D'oro	
Breadsticks, cracked pepper, mini, 1 serving (17 g)	2
Breadsticks, original, 1	1
Breadsticks, original, mini, 1 serving (16 g)	1
Breadsticks, sesame, 1	1
Breadsticks, sesame, mini, 1 serving (18 g)	2
Breadsticks, sodium free, 1	1

Brownies

	POINTS VALUE
Baker's Organic Brownie Bites	
Chocolate chip mint, 1	2
Double chocolate chip, 1	2
Entenmann's	
Little bites - soft baked fudge brownies, 1 pouch	6
Hostess	
Plain brownie bites, 1 pouch	7
Joseph's Sugar Free Cookies	
Pecan walnut brownies, 9	2
Lance	
Fudge brownie with nuts, 1	7
Otis Spunkmeyer	
Double chocolate, 1	6

	POINTS VALUE
Otis Spunkmeyer Café Collection	
Café au lait brownie, 2 oz	6
Turtle brownie, 2 oz	6
Pillsbury Brownie Batter	
Traditional chocolate fudge brownies, 1 serving (1/12 package)	3
Triple chocolate chunk brownie, 1 serving (1/12 package)	4
VitaMuffin Brownie	
Chocolate brownie, 1	1
Weight Watchers Smart Ones	
Brownie a la mode, 1 serving (89 g)	4

Cakes

	POINTS VALUE
Bluebird	
100 calorie chocolate cupcake, 1 package	1
100 calorie golden cupcake, 1 package	1
Drake's	
Coffee cakes, 2	6
Devil dogs, 1	4
Funny bones, 2	7
Ring dings, 2	8
Sunny doodles, 2	5
Yankee doodles, 2	5
Yodels, 2	7
El Torito	
Sweet corn cake mix, 1/2 cup	2

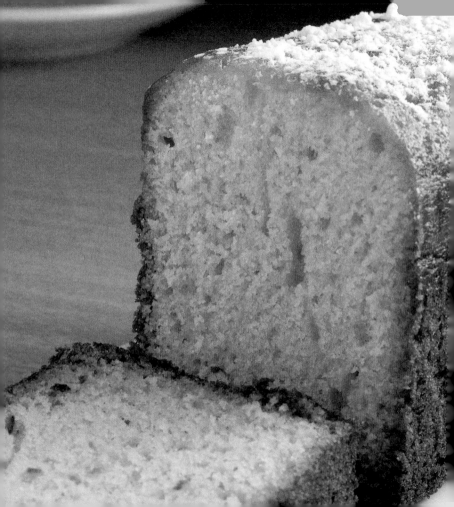

Cakes (con't)	POINTS VALUE
Hostess	
Chocolate cup cakes, 1	4
Cinnamon streusel cakes, 1	4
Devil's food zingers cake, 1	3
Ding dongs, 1	4
Ho hos, 1	3
Raspberry zingers, 1	4
Sno balls, 1	4
Suzy Q's, 1	5
Twinkies, 1	3
Vanilla zingers, 1	4
Hostess 100 Calorie	
Carrot mini cakes, 3	1
Chocolate mini cakes, 3	1
Golden mini cakes, 3	2
Lance	
Fig cake, 1 package	2
Little Debbie	
Christmas tree cakes (chocolate), 2	4
Christmas tree cakes (vanilla), 2	5
Coffee cake, apple streusel, single serve, 1	5
Dessert cakes, chocolate, 1	4
Dessert cakes, spice, 1	4
Dessert cakes, yellow, 1	4
Golden crèmes, 1	3
Swiss rolls, 2	6

	POINTS VALUE
Market Day	
Chocolate fudge volcano cakes, 1	11
Chocolate-chocolate chip puddin' cakes, 1 slice	6
Funnel cakes, 1	6
Mrs. Freshleys Snackaway	
Crème filled chocolate cupcakes, 1	2
Yogurt filled crème cakes, 1	2
Mrs. Smith's	
Carrot cake, 1 serving (1/6 cake)	6
Otis Spunkmeyer	
Apple crumb cake, 1 cake	9
Banana cake, 1 square	8
Blueberry crumb cake, 1 cake	9
Carrot cake, 1 square	8
Cheese crumb cake, 1 cake	10
Chocolate cake, 1 square	8
Pound cake, 1 cake	9
Otis Spunkmeyer Café Collection	
Apple cinnamon coffee cake, 1 serving (3.25 oz)	9
Cheese coffee cake, 1 serving (3.25 oz)	8
Chocolate truffle cake, 1 serving (2.65 oz)	8
Thomas'	
Toast-r-cake corn, 1	2
VitaMuffin Cakes	
Dreamy drizzles chocolate cake, 1 slice	1

Cakes (con't) | POINTS VALUE

Weight Watchers

Caramel cake with caramel icing, 1 cake	1
Carrot cake with cream cheese icing, 1 cake	1
Chocolate cake with chocolate icing, 1 cake	1
Golden sponge cake with creamy filling, 1 cake	1
Lemon cake with lemon icing, 1 cake	1

Weight Watchers Smart Ones

Double fudge cake, 1 serving (77 g)	4
Strawberry shortcake, 1 serving (94 g)	4

Croutons
Chatham Village

Caesar, 2 Tbsp	1
Fat free garlic and onion crouton, 2 Tbsp	1
Garden herb, 2 Tbsp	1
Large cut Caesar crouton, 2 Tbsp	1
Large cut cheese & garlic, 2 Tbsp	1
Large cut garlic and butter flavored crouton, 2 Tbsp	1
Ranch, 2 Tbsp	1
Sea salt & pepper croutons, 2 Tbsp	1

Marzetti

Fat free garlic and onion, 2 Tbsp	1
Garlic & butter flavored, 2 Tbsp	1
Large cut Caesar croutons, 2 Tbsp	1
Large cut cheese & garlic croutons, 2 Tbsp	1

	POINTS VALUE
Large cut ranch crouton, 2 Tbsp	1
Large cut sea salt & pepper croutons, 2 Tbsp	1
Large cut whole grain croutons, 2 Tbsp	1

Doughnuts
Entenmann's

Cinnamon donuts, 1	7
Crumb topped donuts (classic variety pack), 1	6
Crumb topped donuts (softee variety pack), 1	6
Glazed donuts (classic variety), 1	6
Glazed popems (softee variety pack), 4 pieces	5
Plain donuts (softee variety), 1	5
Plain old fashioned donuts (classic variety), 1	5
Powdered donuts (softee variety), 1	5
Rich frosted donuts (classic variety pack), 1	7
Rich frosted donuts (softee variety pack), 1	7

Krispy Kreme Doughnuts

Chocolate glazed mini cruller, 2 pieces	7
Cinnamon sugar mini cake (junior), 4 pieces	6
Glazed honey bun, 1	8
Glazed mini cruller, 2 pieces	7

SENSIBLE

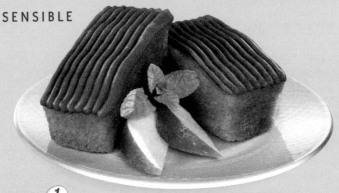

Caramel
Cake

1 POINTS value
Per Cake

yumminess.

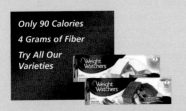

It is possible to eat what you like and be
smart too. We have the treat to prove it.

WeightWatchers

**Go to WeightWatchers.com/cookies
for more information.**

BREAD & BAKED GOODS

Doughnuts, Krispy Kreme Doughnuts (con't)	POINTS VALUE
Iced honey bun, 1	8
Plain mini cake (junior), 5 pieces	5
Powdered mini cake (junior), 4 pieces	6
Little Debbie	
Frosted mini donuts, 4	7
Glazed mini donuts, 1	5
Powdered mini donuts, 4	5

Flatbread/Pita

Azumaya	POINTS VALUE
Large square wrappers, 3	4
Round wraps, 10	3
Square wraps, 8	3
Boca	
Breakfast wraps - original, 1	4
Breakfast wraps - Southwestern flavor, 1	4
Flatout	
100% stone ground whole wheat-mini, 1	1
French toast-mini, 1	1
Garden spinach light, 1	1
Mediterranean herb-mini, 1	1
Southwest chipotle-mini, 1	1
Food for Life	
Organic Ezekiel 4:9 pocket bread, 1	1
Kangaroo	
Salad pockets, 1	2
Wheat 'n honey pita pocket bread, 1/2	1

	POINTS VALUE
Wheat salad pockets, 1	1
White pita pocket bread, 1/2	2
Whole grain sandwich pockets, 1	1
LaTortilla Factory Smart & Delicious	
Multigrain softwraps, 1 (9 1/2")	1
Rosemary softwraps, 1 (9 1/2")	1
Tomato basil softwraps, 1 (9 1/2")	1
Whole grain softwraps, 1 (9 1/2")	3
LaTortilla Factory Sonoma	
Organic traditional wraps, 1(9 1/2")	4
Organic wheat wraps, 1 (9 1/2")	4
Nasoya	
Wrappers, egg roll, 3	3
Wrappers, won ton, 8	3
Thomas'	
Sahara (mini) white pita bread, 1 loaf	1
Sahara 100% whole wheat (mini) pita bread, 1 loaf	1
Sahara 100% whole wheat pita bread, 1 loaf	2
Sahara 100% whole wheat wrap, 1	3
Sahara multigrain pita, 1 loaf	2
Sahara original style white pita bread, 1 loaf	3
Sahara spinach wraps, 1	4
Sahara tomato basil wraps, 1	4
Sahara white (plain) wrap, 1	4
Sahara white pita bread, 1 loaf	3

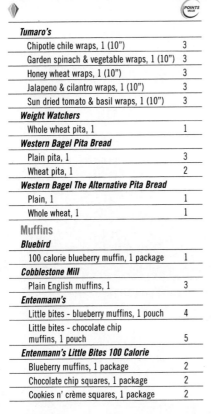

	POINTS VALUE
Tumaro's	
Chipotle chile wraps, 1 (10")	3
Garden spinach & vegetable wraps, 1 (10")	3
Honey wheat wraps, 1 (10")	3
Jalapeno & cilantro wraps, 1 (10")	3
Sun dried tomato & basil wraps, 1 (10")	3
Weight Watchers	
Whole wheat pita, 1	1
Western Bagel Pita Bread	
Plain pita, 1	3
Wheat pita, 1	2
Western Bagel The Alternative Pita Bread	
Plain, 1	1
Whole wheat, 1	1
Muffins	
Bluebird	
100 calorie blueberry muffin, 1 package	1
Cobblestone Mill	
Plain English muffins, 1	3
Entenmann's	
Little bites - blueberry muffins, 1 pouch	4
Little bites - chocolate chip muffins, 1 pouch	5
Entenmann's Little Bites 100 Calorie	
Blueberry muffins, 1 package	2
Chocolate chip squares, 1 package	2
Cookies n' crème squares, 1 package	2

	POINTS VALUE
Hostess	
Banana walnut mini muffins, 1 pouch	6
Blueberry mini muffins, 1 pouch	6
Chocolate chip mini muffins, 1 pouch	6
Kellogg's Eggo	
Muffin tops, mini blueberry, 1 serving (1 set of 4 tops)	3
Muffin tops, mini chocolate chip, 1 serving (1 set of 4)	3
Mrs. Freshleys Snackaway	
Wild blueberry muffins, 1	3
Otis Express	
Banana caramel muffin, 1	5
Banana nut, 1	5
Chocolate chocolate chip muffin, 1	5
Cinnamon crumb coffeecake, 1	5
Strawberry shortcake muffin, 1	5
Wild blueberry muffin, 1	5
Otis Express Delicious Essentials	
Chocolate chocolate chip muffin, 1	7
Otis Express Delicious Essentials Reduced Fat	
Apple cinnamon muffin, 1	7
Banana muffin, 1	7
Wild blueberry muffin, 1	7
Otis Spunkmeyer	
Almond poppy seed, 1/2 (2 oz)	6
Apple cinnamon, 1 (2.25 oz)	6

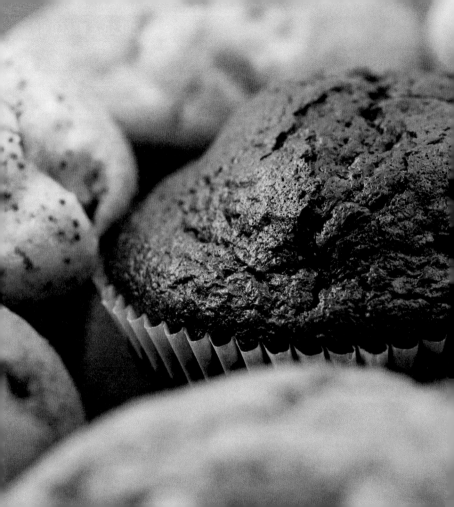

Muffins, Otis Spunkmeyer (con't)	POINTS VALUE
Apple cinnamon, 1/2 small (2 oz)	5
Apple, 1 (1.8 oz)	4
Apple orchard, 1/2 (2 oz)	5
Banana, 1/2 (3.25 oz)	9
Banana mini muffins, 2 (1.8 oz)	5
Banana, 1(1.8 oz)	4
Banana, 1 (2 oz)	5
Banana nut, 1 (2.25 oz)	6
Banana nut, 1/2 small (2 oz)	5
Banana nut (sugar free), low carb, 1 (2 oz)	5
Banana nut, low fat, 1/2 small (2 oz)	3
Banana nut, low fat, 1 (2.25 oz)	4
Blueberry, 1/2 (3.25 oz)	8
Blueberry mini muffins, 2 (1.8 oz)	5
Blueberry, 1/2 (2 oz)	5
Blueberry, 1 (1.8 oz)	4
Blueberry streusel, 1/2 (2 oz)	5
Caramel apple, 1/2 (2 oz)	5
Cheese streusel, 1/2 (3.25 oz)	8
Cheese streusel, 1/2 small (2 oz)	5
Cheese streusel, 1 (2.25 oz)	5
Chocolate chip, 1/2 small (2 oz)	5
Chocolate chip, 1 (2.25 oz)	6
Chocolate chocolate chip, 1/2 (3.25 oz)	8
Chocolate chocolate chip, 1 (2.25 oz)	6
Chocolate chocolate chip, 1/2 small (2 oz)	5
Chocolate chocolate chip mini muffins, 2 (1.8 oz)	5

	POINTS VALUE
Chocolate chocolate chip, low-fat, 1 (2.25 oz)	4
Chocolate chocolate chip, low-fat, 1/2 small (2 oz)	3
Chocolate, 1 (1.8 oz)	4
Chocolate raspberry, 1/2 (2 oz)	5
Corn, 1/2 (3.25 oz)	9
Corn, 1/2 small (2 oz)	5
Corn, 1 (2.25 oz)	6
Cranberry orange, 1/2 (2 oz)	5
Harvest bran, 1 (2.25 oz)	5
Harvest bran, 1/2 small (2 oz)	4
Lemon, 1/2 (2 oz)	5
Orange, 1/2 (2 oz)	6
Orange, 1 small (2 oz)	5
Orange, 1/2 (2 oz)	5
Pumpkin walnut, 1/2 (2 oz)	5
Raspberry cheese streusel, 1/2 (2 oz)	4
Strawberry shortcake, 1/2 (2 oz)	5
Triple berry, 1/2 (2 oz)	5
Triple berry, 1/2 (3.25 oz)	8
Wild blueberry, 1 (2.25 oz)	6
Wild blueberry, 1/2 small (2 oz)	5
Wild blueberry (no sugar added), low carb, 1 (2 oz)	4
Wild blueberry, low-fat, 1/2 small (2 oz)	3
Wild blueberry, low-fat, 1 (2.25 oz)	4

199

BREAD & BAKED GOODS

Muffins (con't)	POINTS VALUE
Otis Spunkmeyer Café Collection	
Banana walnut muffin, 1/2	9
Chocolate chocolate chip muffin, 1/2	8
Wild blueberry muffin, 1/2	8
Otis Spunkmeyer Delicious Essentials	
Reduced fat apple cinnamon, 1	3
Reduced fat banana, 1	4
Reduced fat chocolate chocolate chip, 1	4
Reduced fat wild blueberry, 1	4
Whole grain reduced fat apple cinnamon, 1	4
Whole grain reduced fat banana, 1	4
Whole grain reduced fat chocolate chocolate chip, 1	4
Whole grain reduced fat wild blueberry, 1	3
VitaMuffin	
Appleberrybran, 1 small	1
Bluebran, 1 small	1
Cranbran, 1 small	1
Deep chocolate, 1 small	1
Multibran, 1 small	1
Sugar free velvety chocolate, 1	1
Sugar-free banana nut, 1	1
VitaMuffin VitaTops	
Appleberrybran, 1	1
Bluebran, 1	1
Cranbran, 1	1
Dark chocolate with pomegranate, 1	1

	POINTS VALUE
Double chocolate dream, 1	1
Fudgy peanut butter chip, 1	1
Golden corn, 1	1
Multibran, 1	1
Sugar free velvety chocolate, 1	1
Sugar-free banana nut, 1	1
Weight Watchers	
Berries and crème muffin, 1 muffin	3
Blueberry muffin, 1 muffin	3
Caramel apple muffin, 1 muffin	3
Double chocolate muffin, 1 muffin	3
Nori	
Eden	
Nori (10 sheets), 1 sheet	0
Sushi nori (7 sheets), toasted, 1 sheet	0
Pastries	
Entenmann's	
Pecan danish ring, 1 serving (1/8 danish)	6
Raspberry danish twist (softee variety pack), 1 serving (1/8 danish)	5
Walnut danish ring, 1 serving (1/8 danish)	6
Kellogg's Eggo	
Toaster swirlz mini rolls - cinnamon, 1 serving (1 set of 4 rolls)	2
Lance	
Cinnamon roll, 1	8
Honey buns (glazed), 1	9
Honey buns (iced), 1	9

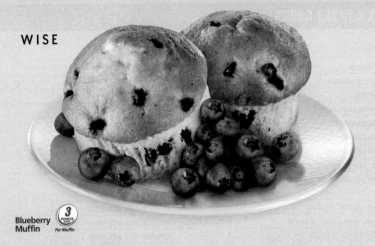

WISE

Blueberry Muffin **(3 POINTS value Per Muffin)**

deliciousness.

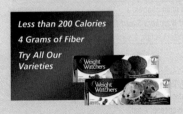

Less than 200 Calories

4 Grams of Fiber

Try All Our Varieties

Delicious proof that sensible and sweet can live in harmony.

WeightWatchers

Go to WeightWatchers.com/muffins for more information.

BREAD & BAKED GOODS

Pastries (con't)	POINTS VALUE
Little Debbie	
Pecan spinwheels, 1	2
Market Day	
Gourmet cinnamon rolls, 1 (3 oz)	7
Otis Spunkmeyer	
Apple danish, 1 pastry	7
Apple demi danish, 1 pastry	3
Bear claw, 4-pack, 1 pastry	6
Breakfast claw, 8-pack, 1 pastry	6
Buttercrumb danish, 4-pack, 1 pastry	6
Cheese danish, 1 pastry	7
Cheese demi danish, 1 pastry	3
Cherry danish, 1 pastry	7
Cinnamon danish, 4-pack, 1 pastry	6
Cinnamon roll, 1 roll	8
Cinnamon roll, 4- pack, 1 roll	3
Cinnamon roll, 8-pack, 1 roll	3
Cinnamon twist, 1 pastry	5
Fruit danish, 8-pack, 1 pastry	5
Giant cinnamon roll, 1/2	6
Raisin danish, 8-pack, 1 pastry	5
Raspberry danish, 1 pastry	5
Raspberry demi danish, 1 pastry	3
Otis Spunkmeyer Café Collection	
Cinnamon chip scone, 1	8
Cinnamon swirl, 1/2 roll	4
Maple pecan scone, 1	8
Wild blueberry scone, 1	7

	POINTS VALUE
Pillsbury	
Apple turnover, 1	4
Caramel rolls, 1	4
Cherry turnover, 1	4
Cinnamon bites with icing packets, 4	4
Cinnamon rolls with cream cheese icing, 1	3
Cinnamon rolls with icing, 1	3
Cinnamon rolls with icing, reduced fat, 1	3
Orange sweet rolls with icing, 1	4
Pillsbury Grands!	
Cinnamon rolls with butter cream icing, 1	7
Cinnamon rolls with cream cheese icing, 1	7
Cinnamon rolls with icing, 1	9
Cinnamon rolls with icing, reduced fat, 1	6
Flaky supreme cinnamon roll, 1	9
Sugar free cinnamon roll, 1	2
Pillsbury Oven Baked	
Cinnamon, 1	6
Tio Pepe's	
Cinnamon churros, 1	2
Weight Watchers Smart Ones	
Chocolate eclair, 1 serving (59 g)	3

Rolls

Alexia	
Ciabatta, 1 roll	2
Classic French rolls, 1 roll	2
Three cheese, 1 roll	2
Whole grain, 1 roll	1

	POINTS VALUE
Alvarado	
Sprouted wheat burger bun, 1	2
Sprouted wheat hot dog bun, 1	2
Sprouted wheat rolls, 1	1
Bluebird	
Pecan spins, 1	2
Cobblestone Mill	
100% whole grain hot dog buns, 1	1
100% whole grain sandwich buns, 1	2
Honey wheat baguettes, 1/4	3
Wheat sub rolls, 1	4
Food for Life	
Organic Ezekiel 4:9 sesame sprouted grain burger bun, 1	3
Organic Ezekiel 4:9 sprouted grain burger bun, 1	3
Organic Ezekiel 4:9 sprouted grain hot dog buns, 1	3
Organic sprouted burger bun, 1	2
Organic sprouted hot dog buns, 1	2
French Meadow Bakery	
Ciabatta roll, 1	0
Hemp roll, 1	3
Peasant rolls, 1	2
Sprouted peasant roll, 1	2
Healthy Life Original	
Sandwich wheat buns, 1	1
Sandwich white buns, 1	1

	POINTS VALUE
Wheat hot dog buns, 1	1
White hot dog buns, 1	1
Healthy Life Southern Country Style	
100% whole wheat dinner rolls, 1	1
100% whole wheat hot dog buns, 1	2
100% whole wheat sandwich buns, 1	2
Mrs. Freshleys Snackaway	
Pecan twirls, 1	2
Nature's Own	
Honey wheat buns, 1	3
Sugar free 100% whole grain wheat hamburger bun, 1	2
Sugar free 100% whole grain wheat hot dog bun, 1	1
Wheat 'n double fiber hamburger rolls, 1	1
Wheat 'n double fiber hot dog rolls, 1	1
Whitewheat hamburger buns, 1	1
Whitewheat hot dog buns, 1	1
Paraclete	
12" hoagie roll, 1/2	3
Dinner rolls, 1	0
Sandwich rolls, 1	1
Pillsbury	
Big and buttery crescent, 1	4
Butter flake crescent, 1	3
Crusty French roll, 1	2
Garlic butter crescent, 1	3

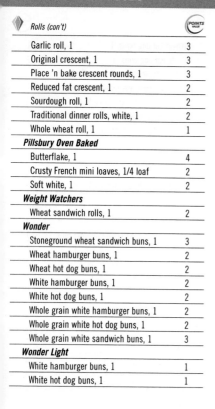

Rolls (con't)	POINTS VALUE
Garlic roll, 1	3
Original crescent, 1	3
Place 'n bake crescent rounds, 1	3
Reduced fat crescent, 1	2
Sourdough roll, 1	2
Traditional dinner rolls, white, 1	2
Whole wheat roll, 1	1
Pillsbury Oven Baked	
Butterflake, 1	4
Crusty French mini loaves, 1/4 loaf	2
Soft white, 1	2
Weight Watchers	
Wheat sandwich rolls, 1	2
Wonder	
Stoneground wheat sandwich buns, 1	3
Wheat hamburger buns, 1	2
Wheat hot dog buns, 1	2
White hamburger buns, 1	2
White hot dog buns, 1	2
Whole grain white hamburger buns, 1	2
Whole grain white hot dog buns, 1	2
Whole grain white sandwich buns, 1	3
Wonder Light	
White hamburger buns, 1	1
White hot dog buns, 1	1

	POINTS VALUE
Stuffing Mix	
Kellogg's Croutettes	
Stuffing mix, 1 cup	2
Stove Top	
Chicken flavor, as packaged, 1/2 cup	2
Chicken made with whole wheat, as packaged, 1 serving (1/5 box)	2
Chicken made with whole wheat, as prepared, 1/2 cup	3
Chicken, as prepared, 1/2 cup (96 g)	3
Chicken, as prepared, 1/2 cup (97 g)	4
Cornbread, as packaged, 1/2 cup	2
Cornbread, as prepared, 1/2 cup	4
Cranberry flavor, as packaged, 1 serving (1/6 box)	2
Cranberry flavor, as prepared, 1/2 cup	4
Italian style roasted garlic, as packaged, 1 serving (1/6 box)	2
Italian style roasted garlic, as prepared, 1/2 cup	4
Lower sodium chicken, as packaged, 1/2 cup	2
Lower sodium chicken, as prepared, 1/2 cup	4
Monterey style mushroom & onion, as packaged, 1 serving (1/6 box)	2
Monterey style mushroom & onion, as prepared, 1/2 cup	4
Northern style long grain and wild rice, as packaged, 1 serving (1/6 box)	2

	POINTS VALUE
Northern style long grain and wild rice, as prepared, 1/2 cup	4
Pork flavor, as packaged, 1/2 cup	2
Pork flavor, as prepared, 1/2 cup	4
Savory herb, as packaged, 1 serving (1/6 box)	2
Sourdough San Francisco style, as packaged, 1 serving (1/6 box)	2
Sourdough San Francisco style, as prepared, 1/2 cup	4
Traditional sage, as packaged, 1 serving (1/6 box)	2
Turkey flavor, as packaged, 1/2 cup	2
Turkey flavor, as prepared, 1/2 cup	4
Stove Top Flex Serve	
Chicken, as packaged, 1 oz	2
Homestyle herb, as packaged, 1 oz	2
Stove Top Flexible Serve	
Homestyle herb, prepared, 1/2 cup	3

Taco Shells

Bearitos	
Blue taco shells, 2	3
Yellow taco shells, 2	3
Yellow tostada shells, 2	3
Garden of Eatin'	
Blue taco shells, 2	3
Yellow taco shells, 2	3

	POINTS VALUE
Old El Paso	
Hard taco shells, 3	3
Mini taco shells, 6	3
Soft taco shells (tortillas), 2	4
Stand n stuff nacho style shells, 2	3
Stand n stuff salsa shells, 2	3
Stand 'n stuff taco shells, 2	3
Super stuffer taco shells, 2	4
Taco salad shell, 1	3
Taco shells, 3	3
White corn taco shells, 3	3
Ortega	
Taco shells, 2	3
Taco Bell Home Originals	
Flavored taco shells - nacho, 3	3
Flavored taco shells - ranch, 3	3
Taco shells, 3	3
Zapata	
Blue corn taco shells, 2	3
Premium taco shells, 2	2
Yellow corn taco shells, 2	3

Tortillas

Alvarado	
Sprouted wheat 10" tortilla burrito, 1	3
Sprouted wheat 8" tortilla fajita, 1	3

Taco Shells (con't) POINTS VALUE

 POINTS VALUE

Azteca

Burrito size flour tortillas, 1	3
Corn tortillas, 2	1
Soft taco size flour tortillas, 2	3
Super size flour tortillas, 1	2

Buena Vida

Fat free flour tortillas, 1	2
Whole grain tortillas, 1	2
Whole wheat tortillas, 1	1

Chi-Chi's

Burrito tortillas, 9", 1	3
Corn tortillas, 6", 2	3
Fajita tortillas, 6", 1	1
Flour tortillas, 10", 1	5
Flour tortillas, 6", 1	2
Flour tortillas, 8", 1	3
Soft taco tortillas, 8", 1	3

Don Marcos

Healthy style fat free flour tortillas, 1	0

Food for Life

Ezekiel 4:9 sprouted grain tortilla, 1	2
Organic Ezekiel 4:9 sprouted grain tortilla (6"), 1	1

LaTortilla Factory

Family pack white corn tortillas, 2 (6" diameter)	2
Tostadas, 1	1
Whole wheat low carb, high fiber garlic & herb flavor, 1	0
Whole wheat low carb, high fiber green onion flavor, 1	0

LaTortilla Factory Smart & Delicious

Gluten free dark teff wraps, 1	3
Gluten free ivory teff wraps, 1	3
Low carb, high fiber large size, 1	1
Low carb, high fiber original soft taco size, 1	0
Low fat low sodium burrito size, 1	2
Low fat low sodium soft taco size, 1	2
Pumpernickel softwraps, 1	1
Traditional softwraps, 1	1
Whole grain rye softwraps, 1	1
Whole grain, white whole wheat softwraps, 1	1

LaTortilla Factory Sonoma

All natural carb cutting, 1	1
All natural gluten free dark teff, 1	3
Made with organic Mediterranean wraps, 1 (9 1/2")	3
Made with organic tomato basil wraps, 1 (9 1/2")	3
Organic multi-grain wraps, 1 (9 1/2")	3
Organic traditional wraps, 1	4
Organic yellow corn tortillas, 2 (7")	2

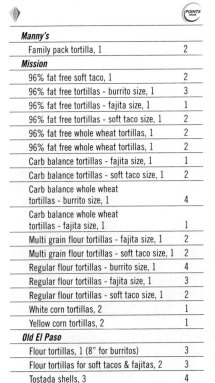

	POINTS VALUE
Manny's	
Family pack tortilla, 1	2
Mission	
96% fat free soft taco, 1	2
96% fat free tortillas - burrito size, 1	3
96% fat free tortillas - fajita size, 1	1
96% fat free tortillas - soft taco size, 1	2
96% fat free whole wheat tortillas, 1	2
96% fat free whole wheat tortillas, 1	2
Carb balance tortillas - fajita size, 1	1
Carb balance tortillas - soft taco size, 1	2
Carb balance whole wheat tortillas - burrito size, 1	4
Carb balance whole wheat tortillas - fajita size, 1	1
Multi grain flour tortillas - fajita size, 1	2
Multi grain flour tortillas - soft taco size, 1	2
Regular flour tortillas - burrito size, 1	4
Regular flour tortillas - fajita size, 1	3
Regular flour tortillas - soft taco size, 1	2
White corn tortillas, 2	1
Yellow corn tortillas, 2	1
Old El Paso	
Flour tortillas, 1 (8" for burritos)	3
Flour tortillas for soft tacos & fajitas, 2	3
Tostada shells, 3	4

	POINTS VALUE
Ortega	
Flour tortillas, 1	3
Rudi's Organic Bakery	
Spelt tortillas, 1	3
Whole spelt tortillas, 1	2
Taco Bell Home Originals	
Flour tortillas, 2	4
Tumaro's Healthy Flour Tortillas	
Chipotle chili & peppers, 1 small (8")	2
Chipotle chili & peppers, 1 large (10")	4
Garden spinach & vegetables, 1 large (10")	3
Garden spinach & vegetables, 1 small (8")	2
Honey wheat, 1 large (10")	3
Honey wheat, 1 small (8")	2
Jalapeño & cilantro, 1 small (8")	2
Jalapeño & cilantro, 1 large (10")	4
Pesto & garlic, 1 (8")	2
Premium white, 1 (8")	2
Tumaro's Low in Carb	
Garden vegetable, 10", 1	2
Garden vegetable, 8", 1	1
Green onion, 10", 1	2
Green onion, 8", 1	1
Multi grain, 10", 1	2
Multi grain, 8", 1	1
Salsa, 10", 1	2
Salsa, 8", 1	1

Tortillas (con't)

Tumaro's Soy-Full Heart

8 grain & soy, 1	1
Apple cinnamon flatbread, 1	1
Wheat, soy & flax flatbread, 1	1

Zapata

Premium tostada shell, 2	2

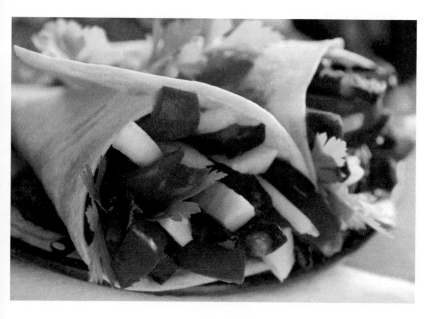

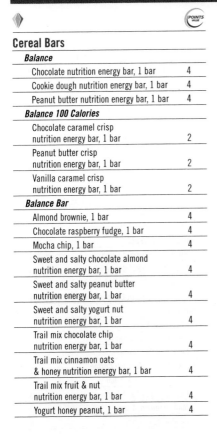

POINTS VALUE

Cereal Bars

Balance

Chocolate nutrition energy bar, 1 bar	4
Cookie dough nutrition energy bar, 1 bar	4
Peanut butter nutrition energy bar, 1 bar	4

Balance 100 Calories

Chocolate caramel crisp nutrition energy bar, 1 bar	2
Peanut butter crisp nutrition energy bar, 1 bar	2
Vanilla caramel crisp nutrition energy bar, 1 bar	2

Balance Bar

Almond brownie, 1 bar	4
Chocolate raspberry fudge, 1 bar	4
Mocha chip, 1 bar	4
Sweet and salty chocolate almond nutrition energy bar, 1 bar	4
Sweet and salty peanut butter nutrition energy bar, 1 bar	4
Sweet and salty yogurt nut nutrition energy bar, 1 bar	4
Trail mix chocolate chip nutrition energy bar, 1 bar	4
Trail mix cinnamon oats & honey nutrition energy bar, 1 bar	4
Trail mix fruit & nut nutrition energy bar, 1 bar	4
Yogurt honey peanut, 1 bar	4

Balance Carbwell

Caramel 'n chocolate nutrition energy bar, 1 bar	4
Chocolate fudge nutrition energy bar, 1 bar	4
Chocolate peanut butter nutrition energy bar, 1 bar	4

Balance Gold

Caramel nut blast, 1 bar	5
Chewy chocolate chip nutrition energy bar, 1 bar	5
Chocolate peanut butter, 1 bar	5
Rocky road, 1 bar	5
Triple chocolate chaos nutrition energy bar, 1 bar	5

Balance Gold Crunch

Chocolate chocolate nutrition energy bar, 1 bar	3
Chocolate mint cookie nutrition energy bar, 1 bar	3
Cookies 'n crème nutrition energy bar, 1 bar	4
Crunchy peanut butter nutrition energy bar, 1 bar	4
S'mores nutrition energy bar, 1 bar	3

Balance Organic

Apricot mango crisp nutrition energy bar, 1 bar	3
Cherry almond crisp nutrition energy bar, 1 bar	3

BREAKFAST, CEREALS & CEREAL BARS

Cereal Bars, Balance Organic (con't)	POINTS VALUE
Cranberry pomegranate crisp nutrition energy bar, 1 bar	3
Barbara's Bakery	
Crunchy granola bar, cinnamon crisp, 2 bars	4
Crunchy granola bar, oats 'n' honey, 2 bars	4
Crunchy granola bar, peanut butter, 2 bars	4
Crunchy granola bar, toasted almond, 2 bars	4
Barbara's Bakery Fruit & Yogurt	
Apple cinnamon, 1 bar	3
Blueberry apple, 1 bar	3
Cherry apple, 1 bar	3
Strawberry apple, 1 bar	3
Bluebird	
Apple cinnamon cereal bars, 1 bar	3
Strawberry cereal bars, 1 bar	3
Cascadian Farm	
Chocolate chip, 1 bar	3
Fruit & nut: raisin, almond sunflower seed & cranberry, 1 bar	3
Granola harvest berry bars, 1 bar	3
Multi-grain bars, 1 bar	3
DrSoy	
Chocolate brownie bar, 1 bar	4
Chocolate peanut bar, 1 bar	4
Iced oatmeal cookie bar, 1 bar	4

	POINTS VALUE
DrSoy Healthy Snacker	
Chocolate caramel crunch, 1 bar	4
Rocky road, 1 bar	4
Entenmann's	
Multigrain real apple cinnamon filled cereal bars, 1 bar	3
Multi-grain real raspberry filled cereal bars, 1 bar	3
Multi-grain real strawberry filled cereal bars, 1 bar	3
EnviroKidz	
Organic crispy rice bar - berry, 1 bar	2
Organic crispy rice bar - chocolate, 1 bar	2
Organic crispy rice bar - peanut butter, 1 bar	2
Estee Smart Treats	
Sugar free chocolate chip, 1	1
Sugar free chocolate crunch, 1	1
Sugar free old fashioned vanilla, 1	1
Sugar free peanut butter crunch, 1	1
Gatorade	
Chocolate, 1 bar	5
Oatmeal raisin, 1 bar	5
Peanut butter, 1 bar	5
General Foods Caribou Coffee	
Caramel high rise, 1 bar	3
Chocolate mocha, 1 bar	3
Mint condition, 1 bar	3
Vanilla latte, 1 bar	3

	POINTS VALUE
General Foods Curves	
Chocolate peanut, 1 bar	1
Strawberries & cream, 1 bar	1
General Foods Fiber One	
Oats & chocolate, 1 bar	2
Oats & peanut butter, 1 bar	3
General Mills Milk 'n Cereal Bar	
Cinnamon toast crunch, 1 bar	4
Cocoa puffs, 1 bar	4
Honey nut cheerios, 1 bar	3
Peanut butter toast crunch, 1 bar	4
Trix, 1 bar	3
GeniSoy	
Café mocha fudge, 1 bar	5
Chocolate caramel, 1 bar	3
Chocolate mint, 1 bar	5
Chunky peanut butter fudge, 1 bar	5
Cookies & cream, 1 bar	5
Honey peanut yogurt, 1 bar	5
Honey peanut yogurt, 1 bar	5
GeniSoy Natural Choice All Natural Protein Bar	
Chocolate peanut butter, 1 bar	4
Cookies & cream, 1 bar	4
Double chocolate, 1 bar	4
Lemon tart, 1 bar	4

	POINTS VALUE
GeniSoy Organic Protein	
Apple cinnamon, 1 bar	3
Mixed berry flavor, 1 bar	3
Rich chocolate, 1 bar	3
GeniSoy Organic Protein Bars	
Apple cinnamon, 1 bar	3
Mixed berry flavor, 1 bar	4
Rich chocolate, 1 bar	3
GeniSoy Ultra Bars	
Chocolate caramel, 1 bar	3
Chocolate raspberry, 1 bar	3
Chocolate raspberry, 1 bar	3
Strawberry, 1 bar	3
Strawberry, 1 bar	3
Tropical, 1 bar	3
Tropical, 1 bar	3
Health Valley	
Apple cobbler cereal bar, 1	3
Baked apple tarts, 1 bar	3
Berry parfait yogurt bar, 1	2
Blueberry chewy granola bar, 1 bar	3
Blueberry cobbler cereal bar, 1	3
Blueberry tarts, 1 bar	3
Café creations cinnamon danish, 1 bar	2
Café creations vanilla crème, 1	3
Chocolate chip chewy granola bar, 1 bar	2
Chocolate tarts, 1 bar	3

211

Cereal Bars, Health Valley (con't)	POINTS VALUE
Double chocolate chip chewy granola bars, 1 bar	3
Dutch apple chewy granola bar, 1 bar	2
Fig cobbler cereal bar, 1	2
French vanilla yogurt bar, 1	2
Peanut butter & chocolate bar, 1 bar	3
Peanut butter & grape bar, 1 bar	3
Peanut butter & strawberry bar, 1 bar	3
Peanut crunch chewy granola bar, 1 bar	2
Raspberry chewy granola bars, 1 bar	3
Raspberry tarts, 1 bar	3
Red cherry tarts, 1 bar	3
Strawberry cobbler cereal bar, 1	3
Strawberry tarts, 1 bar	3
Wild berry chewy granola bar, 1 bar	2
Healthy Snacker Bars	
Chocolate caramel crunch, 1 bar	4
Rocky road, 1 bar	4
Hostess	
Apple fruit & grain cereal bars, 1	2
Banana nut fruit & grain cereal bars, 1	3
Blueberry fruit & grain cereal bars, 1	2
Raspberry fruit & grain cereal bars, 1	2
Strawberry fruit & grain cereal bars, 1	2
Kashi	
Chewy granola bar honey almond flax, 1 bar	2
Chewy granola bar peanut peanut butter, 1 bar	2

	POINTS VALUE
Chewy granola bar trail mix, 1 bar	2
Chewy granola bar, cherry dark chocolate, 1 bar	2
Kashi Crunchy!	
Chocolate pretzel bar, 1 bar	3
Coffee cake bar, 1 bar	3
Kashi GO LEAN Roll!	
Oatmeal walnut bar, 1 bar	3
Kashi GOLEAN	
Original chocolate almond toffee, 1 bar	6
Original cookies 'n cream, 1 bar	6
Original malted chocolate crisp bar, 1 bar	6
Original oatmeal raisin cookie, 1 bar	5
Original Peanut butter & chocolate, 1 bar	6
Kashi GOLEAN Crunchy!	
Chocolate almond, 1 bar	3
Chocolate caramel, 1 bar	2
Chocolate peanut butter bar, 1 bar	3
Kashi GOLEAN Roll!	
Caramel peanut, 1 bar	3
Chocolate peanut, 1 bar	3
Chocolate turtle, 1 bar	3
Kashi TLC	
Crunchy granola bar, honey toasted 7-grain, 2 bars	3
Crunchy granola bar, pumpkin spice flax, 2 bars	3
Crunchy granola bar, roasted almond crunch, 2 bars	3

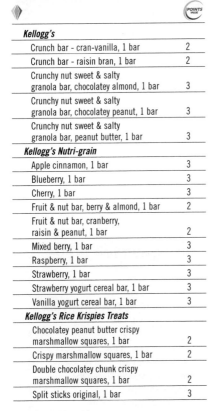

	POINTS VALUE
Kellogg's	
Crunch bar - cran-vanilla, 1 bar	2
Crunch bar - raisin bran, 1 bar	2
Crunchy nut sweet & salty granola bar, chocolatey almond, 1 bar	3
Crunchy nut sweet & salty granola bar, chocolatey peanut, 1 bar	3
Crunchy nut sweet & salty granola bar, peanut butter, 1 bar	3
Kellogg's Nutri-grain	
Apple cinnamon, 1 bar	3
Blueberry, 1 bar	3
Cherry, 1 bar	3
Fruit & nut bar, berry & almond, 1 bar	2
Fruit & nut bar, cranberry, raisin & peanut, 1 bar	2
Mixed berry, 1 bar	3
Raspberry, 1 bar	3
Strawberry, 1 bar	3
Strawberry yogurt cereal bar, 1 bar	3
Vanilla yogurt cereal bar, 1 bar	3
Kellogg's Rice Krispies Treats	
Chocolatey peanut butter crispy marshmallow squares, 1 bar	2
Crispy marshmallow squares, 1 bar	2
Double chocolatey chunk crispy marshmallow squares, 1 bar	2
Split sticks original, 1 bar	3

	POINTS VALUE
Split stix chocolatey, 1 bar	3
Squares chocolatey drizzle, 1 bar	2
Kellogg's Rice Krispies Treats Squares	
Rainbow gems squares, 1 bar	2
Kellogg's Special K Bars	
Blueberry, 1 bar	2
Chocolatey drizzle, 1 bar	2
Cranberry apple, 1 bar	2
Honey nut, 1 bar	2
Peaches & berries, 1 bar	2
Protein meal replacement bar - chocolate peanut butter, 1 bar	3
Protein meal replacement bar - chocolatey chip, 1 bar	3
Protein meal replacement bar - double chocolate, 1 bar	3
Protein meal replacement bar - strawberry, 1 bar	3
Protein snack bar - chocolate delight, 1 bar	2
Protein snack bar - chocolate peanut, 1 bar	2
Strawberry, 1 bar	2
Vanilla crisp, 1 bar	2
Kudos	
M&M's milk chocolate baking bits, 1 bar	2
Milk chocolate granola snickers, 1 bar	2
Whole grain bars - chocolate chip, 1 bar	2
Whole grain bars - peanut butter, 1 bar	3

BREAKFAST, CEREALS & CEREAL BARS

Cereal Bars (con't)	POINTS VALUE
Luna	
Berry almond, 1 bar	3
Caramel nut brownie, 1 bar	4
Chai tea, 1 bar	3
Chocolate raspberry, 1 bar	3
Chocolate pecan pie, 1 bar	3
Chocolate peppermint stick, 1 bar	3
Cookies 'n cream delight, 1 bar	3
Dulce de leche, 1 bar	3
Iced oatmeal raisin, 1 bar	3
Lemonzest, 1 bar	3
Nutz over chocolate, 1 bar	3
Peanut butter cookie, 1 bar	4
S'mores, 1 bar	3
Toasted nuts 'n cranberry, 1 bar	3
Luna Sunrise	
Apple cinnamon, 1 bar	3
Blueberry yogurt, 1 bar	3
Strawberries & crème, 1 bar	3
Vanilla almond, 1 bar	3
Luna Tea Cakes	
Berry pomegranate, 1 bar	3
Mint chocolate, 1 bar	2
Orange blossom, 1 bar	2
Vanilla macadamia, 1 bar	3
Market Day	
Quaker chewy granola bars (3 varieties), 1 bar	2

	POINTS VALUE
Nabisco 100 Calorie	
Chips ahoy, 1 bar	2
Nutter butter, 1 bar	2
Oreo, 1 bar	2
Nabisco Honey Maid	
Oatmeal raisin bar, 1 bar	3
Soft baked blueberry bar, 1 bar	3
Nature Valley	
Granola bites, oats 'n honey, 1 pouch	1
Pecan crunch crunchy granola bar, 2 bars	4
Roasted almond crunchy granola bar, 2 bars	4
Nature Valley Chewy Granola Healthy Heart Bar	
Honey nut, 1 bar	3
Oatmeal raisin, 1 bar	3
Nature Valley Chewy Granola Trail Mix Bar	
Apple cinnamon, 1 bar	3
Fruit 'n nut, 1 bar	3
Mixed berry, 1 bar	3
Nature Valley Chewy Granola Yogurt Coated	
Blueberry yogurt, 1 bar	3
Lemon yogurt, 1 bar	3
Strawberry yogurt, 1 bar	3
Vanilla yogurt, 1 bar	3
Nature Valley Crunchy Granola Bar	
Apple crisp, 2 bars	4
Banana nut, 2 bars	4

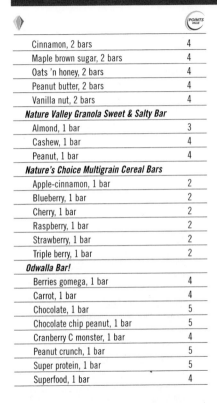

	POINTS VALUE
Cinnamon, 2 bars	4
Maple brown sugar, 2 bars	4
Oats 'n honey, 2 bars	4
Peanut butter, 2 bars	4
Vanilla nut, 2 bars	4

Nature Valley Granola Sweet & Salty Bar

Almond, 1 bar	3
Cashew, 1 bar	4
Peanut, 1 bar	4

Nature's Choice Multigrain Cereal Bars

Apple-cinnamon, 1 bar	2
Blueberry, 1 bar	2
Cherry, 1 bar	2
Raspberry, 1 bar	2
Strawberry, 1 bar	2
Triple berry, 1 bar	2

Odwalla Bar!

Berries gomega, 1 bar	4
Carrot, 1 bar	4
Chocolate, 1 bar	5
Chocolate chip peanut, 1 bar	5
Cranberry C monster, 1 bar	4
Peanut crunch, 1 bar	5
Super protein, 1 bar	5
Superfood, 1 bar	4

Otis Spunkmeyer Café Collection

	POINTS VALUE
Double chocolate caramel bar with snickers, 2 oz	6
Pecan pie bar, 2 oz	6
Raspberry bar, 2 oz	5

Philadelphia Snack Bars

Strawberry cheesecake snack bars, 1	4

Post

Grape nuts trail mix crunch bar, fruit & nut, 1 bar	2
Honey bunches of oats, banana nut, 1 bar	2
Honey bunches of oats, cranberry almond, 1 bar	2
Honey bunches of oats, strawberry, 1 bar	2
Raisin bran, cinnamon, 1 bar	2
Raisin bran, cranberry, 1 bar	2

Quaker Fruit & Oatmeal Bar

Oatmeal on the go, baked apple, 1 bar	3
Oatmeal on the go, cinnamon roll with raisins, 1 bar	3
Oatmeal on the go, wild berry, 1 bar	3

Quaker Oats

Q-smart bar - cranberry almond, 1 bar	2
Q-smart bar - peanut butter chocolate, 1 bar	3

Quaker Oats Baked Fruit Crisp Bars

Apple crisp, 1 bar	3
Mixed berry, 1 bar	3
Strawberry, 1 bar	3

Cereal Bars (con't) **POINTS VALUE**

Quaker Oats Breakfast Bites

Apple crisp, 1 serving (37 g)	2
Raspberry with icing, 1 serving (37 g)	2
Strawberry, 1 serving (37 g)	2
Strawberry with icing, 1 serving (37 g)	2

Quaker Oats Breakfast Cookie

Chocolate chip, 1	3

Quaker Oats Chewy Dipps

Chocolate chip, 1 bar	3
Peanut butter, 1 bar	3

Quaker Oats Chewy Granola Bar

Butterfinger pieces, 1	2
Chocolate chip, 1	2
Chocolate chunk, 1	2
Cookies and cream, 1	2
Peanut butter, 1	2
Peanut butter & chocolate chip, 1	2
Peanut butter & chocolate chunk, 1	2
S'mores, 1	2

Quaker Oats Chewy Granola Bar - 90 Calories

Baked apple, 1 bar	2
Cinnamon sugar, 1 bar	2
Maple brown sugar, 1 bar	2
Oatmeal raisin, 1 bar	2

Real Organic Bars

Real berry, 1 bar	2
Real green, 1 bar	2
Real omega3, 1 bar	3
Real tropical, 1 bar	2

Snickers

Marathon caramel nut surge, 1 bar (singles)	6
Marathon chewy chocolate peanut, 1 bar (singles)	5
Marathon chocolate nut burst, 1 bar (singles)	6
Marathon dark chocolate crunch, 1 (singles)	3
Marathon double chocolate nut, 1 bar (singles)	3
Marathon honey & toasted almond, 1 (singles)	3
Marathon honey nut oat, 1 bar (singles)	2
Marathon multi grain crunch, 1 bar (singles)	5

Sunbelt

Chewy granola chocolate chip chewy granola bar, 1	4
Chewy granola golden almond bar, 1	3
Chewy granola lowfat oatmeal raisin bar, 1	3
Chewy granola oats & honey bar, 1	3
Crunchy granola bars - oats & honey, 1	3
Fruit & grain bars - blueberry, 1	3
Fruit & grain bars - raspberry, 1	3
Fruit & grain bars - strawberry, 1	3
Fruit & grain bars (apple-cinnamon), 1	3

	POINTS VALUE
Granola bars - peanut butter chip, 1	4
S'mores granola treats, 1 bar	3
Sun-Rype Fruit & Veggie	
Tropical, 1 bar	3
Sun-Rype Fruit To Go	
Fruit punch, 1 bar	1
Tropical, 1 bar	1
Uncle Sam	
Cereal bars, 1 bar	3
Weight Watchers Snack Bars	
Blueberry crumbcake, 1 bar	2
Chocolate caramel, 1 bar	2
Lemon dream, 1 bar	2
Double chocolate delight, 1 bar	2
Mint cookie crisp, 1 bar	2
Sweet & salty, 1 bar	2
Weight Watchers Mini Bars	
Chewy oatmeal raisin, 1 bar	1
Chocolate caramel, 1 bar	1
Dark chocolate raspberry, 1 bar	1
Peanut butter bliss, 1 bar	1

Cereal, hot
Hodgson Mill

	POINTS VALUE
Bulgur wheat with soy hot cereal, 1/4 cup	2
Oat bran hot cereal, 1/4 cup	2

Kashi

	POINTS VALUE
7 whole grain pilaf, cooked, 1/2 cup	3

	POINTS VALUE
Kashi GoLean	
Hearty honey and cinnamon, 1 packet	2
Original truly vanilla, 1 packet	2
Quaker Oats	
Multigrain hot cereal, 1/2 cup	2
Oat bran, 1/2 cup	2
Scotch barley, regular & quick cooking, 1/3 cup	2
Whole wheat - hot natural cereal, 1/2 cup	2

Cereal, ready to eat
Alvarado

	POINTS VALUE
Plain grinola, 1/2 cup	4
Raisin grinola, 1/2 cup	4
Annie's Homegrown	
Bunny love toasted whole grain oat breakfast cereal, 3/4 cup	2
Cinna bunnies cinnamon toasted breakfast cereal, 3/4 cup	2
Honey bunnies toasted whole grain oat breakfast cereal, 3/4 cup	2
Arrowhead Mills	
Amaranth flakes, 1 cup	2
Maple buckwheat flakes, 1 cup	3
Oat bran flakes, 1 cup	2
Back To Nature	
Apple blueberry granola, 1/2 cup	3
Apple cinnamon granola, 1/2 cup	3

BREAKFAST, CEREALS & CEREAL BARS

Cereal, ready to eat, Back To Nature (con't)	POINTS VALUE
Apple strawberry granola, 1/2 cup	3
Banana nut multi bran, 3/4 cup	3
Cranberry pecan granola, 1/2 cup	3
Flax & fiber crunch, 1 cup	3
French vanilla granola, 1/2 cup	4
Granola - classic, 1/2 cup	3
Granola - raisin, 1/2 cup	3
Hi protein crunch, 1/2 cup	3
Hi-fiber multibran, 3/4 cup	2
Hi-fiber multibran, 1/2 cup	0
Hi-protein crunch, 1/2 cup	2
Multigrain harvest, 1 cup	4
Oat 'n soy crisp, 3/4 cup	3

Baker's Breakfast Cookies

70% organic homestyle granola, double chocolate chunk, 1/2 cup	4
70% organic homestyle granola, fruit & nut, 1/2 cup	4
70% organic homestyle granola, oatmeal raisin, 1/2 cup	3
70% organic homestyle granola, peanut butter granola, 1/2 cup	4

Barbara's Bakery

Organic apple cinnamon o's, 3/4 cup	2
Organic breakfast o's - fruit juice sweetened, 1 cup	2
Organic brown rice crisps - fruit juice sweetened, 1 cup	2

	POINTS VALUE
Organic caramel wild puffs, 3/4 cup	2
Organic cocoa wild puffs, 1 cup	2
Organic corn flakes - fruit juice sweetened, 1 cup	2
Organic crispy wheats, 3/4 cup	2
Organic fruity punch wild puffs, 1 cup	2
Organic grainshop, 1/2 cup	1
Organic honey crunch'n oats, 2/3 cup	2
Organic honey nut o's, 3/4 cup	2
Organic puffed wheat wild puffs, 1 cup	2
Shredded oats, 1 1/4 cups	4
Shredded spoonfuls, 3/4 cup	2
Shredded wheat, 2 biscuits	2
Ultima flax & granola, 1 cup	4
Ultima high fiber, 1/2 cup	1
Ultima pomegranate, 1/2 cup	1
Vanilla almond shredded oats, 1 cup	4

Barbara's Bakery Puffins

Cinnamon puffins, 3/4 cup	1
Honey rice puffins, 3/4 cup	2
Peanut butter puffins, 3/4 cup	2
Puffins, 3/4 cup	1

Benefit Nutrition

Protein plus cereal with soy, 2/3 cup	2
Simply fiber cereal, 3/4 cup	1
Simply fiber cereal with cinnamon, 3/4 cup	1

	POINTS VALUE
Breadshop	
Blueberry 'n cream granola, 1/2 cup	4
Crunch oat bran, 1/2 cup	4
Gone nuts granola, 1/2 cup	5
Honey gone nuts, 1/2 cup	5
New England supernatural granola, 1/2 cup	5
Pralines 'n crème, 1/2 cup	4
Strawberry 'n cream granola, 1/2 cup	4
Super cereal, 1/2 cup	5
Supernatural granola with almond & raisin, 1/2 cup	5
Cascadian Farm	
Cinnamon raisin granola, 2/3 cup	4
Clifford crunch, 1 cup	1
Great measure, 1 cup	3
Hearty morning, 3/4 cup	3
Honey nut o's, 1 oz	2
Multi-grain squares, 3/4 cup	2
Oats & honey granola, 2/3 cup	5
Purely o's, 1 cup	2
Raisin bran, 1 cup	3
Vanilla almond crunch, 3/4 cup	4
Wheat crunch, 3/4 cup	2
EnviroKidz	
Amazon frosted flakes, 2/3 cup	2
Gorilla munch, 1 cup	2
Koala crisp, 2/3 cup	2

	POINTS VALUE
Orangutan-o's, 3/4 cup	2
Peanut butter panda puffs, 1 cup	3
Food for Life	
Organic Ezekiel 4:9 cereal, almond, 1/2 cup	3
Organic Ezekiel 4:9 cereal, cinnamon raisin, 1/2 cup	3
Organic Ezekiel 4:9 cereal, golden flax, 1/2 cup	3
Organic Ezekiel 4:9 cereal, original, 1/2 cup	3
General Mills	
Basic 4, 1 cup	4
Berry berry kix, 3/4 cup	2
Berry burst cheerios, strawberry banana, 3/4 cup	2
Berry burst cheerios, triple berry, 3/4 cup	2
Berry lucky charms, 1 cup	2
Boo berry, 1 cup	2
Cheerios, 1 cup	2
Chocolate lucky charms, 3/4 cup	2
Cinnamon toast crunch, 3/4 cup	3
Cinnamon toast crunch - reduced sugar, 3/4 cup	2
Cocoa puffs, 3/4 cup	2
Cookie crisp, 3/4 cup	2
Corn chex, 1 cup	2
Count chocula, 3/4 cup	2
Country corn flakes, 1 cup	2

Cereal, ready to eat, General Mills (con't)	POINTS VALUE
Disney's little einsteins fruity stars, 1 cup	2
Disney's mickey mouse clubhouse berry crunch, 1 cup	2
Disney's princesses fairytale flakes, 1 cup	2
Dora the explorer, 3/4 cup	2
Double chocolate cookie crisps, 3/4 cup	3
Fiber one, 1/2 cup	0
Fiber one honey clusters, 1 cup	3
Frankenberry, 1 cup	2
French toast crunch, 3/4 cup	3
Frosted cheerios, 3/4 cup	2
Frosted chex, 3/4 cup	2
Fruity cheerios, 3/4 cup	2
Golden grahams, 3/4 cup	2
Heart healthy blend apple crunch, 1 cup	4
Heart healthy blend with fiber one, 1 cup	3
Honey nut cheerios, 3/4 cup	2
Honey nut chex, 3/4 cup	2
Honey nut clusters, 1 cup	4
Kaboom, 1 1/4 cups	2
Kix, 1 1/4 cups	2
La lechera flakes, 3/4 cup	2
Lucky charms, 3/4 cup	2
Multi-bran chex, 3/4 cup	3
Multi-grain cheerios, 1 cup	2
Oatmeal crisp almond, 1 cup	4
Oatmeal crisp hearty raisin, 1 cup	4

	POINTS VALUE
Oatmeal crisp maple brown sugar, 1 cup	4
Para su familia raisin bran, 1 1/4 cups	3
Peanut butter cookie crisp, 3/4 cup	3
Raisin nut bran, 3/4 cup	3
Reese's puffs, 3/4 cup	2
Rice chex, 1 cup	2
Total corn flakes, 1 1/3 cups	2
Total honey clusters, 3/4 cup	3
Total raisin bran, 1 cup	3
Total vanilla yogurt, 1 cup	3
Total whole grain, 3/4 cup	1
Trix, 1 cup	2
Wheat chex, 3/4 cup	2
Wheaties, 3/4 cup	1
Yogurt burst cheerios, strawberry, 3/4 cup	2
Yogurt burst cheerios, vanilla, 3/4 cup	2
Health Valley	
Cranberry crunch, 3/4 cup	3
Empower cereal, 1 cup	3
Heart wise cereal, 1 cup	3
Organic amaranth flakes, 3/4 cup	1
Organic fiber 7 flakes, 3/4 cup	1
Organic fiber 7 multigrain flakes, 3/4 cup	1
Organic golden flax cereal, 3/4 cup	3
Organic oat bran flakes, 3/4 cup	1
Organic oat bran flakes with raisins, 3/4 cup	1

	POINTS VALUE
Hodgson Mill	
◆ Cracked wheat cereal, 1/4 cup	1
Multi grain cereal with milled flaxseed and soy, 1/3 cup	3
Kashi	
7 whole grain flakes, 1 cup	3
7 whole grain honey puffs, 1 cup	2
7 whole grain nuggets, 1/2 cup	4
7 whole grain puffs, 1 cup	1
Cinna-raisin crunch, 1 cup	3
Golean, 1 cup	2
Good friends, 1 cup	3
Granola - cocoa beach, 1/2 cup	5
Granola - summer berry, 1/2 cup	4
Granola orchard spice, 1/2 cup	4
Heart to heart, 3/4 cup	2
Mighty bites - honey crunch, 1 cup	2
Mountain medley granola, 1/2 cup	4
Vive probiotic cereal - toasted graham & vanilla, 1 1/4 cups	3
Kashi GOLEAN	
Crunch honey almond flax, 1 cup	4
Crunch!, 1 cup	3
Kashi Heart to Heart	
Wild blueberry, 1 1/4 cups	3
Kashi Organic Promise	
Autumn wheat - whole wheat biscuits, 1 cup	3

	POINTS VALUE
Cinnamon harvest - whole wheat cinnamon flavored biscuits, 1 cup	3
Strawberry fields - rice & wheat flakes with strawberries & raspberries, 1 cup	2
Kellogg's	
All-bran apricot bites, 1 cup	2
All-bran yogurt bites, 1- 1/4 cup	3
All-bran, bran buds, 1/3 cup	1
All-bran, extra fiber, 1/2 cup	0
All-bran, original, 1/2 cup	1
All-bran, strawberry medley, 1/2 cup	3
Apple jacks, 1 cup	2
Caramel nut crunch, 1 cup	4
Cinnamon mini swirlz, 1 cup	2
Cocoa krispies cereal straws, 3	3
Cocoa rice krispies, 3/4 cup	2
Cocoa rice krispies coco-nilla, 3/4 cup	2
Complete oat bran flakes, 3/4 cup	1
Complete wheat bran flakes, 3/4 cup	1
Corn flakes, 1 cup	2
Corn pops, 1 cup	2
Cracklin' oat bran, 3/4 cup	4
Crispix, 1 cup	2
Eggo cinnamon toast, 1 cup	2
Eggo crunch maple, 1 cup	2
Froot loops, 1 cup	2
Froot loops - reduced sugar, 1 1/4 cups	2
Froot loops cereal straws, 3	3

BREAKFAST, CEREALS & CEREAL BARS

Cereal, ready to eat, Kellogg's (con't)	POINTS VALUE
Froot loops dark berries, 1 cup	2
Froot loops smoothie with yogurty coated cereal pieces, 1 cup	2
Frosted flakes, 3/4 cup	2
Frosted flakes reduced sugar, 1 cup	2
Frosted rice krispies, 3/4 cup	2
Fruit harvest strawberry blueberry, 3/4 cup	2
Honey crunch toasted, 1- 1/4 cup	4
Honey smacks, 3/4 cup	2
Just right fruit & nut, 3/4 cup	4
Low fat granola with raisins, 2/3 cup	4
Low fat granola without raisins, 1/2 cup	3
Marshmallow froot loops, 1 cup	2
Mini-swirlz peanut butter, 1 cup	3
Mini-wheats frosted bite size, 24 pieces	3
Mini-wheats frosted bite size cinnamon, 24	3
Mini-wheats frosted bite-size strawberry delight, 24 pieces	3
Mini-wheats frosted original, 5 pieces	3
Mini-wheats vanilla crème bite size, 24	3
Mini-wheats, un-frosted bite size, 30	3
Müeslix, 2/3 cup	3
Pops, chocolate peanut butter, 3/4 cup	2
Product 19, 1 cup	2
Raisin bran, 1 cup	3
Raisin bran crunch, 1 cup	3
Rice krispies, 1 1/4 cups	2

	POINTS VALUE
Rice krispies berry, 1 cup	2
Rice krispies treats cereal, 3/4 cup	3
Rice Krispies with strawberries, 1 cup	2
Smart start - antioxidant, 1 cup	3
Smart start - healthy heart, 1 1/4 cups	4
Smart start healthy heart, maple & brown sugar, 1 1/4 cups	4
Smorz, 1 cup	2
Special K, 1 cup	2
Special K chocolatey delight, 3/4 cup	2
Special K cinnamon pecan, 3/4 cup	2
Special K fruit & yogurt cereal, 3/4 cup	2
Special K low carb lifestyle protein plus, 3/4 cup	1
Special K red berries, 1 cup	2
Special K vanilla almond, 3/4 cup	2
Kellogg's Smart Start	
Healthy heart cinnamon raisin, 1 cup	3
Kellogg's Smart Start Healthy Heart	
Maple & brown sugar, 1 1/4 cups	4
Lifestream	
Multigrain honey puffs natural cereal, 1 cup	2
Market Day	
Apple berry breakfast bowl, 1	3
Mother's	
Cinnamon oat crunch, 1 serving (60 g)	4
Cocoa bumpers, 1 serving (33 g)	2

	POINTS VALUE
Graham bumpers, 1 serving (28 g)	2
Honey bumpers, 1 serving (33 g)	2
Peanut butter bumpers, 1 serving (33 g)	3
Nature's Path	
8 grain synergy flakes, 2/3 cup	1
Blueberry almond muesli organic cereal, 1/2 cup	4
Corn puffs, 1 cup	1
Flax plus granola, 1/2 cup	3
Flax plus multibran flakes, 3/4 cup	1
Fruit juice sweet cornflakes, 3/4 cup	2
Ginger zing granola, 2/3 cup	6
Hemp plus granola, 1/2 cup	2
Heritage bites, 3/4 cup	1
Heritage flakes, 3/4 cup	2
Heritage granola, 1/2 cup	2
Heritage muesli, 1/2 cup	4
Heritage o's, 3/4 cup	2
Honey'd cornflakes, 3/4 cup	2
Kamut krisp, 3/4 cup	1
Kamut puffs, 1 cup	1
Mesa sunrise, 3/4 cup	2
Millet puffs, 1 cup	1
Millet rice, 3/4 cup	2
Multigrain flakes, 2/3 cup	2
Multigrain with raisin, 2/3 cup	2
Oaty bites, 3/4 cup	2

	POINTS VALUE
Optimum power cereal, 1 cup	3
Optimum slim cereal, 1 cup	3
Optimum zen, 3/4 cup	3
Rice puffs, 1 cup	1
Soy plus granola, 1/2 cup	2
Spelt flakes cereal, 3/4 cup	2
Wheat puffs, 1 cup	1
Whole grain crispy rice cereal, 3/4 cup	2
Nutritious Living	
Dr. Sears zone cereal, 3/4 cup	3
Heartmates cereal, 3/4 cup	1
Nutritious Living Hi-Lo	
Hi-lo cereal, 1/2 cup	1
Maple pecan, 1/2 cup	1
Maple pecan cereal cup, 1 container	2
Vanilla almond, 1/2 cup	1
Vanilla almond cereal cup, 1 container	2
With strawberries, 1/2 cup	1
Post	
Bamm bamm mixed berry pebbles, 3/4 cup	2
Bran flakes, 3/4 cup	1
Cocoa pebbles, 3/4 cup	2
Fiesta fruity pebbles, 3/4 cup	2
Frosted shredded wheat spoon size, 1 cup	3
Fruity pebbles, 3/4 cup	2
Fruity pebbles reduced sugar, 3/4 cup	2
Golden crisp, 3/4 cup	2

Cereal, ready to eat, Post (con't)

	POINTS VALUE
Grape-nut flakes, 3/4 cup	2
Grape-nut o's, 1 cup	2
Grape-nuts, 1/2 cup	3
Grape-nuts trail mix, crunch raisin almond, 1/2 cup	3
Honey bunches of oats cinnamon, 3/4 cup	2
Honey bunches of oats honey roasted, 3/4 cup	2
Honey bunches of oats with almonds, 3/4 cup	2
Honey bunches of oats with real peaches cereal, 1 serving (31 g)	2
Honey bunches of oats with real strawberries cereal, 1 serving (31 g)	2
Honey nut shredded wheat spoon size, 1 cup	3
Honeycomb, 1 1/2 cups	2
Oreo o's with marshmallow bits cereal, 1 serving (27 g)	2
Organic grape-nuts, 1/2 cup	3
Organic honey bunches of oats honey roasted, 3/4 cup	2
Raisin bran, 1 cup	3
Shredded wheat cinnamon, 1 cup	3
◆ The original shredded wheat, 2 biscuits	2
◆ The original shredded wheat 'n bran spoon size, 1 1/4 cup	3
◆ The original shredded wheat spoon size, 1 cup	3

	POINTS VALUE
Toasties, 1 cup	2
Waffle crisp, 1 cup	2
Post Select	
Banana nut crunch, 1 cup	5
Blueberry morning, 1 1/4 cups	4
Cranberry almond crunch, 3/4 cup	4
Great grains crunchy pecan, 1/2 cup	4
Great grains raisins, dates & pecans, 1/2 cup	4
Maple pecan crunch cereal, 1 serving (52 g)	4
Organic apple cinnamon harvest, 1 cup	3
Quaker Oats	
Cap'n crunch, peanut butter, 3/4 cup	2
Cap'n crunch, peanut butter chocolate, 3/4 cup	2
Cap'n crunch, regular, 3/4 cup	2
Cap'n crunch, with crunchberries, 3/4 cup	2
Cap'n crunch's choco crunch cereal, 3/4 cup	1
Cinnamon life, 3/4 cup	2
Cinnamon oatmeal squares, 1 cup	4
Crunchy bran, 3/4 cup	1
King vitamin, 1 1/2 cups	2
Life, 3/4 cup	2
Life cereal, chocolate oat clusters, 1 cup	4
Life cereal, vanilla yogurt crunch, 1 1/4 cups	4

	POINTS VALUE
Natural granola oats, honey & raisins, 1/2 cup	4
Natural granola, low fat, 2/3 cup	4
Natural granola, oats & honey, 1/2 cup	4
Oat bran cereal, 1 1/4 cups	4
Oatmeal squares, 1 cup	4
Oh!s - honey graham, 3/4 cup	2
♦ Puffed rice, 1 cup	1
♦ Puffed wheat, 1 1/4 cups	1
Quisp, 1 cup	2
♦ Shredded wheat, 3 biscuits	4
Toasted oatmeal cereal - honey nut, 1 cup	3
Toasted oatmeal cereal - original, 1 cup	3

Quaker Oats Simple Harvest

Banana honey pecan cereal, 1 serving (50 g)	3
Cinnamon & honey cereal, 1 serving (52 g)	3

Sunbelt

Berry basic whole grain flakes with real fruit pieces, 1/2 cup	5
Granola (low fat) with cinnamon & raisins, 1/2 cup	5

Uncle Sam

Cereal, 3/4 cup	3
Cereal with mixed berries, 1 cup	3

Weetabix

Alpen - no sugar, no salt added muesli-style cereal, 2/3 cup	3
Alpen original muesli-style cereal, 2/3 cup	3
Organic crispy flakes, 3/4 cup	1
Organic crispy flakes & fiber, 1 1/4 cups	3
Organic weetabix, 2 biscuits	2

Cream of Wheat, Rice

Amy's

Cream of rice hot cereal bowl, 1	3

Arrowhead Mills

Instant rice cereal, 1 packet	2

Cream of Wheat

♦ Cream of wheat, 1 minute, 1 cup	2
♦ Cream of wheat, 10 minute, 1 cup	2
♦ Cream of wheat, 2 1/2 minute, 1 cup	2
Instant cream of wheat, apples 'n cinnamon, 1 packet	2
Instant cream of wheat, cinnamon swirl, 1 packet	2
Instant cream of wheat, maple brown sugar, 1 packet	2
♦ Instant cream of wheat, original, 1 packet	2
Instant cream of wheat, peaches 'n cream, 1 packet	3
Instant cream of wheat, strawberries 'n cream, 1 packet	2

Manischewitz

♦ Creamy hot wheat cereal, 1/4 cup	2

Nabisco

Cream of rice, 1 serving (46 g)	3

Farina
Cream of Wheat

Instant cream of wheat enriched farina (1 minute), 3 Tbsp	2

H-O

Cream farina, 3 Tbsp	2

French Toast
Ian's

Banana French toast sticks, 1 serving (92 g)	5
Cinnamon & honey French toast sticks, 1 serving (91 g)	5
Triple berry French toast sticks, 1 serving (91 g)	5
Wheat free, gluten free French toast sticks, 1 serving (56 g)	5

Kellogg's Eggo

French toaster sticks - cinnamon, 2 sticks	5
French toaster sticks - original, 2 sticks	5
French toaster sticks maple, 1 piece	3

Market Day

Cinnamon crunch French toast bites, 6 pieces	7
French toast sticks, 4 pieces	6

Pillsbury

French toast sticks - original, 6	5

Grits
Quaker Oats

♦ Enriched hominy quick golden grits, 1/4 cup	2
♦ Enriched white hominy grits, 1/4 cup	2
♦ Enriched white hominy quick grits, 1/4 cup	2
Instant grits - American cheese flavor, 1 packet	2
Instant grits - butter express, 1 cup	3
Instant grits - butter flavor, 1 packet	2
Instant grits - cheddar blend, 1 packet	2
Instant grits - cheddar cheese flavor, 1 packet	2
Instant grits - country bacon, 1 packet	2
Instant grits - ham 'n cheese flavor, 1 packet	2
♦ Instant grits - original flavor, 1 packet	2
Instant grits - three cheese, 1 packet	2

Oatmeal
Amy's

Multi-grain hot cereal bowl, 1	1
Rolled oats hot cereal bowl, 1	4
Steel-cut oats hot cereal bowl, 1	4

Arrowhead Mills

Instant oatmeal - maple apple spice, 1 packet	2
♦ Instant oatmeal original plain, 1 packet	2

◆	POINTS VALUE
H-O	
◆ Instant oats, 1/2 cup	2
Hodgson Mill	
◆ Steel cut oats, 1/4 cup (dry)	2
Kashi Heart to Heart	
Instant oatmeal raisin spice, 1 packet	2
Instant oatmeal, apple cinnamon, 1 packet	3
Instant oatmeal, maple, 1 packet	3
Nature's Path	
Organic instant hot oatmeal, apple cinnamon, 1 packet	4
Organic instant hot oatmeal, flax 'n oats, 1 packet	4
Organic instant hot oatmeal, maple nut, 1 packet	4
◆ Organic instant oatmeal, original, 1 packet	3
Quaker	
Oatmeal, lower sugar apples & cinnamon, 1 packet	2
Oatmeal, lower sugar maple & brown sugar, 1 packet	2
Quaker Oats	
Instant oatmeal - apples and cinnamon, 1 packet	2
Instant oatmeal - baked apple flavor, 1 packet	3
Instant oatmeal - baked cinnamon roll, 1 packet	3

◆	POINTS VALUE
Instant oatmeal - cinnamon & spice, 1 packet	3
Instant oatmeal - cinnamon & spice, 1 packet	3
Instant oatmeal - crunchy apples & cinnamon, 1 packet	3
Instant oatmeal - crunchy maple brown sugar, 1 packet	3
Instant oatmeal - crunchy mixed berry, 1 packet	3
Instant oatmeal - dinosaur eggs - brown sugar cinnamon, 1 packet	3
Instant oatmeal - French toast, 1 packet	3
Instant oatmeal - honey nut, 1 packet	3
Instant oatmeal - magicolor crunch, 1 packet	3
Instant oatmeal - maple & brown sugar, 1 packet	3
Instant oatmeal - peaches & cream, 1 packet	3
Instant oatmeal - raisin-spice, 1 packet	3
◆ Instant oatmeal - regular flavor, 1 packet	2
Instant oatmeal - strawberries & cream, 1 packet	3
Instant oatmeal express - baked apple, 1 cup	3
Instant oatmeal express - cinnamon roll, 1 cup	3
Instant oatmeal express - golden brown sugar, 1 cup	4

BREAKFAST, CEREALS & CEREAL BARS

Oatmeal, Quaker Oats (con't)	POINTS VALUE
Instant oatmeal nutrition for women - apple cinnamon, 1 packet	3
Instant oatmeal nutrition for women - golden brown sugar, 1 packet	3
Instant oatmeal nutrition for women - vanilla cinnamon, 1 packet	3
Instant oatmeal weight control - banana bread, 1 packet	3
Instant oatmeal weight control - cinnamon toast, 1 packet	3
Instant oatmeal weight control - maple brown sugar, 1 packet	3
◆ Old fashioned oats, 1/2 cup	2
Organic instant - maple brown sugar, 1 packet	3
◆ Organic instant - regular, 1 packet	2
◆ Quick oats, 1/2 cup	2
Quaker Oats Simple Harvest	
Apple & cinnamon oatmeal, 1 packet	2
Maple brown sugar oatmeal, 1 packet	3
Plain oatmeal, 1 packet	2
Vanilla, almond, honey oatmeal, 1 packet	3
Uncle Sam	
Instant oatmeal, 1 packet	2
Instant oatmeal with soymilk - cinnamon raisin, 1 packet	3
Instant oatmeal with soymilk - French vanilla, 1 packet	3

	POINTS VALUE
Weight Watchers	
Maple brown sugar oatmeal, 1 serving (39 g)	2
Pancake Syrup	
Aunt Jemima	
Lite syrup, 1/4 cup	2
Pancakes	
Aunt Jemima	
Buckwheat pancake mix, 1/4 cup	1
Buttermilk complete mix, 1/3 cup	2
Buttermilk pancake mix, 1/4 cup	2
Complete pancake mix, 1/3 cup	3
Original pancake mix, 1/3 cup	3
Reduced calorie buttermilk complete mix, 1/3 cup	2
Whole wheat mix, 1/4 cup	2
Betty Crocker	
Complete buttermilk mix (box), prepared, 3	4
Complete buttermilk mix (pouch), prepared, 3	4
Complete original mix (box), prepared, 3	4
Bisquick	
Buttermilk pancakes, 3	6
Heart smart pancakes, 3	4
Original pancakes, 3	6
Bisquick Shake 'N Pour	
Buttermilk, 1/2 cup	4

	POINTS VALUE
Cherrybrook Kitchen	
Gluten free pancake and waffle mix, 1 serving (mix for 1 4" pancake)	2
Original pancake mix, 1 serving (mix for 1 4" pancake)	2
Whole grain pancake mix, 1 serving (mix for 1 4" pancake)	1
Heidi's	
Cottage cheese pancake mix (original), 1/4 cup	3
Grainy day pancake mix, 1/3 cup	3
Oats n' apple pancake mix, 1/3 cup	4
Sourdough pancake mix, 1/3 cup	4
Whole wheat cottage cheese pancake mix, 1/4 cup	3
Hodgson Mill	
Buckwheat pancake mix, 1/3 cup	2
Multi grain buttermilk pancake mix with milled flaxseed, 1/3 cup	2
Whole wheat buttermilk pancake mix, 1/3 cup	2
Kellogg's Eggo	
Blueberry pancakes, 3	6
Buttermilk, 3	6
Buttermilk mini-pancakes, 11	6
Nutrigrain pancakes, 3	5
Pancakes jungle, 3	6

	POINTS VALUE
Maple Grove	
Blueberry pancake mix, dry, 1/3 cup	3
Blueberry pancake mix, prepared, 1 serving (110 g)	5
Buttermilk & honey pancake mix, dry, 1/3 cup	3
Buttermilk & honey pancake mix, prepared, 1 serving (110 g)	5
Gluten free pancake mix, dry, 1/4 cup	2
Gluten free pancake mix, prepared, 1 serving (110 g)	5
Honey buckwheat pancake mix, dry, 1/3 cup	3
Honey buckwheat pancake mix, prepared, 1 serving (110 g)	5
Sugar free pancake mix, 1/3 cup	1
Market Day	
Banana mini pancakes, 6	2
Chocolate chip mini pancakes, 6 pieces	3
Microwave pancakes, 3	4
Pillsbury	
Blueberry, 3	4
Buttermilk, 3	5
Buttermilk mini's, 11	5
Chocolate burst, 3	6
Maple burst, 3	6
Mini buttermilk pancakes, 16	4
Original, 3	5

BREAKFAST, CEREALS & CEREAL BARS

Pancakes (con't)	POINTS VALUE
Pillsbury Mini Pancakes with Dippin' Cups	
Blueberry, 14	9
Buttermilk, 14	9
Sweet 'N Low	
Pancake mix, prepared, 1 serving (45 g)	3

Pastries
Little Debbie
Honey buns, 1	5

Toaster Pastries
Amy's
Apple toaster pops, 1 piece	3
Cheese pizza toaster pops, 1 piece	3
Strawberry toaster pops, 1 piece	3

Flavor Kist
Toast'em pop-ups, frosted blueberry, 1	4
Toast'em pop-ups, frosted brown sugar cinnamon, 1	4
Toast'em pop-ups, frosted cherry, 1	4
Toast'em pop-ups, frosted chocolate fudge, 1	4
Toast'em pop-ups, frosted strawberry, 1	4
Toast'em pop-ups, frosted wild berry, 1	4

Kellogg's
Apple strudel, 1	4
Brown sugar cinnamon made with whole grains, 1	4
Double berry, 1	4

	POINTS VALUE
Hot chocolate, 1	4
Mint chocolate chip, 1	4
Splitz - chocolate vanilla, 1	4
Splitz - strawberry blueberry, 1	4
Splitz, strawberry chocolate, 1	4
Strawberry cheese danish, 1	4
Strawberry made with whole grains, 1	4
Strawberry milkshake, 1	4

Kellogg's Pop-Tarts
Apple cinnamon, 1	5
Blueberry, 1	5
Brown sugar cinnamon, 1	5
Caramel chocolate, frosted, 1	4
Chocolate chip, 1	5
Chocolate chip cookie dough, 1	4
Cinnamon roll, 1	5
French toast, 1	5
Frosted blueberry, 1	4
Frosted brown sugar cinnamon, 1	5
Frosted cherry, 1	4
Frosted chocolate fudge, 1	4
Frosted chocolate vanilla crème, 1	4
Frosted cookies and crème, 1	4
Frosted raspberry, 1	4
Frosted s'mores, 1	4
Frosted strawberry, 1	4
Frosted wild berry, 1	4

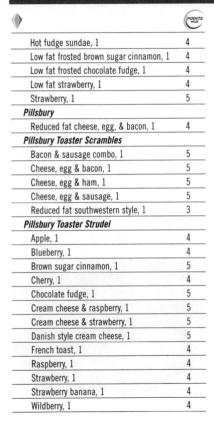

	POINTS VALUE
Hot fudge sundae, 1	4
Low fat frosted brown sugar cinnamon, 1	4
Low fat frosted chocolate fudge, 1	4
Low fat strawberry, 1	4
Strawberry, 1	5
Pillsbury	
Reduced fat cheese, egg, & bacon, 1	4
Pillsbury Toaster Scrambles	
Bacon & sausage combo, 1	5
Cheese, egg & bacon, 1	5
Cheese, egg & ham, 1	5
Cheese, egg & sausage, 1	5
Reduced fat southwestern style, 1	3
Pillsbury Toaster Strudel	
Apple, 1	4
Blueberry, 1	4
Brown sugar cinnamon, 1	5
Cherry, 1	4
Chocolate fudge, 1	5
Cream cheese & raspberry, 1	5
Cream cheese & strawberry, 1	5
Danish style cream cheese, 1	5
French toast, 1	4
Raspberry, 1	4
Strawberry, 1	4
Strawberry banana, 1	4
Wildberry, 1	4

	POINTS VALUE
Waffles	
Bisquick	
Buttermilk waffles, 2	4
Heart smart waffles, 2	3
Original waffles, 2	4
EnviroKidz	
Gorilla banana waffles, 2	4
Koala choco waffles, 2	4
Kashi GOLEAN	
Blueberry, 2	3
Original, 2	3
Strawberry waffles, 2	3
Kashi Heart to Heart	
Honey oat waffle, 2	3
Kellogg's	
Nutri-grain blueberry waffles, 2	3
Kellogg's Eggo	
Apple cinnamon, 2	4
Banana bread, 2	4
Blueberry, 2	4
Brown sugar & cinnamon flip flop waffles, 2	4
Buttermilk, 2	4
Buttery syrup mini waffles, 3	5
Choco-nilla flip flop waffles, 2	4
Chocolate chip, 2	5
Cinnamon toast mini waffles, 1 serving (3 sets of 4 waffles)	6

Waffles, Kellogg's Eggo (con't)	POINTS VALUE
French vanilla, 2	4
Homestyle, 2	4
Homestyle mini waffles, 1 serving (3 sets of 4 waffles)	5
Nutri-grain, 2	4
Nutri-grain cinnamon, 2	3
Nutri-grain low fat, 2	2
Shrek homestyle, 2	4
Special K - low fat waffles, 2	3
Strawberry, 2	4
Waffles - French toast, 1	3
Waffles - special k red berries low fat, 2	3
Waf-fulls - strawberry, 1 piece	4
Lifestream	
8 grain sesame, 2	5
Buckwheat wildberry, 2	5
Flax plus, 2	5
Hemp plus, 2	4
Mesa sunrise, 2	4
Soy plus, 2	4
Maple Grove	
Belgian waffle mix, dry, 1/4 cup	2
Belgian waffle mix, prepared, 1 serving (85 g)	2
Nature's Path	
Optimum power waffles, 2	3

Pillsbury	POINTS VALUE
Blueberry, 2	4
Buttermilk, 2	4
Homestyle, 2	4
Waffle sticks - homestyle, 6	5

Wheat Germ
Hodgson Mill

100% untoasted wheat germ, 2 Tbsp (dry)	0
Wheat germ with milled flaxseed & cinnamon, 2 Tbsp	1

Kretschmer

Honey crunch wheat germ, 1 2/3 Tbsp	1
Wheat germ - regular, 2 Tbsp	1

Tree of Life

Wheat germ, toasted, 3 Tbsp	2

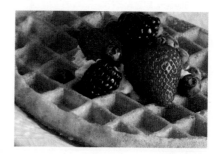

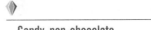

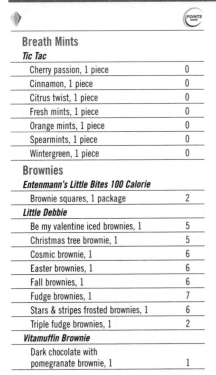

Breath Mints

Tic Tac

Cherry passion, 1 piece	0
Cinnamon, 1 piece	0
Citrus twist, 1 piece	0
Fresh mints, 1 piece	0
Orange mints, 1 piece	0
Spearmints, 1 piece	0
Wintergreen, 1 piece	0

Brownies

Entenmann's Little Bites 100 Calorie

Brownie squares, 1 package	2

Little Debbie

Be my valentine iced brownies, 1	5
Christmas tree brownie, 1	5
Cosmic brownie, 1	6
Easter brownies, 1	6
Fall brownies, 1	6
Fudge brownies, 1	7
Stars & stripes frosted brownies, 1	6
Triple fudge brownies, 1	2

Vitamuffin Brownie

Dark chocolate with pomegranate brownie, 1	1

Candy, non-chocolate

Be Happy & Healthy

Yummy gummy in my tummy, 18 pieces	3

Brookside

Macaroons, 11 pieces	4
Starbuds, 11 pieces	4
Vanilla clodhoppers, 1 package	3
X-treme fruit bites, atomic apple, 1 package	1
X-treme fruit bites, charg-n cherry, 1 package	1
X-treme fruit bites, chili lime fusion, 1 package	1
X-treme fruit bites, citrus cyclone, 1 package	1

Cambridge Brands

Sugar daddy, junior pop, 3	3
Sugar daddy, large pop, 1	4

Campino

Peach, 4 pieces	1
Strawberry, 4 pieces	1

Charm's

Blow pop, junior, 1	1
Blow pop, regular, 1	1
Blow pop, super, 1	3
Charm's way 2 sour blow pop, junior, 1	1
Charm's way 2 sour blow pop, regular, 1	1

CANDY, COOKIES & DESSERTS

Candy, non-chocolate, Charm's (con't)	POINTS VALUE
Charm's way 2 sour blow pop, super, 1	3
Fluffy stuff, 1 bag (1.06 oz)	2
Fluffy stuff, 1 small bag (0.6 oz)	1
Sour pop, regular flat pop, 1	1
Squares, 2 pieces	0
Sweet pop, junior flat pop, 1	1
Sweet pop, regular flat pop, 1	1
Sweet/sour pop, regular flat pop, 1	1
Zip-a-dee-doo-da pop, 3	1
Estee	
No sugar added caramels, 5 pieces	3
Peanut brittle - no sugar added, 1 1/2 oz	5
Sugar free assorted fruit hard, 3 pieces	0
Sugar free hard butterscotch, 3 pieces	0
Sugar free hard peppermint, 3 pieces	0
Sugar free hard tropical fruit, 3 pieces	0
Sugar free toffee hard, 3 pieces	0
Estee Smart Treats	
Sugar free cookie dough candy bar, 1	1
Sugar free gourmet jelly beans, 26 pieces	2
Sugar free gummy bears, 17 pieces	1
Sugar free sour citrus slices, 15 pieces	2
Flat Earth	
Crispy apple crunchy fruit snacks, 22 pieces	3
Luscious pineapple flavored crunchy fruit snacks, 35 pieces	3

	POINTS VALUE
Hershey's	
Good & plenty, 1 box	4
Payday, 1 bar	5
Zagnut, 1 bar	5
Jelly Belly	
Jelly beans, 35 pieces	3
Jolly Rancher	
Gummis, 9 pieces	3
Hard candy twists assortment, 3 pieces	1
Jelly beans, 25 pieces	2
Kellogg's Yogos	
Yogurty covered fruit bits, berry berry banana, 1 pouch	2
Yogurty covered fruit snack bitin' berry blast, 1 pouch	2
Yogurty covered fruit snack, sour apple, 1 pouch	2
Yogurty covered fruit snack, watermelon splash, 1 pouch	2
Yogurty covered fruit snacks, berry berry banana, single serve, 1 pouch	4
Yogurty covered fruity dots, crazy berries, 1 pouch	4
Yogurty covered fruity dots, island explosion, single serve, 1 pouch	4
Yogurty covered fruity dots, strawberry slam, single serve, 1 pouch	4
Kraft	
Caramels, 5 pieces	3

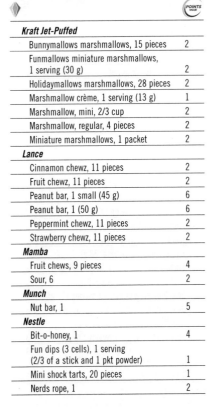

	POINTS VALUE
Kraft Jet-Puffed	
Bunnymallows marshmallows, 15 pieces	2
Funmallows miniature marshmallows, 1 serving (30 g)	2
Holidaymallows marshmallows, 28 pieces	2
Marshmallow crème, 1 serving (13 g)	1
Marshmallow, mini, 2/3 cup	2
Marshmallow, regular, 4 pieces	2
Miniature marshmallows, 1 packet	2
Lance	
Cinnamon chewz, 11 pieces	2
Fruit chewz, 11 pieces	2
Peanut bar, 1 small (45 g)	6
Peanut bar, 1 (50 g)	6
Peppermint chewz, 11 pieces	2
Strawberry chewz, 11 pieces	2
Mamba	
Fruit chews, 9 pieces	4
Sour, 6	2
Munch	
Nut bar, 1	5
Nestle	
Bit-o-honey, 1	4
Fun dips (3 cells), 1 serving (2/3 of a stick and 1 pkt powder)	1
Mini shock tarts, 20 pieces	1
Nerds rope, 1	2

	POINTS VALUE
Nips, butter rum, 2 pieces	1
Nips, caramel, 2 pieces	1
Nips, coffee, 2 pieces	1
Nips, peanut butter parfait, 2 pieces	1
Pixy stix (3 pack), 3	1
Spree - mini chewy, 16 pieces	1
Spree - regular, 8 pieces	1
SweeTarts - mini chewy, 23 pieces	1
SweeTarts - regular, 8 pieces	1
Wonderball, 1	3
Odense	
Marzipan, 2 Tbsp	4
Planters	
Original peanut bar, 1 package	5
Pull 'N' Peel	
Pink lemonade, 1 piece	2
Reed's	
Rootbeer, 1 piece	1
Skittles	
Original bite size candies, 1 1/2 oz (about 1/4 cup)	4
Original bite size candies, 1 small bag (15 g)	1
Original bite size candies, 1 single bag (singles)	5
Original bite size candies, 1 bag (fun size)	2
Skittles sour, 1 bag (51 g)	4
Skittles sour, 1 1/2 oz	3

CANDY, COOKIES & DESSERTS

Candy, non-chocolate, Skittles (con't)	POINTS VALUE
Skittles sour, 1 small bag (fun size)	2
Tropical bite size candies, 1 bag (fun size)	2
Tropical bite size candies, 1 1/2 oz (about 1/4 cup)	4
Tropical bite size candies, 1 single bag (singles)	5
Wild berry bite size candies, 1 single bag (singles)	5
Wild berry bite size candies, 1 1/2 oz (about 1/4 cup)	4
Wild berry bite size candies, 1 bag (fun size)	2
Starburst	
Fruit chews, California fruits, 8 pieces	4
Fruit chews, California fruits, 1 package	5
Fruit chews, fruit & crème, 8 small (fun size)	3
Fruit chews, fruit & crème, 8	3
Fruit chews, fruit & crème, 1 package	5
Fruit chews, original fruits, 1 package	5
Fruit chews, original fruits, 8 pieces	4
Fruit chews, tropical fruits, 1 package	5
Fruit chews, tropical fruits, 8 pieces (fun size)	3
Fruit chews, tropical fruits, 8 pieces (40 g)	4
Jelly beans original fruits, 1/4 cup (1.5 oz)	3
Sunbelt	
Fruit jammers gummy bears, 13 pieces	2

	POINTS VALUE
Tootsie Roll	
Caramel apple pops, 1	1
Crows, 12 pieces	3
Mason dots, 12 pieces	3
Tootsie frooties, 12 pieces	3
Tootsie fruit rolls, 6 pieces	3
Tootsie pops, 1 regular	1
Tootsie pops, 3 miniature	1
Tootsie pops, 1 small	1
Wild berry dots, 12	3
Trolli Gummy Candy	
Classic bears, 1 serving (40 g)	3
Melon-o's, 1 serving (39 g)	3
Peachie-o's, 1 serving (39 g)	3
Peachie-o's, 1 bag (35 g)	3
Road kill, 1 serving (39 g)	3
Rocket racers, 1 serving (38 g)	3
Small brite crawlers, 1 serving (39 g)	2
Sour apple-o's, 1 serving (39 g)	3
Sour brite crawler eggs, 1 serving (40 g)	3
Sour brite crawlers, 1 serving (36 g)	3
Sour brite crawlers, 1 bag (43 g)	3
Sour brite octopus, 1 serving (36 g)	3
Squiggles, 1 serving (38 g)	3
Stingin' red ants hot cinnamon, 1 serving (39 g)	3

	POINTS VALUE
Stingin' red ants hot cinnamon, 1 bag (35 g)	2
Strawberry puffs, 1 serving (39 g)	3
Twizzlers	
Cherry bites, 17 pieces	3
Pull-n-peel, 2 pieces	3
Sourz assortment, 1 package	3
Strawberry, 1 package	5
Twerpz, 1 package	4
Weight Watchers Fruities	
Blackberry, 3 pieces	0
Cherry, 3 pieces	0
Strawberry, 3 pieces	0
Welch's	
Cranberries & spiced apples, 1 serving (1.4 oz)	3
Welch's Fruit 'n Yogurt Snacks	
Blueberry, 1 pouch	2
Cherry, 1 pouch	2
Strawberry, 1 pouch	2
Welch's Fruit Snacks	
Berries n cherries, 1 pouch	2
Concord grape, 1 pouch	2
Fruit punch, 1 pouch	2
Mixed fruit, 1 pouch	2
Strawberry, 1 pouch	2

	POINTS VALUE
Welch's Reduced Sugar Fruit Snacks	
Mixed fruit, 20 pieces	2
Werther's Original	
Caramel coffee, 3 pieces	1
Caramel coffee sugar free, 5 pieces	1
Caramel mint, 4 pieces	1
Chewy caramels, 6 pieces	4
Hard candies, 3 pieces	1
Sugar free caramel mint, 5 pieces	1
Sugar free hard candies, 5 pieces	1
Wonka	
Bottle caps, 8 pieces	1
Chewy gobs, 9 pieces	1
Chewy runts, 13 pieces	1
Chewy tart n tinys, 1 Tbsp	1
Egg breakers, 6 pieces	1
Freckled eggs, 9 pieces	1
Fruit runts, 12 pieces	1
Gobstopper, 9 pieces	1
Heartbreaker, 8 pieces	1
Laffy taffy, 5 bars	3
Merry mix, 11 pieces	1
Nerds, 1 Tbsp	1
Nerds gum ball, 1	1
Oompas, 1 serving (52 g)	4
Runts, hearts, 1 serving (15 g)	1

Candy, non-chocolate, Wonka (con't)	POINTS VALUE
Shock tarts, 8 pieces	1
Shock tarts gum ball, 1	1
Snowball gobs, 6 pieces	1
Tangy taffy, 1 bar	4
Tart n tinys, 1 Tbsp	1

Chocolate Candy
3 Musketeers

3 musketeers bar, 1 bar (60.4 g)	6
3 musketeers bar, 1 bar (fun size)	1
3 musketeers bar, 1 piece (41 g)	4
3 musketeers bar - mint, 1 bar (fun size)	2
3 musketeers bar - mint, 2 pieces (35 g)	4

Andes

Cherry jubilee thins, 8 pieces	5
Creme de menthe changemaker, 3 pieces	5
Creme de menthe thins, 8 pieces	5
Mint parfait thins, 8 pieces	5
Toffee crunch thins, 8 pieces	5

Annabelle Candy Company

Big hunk candy bar, 1 bar	5

Brookside

Cocoa clodhoppers, 1 package	3

Cadbury's

Caramello, 1 bar	5
Dairy milk chocolate bar, 10 pieces	5
Fruit & nut chocolate bar, 10 pieces	5

	POINTS VALUE
Mini-eggs, 12 pieces	4
Royal dark chocolate bar, 10 pieces	5

Cambridge Brands

Charleston chew, chocolate, 1	5
Charleston chew, strawberry, 1	5
Charleston chew, vanilla, 13 pieces	4
Chocolate sugar babies, 19 pieces	4
Junior caramels, 2 boxes (24 g)	2
Junior caramels, 13 pieces	4
Junior mints, 16 pieces	3
Junior mints, 1 box (18 g)	2
Junior mints deluxe, 3 pieces	4
Junior mints inside-out, 15 pieces	4
Junior mints minis, 54 pieces	4
Sugar babies, 30 pieces	4
Sugar babies, 2 boxes (35 g)	3
Sugar mama, 7 pieces	3

Cella's

Dark chocolate covered cherries, 2 pieces	2
Milk chocolate covered cherries, 2 pieces	3

CocoaVia

Chocolate almond crunch bar, 1 bar (singles)	2
Chocolate bar, 1 bar (singles)	2
Chocolate blueberry crunch bar, 1 bar (singles)	2
Chocolate covered almonds, 1 bag (singles)	3

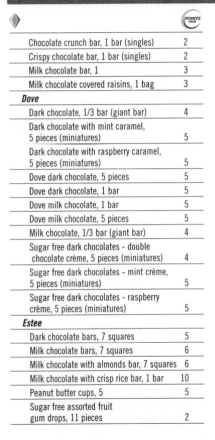

	POINTS VALUE
Chocolate crunch bar, 1 bar (singles)	2
Crispy chocolate bar, 1 bar (singles)	2
Milk chocolate bar, 1	3
Milk chocolate covered raisins, 1 bag	3
Dove	
Dark chocolate, 1/3 bar (giant bar)	4
Dark chocolate with mint caramel, 5 pieces (miniatures)	5
Dark chocolate with raspberry caramel, 5 pieces (miniatures)	5
Dove dark chocolate, 5 pieces	5
Dove dark chocolate, 1 bar	5
Dove milk chocolate, 1 bar	5
Dove milk chocolate, 5 pieces	5
Milk chocolate, 1/3 bar (giant bar)	4
Sugar free dark chocolates - double chocolate crème, 5 pieces (miniatures)	4
Sugar free dark chocolates - mint crème, 5 pieces (miniatures)	5
Sugar free dark chocolates - raspberry crème, 5 pieces (miniatures)	5
Estee	
Dark chocolate bars, 7 squares	5
Milk chocolate bars, 7 squares	6
Milk chocolate with almonds bar, 7 squares	6
Milk chocolate with crisp rice bar, 1 bar	10
Peanut butter cups, 5	5
Sugar free assorted fruit gum drops, 11 pieces	2

	POINTS VALUE
Estee Smart Treats	
Sugar free chocolate fudge candy bar, 1	2
Sugar free raspberry candy bar, 1	2
Ferrero Rondnoir	
Fine dark chocolates, 1 package	4
Guylian	
Belgian dark chocolate orange, no sugar added, 8 squares	3
Belgian dark chocolate, no sugar added, 8 squares	3
Belgian milk chocolate, no sugar added, 8 squares	3
Extra dark 70% cocoa, no sugar added, 8 squares	4
La trufflina, 3 pieces	5
Opus (assorted Belgian chocolates), 3 pieces	6
Seashells, 4 pieces	6
Guylian Solitaire	
Assorted dark chocolates, 6 pieces	3
Guylian Solitaire Extra Dark	
Extra dark 70% cocoa, 6 pieces	3
Guylian Twists	
Assorted dark, 5 pieces	6
Dark chocolate orange cream, 5 pieces	6
Milk chocolate truffle, 5 pieces	6
Original praline, 4 pieces	5

Chocolate Candy (con't) (POINTS VALUE)

Hershey's

Almond joy bar, 1 bar	5
Chocolate covered marshmallow eggs, 1	2
Dark chocolate nuggets with almonds, 4 pieces	4
Extra dark chocolate bar chocolate bar, 3 pieces	3
Heath milk chocolate English toffee bar, 1 package	5
Hersey-ets (pastel), 42 pieces	4
Kissables, 1 package	5
Kisses brand milk chocolates, 9 pieces	5
Kisses brand milk chocolates filled with caramel, 9 pieces	5
Kisses brand milk chocolates filled with peanut butter, 9 pieces	6
Kisses with almonds, 9 pieces	5
Milk chocolate, 1 bar	5
Milk chocolate nuggets, 4 pieces	5
Milk chocolate with almond nuggets, 4 pieces	5
Milk chocolate with almonds, 1 bar	5
Milk duds, 1 box (52 g)	5
Mini robin eggs, 1 package	5
Miniatures, 5 pieces	4
Nuggets chocolates with raisins and almonds, 4 pieces	5
Nuggets chocolates with toffee and almonds, 4 pieces	5

(POINTS VALUE)

Rolo, 1 package	5
Symphony almond and toffee, 1 bar	5
Symphony milk chocolate, 1 bar	5
Take 5 candy bar, 1 package	5
Whatchamacallit, 1 bar	6

Hershey's Sugar Free

York peppermint pattie, bite sized, 3 pieces	3

Kit Kat

Kit kat, 1 (4-piece bar)	5
Wafer bar, 4-piece, white chocolate, 1 bar	5

M&M's

Dark chocolate candies, 1 bag (47.9 g)	5
Dark chocolate candies, 1/3 cup (1.5 oz)	5
M&M's almond chocolate candies, 1 bag (37.1 g)	5
M&M's almond chocolate candies, 1 1/2 oz	5
M&M's peanut butter chocolate candies, 1 bag (46.2 g)	6
M&M's peanut butter chocolate candies, 1 1/2 oz	5
M&M's peanut chocolate candies, 1 small bag (fun size)	2
M&M's peanut chocolate candies, 1 1/2 oz	5
M&M's peanut chocolate candies, 1 bag (49.3 g)	6
M&M's plain milk chocolate, 1 bag (47.9 g)	5
M&M's plain milk chocolate, 1 1/2 oz	5
M&M's plain milk chocolate, 1 small bag (fun size)	2

	POINTS VALUE
M&M's Minis	
Milk chocolate candies, 1 pack	3
Milk chocolate candies, 1 tube	4
M-AZING	
Chocolate bar with m&m's mini's crunchy chocolate candies, 1 bar	5
Chocolate bar with m&m's minis peanut butter chocolate candies, 1 bar	5
Merci	
Assortment of European chocolates, 3 pieces	6
Milka	
Milk chocolate, 1 serving (33 g)	4
Truffle bar cookies & crème, 1 serving (33 g)	4
Milky Way	
Midnight bar, 5 pieces (miniatures)	4
Midnight bar, 1 bar (singles)	5
Milky way bar, 1 bar (58.1 g)	6
Milky way bar, 1 bar (fun size)	2
Milky way bar, 5 pieces (miniatures)	4
Nestle	
100 grand, 1 bar	4
Baby Ruth, 1	7
Baby Ruth - fun size, 2	3
Baby Ruth sugar free, 1 bar	3
Buncha crunch, 1 bag	4

	POINTS VALUE
Butterfinger, 1	6
Butterfinger - fun size, 1	2
Butterfinger BB's, 1 bag	5
Butterfinger bunny, 1 serving (1.5 oz)	5
Butterfinger crisp mini, 4 bars	5
Butterfinger crisp single, 1 bar	6
Butterfinger heart bag, 5 pieces	4
Butterfinger heart singles, 1 piece	4
Butterfinger pieces in milk chocolate, 1 serving (1/5 bar)	4
Butterfinger pumpkins, 5 pieces	5
Chunky bar, 1	5
Creme eggs - baby ruth, 1	4
Crunch, 1	5
Crunch - fun size, 4	5
Crunch assorted minis, 4 pieces	5
Crunch bunny, 1 serving (1.5 oz)	5
Crunch dark, 1 bar	4
Crunch dark heart, 1 piece	3
Crunch dark stixx, 1 stick	2
Crunch dark with caramel, 1 bar	5
Crunch disk (Easter/Xmas), 1	4
Crunch harvest pumpkins, 5 pieces	4
Crunch heart bag, 5 pieces	4
Crunch heart singles, 1 piece	3
Crunch stixx, 1 stick	2
Crunch sugar free, 4 bars	4

Chocolate Candy, Nestle (con't)	POINTS VALUE
Crunch sugar free, 1 bar	4
Crunch with caramel, 1 bar	5
Crunch with caramel, 2 bars (fun size)	4
Goobers, 1 bag	5
Jingles crunch, 5 pieces	4
Jingles dark chocolate, 5 pieces	5
Jingles milk chocolate, 5 pieces	5
Jingles milk chocolate with butterfingers, 5 pieces	4
Milk chocolate, 1	5
Nesteggs caramel, 5 pieces	5
Nesteggs crunch, 5 pieces	4
Nesteggs dark chocolate, 6 pieces	5
Nesteggs milk chocolate, 5 pieces	5
Nesteggs milk chocolate with butterfingers, 5 pieces	5
Nesteggs peanut butter, 5 pieces	5
Nips, chocolate parfait, 2 pieces	1
Oh Henry!, 1	3
Raisinets, 1 bag	4
Sno caps, 1/4 cup	4
Treasures - chocolate crème, 3 pieces	4
Treasures - peanut butter, 3 pieces	4
Treasures - w/caramel, 3 pieces	4
Turtles, 2 pieces	4
White crunch, 1	5

	POINTS VALUE
Pangburn's	
Millionaires, 2 pieces	4
Peter Paul	
Mounds, 1 package	5
Reese's	
Peanut butter cup, 1 package (2 cups)	5
Pieces, 1 package	5
Reesesticks, 1 package	5
Reese's Sugar Free	
Peanut butter cups, miniature, 5 pieces	3
Riesen	
Chewy chocolate caramel, 4 pieces	4
Russell Stover	
Assorted chocolates, 2 pieces	3
Bite size pecan delight, 3 pieces	4
Cherry cordials, 3 pieces	4
Chocolate covered nuts, 3 pieces	6
Double pecan delight, 2 pieces	5
French chocolate mint bar, 1 piece	6
French chocolate mint box, 4 pieces	5
Milk chocolate butternut toffee sticks, 5 pieces	5
Milk chocolate toffee sticks, 4	6
Mint patties, 3 pieces	4
Pecan delight, 2 pieces	6
Pecan delight bars, 3 pieces	5
Truffle assortment, 3 pieces	6

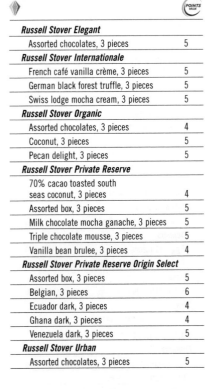

	POINTS VALUE
Russell Stover Elegant	
Assorted chocolates, 3 pieces	5
Russell Stover Internationale	
French café vanilla crème, 3 pieces	5
German black forest truffle, 3 pieces	5
Swiss lodge mocha cream, 3 pieces	5
Russell Stover Organic	
Assorted chocolates, 3 pieces	4
Coconut, 3 pieces	5
Pecan delight, 3 pieces	5
Russell Stover Private Reserve	
70% cacao toasted south seas coconut, 3 pieces	4
Assorted box, 3 pieces	5
Milk chocolate mocha ganache, 3 pieces	5
Triple chocolate mousse, 3 pieces	5
Vanilla bean brulee, 3 pieces	4
Russell Stover Private Reserve Origin Select	
Assorted box, 3 pieces	5
Belgian, 3 pieces	6
Ecuador dark, 3 pieces	4
Ghana dark, 3 pieces	4
Venezuela dark, 3 pieces	5
Russell Stover Urban	
Assorted chocolates, 3 pieces	5

	POINTS VALUE
Snickers	
Snickers almond, 1 bar	5
Snickers almond bar, 1 (fun size)	2
Snickers almond bar, 4 pieces (miniatures)	4
Snickers bar, 4 miniatures	4
Snickers bar, 1 bar (fun size)	2
Snickers bar, 1 bar	7
Snickers bar - dark, 4 pieces (miniatures)	4
Snickers bar - dark, 1 bar (fun size)	2
Snickers bar - dark, 1 bar	6
Terry's	
Milk chocolate orange, 1 serving (44 g)	5
Pure milk chocolate, 1 serving (44 g)	6
Toblerone	
Swiss bittersweet chocolate with honey & almond nougat, 1 serving (33 g)	4
Swiss milk chocolate with honey & almond nougat, 1 serving (33 g)	4
Swiss milk chocolate with honey & almond nougat, 1 serving (40 g)	5
Swiss milk chocolate with honey & almond nougat, 1 (50 g)	6
Swiss milk chocolate with honey & almond nougat, 1 small (35 g)	4
Swiss minis milk chocolate with honey & almond nougat, 1 serving (38 g)	5
Swiss white confection with honey & almond nougat, 1 serving (33 g)	4

Chocolate Candy (con't)	POINTS VALUE

Toffifay	
Caramel/hazelnut/chocolate candy, 5 pieces	5
Tootsie Roll	
Fruit smoothie pops, 1	1
Mini chews, 30 pieces	4
Tootsie roll, 1/2 regular	2
Tootsie roll, 12 small (midgees)	3
Tootsie roll, 6 regular (midgees)	3
Tootsie roll, 1/2 large	3
Tootsie roll, 2 snack bars	2
Tree of Life	
Carob malt balls, 1 serving (40 g)	5
Twix	
Caramel cookie bar, 1 bar (family pack)	3
Caramel cookie bar, 2 bars	7
Caramel cookie bar, 1 bar (fun size)	2
Caramel cookie bar, 3 pieces	3
Peanut butter cookie bar, 2 bars	7
Peanut butter cookie bar, 1 bar (fun size)	2
Peanut butter cookie bar, 1 bar (family pack)	3
Weight Watchers by Whitman's	
Almond nougat, 1 piece	1
Caramel drops, 7 pieces	3
Caramel medallions, 1 piece	1
Coconut, 1 piece	1
Crispy butter cream caramel, 1 piece	1

	POINTS VALUE
Double chocolate mousse, 1 piece	1
English toffee squares, 1 piece	1
Mint patties, 1 piece	1
Nougienuttychew, 1 piece	1
Peanut butter cups, 1 piece	2
Peanut butter crunch, 1 piece	1
Pecan crowns, 1 piece	1
Werther's Original	
Caramel chocolate, 6 pieces	6
Caramel chocolate, dark with 42% cacao, 6 pieces	6
Whitman's	
Assorted sampler, 4 pieces	5
Whitman's Soho	
Assorted chocolates, 3 pieces	5
Whoppers	
Eggs, 31 pieces	4
Malted milk balls, 1 package	5
Wonka	
Wonka bar, 1 bar	6
York	
Peppermint pattie, 1 pattie	3

Coffee Cakes
Entenmann's
Crumb coffee cake, 1 serving (1/10 cake)	6

Little Debbie
Coffee cake (apple streusel), 1	5

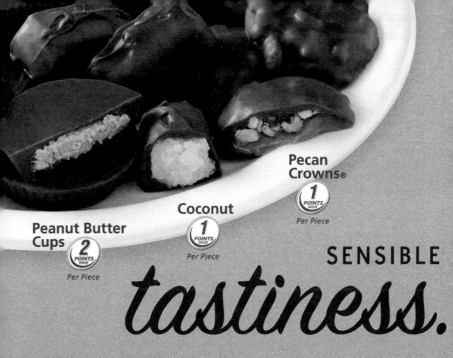

Pecan Crowns®
(1) POINTS VALUE
Per Piece

Coconut
(1) POINTS VALUE
Per Piece

Peanut Butter Cups
(2) POINTS VALUE
Per Piece

SENSIBLE
tastiness.

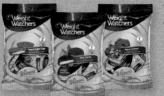

Weight Watchers® by Whitman's® chocolates are deliciou
and a sensible way to satisfy your sweet tooth.

* Individually wrapped
* Made with real *Whitman's* chocolate
* 12 flavors available
* *1-2 POINTS®* value per piece

WeightWatcher
by *Whitman's*

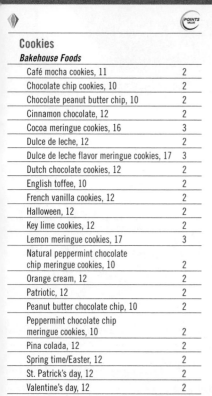

Cookies
Bakehouse Foods

	POINTS VALUE
Café mocha cookies, 11	2
Chocolate chip cookies, 10	2
Chocolate peanut butter chip, 10	2
Cinnamon chocolate, 12	2
Cocoa meringue cookies, 16	3
Dulce de leche, 12	2
Dulce de leche flavor meringue cookies, 17	3
Dutch chocolate cookies, 12	2
English toffee, 10	2
French vanilla cookies, 12	2
Halloween, 12	2
Key lime cookies, 12	2
Lemon meringue cookies, 17	3
Natural peppermint chocolate chip meringue cookies, 10	2
Orange cream, 12	2
Patriotic, 12	2
Peanut butter chocolate chip, 10	2
Peppermint chocolate chip meringue cookies, 10	2
Pina colada, 12	2
Spring time/Easter, 12	2
St. Patrick's day, 12	2
Valentine's day, 12	2

	POINTS VALUE
Vanilla bouquet cookies, 12	2
Vanilla meringue cookies, 17	3
Winter holidays, 12	2

Baker's Breakfast Cookie

Caramel apple, 1	5
Lemon berry, 1	5
Mocha cappuccino, 1	6
Organic breakfast cookie mini, double chocolate chunk, 1	2
Organic breakfast cookie mini, fruit & nut, 1	2
Organic breakfast cookie mini, oatmeal raisin, 1	2
Organic breakfast cookie mini, peanut butter, 1	2

Barbara's Bakery

100 calorie mini cookies, chocolate, 1 package	2
100 calorie mini cookies, ginger, 1 package	2
100 calorie mini cookies, oatmeal, 1 package	2
Fat free wheat free fig bars, 1	1
Fat free wheat free raspberry fig bars, 1	1
Fat free whole wheat apple cinnamon fig bars, 1	1
Fat free whole wheat fig bars, 1	1

	POINTS VALUE
Low fat traditional blueberry fig bars, 1	1
Low fat traditional fig bars, 1	1
Organic animal cookies, vanilla, 10	3
Snackimals animal cookies, chocolate chip, 10	3
Snackimals animal cookies, oatmeal - wheat free, 10	2
Snackimals animal cookies, snickerdoodle, 10	3
Snackimals animal cookies, vanilla, 10	3
Barry's Bakery	
French twist no trans fat American apple pie, 1	1
French twist no trans fat café mocha, 1	1
French twist no trans fat California almond, 1	1
French twist no trans fat chocolate, 1	1
French twist no trans fat chocolate chip, 1	1
French twist no trans fat key lime, 1	1
French twist no trans fat maple French toast, 1	1
French twist no trans fat original, 1	1
French twist no trans fat vanilla, 1	1
French twist no trans fat wild raspberry, 1	1
Merangos, banana, 11	2
Merangos, café mocha, 12	2
Merangos, chocolate, 11	2

	POINTS VALUE
Merangos, chocolate chip, 10	2
Merangos, cinnamon, 11	2
Merangos, coconut, 11	2
Merangos, French vanilla, 12	2
Merangos, mint, 11	2
Merangos, mint chocolate chip, 11	2
Merangos, rainbow, 11	2
Merangos, tropical, 11	2
Merangos, very berry, 11	2
Mini peaks banana, 100 pieces	2
Mini peaks cappuccino, 100 pieces	2
Mini peaks chocolate, 100 pieces	2
Mini peaks chocolate mint, 100 pieces	2
Mini peaks cinnamon, 100 pieces	2
Mini peaks coconut, 100 pieces	2
Mini peaks mint, 100 pieces	2
Mini peaks mint chocolate chip, 100 pieces	2
Mini peaks mocha, 100 pieces	2
Mini peaks rainbow, 100 pieces	2
Mini peaks tropical, 100 pieces	2
Mini peaks vanilla, 100 pieces	2
Mini peaks verry berry, 100 pieces	2
Parisan sweets grande meringues, café mocha, 4	2
Parisan sweets grande meringues, chocolate, 4	2

CANDY, COOKIES & DESSERTS

Cookies, Barry's Bakery (con't)	POINTS VALUE
Parisan sweets grande meringues, key lime, 4	2
Parisan sweets grande meringues, rainbow, 4	2
Parisan sweets grande meringues, vanilla, 4	2
Parisan sweets mini meringues, café mocha, 100	2
Parisan sweets mini meringues, chocolate, 100	2
Parisan sweets mini meringues, key lime, 100	2
Parisan sweets mini meringues, rainbow, 100	2
Parisan sweets mini meringues, vanilla, 100 pieces	2
Parisan sweets petite meringues, café mocha, 12	2
Parisan sweets petite meringues, chocolate, 12	2
Parisan sweets petite meringues, key lime, 12	2
Parisan sweets petite meringues, rainbow, 12	2
Parisan sweets petite meringues, vanilla, 12	2
Breadshop	
Low fat animal cookies, 15	2

	POINTS VALUE
Carr's	
Ginger lemon cremes, 2 pieces	3
Hob nobs, 2 pieces	3
Dove	
Beyond chocolate chunk, 1	3
Chocolate walnut oasis, 1	3
Chocolate walnut rendezvous, 1	3
Milk chocolate moment, 3	4
Mint chocolate seranade, 3	4
Toffee chocolate thrill, 3	4
Dunkaroos	
Cinnamon graham w/vanilla frosting, 1 tray	3
Honey graham cookie with chocolate chips & chocolate frosting, 1 tray	3
Entenmann's	
Original chocolate chip cookies, 3	3
Erin Baker's	
Banana walnut, 1	6
Chocolate chunk raisin, 1	6
Double chocolate chunk, 1	6
Fruit & nut, 1	6
Oatmeal raisin, 1	5
Peanut butter, 1	6
Peanut butter & jelly, 1	6
Vegan peanut butter chocolate chunk, 1	7

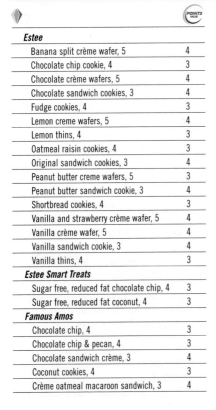

	POINTS VALUE
Estee	
Banana split crème wafer, 5	4
Chocolate chip cookie, 4	3
Chocolate crème wafers, 5	4
Chocolate sandwich cookies, 3	4
Fudge cookies, 4	3
Lemon creme wafers, 5	4
Lemon thins, 4	3
Oatmeal raisin cookies, 4	3
Original sandwich cookies, 3	4
Peanut butter creme wafers, 5	3
Peanut butter sandwich cookie, 3	4
Shortbread cookies, 4	3
Vanilla and strawberry crème wafer, 5	4
Vanilla crème wafer, 5	4
Vanilla sandwich cookie, 3	4
Vanilla thins, 4	3
Estee Smart Treats	
Sugar free, reduced fat chocolate chip, 4	3
Sugar free, reduced fat coconut, 4	3
Famous Amos	
Chocolate chip, 4	3
Chocolate chip & pecan, 4	3
Chocolate sandwich crème, 3	4
Coconut cookies, 4	3
Crème oatmeal macaroon sandwich, 3	4

	POINTS VALUE
Crème vanilla sandwich, 3	4
Lemon, 5	3
Oatmeal chocolate chip & walnut, 4	3
Oatmeal raisin, 4	3
Sandwich crème peanut butter, 3	4
Vanilla animal cookies, 10	3
Gamesa	
Animalitos cookies, 14	2
Arcoiris marshmallow cookies, 1 package	4
Barras de coco coconut cookies, 5	2
Chocolate sugar wafers, 3	4
Chocolatines marshmallow cookies, 2	3
Emperador chocolate crème sandwich cookies, 2	3
Emperador combinado crème sandwich cookies, 2	3
Emperador limon crème sandwich cookies, 3	3
Emperador strawberry crème sandwich cookies, 2	3
Emperador vanilla crème sandwich cookies, 2	3
Grageas cookies with sprinkles, 11	3
Hawaianas coconut cookies, 3	3
Mamut chocolate marshmallow cookies, 1	3
Marias cookies, 8	2
Merengue marshmallow cookies, 3	2

CANDY, COOKIES & DESSERTS

Cookies, Gamesa (con't)	POINTS VALUE
Pineapple fruitbars cookies, 1	2
Piruetas lime sandwich cookies, 3	3
Populares cookies, 4	2
Ricanelas cinnamon graham cookies, 8	3
Roscas cinnamon cookies, 3	3
Strawberry fruitbars cookies, 1	3
Strawberry sugar wafers, 3	3
Vanilla sugar wafers, 3	4
Grandma's	
Homestyle lemon iced big cookies, 1	4
Homestyle sugar big cookies, 1	4
Limited edition holiday cinnamon sugar flavored big cookies, 1	4
Limited edition holiday gingerbread flavored big cookies, 1	3
Peanut butter sandwich crème, 5	5
Rich n' chewy chocolate chip, soft, 1 package	6
Vanilla mini sandwich cookies, 9	3
Vanilla sandwich crème, 5	5
Grandma's Homestyle Big Cookies	
Chocolate chip, 1	5
Fudge chocolate chip, 1	4
Oatmeal raisin, 1	4
Peanut butter, 1	4
Hain Pure Foods	
Low fat vanilla animal cookies, 10	3

	POINTS VALUE
Health Valley	
Chocolate mint sandwich cookies, 2	3
Chocolate sandwich cookies, 2	3
Double chocolate chunk cookies, 1	3
Double chocolate sandwich cookies, 2	3
Low fat healthy chips double chocolate, 3	2
Low fat raisin oatmeal, 3	2
Mini chocolate chip cookies, 4	3
Mini chocolate chocolate chip cookies, 4	3
Mini peanut butter cookies, 4	3
Oatmeal cookies, chocolate chip, 1	2
Oatmeal cookies, peanut, 1	2
Vanilla flavored sandwich cookies, 2	3
Hershey's	
Peanut butter snack barz, 1 bar	6
Ian's	
Organic chocolate chip cookie buttons, 1 serving (23 g)	2
Organic double chocolate chip cookie buttons, 1 serving (23 g)	2
Wheat free/gluten free chocolate chip cookie buttons, 1 serving (30 g)	3
Wheat free/gluten free crunchy cinnamon cookie buttons, 1 serving (30 g)	3
Joseph's Sugar Free Cookies	
Almond, 4	2
Chocolate chip, 4	2

	POINTS VALUE
Chocolate peanut butter, 4	2
Chocolate raspberry bite size cake, 4	2
Chocolate walnut, 4	2
Coconut, 4	2
Lemon, 4	2
Oatmeal, 4	2
Oatmeal chocolate chip with pecans, 4	2
Peanut butter, 4	2
Pecan chocolate chip, 4	2
Pecan shortbread, 4	2
Kashi	
Happy trail mix, 1	2
Oatmeal dark chocolate, 1	2
Oatmeal raisin flax, 1	2
Keebler	
Animal cookies - frosted, 8	4
Bug bites cinnamon grahams, 13	3
Chips deluxe chocolate lovers, 1	2
Chips deluxe coconut, 2	4
Chips deluxe fudge striped caramel chip, 1	3
Chips deluxe fudge striped original, 1	3
Chips deluxe original, 2	4
Chips deluxe peanut butter chocolate, 1	2
Chips deluxe peanut butter cups, 1	2
Chips deluxe rainbow, 1	2
Chips deluxe rainbow, bite size, 1 package	5

	POINTS VALUE
Chips deluxe soft n' chewy, 1	2
Country style oatmeal with raisins, 2	3
Dunking delights chocolate sandwich with vanilla crème, 1	2
Dunking delights graham sandwich with cheesecake crème, 1	2
E.L. fudge butter fudge crème, 1	2
EL fudge, original double stuffed, 2	4
Fudge shoppe caramel filled, 2	4
Fudge shoppe deluxe grahams, 3 pieces	3
Fudge shoppe fudge sticks, 3	4
Fudge shoppe fudge stripes, 3	3
Fudge shoppe fudge stripes white, 3	4
Fudge shoppe fudge stripes, mini, 1 package	5
Fudge shoppe grasshopper fudge mint, 4	3
Fudge shoppe merry mint patties holiday, 2	3
Fudge shoppe mint crème filled, 2	4
Fudge shoppe peanut butter filled, 2	4
Fudge shoppe, filled triple fudge, 2	4
Gripz chips deluxe chocolate chip cookies, 1 pouch	3
Gripz chips deluxe cookies, 1 pouch	3
Gripz double chocolate chip bites, 1 pouch	3
Honey grahams scooby-doo bones, 9	3
Right bites chips deluxe, 1 pouch	2
Right bites cinnamon grahams, 1 pouch	2

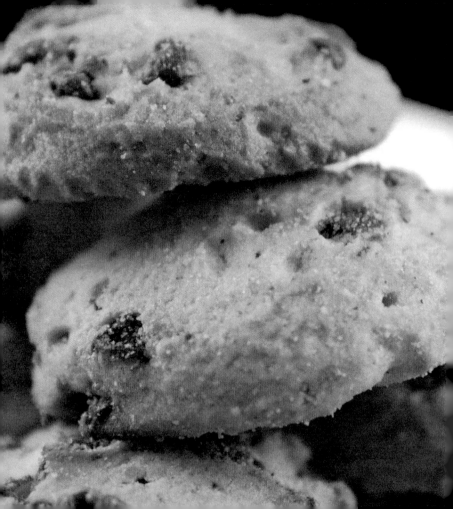

Cookies, Keebler (con't)

	POINTS VALUE
Right bites mini fudge stripes, 1 pouch	2
Right bites mini mints grasshopper, 1 pouch	2
Right bites sandies shortbread, 1 pouch	2
Sandies butter pecan drops, 4	3
Sandies fudge drops, 4	3
Sandies, chocolate chip and pecan shortbread, 2	4
Sandies, pecan shortbread, 2	4
Sandies, reduced fat pecan shortbread, 2	4
Sandies, simply shortbread, 2	4
Scooby-doo bones, graham cracker sticks cinnamon, 9	3
Soft batch chocolate chunk, 1	7
Soft batch oatmeal raisin, 1	2
Soft batch peanut butter, 1	2
Soft batch, chocolate chip, 1	2
Vanilla wafers, 8	3
Vanilla wafers mini, 18	3
Vienna fingers, 2	3
Vienna fingers, reduced fat, 2	3

Kraft

	POINTS VALUE
Cameo crème sandwich cookies, 1 serving (31 g)	4
Cameo crème sandwich cookies, 1 package (4-count)	6
Cameo crème sandwich cookies - mini, 9	3
Cameo crème sandwich cookies - mini, 1 package	4

	POINTS VALUE
South beach diet cookies - oatmeal chocolate chip, 2	2
South beach diet cookies - oatmeal chocolate chip, 1 package	2
South beach diet cookies - peanut butter, 2	2
South beach diet cookies - peanut butter, 1 package	2

Kraft Handi-Snacks

	POINTS VALUE
Teddy grahams bearwiches - honey, 1 serving (26 g)	3

Lance

	POINTS VALUE
Bite size chocolate chip cookies, 4	3
Choc-o-lunch, 6	4
Choc-o-lunch, 5 small	4
Lem-o-lunch, 5	5
Malt, 6	4
Nut-o-lunch, 5	4
Oatmeal crèmes, 1 small	5
Oatmeal crèmes, 1	7
Peanut butter crème filled wafer, 1 package	7
Peanut butter crème filled wafer, 1 bar	5
Peanut butter nekot, 6	6
Strawberry creme filled vanilla cookies, 5	5
Strawberry crème filled wafers, 4	4
Vanilla crème filled wafers, 4	4
Van-o-lunch, 5 small	5
Van-o-lunch, 6	5

CANDY, COOKIES & DESSERTS

Cookies (con't)	POINTS VALUE
Little Debbie	
Apple flips, 1	3
Caramel cookie bars, 1	4
Cherry cordials (Christmas & Valentine), 1	4
Chocolate chip creme pies, 1	4
Christmas gingerbread cookies, 1	2
Cookie wreaths cookies, 1	2
Easter marshmallow treats, 1 bar	2
Easter puffs cookies, 1	3
Fall marshmallow treats, 1 bar	2
Fig bars, 1	3
Fudge rounds, 1	3
German chocolate cookie rings with caramel & coconut, 1	3
Gingerbread cookies, 1	2
Holiday marshmallow treats, 1 bar	2
Jelly crème pies, 1	4
Marshmallow pie, banana, 1	4
Marshmallow pie, banana, single serve, 1	4
Marshmallow pie, chocolate, single serve, 1	4
Marshmallow pie, chocolate flavored, 1	4
Marshmallow supremes, 1	3
Marshmallow treat, single serve, 1 bar	4
Marshmallow treats, 1 bar	2
Nutty bar singles, 1	3
Nutty bar thins, 2	5

	POINTS VALUE
Nutty bars wafer bars, 2	8
Oatmeal creme pies, 1	4
P.b. & j. oatmeal pies, 1	3
Pumpkin delights filled cookies, 1	3
Raisin crème pies, 1	4
Smores cookie, 1	4
Snow puffs, 1	2
Spirit of America marshmallow treats, 1 bar	2
Star crunch cosmic snacks, 1	3
Stars & stripes marshmallow puffs, 1	4
Sugar free wafers (chocolate crème filled), 3	4
Sugar free wafers (crème filled), 3	4
Sugar free wafers (strawberry crème filled), 3	4
Manischewitz	
Almond biscotti, 2	2
Coconut macaroons - sugar free, 2	1
Market Day	
Chocolate chip cookie dough, 2	3
Chocolate chip cookie meltdown, 1	12
Trail mix breakfast cookies, 1	4
Mi-Del	
Arrowroot cookies, 14	2
Chocolate chip, 4	3
Chocolate mint, 3	3
Chocolate snaps, 5	3

	POINTS VALUE		POINTS VALUE
Double chocolate, 3	3	Creamsicle, 13	2
Ginger snaps, 4	2	Fat free chocolate mini cookies, 13	2
Gluten free cinnamon snaps, 4	3	Fat free vanilla, 13	2
Gluten free ginger snaps, 5	3	Low fat mint chocolate chip, 12	2
Lemon snaps, 5	3	Peppermint crush, 9	2
Mini pecan cookies, 4	3	Rainbow vanilla, 13	2
Oatmeal raisin snaps, 4	3	Watermelon, 13	2
Organic ginger snaps, 5	3	**Miss Meringue Sugar Free**	
Organic vanilla snaps, 5	3	Chocolate meringue cookies, 13	0
Royal vanilla, 3	3	Vanilla meringue cookies, 13	0
Vanilla snaps, 5	3	**Mrs. Denson's**	
Wheat free chocolate sandwich cookies, 3	3	Organic chocolate chip cookies, 1	2
Miss Meringue		Organic oatmeal raisin cookies, 1	2
Fat free cappuccino, 4	2	Wheat free chocolate chip macaroon, 1	3
Fat free vanilla, 4	2	Wheat free oatmeal raisin cookies, 1	2
Fat free vanilla rainbow, 4	2	Wheat free quinoa macaroon, 1	2
Low fat chocolate chip, 4	2	**Mrs. Freshleys Snackaway**	
Low fat mint chocolate chip, 4	2	Peanut butter wafer bars, 1	3
Low fat triple chocolate chip, 4	2	Yogurt filled oatmeal crème cookies, 1	2
Miss Meringue Chocolettes		**Murray**	
Chocolaty crunch, 8	3	Sugar free chocolate chip, 3	4
Mint, 10	3	Sugar free chocolate chip with pecans, 3	4
Strawberry vanilla, 10	3	Sugar free double fudge, 3	4
Vanilla, 10	3	Sugar free fudge dipped grahams, 4	3
Miss Meringue Minis		Sugar free fudge dipped mint, 4	3
Apple spice, 13	2	Sugar free fudge dipped shortbread, 5	3
Chocolate chip, 12	3	Sugar free fudge dipped wafers, 4	3

CANDY, COOKIES & DESSERTS

Cookies, Murray (con't) POINTS VALUE

Sugar free gingersnaps, 7	3
Sugar free oatmeal, 3	3
Sugar free peanut butter, 3	4
Sugar free pecan shortbread, 3	4
Sugar free sandwich crème chocolate, 3	3
Sugar free sandwich crème lemon, 3	3
Sugar free sandwich crème vanilla, 3	3
Sugar free shortbread, 8	3
Sugar free vanilla wafer, 9	3
Sugar free wafer duplex, 5	3
Sugar free wafers - lemon, 4	2
Sugar free wafers - vanilla, 4	2
Sugar wafers - peanut butter, 5	4
Sugar wafers - strawberry, 5	3
Sugar wafers - vanilla, 5	3

Nabisco

Biscos sugar wafers, 1 serving (28 g)	3
Biscos waffle cremes, 4 (34 g)	4
Chips ahoy, 3	4
Chips ahoy cookie barz, 1	4
Chips ahoy, candy blasts, 1 serving (15 g)	2
Chips ahoy, chewy real chocolate chip, 1 serving (27 g)	3
Chips ahoy, mini chocolate chip bite-size go-pak, 1 package (35 g)	4
Chips ahoy, mini chocolate chip bite-size go-pak, 1 serving (31 g)	3

POINTS VALUE

Chips ahoy, reduced-fat, 3	3
Chips ahoy, soft baked chunky chocolate chip, 1 serving (28 g)	3
Famous chocolate wafers, 1 serving (32 g)	3
Fig newtons, 2	2
Fig newtons fat free fruit chewy cookies, 2	2
Ginger snaps, 1 serving (28 g)	3
Golden oreo crème sandwich cookies - original crème, 1 package (51 g)	6
Honey maid cookies - oatmeal, 3	3
Honey maid cookies - oatmeal raisin, 3	3
Honey maid cookies - oatmeal raisin mini, 1 package (56 g)	5
Honey maid graham bars - banana flavored, 1	3
Lorna doone shortbread cookies, 1 serving (29 g)	3
Lorna doone shortbread cookies, 1 package (28 g)	3
Lorna doone shortbread cookies, 1 package (42 g)	5
Mallomars pure chocolate cookies, 1 serving (28 g)	3
Newtons fruit chewy cookies - fig, 1 package (28 g)	2
Newtons fruit chewy cookies – fig, fat free, 1 (30 g)	2
Newtons fruit chewy cookies - fig, 100% whole grain, 2 (31 g)	2

	POINTS VALUE
Newtons snackable dessert cookies - strawberry shortcake, 2 (36 g)	3
Nilla wafers, 1 serving (30 g)	3
Nutter butter bites sandwich cookies - peanut butter, 1 package (42 g)	5
Nutter butter patties - peanut crème, 5	4
Nutter butter sandwich bites, 1 serving (35 g)	4
Nutter butter sandwich bites go-pak, 1 serving (30 g)	3
Nutter butter sandwich bites snak saks, 1 serving (49 g)	5
Nutter butter sandwich cookies, 1 serving (28 g)	3
Nutter butter sandwich cookies, 1 package (53 g)	6
Oreo, 3	4
Oreo chocolate crème mini, 1 serving (35 g)	4
Oreo chocolate crème mini, 1 serving (43 g)	5
Oreo chocolate crème mini snak saks, 1 serving (29 g)	3
Oreo chocolate fudge covered sandwich cookies, 1 serving (19 g)	2
Oreo chocolate mini bite size, 1 serving (35 g)	4
Oreo chocolate mini bite size go-pak, 1 serving (29 g)	3

	POINTS VALUE
Oreo chocolate mini bite size packs 2 go, 1 serving (42 g)	4
Oreo chocolate sandwich cookies, 1 package (2 count)	2
Oreo chocolate sandwich cookies, 1 serving (57 g)	6
Oreo chocolate sandwich cookies - double delight peanut butter 'n, 2 (29 g)	3
Oreo chocolate sandwich cookies - double stuff smilin', 2 (29 g)	3
Oreo chocolate sandwich cookies - mini chocolate crème, 1 package (50 g)	5
Oreo chocolate sandwich cookies - mini white crème, 1 package (49 g)	5
Oreo chocolate sandwich cookies - sugar free, 2	2
Oreo cookie barz, 1	4
Oreo double delight mint'n crème sandwich cookies, 1 serving (29 g)	3
Oreo double stuff packs 2 go, 1 serving (42 g)	5
Oreo double stuff sandwich cookies, 1 serving (29 g)	3
Oreo double stuff sandwich cookies- chocolate crème, 1 package	2
Oreo double stuff sandwich cookies- chocolate crème, 2	3
Oreo golden original sandwich cookies, 1 serving (35 g)	4

CANDY, COOKIES & DESSERTS

Cookies, Nabisco (con't)	POINTS VALUE
Oreo golden with chocolate creme sandwich cookies, 1 serving (35 g)	4
Oreo Halloween orange creme sandwich cookies, 1 serving (29 g)	3
Oreo mini bite size snak saks, 1 serving (28 g)	3
Oreo spring purple creme sandwich cookies, 1 serving (29 g)	3
Raspberry newtons, 2	2
Social tea biscuits, 1 serving (31 g)	3
Soft cookies - chips ahoy, 1	4
Strawberry newtons, 2	2
Twirls, marshmallow fudge, 1 serving (30 g)	3
Nabisco 100 Calorie Packs	
Chips ahoy, thin crisps, 1 package	2
Oreo thins, 1 package	2
Nabisco SnackWell's	
Chocolate chip, 3	3
Crème sandwich, 1 package	5
Crème sandwich, 2	2
Sandwich cookies - crème, 1 package	2
Sugar free lemon creme, 3	3
Sugar free shortbread, 3	3
Nabisco Teddy Grahams	
Graham snacks - chocolate, 1 package	2
O'coco's	
Cinnamon organic chocolate crisps, 1 container	2

	POINTS VALUE
Mocha organic chocolate crisps, 1 container	2
Original organic chocolate crisps, 1 container	2
Organica Foods	
Double chocolate coffee toffee, 2	3
Ginger snaps, 3	2
Gingered walnut cherry chocolate chip, 2	3
Iced shortbread, lemon shortbread with lemon tangerine icing, 3	3
Lemon poppyseed snaps, 3	2
Oatmeal coconut cranberry chocolate chip, 2	2
Peanut butter almond chocolate chip, 2	3
Snickerdoodle snaps, 3	2
Otis Express Supreme Indulgence	
Honey nut chocolate buzz, 1/2	4
Lemon white chunk, 1/2	4
Otis Express Sweet Discovery	
All American, 1	4
Boo-licious, 1	3
Yogurt raisin sensation, 1	4
Otis Express Sweet Discovery Reduced Fat	
Butter sugar cookie, 1	3
Carnival cookie, 1	3
Oatmeal raisin, 1	3
Otis Express Value Zone Reduced Fat	
100% whole grain chocolate brownie cookie, 1	4

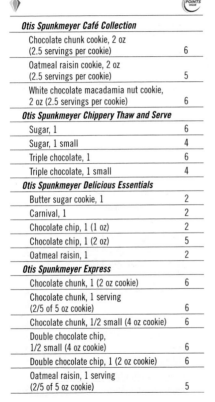

	POINTS VALUE
Otis Spunkmeyer Café Collection	
Chocolate chunk cookie, 2 oz (2.5 servings per cookie)	6
Oatmeal raisin cookie, 2 oz (2.5 servings per cookie)	5
White chocolate macadamia nut cookie, 2 oz (2.5 servings per cookie)	6
Otis Spunkmeyer Chippery Thaw and Serve	
Sugar, 1	6
Sugar, 1 small	4
Triple chocolate, 1	6
Triple chocolate, 1 small	4
Otis Spunkmeyer Delicious Essentials	
Butter sugar cookie, 1	2
Carnival, 1	2
Chocolate chip, 1 (1 oz)	2
Chocolate chip, 1 (2 oz)	5
Oatmeal raisin, 1	2
Otis Spunkmeyer Express	
Chocolate chunk, 1 (2 oz cookie)	6
Chocolate chunk, 1 serving (2/5 of 5 oz cookie)	6
Chocolate chunk, 1/2 small (4 oz cookie)	6
Double chocolate chip, 1/2 small (4 oz cookie)	6
Double chocolate chip, 1 (2 oz cookie)	6
Oatmeal raisin, 1 serving (2/5 of 5 oz cookie)	5

	POINTS VALUE
Oatmeal raisin, 1/2 small (4 oz cookie)	5
Oatmeal raisin, 1 (2 oz cookie)	5
Peanut butter, 1/2 small (4 oz cookie)	6
Peanut butter, 1 (2 oz cookie)	6
White chunk macadamia nut, 1 (2 oz cookie)	6
White chunk macadamia nut, 1/2 small (4 oz cookie)	6
White chunk macadamia nut, 1 serving (2/5 of 5 oz cookie)	6
Otis Spunkmeyer Otis Express	
Chocolate chunk, 1	6
Double chocolate chip, 1	6
Oatmeal raisin, 1	5
Peanut butter, 1	6
Otis Spunkmeyer Spunkies Sweet Discovery	
Chocolate chip, 4	3
Peanut butter, 4	3
Otis Spunkmeyer Sugar Free	
Chocolate chip cookie, 1	3
Double chocolate cookie, 1	2
Lemon cookie, 1	3
Otis Spunkmeyer Supreme Indulgence	
Buttery pecan decadence, 1/2 (1.5 oz)	4
Buttery pecan decadence, 1/2 (2 oz)	6
Chocolate peanut butter flutter, 1 (2 oz)	6
Chocolate peanut butter flutter, 1/2 (1.5 oz)	4

Cookies, Otis Spunkmeyer Supreme Indulgence (con't)	POINTS VALUE
Chunky chocolate supreme, 1/2 (2 oz)	6
Chunky chocolate supreme, 1(2 oz)	6
Chunky chocolate supreme, 1/2 (1.5 oz)	4
Cranberry white chocolate duo, 1/2 (1.5 oz)	4
Double chunky chocolate dream, 1/2 (1.5 oz)	4
Lemon white chunk, 1/2 (2 oz)	6
Nutty white chocolate delight, 1/2 (1.5 oz)	5
Nutty white chocolate delight, 1 (2 oz)	6
Oatmeal cinnaraisin cravin', 1/2 (1.5 oz)	4
Oatmeal cinnaraisin cravin', 1/2 (2 oz)	5
Oatmeal cinnaraisin cravin', 1 (2 oz)	5
Shortbread, 1/2 (1.5 oz)	10

Otis Spunkmeyer Sweet Discovery

	POINTS VALUE
All American, 1	4
Apple cinnamon raisin breakfast cookie, 1	3
Apple cinnamount, 1	4
Boo-licious, 1	3
Butter sugar, 1 (2 oz)	6
Butter sugar, 1 bite size	2
Butter sugar, 1 (1.3 oz)	4
Butter sugar, 1/2 (2 oz)	6
Buttercrunch toffee, 1 (1.3 oz)	4
Buttercrunch toffee, 1(2 oz)	6
Buttercrunch toffee, 1/2 small (2 oz)	6
Café vienna, 1	4
Carnival, 1(1.3 oz)	4

	POINTS VALUE
Carnival, 1(2 oz)	6
Carnival, 1/2 (2 oz)	6
Chocolate chip, 1 (1.3 oz)	4
Chocolate chip, 1/2 (2 oz)	6
Chocolate chip, 1 bite size	2
Chocolate chip, 1 (2 oz)	6
Chocolate chip, 1 (3 oz)	8
Chocolate chip pecan, 1	4
Chocolate chip walnut, 1 (2 oz)	6
Chocolate chip walnut, 1 (1.3 oz)	4
Chocolate obsession, 1	4
Chocolate with reese's pieces, 1	4
Cranberry oatmeal, 1	3
Double chocolate brownie cookie, 1	4
Double chocolate chip, 1/2	6
Double chocolate chip, 1 (1.3 oz)	4
Double chocolate chip, 1 bite size	2
Double chocolate chip, 1 (2 oz)	6
Holiday carnival, 1	4
Milk chocolate chunk, 1 (1.3 oz)	4
Milk chocolate chunk, 1 (2 oz)	6
Oatmeal raisin, 1 (85 g)	7
Oatmeal raisin, 1 bite size	2
Oatmeal raisin, 1 (1.3 oz)	3
Oatmeal raisin, 1/2 (2 oz)	5
Oatmeal raisin, 1 (2 oz)	5
Peanut butter, 1 (85 g)	9

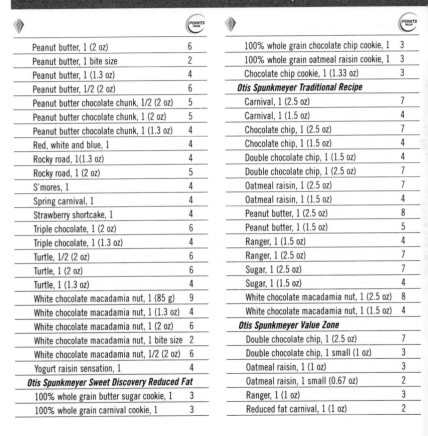

	POINTS VALUE
Peanut butter, 1 (2 oz)	6
Peanut butter, 1 bite size	2
Peanut butter, 1 (1.3 oz)	4
Peanut butter, 1/2 (2 oz)	6
Peanut butter chocolate chunk, 1/2 (2 oz)	5
Peanut butter chocolate chunk, 1 (2 oz)	5
Peanut butter chocolate chunk, 1 (1.3 oz)	4
Red, white and blue, 1	4
Rocky road, 1(1.3 oz)	4
Rocky road, 1 (2 oz)	5
S'mores, 1	4
Spring carnival, 1	4
Strawberry shortcake, 1	4
Triple chocolate, 1 (2 oz)	6
Triple chocolate, 1 (1.3 oz)	4
Turtle, 1/2 (2 oz)	6
Turtle, 1 (2 oz)	6
Turtle, 1 (1.3 oz)	4
White chocolate macadamia nut, 1 (85 g)	9
White chocolate macadamia nut, 1 (1.3 oz)	4
White chocolate macadamia nut, 1 (2 oz)	6
White chocolate macadamia nut, 1 bite size	2
White chocolate macadamia nut, 1/2 (2 oz)	6
Yogurt raisin sensation, 1	4

Otis Spunkmeyer Sweet Discovery Reduced Fat

	POINTS VALUE
100% whole grain butter sugar cookie, 1	3
100% whole grain carnival cookie, 1	3
100% whole grain chocolate chip cookie, 1	3
100% whole grain oatmeal raisin cookie, 1	3
Chocolate chip cookie, 1 (1.33 oz)	3

Otis Spunkmeyer Traditional Recipe

	POINTS VALUE
Carnival, 1 (2.5 oz)	7
Carnival, 1 (1.5 oz)	4
Chocolate chip, 1 (2.5 oz)	7
Chocolate chip, 1 (1.5 oz)	4
Double chocolate chip, 1 (1.5 oz)	4
Double chocolate chip, 1 (2.5 oz)	7
Oatmeal raisin, 1 (2.5 oz)	7
Oatmeal raisin, 1 (1.5 oz)	4
Peanut butter, 1 (2.5 oz)	8
Peanut butter, 1 (1.5 oz)	5
Ranger, 1 (1.5 oz)	4
Ranger, 1 (2.5 oz)	7
Sugar, 1 (2.5 oz)	7
Sugar, 1 (1.5 oz)	4
White chocolate macadamia nut, 1 (2.5 oz)	8
White chocolate macadamia nut, 1 (1.5 oz)	4

Otis Spunkmeyer Value Zone

	POINTS VALUE
Double chocolate chip, 1 (2.5 oz)	7
Double chocolate chip, 1 small (1 oz)	3
Oatmeal raisin, 1 (1 oz)	3
Oatmeal raisin, 1 small (0.67 oz)	2
Ranger, 1 (1 oz)	3
Reduced fat carnival, 1 (1 oz)	2

CANDY, COOKIES & DESSERTS

Cookies, Otis Spunkmeyer Value Zone (con't)	POINTS VALUE
Reduced fat chocolate chip, 1 (1 oz)	2
Reduced fat oatmeal raisin, 1 (1 oz)	2
Reduced fat sugar, 1 (1 oz)	2
Otis Spunkmeyer Value Zone Reduced Fat	
100% whole grain chocolate brownie cookie, 1	2
100% whole grain chocolate chip cookie, 1	2
100% whole grain oatmeal raisin cookie, 1	2
Payaso	
Animal cookies, 15	2
Maria cookies, 8	3
Peek Freans	
Cinnamon crisp, 3	4
Crème biscuits - bourbon, 2	3
Digestive, 3	4
Digestive family, 2	4
Family shortcake (fudge covered shortcake), 2	3
Garden, 2	4
Orange blossom, 3	3
Pecan passion, 2	4
Toffee crisp, 3	4
Pepperidge Farm	
Bordeaux cookies, 4	3
Brussels cookies, 3	3
Butter chessmen cookies, 3	3
Chocolate hazelnut creme-filled pirouettes, 2	3

	POINTS VALUE
Dark chocolate chunk soft baked Nantucket cookies, 1	4
Milano cookies, 3	4
Milk chocolate macadamia soft baked cookies, 1	4
Mini Milano cookies, 6	4
Mini mint Milano cookies, 6	4
Mini Sausalito cookies, 4	4
Mint milano cookies, 2	3
Nantucket chocolate chunk cookies, 1	3
Sausalito chocolate chunk cookies, 1	3
Perfect Bite Cookies	
Sugar free chocolate chip, 3	2
Sugar free lemon, 3	2
Sugar free oatmeal, 3	2
Sugar free peanut butter, 3	2
Pillsbury	
Holiday shapes (sugar), 2	3
Sugar cookie dough sheets, 1 serving (1/12 package)	4
Pillsbury Create 'N Bake	
Chocolate chip cookies, 1 ball	3
Chocolate chip walnut cookies, 1 ball	3
Double chocolate chip & chip cookies, 1 ball	3
Oatmeal chocolate chip cookies, 1 ball	3
Peanut butter cookies, 1 ball	3
Sugar cookies, 1 slice	3

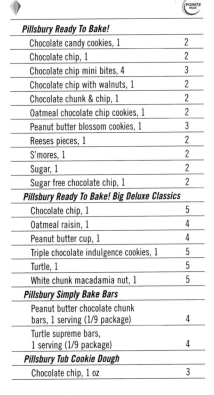

	POINTS VALUE
Pillsbury Ready To Bake!	
Chocolate candy cookies, 1	2
Chocolate chip, 1	2
Chocolate chip mini bites, 4	3
Chocolate chip with walnuts, 1	2
Chocolate chunk & chip, 1	2
Oatmeal chocolate chip cookies, 1	2
Peanut butter blossom cookies, 1	3
Reeses pieces, 1	2
S'mores, 1	2
Sugar, 1	2
Sugar free chocolate chip, 1	2
Pillsbury Ready To Bake! Big Deluxe Classics	
Chocolate chip, 1	5
Oatmeal raisin, 1	4
Peanut butter cup, 1	4
Triple chocolate indulgence cookies, 1	5
Turtle, 1	5
White chunk macadamia nut, 1	5
Pillsbury Simply Bake Bars	
Peanut butter chocolate chunk bars, 1 serving (1/9 package)	4
Turtle supreme bars, 1 serving (1/9 package)	4
Pillsbury Tub Cookie Dough	
Chocolate chip, 1 oz	3

	POINTS VALUE
Quaker Oats Breakfast Cookie	
Apple cinnamon, 1	3
Oatmeal raisin, 1	3
Rocks n' Rolls	
Almond French munching cookies, 1 serving (30 g)	2
Chocolate French munching cookies, 1 serving (30 g)	2
Cinnamon French munching cookies, 1 serving (30 g)	2
Lemon & vanilla French munching cookies, 1 serving (30 g)	2
Orange chocolate chip French munching cookies, 1 serving (30 g)	2
Praline French munching cookies, 1 serving (30 g)	2
Raspberry chocolate chip French munching cookies, 1 serving (30 g)	2
Santa Fe Farms Fat Free Cookies	
Chocolate chocolate chip, 4	1
Chocolate mint chip, 4	1
Ginger, 4	1
Stella D'oro	
Almond delight cookies, 1 serving (30 g)	4
Almond toast cookies, 1 serving (27 g)	2
Angel wings cookies, 1 serving (30 g)	4
Anginetti cookies, 1 serving (30 g)	3

Cookies, Stella D'oro (con't)	POINTS VALUE
Anisette sponge cookies, 1 serving (25 g)	2
Anisette toast, 1 serving (34 g)	3
Banana walnut toast cookies, 1 serving (26 g)	2
Biscotti, almond, 1 serving (20 g)	2
Biscotti, chocolate almond, 1 serving (20 g)	2
Biscotti, chocolate chunk, 1 serving (20 g)	2
Biscotti, French vanilla, 1 serving (20 g)	2
Blueberry toast cookies, 1 serving (26 g)	2
Breakfast treats, chocolate, 1 serving (23 g)	2
Breakfast treats, mini, original, 1 serving (28 g)	3
Breakfast treats, original, 1 serving (23 g)	2
Cinnamon raisin toast cookies, 1 serving (26 g)	2
Egg jumbo cookies, 1 serving (33 g)	3
Holiday fruit slices, 2 (33 g)	3
Lady stella cookie assortment, 3 (28 g)	3
Margherite, 2 (29 g)	3
Margherite cookies, mini, 1 serving (34 g)	3
Mini anisette toast cookies, 1 serving (34 g)	3
Roman egg biscuits, 1 serving (32 g)	3
Swiss fudge, 3 (34 g)	4
Viennese cinnamon breakfast treats, 1 serving (22 g)	2

	POINTS VALUE
Stella D'oro Holiday	
Pfeffernusse spice drops, 1 serving (25 g)	2
Tree of Life	
Coconut macaroon, unsulphured, 1 oz	4
Walkers	
Pure butter chocolate chip shortbread, 2 pieces	3
Pure butter shortbread, 1 piece	3
Pure butter shortbread rounds, 1 piece	2
Pure butter shortbread triangles, 2 pieces	3
Weight Watchers	
Chocolate chip soft cookies, 1	1
Oatmeal raisin soft cookies, 1	1
Whitman's	
Chocolate chip cookies, 1	1
Oatmeal raisin cookies, 1	1

Crackers
Nabisco Teddy Grahams

Graham snacks - chocolate, 1 package	3
Graham snacks - chocolate, 24 pieces	3
Graham snacks - cinnamon, 1 package	2
Graham snacks - honey, 2 packages	3

Peek Freans

Signature ovals - sesame, 5	1

SMART

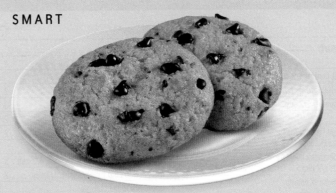

Chocolate Chip
Soft Cookies

1 POINTS value Per Cookie

sweetness.

Under 100
Calories

Good Source
of Fiber

Two Great
Flavors

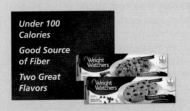

It's true! These tasty cookies filled
with real chocolate chips are a
smart and sensible snack choice.

WeightWatchers

**Go to WeightWatchers.com/cookies
for more information.**

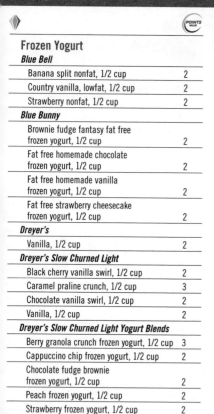

	POINTS VALUE
Frozen Yogurt	
Blue Bell	
Banana split nonfat, 1/2 cup	2
Country vanilla, lowfat, 1/2 cup	2
Strawberry nonfat, 1/2 cup	2
Blue Bunny	
Brownie fudge fantasy fat free frozen yogurt, 1/2 cup	2
Fat free homemade chocolate frozen yogurt, 1/2 cup	2
Fat free homemade vanilla frozen yogurt, 1/2 cup	2
Fat free strawberry cheesecake frozen yogurt, 1/2 cup	2
Dreyer's	
Vanilla, 1/2 cup	2
Dreyer's Slow Churned Light	
Black cherry vanilla swirl, 1/2 cup	2
Caramel praline crunch, 1/2 cup	3
Chocolate vanilla swirl, 1/2 cup	2
Vanilla, 1/2 cup	2
Dreyer's Slow Churned Light Yogurt Blends	
Berry granola crunch frozen yogurt, 1/2 cup	3
Cappuccino chip frozen yogurt, 1/2 cup	2
Chocolate fudge brownie frozen yogurt, 1/2 cup	2
Peach frozen yogurt, 1/2 cup	2
Strawberry frozen yogurt, 1/2 cup	2

	POINTS VALUE
Edy's	
Vanilla, 1/2 cup	2
Edy's Slow Churned Light	
Black cherry vanilla swirl, 1/2 cup	2
Caramel praline crunch, 1/2 cup	3
Chocolate vanilla swirl, 1/2 cup	2
Vanilla, 1/2 cup	2
Edy's Slow Churned Light Yogurt Blends	
Berry granola crunch frozen yogurt, 1/2 cup	3
Cappuccino chip frozen yogurt, 1/2 cup	2
Chocolate fudge brownie frozen yogurt, 1/2 cup	2
Peach frozen yogurt, 1/2 cup	2
Strawberry frozen yogurt, 1/2 cup	2
Fruitfull	
Blueberry, 1 bar	2
Chocolate yogurt bar, 1 bar	3
Vanilla, 1 bar	3
Schwan's LiveSmart	
Black cherry frozen yogurt, 1/2 cup	3
Blueberry frozen yogurt, 1/2 cup	3
Caramel frozen yogurt, 1/2 cup	3
Chocolate frozen yogurt, 1/2 cup	2
Chocolate fudge brownie frozen yogurt, 1/2 cup	3
Peach frozen yogurt, 1/2 cup	2
Raspberry swirl frozen yogurt, 1/2 cup	3

	POINTS VALUE
Strawberry supreme frozen yogurt, 1/2 cup	3
Triple lemon frozen yogurt, 1/2 cup	3
Vanilla frozen yogurt, 1/2 cup	2
Wild berry frozen yogurt, 1/2 cup	3
Turkey Hill	
Blueberry muffin, 1/2 cup	3
Chocolate cherry cordial, fat free, 1/2 cup	2
Chocolate chip cookie dough, 1/2 cup	2
Chocolate marshmallow, fat free, 1/2 cup	2
Fudge ripple, fat free, 1/2 cup	2
Green tea mango, 1/2 cup	2
Mint cookies 'n cream, low fat, 1/2 cup	2
Neapolitan, fat free, 1/2 cup	2
Orange cream swirl, 1/2 cup	2
Peach mango, 1/2 cup	2
Peanut butter marshmallow, 1/2 cup	3
Pom blue acia smoothie, 1/2 cup	2
Raspberry lemonade, 1/2 cup	2
Southern lemon pie, 1/2 cup	2
Strawberry kiwi/passion fruit, 1/2 cup	2
Vanilla bean, low fat, 1/2 cup	2

Fruit Cobblers
Mrs. Smith's

Apple cobbler, 1 serving (1/8 cobbler)	5
Blackberry cobbler, 1 serving (1/8 cobbler)	5
Cherry cobbler, 1 serving (1/8 cobbler)	5

	POINTS VALUE
Peach cobbler, 1 serving (1/8 cobbler)	5

Gelatins
Del Monte

Mango chiller, 1 cup	3
Peaches in peach flavored gel, 1 cup	2
Peaches in strawberry banana flavored gel-lite, 1 cup	1
Raspberry chiller, 1 cup	3
Strawberry chiller, 1 cup	3

Jell-O

Apple, 1/4 package	2
Apricot, prepared, 1/2 cup	2
Berry blue, prepared, 1/2 cup	2
Black cherry, prepared, 1/2 cup	2
Cherry, prepared, 1/2 cup	2
Color changing grape flavor extreme, 1/4 package	2
Cranberry raspberry, prepared, 1/2 cup	2
Cranberry, prepared, 1/2 cup	2
Grape, prepared, 1/2 cup	2
Lemon, prepared, 1/2 cup	2
Lime, prepared, 1/2 cup	2

CANDY, COOKIES & DESSERTS

Gelatins, Jell-O (con't)	**POINTS VALUE**
Mexican gelatina lime, 1/8 package	1
Mexican gelatina orange, 1/8 package	1
Mexican gelatina pineapple, 1/8 package	1
Mexican gelatina strawberry, 1/8 package	1
Mixed fruit, prepared, 1/2 cup	2
Orange, prepared, 1/2 cup	2
Peach, prepared, 1/2 cup	2
Pineapple, prepared, 1/2 cup	2
Raspberry, prepared, 1/2 cup	2
Strawberry banana, prepared, 1/2 cup	2
Strawberry, prepared, 1/2 cup	2
Sugar free gelatin strawberry, 1/8 package	0
Sugar-free black cherry, 1/4 package	0
Sugar-free cherry, prepared, 1/2 cup	0
Sugar-free cranberry, prepared, 1/2 cup	0
Sugar-free lemon, prepared, 1/2 cup	0
Sugar-free lime, prepared, 1/2 cup	0
Sugar-free mixed fruit, prepared, 1/2 cup	0
Sugar-free orange, prepared, 1/2 cup	0
Sugar-free raspberry, prepared, 1/2 cup	0
Sugar-free strawberry banana, prepared, 1/2 cup	0
Sugar-free strawberry kiwi, prepared, 1/2 cup	0
Sugar-free strawberry, prepared, 1/2 cup	0
Summer breezes pina colada, 1/4 package	2

	POINTS VALUE
Summer breezes strawberry daquiri, 1/4 package	2
Watermelon, prepared, 1/2 cup	2
Wild strawberry, prepared, 1/2 cup	2
Jell-O Fruit Passions	
Peaches & pineapple 'n orange, 1 serving (6 oz)	1
Peaches 'n strawberry, 1 serving (6 oz)	1
Pineapple & peaches 'n lemon-lime, 1 serving (6 oz)	1
Pineapple 'n raspberry, 1 serving (6 oz)	1
Tropical fruit 'n peach, 1 serving (6 oz)	1
Jell-O Gel Cups X-Treme	
Cherry & blue raspberry, 1	1
Jell-O Gelatin Snacks	
Orange, 1	1
Raspberry, 1	1
Strawberry, 1	1
Strawberry/orange, 1	1
Strawberry/raspberry, 1	1
Sugar free lemon lime, 1	0
Jell-O Sugar Free Low Calorie Gelatin Snacks	
Cherry/black-cherry, 1	0
Orange, 1	0
Orange lemon-lime, 1	0
Peach, 1	0

	POINTS VALUE
Peach & watermelon, 1	0
Raspberry, 1	0
Raspberry/orange, 1	0
Strawberry, 1	0
Strawberry-kiwi, 1	0
Strawberry-kiwi & tropical berry, 1	0
Tropical berry, 1	0
Jell-O Sugar-Based Gelatin Snacks	
Watermelon & green apple, 1	1
Knox	
Unflavored gelatin, 1/4 envelope	0
Kool-Aid Gels	
Cherry tropical punch, 1 container	1
Grape, 1 container	1
Ice blue raspberry, 1 container	1
Oh yea orange, 1 container	1
Orange, 1 container	1
Soarin' strawberry, 1 container	1
Payaso	
Strawberry gelatin dessert, 1/8 package	2

Gum, chewing
Big League Chew

	POINTS VALUE
Grape, 8 pieces	0
Original, 8 pieces	0
Sour apple, 8 pieces	0
Strawberry, 8 pieces	0
Watermelon, 8 pieces	0

	POINTS VALUE
Extra	
Cool green apple, 1 stick	0
Hubba Bubba Bubble Jug	
Tropical fruit, 1 tsp	1
Watermelon, 1 tsp	1
Hubba Bubba Bubble Tape	
Awesome original, 1 piece	0
Cotton candy, 1 piece	0
Gushing grape, 1 piece	0
Sour apple, 1 piece	0
Sour blue raspberry, 1 piece	0
Sour watermelon, 1 piece	0
Triple treat, 1 piece	0
Hubba Bubba Max	
Cherry-lemonade, 1 piece	1
Grape-berry, 1 piece	1
Sour double berry, 1 piece	1
Strawberry-watermelon, 1 piece	1
Hubba Bubba Ouch Multiflavor	
Grape, 1 stick	0
Sour watermelon, 1 stick	0
Strawberry, 1 stick	0
Juicy Fruit	
Tropikiwi kick, 2 pellets	0
Orbit	
Bubblemint, 1 piece	0
Cinnamint, 1 piece	0

CANDY, COOKIES & DESSERTS

Gum, chewing, Orbit (con't)

	POINTS VALUE
Citrusmint, 1 piece	0
Peppermint, 1 piece	0
Spearmint, 1 piece	0
Sweet mint, 1 piece	0
Wintermint, 1 piece	0
Orbit White	
Bubblemint, 2 pieces	0
Peppermint, 2 pieces	0
Spearmint, 2 pieces	0
Skittles	
Bubble gum extreme fruit, 2 pieces	0
Bubble gum original, 2 pieces	0
Trident Splash	
Apple with raspberry, 1 piece	0
Strawberry with lime, 1 piece	0
Wrigley's	
Big red, 1 stick	0
Doublemint, 1 stick	0
Juicy fruit, 1 stick	0
Juicy fruit grapermelon, 2 pieces	0
Juicy fruit strappleberry, 2 pieces	0
Spearmint, 1 stick	0
Winterfresh, 1 stick	0
Wrigley's Eclipse	
Cherry chill, 2 pieces	0
Cinnamon, 3 pieces	0
Lemon burst, 2 pieces	0

	POINTS VALUE
Peppermint, 2 pieces	0
Peppermint, 3 pieces	0
Polar ice, 2 pieces	0
Spearmint, 2 pieces	0
Winterfresh, 2 pieces	0
Winterfrost, 3 pieces	0
Wrigley's Extra Sugarfree	
Cinnamon, 1 stick	0
Classic bubble gum, 1 stick	0
Peppermint, 1 stick	0
Polar ice, 1 piece	0
Spearmint, 1 stick	0
Wildberry frost, 1 stick	0
Winterfresh, 1 stick	0
Wrigley's Freedent	
Peppermint, 1 stick	0
Spearmint, 1 stick	0
Winterfresh, 1 stick	0

Ice Cream
Barq's Floatz

	POINTS VALUE
Frozen root beer & vanilla ice cream float, 1 cup	3

Blue Bell

	POINTS VALUE
Almond bar, 1 bar	5
Banana pudding, 1/2 cup	4
Banana split, 1/2 cup	4
Banana split no sugar added lowfat, 1/2 cup	1

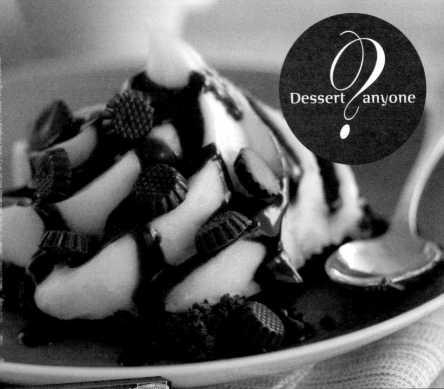

Dessert ?anyone

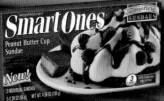

CANDY, COOKIES & DESSERTS

Ice Cream, Blue Bell (con't)	POINTS VALUE
Belle bar, 1 bar	5
Birthday cake, 1/2 cup	5
Buttered pecan, 1/2 cup	5
Buttered pecan no sugar added lowfat, 1/2 cup	1
Caramel turtle fudge ice cream, 1/2 cup	5
Century sundae ice cream, 1/2 cup	5
Cherry vanilla, 1/2 cup	4
Chocolate chip, 1/2 cup	4
Chocolate chip cookie dough, 1/2 cup	5
Chocolate chip country cookie, 1	6
Chocolate covered cherries, 1/2 cup	5
Chocolate overload bar, 1 bar	6
Coffee, 1/2 cup	4
Cookies n cream, 1/2 cup	4
Cookies 'n cream bars, 1 bar	5
Cookies 'n cream sandwich, 1	4
Country cone, cookies 'n cream, 1	6
Country cone, vanilla, 1	7
Country vanilla no sugar added lowfat, 1/2 cup	1
Créme pops, 1 bar	1
Double banana bar, 1 bar	4
Double fudge bar, 1 bar	6
Double vanilla ice cream sandwich, 1	4
Dutch chocolate, 1/2 cup	4
Dutch chocolate, no sugar added lowfat, 1/2 cup	1

	POINTS VALUE
French vanilla, 1/2 cup	4
Fudge blast, 1 bar	4
Fudge bombstik, 1 bar	5
Fudge brownie nut, 1/2 cup	4
Great divide bars, 1 bar	5
Great divide ice cream cone, 1 cone	6
Homemade vanilla, 1/2 cup	4
Hot fudge sundae, 1/2 cup	4
Ice cream sandwich, 1	4
Key lime pie, 1/2 cup	4
Krunch bar, 1 bar	6
Milk chocolate, 1/2 cup	4
Mini krunch bars, 2 bars	6
Mini krunch bars, 1 bar	3
Mini sandwiches, 1	1
Mini sandwiches, 2	2
Mini vanilla country cones, 2 cones	4
Mini vanilla country cones, 1 cone	2
Mint chocolate chip, 1/2 cup	4
Mooo bar, 1 bar	5
Natural vanilla bean, 1/2 cup	4
Neapolitan ice cream sandwich, 1	4
No sugar added fudge bars, 1 bar	1
No sugar added krunch bars, 1 bar	2
No sugar added mooo bars, 1 bar	2
Oatmeal country cookie, 1	7
Peaches & homemade vanilla, 1/2 cup	4

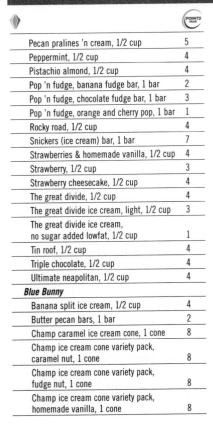

	POINTS VALUE
Pecan pralines 'n cream, 1/2 cup	5
Peppermint, 1/2 cup	4
Pistachio almond, 1/2 cup	4
Pop 'n fudge, banana fudge bar, 1 bar	2
Pop 'n fudge, chocolate fudge bar, 1 bar	3
Pop 'n fudge, orange and cherry pop, 1 bar	1
Rocky road, 1/2 cup	4
Snickers (ice cream) bar, 1 bar	7
Strawberries & homemade vanilla, 1/2 cup	4
Strawberry, 1/2 cup	3
Strawberry cheesecake, 1/2 cup	4
The great divide, 1/2 cup	4
The great divide ice cream, light, 1/2 cup	3
The great divide ice cream, no sugar added lowfat, 1/2 cup	1
Tin roof, 1/2 cup	4
Triple chocolate, 1/2 cup	4
Ultimate neapolitan, 1/2 cup	4
Blue Bunny	
Banana split ice cream, 1/2 cup	4
Butter pecan bars, 1 bar	2
Champ caramel ice cream cone, 1 cone	8
Champ ice cream cone variety pack, caramel nut, 1 cone	8
Champ ice cream cone variety pack, fudge nut, 1 cone	8
Champ ice cream cone variety pack, homemade vanilla, 1 cone	8

	POINTS VALUE
Chocolate chip cookie dough ice cream, 1/2 cup	4
Chocolate chip ice cream, 1/2 cup	3
Chocolate chocolate bar, 1 bar	3
Chocolate fudge bars, 2 bars	3
Chocolate ice cream, 1/2 cup	3
Chocolate lovers' champ ice cream cones, 1 cone	7
Chocolate malt cups, 1 cup	5
Chocolate raspberry cheesecake light ice cream, 1/2 cup	2
Chocolate sundae crunch bar, 1 bar	4
Chocolate sundae cups, 1 cup	3
Chocolate/vanilla flavored ice cream, 1/2 cup	3
Classic vanilla sundae cones, 1 cone	6
Cookies & cream ice cream, 1/2 cup	3
Crunch bar, 1 bar (48 g)	4
Crunch bar, 1 bar (59 g)	5
Double fudge bars, 2 bars	3
Double strawberry light ice cream, 1/2 cup	2
English toffee bars, 1 bar	3
French vanilla flavored ice cream, 1/2 cup	3
Fudge bar, 1 bar	2
Fudge ice cream bar, 1 bar	1
Fudge twirl ice cream, 1/2 cup	3
Goin' bananas bar, 2 bars	3

273

CANDY, COOKIES & DESSERTS

Ice Cream, Blue Bunny (con't)

	POINTS VALUE
Homemade vanilla ice cream bars, 1 bar	4
Homemade vanilla ice cream sandwiches, 1	4
Ice cream sandwich, 1	4
Mint bon bon ice cream, 1/2 cup	3
Mississippi mud ice cream sandwich, 1	4
Neapolitan ice cream, 1/2 cup	3
Neapolitan ice cream sandwich, 1	4
New York vanilla flavored ice cream, 1/2 cup	3
Orange and vanilla low fat ice cream bar, 1 bar	2
Orange dream bar, 1 bar	2
Original banana split ice cream, 1/2 cup	3
Original bunny tracks ice cream, 1/2 cup	4
Original butter pecan ice cream, 1/2 cup	4
Original chocolate caramel commotion ice cream, 1/2 cup	4
Original chocolate chip cookie dough ice cream, 1/2 cup	4
Original chocolate chip ice cream, 1/2 cup	3
Original chocolate ice cream, 1/2 cup	3
Original cookies & cream ice cream, 1/2 cup	4
Original French vanilla flavored ice cream, 1/2 cup	3
Original homemade vanilla flavored ice cream, 1/2 cup	3

	POINTS VALUE
Original hot fudge sundae ice cream, 1/2 cup	4
Original mint chip ice cream, 1/2 cup	3
Original neapolitan ice cream, 1/2 cup	3
Original orange dream, 1/2 cup	3
Original Ozark black walnut ice cream, 1/2 cup	4
Original peanut butter brownie sensation ice cream, 1/2 cup	4
Original strawberry cheesecake ice cream, 1/2 cup	3
Original strawberry ice cream, 1/2 cup	3
Original tin roof sundae ice cream, 1/2 cup	4
Original vanilla flavored ice cream, 1/2 cup	3
Peanut butter fudge light ice cream, 1/2 cup	2
Rainbow sherbet cups, 1 cup	2
Raspberry and vanilla low fat ice cream bars, 1 bar	2
Rocky road ice cream sandwich, 1	4
Root beer float bars, 1 bar	2
Star bar, 1 bar	3
Strawberry cheesecake ice cream sandwiches, 1	4
Strawberry marble ice cream, 1/2 cup	3
Strawberry sundae crunch bar, 1 bar	4
Strawberry sundae cups, 1 cup	3
Strawberry vanilla bar, 1 bar	3

	POINTS VALUE
Super chunky cookie dough ice cream, 1/2 cup	4
Super fudge brownie light ice cream, 1/2 cup	2
The champ ice cream cone, 1 cone	8
Toffee bars, 1 bar	2
Vanilla flavored ice cream, 1/2 cup	3
Vanilla flavored ice cream cups, 1 cup	3
Vanilla fudge, 1 bar	1
Vanilla light ice cream, 1/2 cup	2
Vanilla nutty sundae cones, 1 bar	5
Yogurt smoothie fat free frozen yogurt bar, peach, 1 bar	1
Yogurt smoothie fat free frozen yogurt bar, strawberry, 1 bar	1
Blue Bunny Champ	
Strawberry cone, 1 cone	5
Blue Bunny Fat Free No Sugar Added	
Caramel toffee crunch ice cream, 1/2 cup	1
Vanilla flavored ice cream, 1/2 cup	1
Blue Bunny FrozFruit	
Coconut cream bar, 1 bar	4
Blue Bunny Hi Lite	
Chocolate lite ice cream, 1/2 cup	2
Cookies & cream lite ice cream, 1/2 cup	3
Fudge nut sundae lite ice cream, 1/2 cup	3
Homemade vanilla lite ice cream, 1/2 cup	3

	POINTS VALUE
Mint chip lite ice cream, 1/2 cup	3
Vanilla flavored lite ice cream, 1/2 cup	2
Blue Bunny Light	
Cookies 'n cream bar, 1 bar	3
Ice cream cone, caramel, 1	6
Ice cream cone, fudge, 1	6
Ice cream cone, vanilla, 1	5
Triple chocolate sandwiches, 1	3
Blue Bunny No Sugar Added	
Banana split reduced fat ice cream, 1/2 cup	2
Blue Bunny Personals	
Banana split ice cream, 1/2 cup	4
Bunny tracks light ice cream, 1/2 cup	2
Chocolate gelato, 1/2 cup	4
Double strawberry light ice cream, 1/2 cup	2
Espresso gelato, 1/2 cup	4
Hazelnut gelato, 1/2 cup	4
Italian chocolate chip gelato, 1/2 cup	5
Peanut butter fudge light, 1/2 cup	2
Peanut butter panic ice cream, 1/2 cup	5
Pistachio gelato, 1/2 cup	4
Premium bunny tracks light ice cream, 1/2 cup	2
Premium chocolate raspberry cheesecake light ice cream, 1/2 cup	2
Premium double strawberry ice cream, 1/2 cup	3

CANDY, COOKIES & DESSERTS

Ice Cream, Blue Bunny Personals (con't)	POINTS VALUE
Premium turtle sundae, 1/2 cup	4
Super chunky cookie dough ice cream, 1/2 cup	4
Super fudge brownie ice cream, 1/2 cup	4
Super fudge brownie light ice cream, 1/2 cup	2
Blue Bunny Premium	
All natural vanilla bean ice cream, 1/2 cup	4
Bordeaux cherry chocolate ice cream, 1/2 cup	4
Bunny tracks ice cream, 1/2 cup	5
Bunny tracks ice cream (pint), 1/2 cup	5
Bunny tracks light ice cream, 1/2 cup	2
Butter pecan ice cream, 1/2 cup	4
Butter Pecan ice cream (pint), 1/2 cup	4
Butter pecan light ice cream, 1/2 cup	2
Coffee break ice cream, 1/2 cup	3
Cookies & cream ice cream (pint), 1/2 cup	4
Cookies and cream ice cream, 1/2 cup	4
Double strawberry ice cream, 1/2 cup	3
Double strawberry ice cream (pint), 1/2 cup	3
Fat free no sugar added brownie sundae ice cream, 1/2 cup	1
French vanilla flavored ice cream, 1/2 cup	4
Homemade chocolate ice cream, 1/2 cup	4
Homemade chocolate ice cream (pint), 1/2 cup	4
Homemade turtle sundae ice cream, 1/2 cup	4

	POINTS VALUE
Homemade turtle sundae ice cream (pint), 1/2 cup	6
Homemade vanilla flavored ice cream, 1/2 cup	4
Homemade vanilla flavored ice cream (pint), 1/2 cup	4
Mint chocolate chunk ice cream, 1/2 cup	4
No sugar added bunny tracks ice cream, 1/2 cup	3
No sugar added butter pecan ice cream, 1/2 cup	3
No sugar added cherry vanilla flavored ice cream, 1/2 cup	2
No sugar added double strawberry ice cream, 1/2 cup	2
No sugar added rocky road ice cream, 1/2 cup	3
No sugar added turtle sundae ice cream, 1/2 cup	3
No sugar added vanilla flavored ice cream, 1/2 cup	2
Peanut butter panic ice cream, 1/2 cup	5
Pistachio almond ice cream, 1/2 cup	3
Rocky road ice cream, 1/2 cup	4
Super fudge brownie ice cream, 1/2 cup	4
Toasted almond fudge ice cream, 1/2 cup	4
Vanilla flavored ice cream, 1/2 cup	3
Vanilla flavored ice cream (pint), 1/2 cup	4

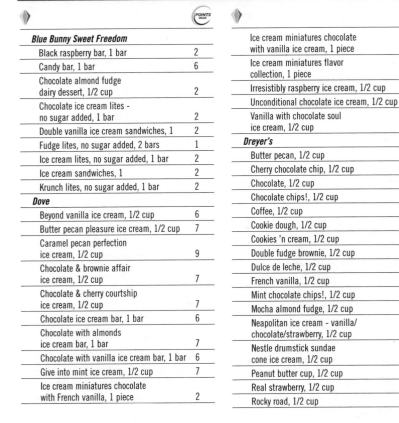

	POINTS VALUE
Blue Bunny Sweet Freedom	
Black raspberry bar, 1 bar	2
Candy bar, 1 bar	6
Chocolate almond fudge dairy dessert, 1/2 cup	2
Chocolate ice cream lites - no sugar added, 1 bar	2
Double vanilla ice cream sandwiches, 1	2
Fudge lites, no sugar added, 2 bars	1
Ice cream lites, no sugar added, 1 bar	2
Ice cream sandwiches, 1	2
Krunch lites, no sugar added, 1 bar	2
Dove	
Beyond vanilla ice cream, 1/2 cup	6
Butter pecan pleasure ice cream, 1/2 cup	7
Caramel pecan perfection ice cream, 1/2 cup	9
Chocolate & brownie affair ice cream, 1/2 cup	7
Chocolate & cherry courtship ice cream, 1/2 cup	7
Chocolate ice cream bar, 1 bar	6
Chocolate with almonds ice cream bar, 1 bar	7
Chocolate with vanilla ice cream bar, 1 bar	6
Give into mint ice cream, 1/2 cup	7
Ice cream miniatures chocolate with French vanilla, 1 piece	2

	POINTS VALUE
Ice cream miniatures chocolate with vanilla ice cream, 1 piece	2
Ice cream miniatures flavor collection, 1 piece	2
Irresistibly raspberry ice cream, 1/2 cup	6
Unconditional chocolate ice cream, 1/2 cup	7
Vanilla with chocolate soul ice cream, 1/2 cup	7
Dreyer's	
Butter pecan, 1/2 cup	4
Cherry chocolate chip, 1/2 cup	4
Chocolate, 1/2 cup	4
Chocolate chips!, 1/2 cup	4
Coffee, 1/2 cup	3
Cookie dough, 1/2 cup	4
Cookies 'n cream, 1/2 cup	4
Double fudge brownie, 1/2 cup	4
Dulce de leche, 1/2 cup	4
French vanilla, 1/2 cup	4
Mint chocolate chips!, 1/2 cup	4
Mocha almond fudge, 1/2 cup	4
Neapolitan ice cream - vanilla/ chocolate/strawberry, 1/2 cup	3
Nestle drumstick sundae cone ice cream, 1/2 cup	4
Peanut butter cup, 1/2 cup	4
Real strawberry, 1/2 cup	3
Rocky road, 1/2 cup	4

CANDY, COOKIES & DESSERTS

Ice Cream, Dreyer's (con't)	POINTS VALUE
Spumoni, 1/2 cup	4
Vanilla, 1/2 cup	4
Vanilla bean, 1/2 cup	3
Vanilla chocolate, 1/2 cup	3
Vanilla fudge swirl, 1/2 cup	4
Dreyer's Fat Free, No Sugar Added	
Chocolate fudge, 1/2 cup	1
Dreyer's Grand	
Double vanilla, 1/2 cup	3
Girl scout samoas cookie, 1/2 cup	4
Girl scouts tagalongs cookie, 1/2 cup	4
Girl scouts thin mint cookie, 1/2 cup	3
Nestle ice cream sandwich ice cream, 1/2 cup	3
Dreyer's Grand Limited Edition	
Apple pie ice cream, 1/2 cup	3
Egg nog ice cream, 1/2 cup	2
Peppermint ice cream, 1/2 cup	2
Pumpkin ice cream, 1/2 cup	3
Root beer float ice cream, 1/2 cup	4
Dreyer's Loaded	
Chocolate fudge brownie ice cream, 1/2 cup	3
Chocolate peanut butter cup ice cream, 1/2 cup	3
Cookies 'n cream ice cream, 1/2 cup	2
Nestle butterfinger frozen dairy dessert, 1/2 cup	3

	POINTS VALUE
Nestle toll house chocolate chip cookie dough ice cream, 1/2 cup	3
Nestle toll house chocolate chip mint brownie ice cream, 1/2 cup	3
Dreyer's No Sugar Added	
Fudge tracks, 1/2 cup	2
Dreyer's No Sugar Added Light	
Butter pecan, 1/2 cup	2
Chocolate, 1/2 cup	1
Coffee, 1/2 cup	2
Cookie dough, 1/2 cup	2
Cookies n cream, 1/2 cup	2
Mint chocolate chips!, 1/2 cup	2
Neapolitan, 1/2 cup	2
Triple chocolate, 1/2 cup	2
Vanilla, 1/2 cup	2
Dreyer's Slow Churned Light	
Butter pecan, 1/2 cup	3
Caramel delight, 1/2 cup	3
Chocolate, 1/2 cup	2
Chocolate chip, 1/2 cup	3
Chocolate fudge chunk, 1/2 cup	3
Coffee, 1/2 cup	2
Cookie dough, 1/2 cup	3
Cookies 'n cream, 1/2 cup	3
Double fudge brownie ice cream, 1/2 cup	3
French silk, 1/2 cup	3

	POINTS VALUE		POINTS VALUE
French vanilla, 1/2 cup	2	Cookies 'n cream, 1/2 cup	4
Fudge tracks, 1/2 cup	3	Double fudge brownie, 1/2 cup	4
Mint chocolate chip, 1/2 cup	3	Dulce de leche, 1/2 cup	4
Neapolitan, 1/2 cup	2	French vanilla, 1/2 cup	4
Peanut butter cup, 1/2 cup	3	Mint chocolate chips!, 1/2 cup	4
Raspberry chip royale, 1/2 cup	3	Neapolitan ice cream - vanilla/ chocolate/strawberry, 1/2 cup	3
Rocky road, 1/2 cup	3	Nestle drumstick sundae cone ice cream, 1/2 cup	4
Strawberry, 1/2 cup	2	Nestle ice cream sandwich, 1/2 cup	3
Take the cake ice cream, 1/2 cup	3	Peanut butter cup, 1/2 cup	4
Vanilla, 1/2 cup	2	Real strawberry, 1/2 cup	3
Vanilla bean, 1/2 cup	2	Rocky road, 1/2 cup	4
Vanilla chocolate, 1/2 cup	2	Spumoni, 1/2 cup	4
Dreyer's Slow Churned Light Limited Edition		Vanilla, 1/2 cup	4
Cheesecake diva ice cream, 1/2 cup	3	Vanilla bean, 1/2 cup	3
Cookies 'n dreamz ice cream, 1/2 cup	3	Vanilla chocolate, 1/2 cup	3
Mint karaoke cookie ice cream, 1/2 cup	3	Vanilla fudge swirl, 1/2 cup	4
Most-orange-inal, 1/2 cup	2	***Edy's Fat Free, No Sugar Added***	
One split wonder, 1/2 cup	3	Chocolate fudge, 1/2 cup	2
Dreyer's Slow Churned Light No Sugar Added		***Edy's Grand***	
French vanilla, 1/2 cup	2	Double vanilla, 1/2 cup	3
Edy's		Girl scouts samoas cookie, 1/2 cup	4
Butter pecan, 1/2 cup	4	Girl scouts tagalongs cookie, 1/2 cup	4
Cherry chocolate chip, 1/2 cup	4	Girl scouts thin mint cookie, 1/2 cup	3
Chocolate, 1/2 cup	4	Mocha almond fudge ice cream, 1/2 cup	4
Chocolate chips!, 1/2 cup	4		
Coffee, 1/2 cup	3		
Cookie dough, 1/2 cup	4		

CANDY, COOKIES & DESSERTS

 Ice Cream (con't)

	POINTS VALUE
Edy's Grand Limited Edition	
Apple pie ice cream, 1/2 cup	3
Egg nog ice cream, 1/2 cup	2
Peppermint ice cream, 1/2 cup	2
Pumpkin ice cream, 1/2 cup	3
Root beer float ice cream, 1/2 cup	4
Edy's Loaded	
Chocolate fudge brownie ice cream, 1/2 cup	3
Chocolate peanut butter cup ice cream, 1/2 cup	3
Cookies 'n cream ice cream, 1/2 cup	2
Nestle butterfinger frozen dairy dessert, 1/2 cup	3
Nestle toll house chocolate chip cookie dough ice cream, 1/2 cup	3
Nestle toll house chocolate chip mint brownie ice cream, 1/2 cup	3
Edy's No Sugar Added	
Fudge tracks, 1/2 cup	2
Edy's No Sugar Added Light	
Butter pecan, 1/2 cup	2
Coffee, 1/2 cup	2
Cookie dough, 1/2 cup	2
Cookies n cream, 1/2 cup	2
Mint chocolate chips!, 1/2 cup	2
Neapolitan, 1/2 cup	2
Triple chocolate, 1/2 cup	2
Vanilla, 1/2 cup	2

	POINTS VALUE
Edy's Slow Churned Light	
Caramel delight, 1/2 cup	3
Chocolate, 1/2 cup	2
Chocolate chip, 1/2 cup	3
Chocolate fudge chunk, 1/2 cup	3
Coffee, 1/2 cup	2
Cookie dough, 1/2 cup	3
Cookies 'n cream, 1/2 cup	3
Double fudge brownie ice cream, 1/2 cup	3
French silk, 1/2 cup	3
French vanilla, 1/2 cup	2
Fudge tracks, 1/2 cup	3
Mint chocolate chip, 1/2 cup	3
Neapolitan, 1/2 cup	2
Peanut butter cup, 1/2 cup	3
Raspberry chip royale, 1/2 cup	3
Rocky road, 1/2 cup	3
Strawberry, 1/2 cup	2
Take the cake ice cream, 1/2 cup	3
Vanilla, 1/2 cup	2
Vanilla bean, 1/2 cup	2
Vanilla bean, 1/2 cup	2
Vanilla chocolate, 1/2 cup	2
Edy's Slow Churned Light Limited Edition	
Cheesecake diva ice cream, 1/2 cup	3
Cookies 'n dreamz ice cream, 1/2 cup	3
Mint karaoke cookie ice cream, 1/2 cup	3

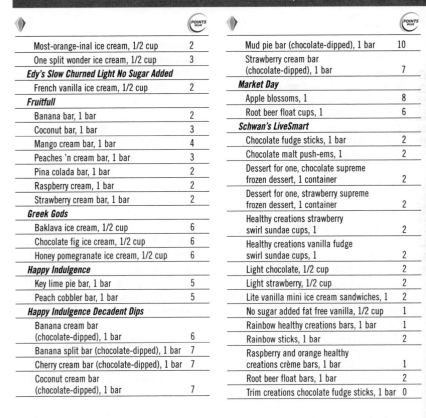

	POINTS VALUE
Most-orange-inal ice cream, 1/2 cup	2
One split wonder ice cream, 1/2 cup	3
Edy's Slow Churned Light No Sugar Added	
French vanilla ice cream, 1/2 cup	2
Fruitfull	
Banana bar, 1 bar	2
Coconut bar, 1 bar	3
Mango cream bar, 1 bar	4
Peaches 'n cream bar, 1 bar	3
Pina colada bar, 1 bar	2
Raspberry cream, 1 bar	2
Strawberry cream bar, 1 bar	2
Greek Gods	
Baklava ice cream, 1/2 cup	6
Chocolate fig ice cream, 1/2 cup	6
Honey pomegranate ice cream, 1/2 cup	6
Happy Indulgence	
Key lime pie bar, 1 bar	5
Peach cobbler bar, 1 bar	5
Happy Indulgence Decadent Dips	
Banana cream bar (chocolate-dipped), 1 bar	6
Banana split bar (chocolate-dipped), 1 bar	7
Cherry cream bar (chocolate-dipped), 1 bar	7
Coconut cream bar (chocolate-dipped), 1 bar	7

	POINTS VALUE
Mud pie bar (chocolate-dipped), 1 bar	10
Strawberry cream bar (chocolate-dipped), 1 bar	7
Market Day	
Apple blossoms, 1	8
Root beer float cups, 1	6
Schwan's LiveSmart	
Chocolate fudge sticks, 1 bar	2
Chocolate malt push-ems, 1	2
Dessert for one, chocolate supreme frozen dessert, 1 container	2
Dessert for one, strawberry supreme frozen dessert, 1 container	2
Healthy creations strawberry swirl sundae cups, 1	2
Healthy creations vanilla fudge swirl sundae cups, 1	2
Light chocolate, 1/2 cup	2
Light strawberry, 1/2 cup	2
Lite vanilla mini ice cream sandwiches, 1	2
No sugar added fat free vanilla, 1/2 cup	1
Rainbow healthy creations bars, 1 bar	1
Rainbow sticks, 1 bar	2
Raspberry and orange healthy creations crème bars, 1 bar	1
Root beer float bars, 1 bar	2
Trim creations chocolate fudge sticks, 1 bar	0

281

Ice Cream (con't)

 POINTS VALUE

The Skinny Cow Ice Cream Bars	
Low fat fudge bars, 1 bar	1
Mini fudge bars, 1 bar	2
The Skinny Cow Low Fat Ice Cream Cones	
Low fat chocolate fudge, 1	3
Low fat mint, 1	3
Low fat vanilla/caramel, 1	3
The Skinny Cow Low Fat Ice Cream Sandwiches	
Low fat chocolate peanut butter, 1	3
Low fat cookies n' cream, 1	3
Low fat mint, 1	2
Low fat strawberry, 1	2
Low fat vanilla, 1	2
Low fat vanilla/chocolate combo, 1	2
No sugar added vanilla, 1	2
Turkey Hill	
Ice cream sandwich double decker, 1	4
Ice cream sandwich, vanilla bean, 1	4
Vanilla fudge sundae cone, 1	8
Turkey Hill Carb-IQ Ice Cream	
Choco mint chip, 1/2 cup	2
Chocolate, 1/2 cup	2
Peanut butter paradise, 1/2 cup	3
Vanilla bean, 1/2 cup	2

 POINTS VALUE

Turkey Hill Creamy Commotions	
Chocolate cupcake, 1/2 cup	4
Chocolate malt chip, 1/2 cup	4
Chocolate pretzel, 1/2 cup	4
Moose tracks, 1/2 cup	4
Peanut butter kandy kake, 1/2 cup	5
Strawberry cheesecake, 1/2 cup	4
Turkey Hill Duetto	
Cherry, 1/2 cup	3
Chocolate coconut, 1/2 cup	3
Lemon, 1/2 cup	3
Mango, 1/2 cup	2
Raspberry, 1/2 cup	3
Rootbeer, 1/2 cup	3
Turkey Hill Fat Free No Sugar Added	
Cherry fudge ripple, 1/2 cup	1
Dutch chocolate, 1/2 cup	1
Vanilla bean, 1/2 cup	1
Turkey Hill Light Recipe	
Banana split, 1/2 cup	2
Chocolate, 1/2 cup	4
Chocolate chip, 1/2 cup	3
Chocolate chip cookie dough, 1/2 cup	2
Chocolate nutty moose tracks, 1/2 cup	3
Choco malt chip, 1/2 cup	2

	POINTS VALUE		POINTS VALUE
Chocolate pretzel, 1/2 cup	2	Chocolate marshmallow, 1/2 cup	4
Coffee, 1/2 cup	3	Chocolate peanut butter cup, 1/2 cup	4
Dulce de chocolate, 1/2 cup	3	Coconut cream pie, 1/2 cup	4
Extreme cookies n' cream, 1/2 cup	3	Colombian coffee, 1/2 cup	3
Ice cream sandwich, 1	3	Cookies n' cream, 1/2 cup	4
Mint chocolate chip, 1/2 cup	4	Dutch chocolate, 1/2 cup	3
Moose tracks, 1/2 cup	3	Eagles touchdown sundae, 1/2 cup	4
Neapolitan, 1/2 cup	3	Egg nog, 1/2 cup	3
Nutty neapolitan, 1/2 cup	4	French vanilla, 1/2 cup	3
Peanut butter mania, 1/2 cup	3	Fried ice cream, 1/2 cup	4
Raspberry chocolate chunk, 1/2 cup	3	Fudge ripple, 1/2 cup	3
Skinny minty, 1/2 cup	3	German chocolate cake, 1/2 cup	4
Strawberry cheesecake, 1/2 cup	3	Neapolitan, 1/2 cup	3
Vanilla bean, 1/2 cup	3	Orange cream swirl, 1/2 cup	3
Turkey Hill No Sugar Added		Original vanilla, 1/2 cup	3
Peanut brittle, low fat, 1/2 cup	2	Party cake, 1/2 cup	4
Turkey Hill Premium		Peaches n' cream, 1/2 cup	3
Baked apple dumpling, 1/2 cup	4	Peanut Butter Ripple, 1/2 cup	4
Banana split, 1/2 cup	3	Phillies graham slam, 1/2 cup	5
Bill's stampede sundae, 1/2 cup	4	Rocky road, 1/2 cup	4
Black cherry, 1/2 cup	3	Rum raisin, 1/2 cup	3
Black raspberry, 1/2 cup	3	Southern lemon pie, 1/2 cup	4
Butter pecan, 1/2 cup	4	Strawberries and cream, 1/2 cup	3
Choco mint chip, 1/2 cup	4	Tin roof sundae, 1/2 cup	4
Chocolate chip cookie dough, 1/2 cup	4	Vanilla and chocolate, 1/2 cup	3
		Vanilla bean, 1/2 cup	3

CANDY, COOKIES & DESSERTS

Ice Cream (con't)

	POINTS VALUE
Weight Watchers	
Chocolate chip cookie dough, 1 cup	2
Chocolate fudge brownie, 1 cup	2
Chocolate mousse bar, 1	1
Chocolate round ice cream sandwiches, 1	2
English toffee crunch bar, 1 bar	2
Giant chocolate cookies & cream bar, 1 bar	2
Giant chocolate fudge sundae cone, 1 cone	2
Giant cookies & cream bar, 1 bar	2
Giant fudge bar, 1 bar	1
Giant latte bars, 1 bar	1
Giant orange sorbet & ice cream bar, 1 bar	2
Giant vanilla fudge sundae cone, 1 cone	2
Giant wildberry sorbet & ice cream bar, 1 bar	2
Key lime sherbet & ice cream bar, 1 bar	1
Mint chocolate chip, 1 cup	2
Passion fruit sherbet & ice cream bar, 1 bar	1
Strawberry sherbet & ice cream bar, 1 bar	1
Turtle sundae, 1 cup	3
Vanilla ice cream sandwich, 1	2
Vanilla round ice cream sandwiches, 1	2
Weight Watchers Smart Ones	
Chocolate chip cookie dough sundae, 1 serving (75 g)	3

	POINTS VALUE
Mint chocolate chip sundae, 1 serving (69 g)	3
Mocha fudge sundae, 1 serving (69 g)	3
Peanut butter cup sundae, 1 serving (65 g)	3

Ice Cream Cones and Toppings

	POINTS VALUE
Blue Bunny	
Chocolate ice cream cups, 1	2
Cool Whip	
Chocolate, 2 Tbsp	1
Extra creamy whipped topping, 2 Tbsp	1
Free whipped topping, 2 Tbsp	0
French vanilla, 2 Tbsp	1
Lite whipped topping, 2 Tbsp	0
Strawberry, 2 Tbsp	1
Sugar free whipped topping, 2 Tbsp	0
Whipped topping, 2 Tbsp	1
Dream Whip	
Whipped topping mix, 1 serving (1/16 envelope)	0
Whipped topping mix, prepared as directed, 2 Tbsp	0
Fisher Chef's Naturals	
Nut topping, 1 oz	4
Flavia	
Creamy topping, 1 sachet	1

Giant Chocolate Fudge Ice Cream Bar 1 POINTS VALUE Per Bar

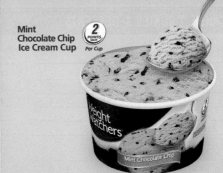

Mint Chocolate Chip Ice Cream Cup 2 POINTS VALUE Per Cup

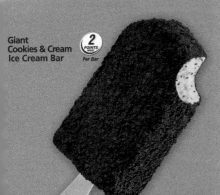

Giant Cookies & Cream Ice Cream Bar 2 POINTS VALUE Per Bar

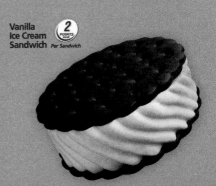

Vanilla Ice Cream Sandwich 2 POINTS VALUE Per Sandwich

Weight Watchers® frozen treats bring GIANT size indulgence and unique, exciting flavors with *POINTS*® values of just 1 or 2 per serving!

WeightWatchers®

Go to WeightWatchers.com/icecream to find a store near you.

Ice Cream Cones and Toppings (con't)

	POINTS VALUE
Hershey's Shell Topping	
Chocolate, 2 Tbsp	6
Heath, 2 Tbsp	6
Reese, 2 Tbsp	5
Keebler	
Ice cream cup fudge-dipped fudge shoppe, 1 cup	1
Ice cream cup, vanilla, 1 cup	0
Ice cream waffle bowl, 1 bowl	1
Ice cream waffle cone, 1 cone	1
Sugar cones, 1	1
Nabisco	
Oreo chocolate ice cream cones, 1	1
Oreo crunchies, 1 serving (11 g)	1
Nabisco Comet	
Ice cream cups, 1	0
Ice cream cups rainbow, 1	0
Sugar cones, 1	1
Planters	
Nut topping, 2 Tbsp	3
Polaner Sugar Free Topping	
Blueberry, 2 Tbsp	1
Seedless raspberry, 2 Tbsp	0
Strawberry, 2 Tbsp	1
Smucker's	
Light hot fudge topping, 2 Tbsp	1
Sugar free hot fudge topping, 2 Tbsp	2

Ices, Sherbets, Sorbets, Frozen Fruit Bars

	POINTS VALUE
Blue Bell	
Bullets, 1 bar	1
Kid pop, 1 bar	1
Lime sherbet, 1/2 cup	3
Megabite, 1 bar	3
Mini rainbows, 1 bar (40 g)	1
Mini rainbows, 2 bars (81 g)	1
Orange sherbet, 1/2 cup	3
Pineapple sherbet, 1/2 cup	2
Rainbow, 1/2 cup	3
Rainbow freeze, 1 bar	2
Sugar free bullets, 1 bar	0
Blue Bunny	
Banana pop, 1 bar	1
Cool tubes orange sherbet push ups, 1 tube	2
Jarritos bomb pop, 1 bar	1
Lemonade bomb pop, 1 bar	1
Lime fat free sherbet, 1/2 cup	2
Lucas chamoy bar, 1 bar	1
Lucas pelucas bar, 1 bar	1
Orange fat free sherbet, 1/2 cup	2
Pineapple fat free sherbet, 1/2 cup	2
Polar pops, all flavors, 1 bar	1

	POINTS VALUE		POINTS VALUE
Rainbow fat free sherbet, 1/2 cup	2	Tangerine whole fruit bar, 1 bar	1
Raspberry fat free sherbet, 1/2 cup	2	Tropical rainbow - pineapple/orange/key lime, 1/2 cup	3
Slush pops (grape, cherry, orange), 1 bar	1		
Sour bomb pops (watermelon, orange blast, green apple), 1 bar	1	***Dreyer's Fruit Bars***	
		Strawberry banana, 1 bar	1
Sugar free bomb pops, 1 bar	0	***Edy's***	
The original bomb pop (cherry, lime, blue raspberry), 1 bar	1	Berry rainbow - blackberry/raspberry/orange, 1/2 cup	3
Twin pops, all flavors, 1 bar	1	Creamy coconut whole fruit bar, 1 bar	2
Blue Bunny FrozFruit		Grape whole fruit bar, 1 bar	2
No sugar added strawberry fruit bar, 1 bar	0	Lemonade whole fruit bar, 1 bar	2
Pomegranate cherry fruit bar, 1 bar	2	Lime whole fruit bar, 1 bar	2
Raspberry acai fruit bar, 1 bar	1	Orange & cream whole fruit bar, low fat, 1 bar	2
Strawberry fruit bar, 1 bar	1	Orange cream, 1/2 cup	3
Tropical fruit bar, 1 bar	1	Strawberry whole fruit bar, 1 bar	2
Dreyer's		Swiss orange, 1/2 cup	3
Berry rainbow - blackberry/raspberry/orange, 1/2 cup	3	Tangerine whole fruit bar, 1 bar	1
Creamy coconut whole fruit bar, 1 bar	2	Tropical rainbow - pineapple/orange/key lime, 1/2 cup	3
Grape whole fruit bar, 1 bar	2	***Edy's Fruit Bars***	
Lemonade whole fruit bar, 1 bar	2	Strawberry banana, 1 bar	1
Lime whole fruit bar, 1 bar	2	***Fruitfull***	
Orange & cream whole fruit bar, low fat, 1 bar	2	Fuzzynavel bar, 1 bar	1
Orange cream, 1/2 cup	3	Green tea melon, 1 bar	2
Strawberry whole fruit bar, 1	2	Guava bar, 1 bar	1
Swiss orange, 1/2 cup	3	Lemon bar, 1 bar	2
		Lime bar, 1 bar	2

CANDY, COOKIES & DESSERTS

Ices, Sherbets, Sorbets, Frozen Fruit Bars, Fruitfull (con't)	POINTS VALUE
Passionate cherry bar, 1 bar	2
Pineapple bar, 1 bar	2
Raspberry bar, 1 bar	1
Strawberry bar, 1 bar	1
Tamarind, 1 bar	2
Tropical splash bar, 1 bar	2
Watermelon bar, 1 bar	1
Icee M-Paks	
Blue raspberry, 2 1/4 oz	1
Cherry, 2 1/4 oz	1
Cherry cola, 2 1/4 oz	1
Sour apple, 2 1/4 oz	1
Kool-Aid	
Kool pops freezer bars, 1	1
Luigi's Real Italian Ice	
Cherry, 1 cup	2
Grape, 1 cup	2
Lemon, 1 cup	2
Squeeze-up tube, cherry, 1 tube	1
Squeeze-up tube, lemon, 1 tube	1
Squeeze-up tube, strawberry, 1 tube	1
Strawberry, 1 cup	2
Variety pack (lemon/strawberry), 1 cup	2
Variety pack, mango, 1 cup	3
Variety pack, pina colada, 1 cup	3
Luigi's Swirl Real Italian Ice	
Blue razzin' lemonade, 1 cup	3
Bubble gum burst, 1 cup	3

	POINTS VALUE
Cherry lime chiller, 1 cup	3
Strawberry banana blast, 1 cup	3
Minute Maid	
Soft frozen cherry limeade, 1 tube	2
Soft frozen lemonade, 1 tube	2
Soft frozen limeade, 1 tube	2
Soft frozen raspberry lemonade, 1 tube	2
Schwan's LiveSmart	
Bomb pop jr., 1	1
Cherry freeze cups, 1/2 cup	3
Lemon freeze cups, 1/2 cup	3
Mike & ike tropical typhoon pops, 1 bar	1
Orange sherbet, 1/2 cup	2
Orange sherbet push-ems, 1	2
Passion punch sherbet, 1/2 cup	3
Peach mango fruit bars, 1 bar	1
Push-ems rainbow sherbet, 1	2
Rainbow sherbet, 1/2 cup	2
Schwan's pops, 1	0
Strawberry daiquiri sorbet, 1/2 cup	3
Strawberry fruit bars, 1 bar	1
Twin pops, 1	1
Watermelon sherbet, 1/2 cup	3
Z-bops sour cherry blue raz, 1	2
Sharon's	
Blueberry sorbet, 1/2 cup	1
Chocolate, 1/2 cup	3

◆	POINTS VALUE
Coconut, 1/2 cup	4
Lemon, 1/2 cup	2
Mango, 1/2 cup	1
Mixed berry, 1/2 cup	2
Passion fruit, 1/2 cup	2
Raspberry, 1/2 cup	1
Strawberry sorbet, 1/2 cup	2
Turkey Hill	
Cherry orchard, 1/2 cup	3
Fruit rainbow sherbet, 1/2 cup	2
Orange grove sherbet, 1/2 cup	2
Turkey Hill Venice Ice	
Lemon & cherry, 1/2 cup	2
Mango, 1/2 cup	2
Pomegranate blueberry with acai, 1/2 cup	2
Raspberry, 1/2 cup	2

Mousses

Sans Sucre Sugar Free

	POINTS VALUE
Cheesecake mousse mix (low fat), 1/2 cup	2
Chocolate cheesecake mousse mix (low fat), 1/2 cup	2
Chocolate mousse mix (low fat), 1/2 cup	1
French vanilla mousse mix (low fat), 1/2 cup	2
Key lime pie & mousse mix (low fat), 1/2 cup	2
Lemon mousse mix (low fat), 1/2 cup	2

◆	POINTS VALUE
Mocha cappuccino mousse mix (low fat), 1/2 cup	1
Strawberry mousse mix (low fat), 1/2 cup	2
Weight Watchers Smart Ones	
Chocolate mousse, 1 serving (77 g)	3

Pies

Amy's

	POINTS VALUE
Apple pie, 1/2	5
Lance	
Pecan pie, 1	8
Market Day	
Apple deep dish pie, 1 serving (1/12 pie)	8
No sugar added apple pie, 1 slice	7
Mrs. Smith's	
Apple pie, 1 serving (1/8 pie)	8
Apple pie, no sugar added, 1 serving (1/6 pie)	4
Blueberry pie, 1 serving (1/8 pie)	7
Boston cream pie, 1 serving (1/8 pie)	4
Cherry pie, 1 serving (1/8 pie)	8
Chocolate cream pie, 1 serving (1/4 pie)	8
Coconut cream pie, 1 serving (1/4 pie)	8
Coconut custard pie, 1 serving (1/8 pie)	6
Dutch apple crumb pie, 1 serving (1/8 pie)	7
Hearty pumpkin pie, 1 serving (1/8 pie)	5
Key lime pie, 1 serving (1/9 pie)	10
Lemon meringue pie, 1 serving (1/8 pie)	7

CANDY, COOKIES & DESSERTS

Pies, Mrs. Smith's (con't)	POINTS VALUE
Mince pie, 1 serving (1/8 pie)	9
Peach pie, 1 serving (1/8 pie)	7
Pecan pie, 1 serving (1/5 pie)	12
Pumpkin custard pie, 1 serving (1/8 pie)	5
Red raspberry pie, 1 serving (1/8 pie)	8
Sweet potato pie, 1 serving (1/8 pie)	7
Mrs. Smith's Restaurant Classics	
French silk chocolate pie, 1 serving (1/9 pie)	14
Mrs. Smith's Special Recipe	
Deep dish apple pie, 1 serving (1/12 pie)	7
Deep dish cherry pie, 1 serving (1/12 pie)	8
Deep dish peach pie, 1 serving (1/12 pie)	7
Homemade pumpkin pie, 1 serving (1/10 pie)	6
Mrs. Smith's Traditional Recipe Slices	
Apple pie slices sweetened with splenda, 1 slice	6
Mixed berry pie slices sweetened with splenda, 1 slice	5
Weight Watchers Smart Ones	
Key lime pie, 1 serving (79 g)	4

Puddings
Jell-O

	POINTS VALUE
Flan mix, 1/4 package	2
Lemon, prepared, 1/2 cup	3
Milk chocolate, prepared, 1/2 cup	3

	POINTS VALUE
Sugar free chocolate mint fudge sundae, 1	1
Sugar free dulce de leche vanilla caramel sundae, 1	1
Sugar free mochaccino chocolate coffee sundae, 1	1
Vanilla, prepared, 1/2 cup	3
Jell-O 100 Calorie Packs	
Smoothies, 1	2
Jell-O Americana	
Custard dessert, prepared, 1/2 cup	3
Jell-O Cook & Serve	
Americana custard mix, 1 serving (1/6 package)	2
Banana cream mix, 1 serving (22 g)	2
Banana cream, prepared, 1/2 cup	3
Butterscotch mix, 1/4 package	2
Butterscotch, prepared, 1/2 cup	3
Chocolate fudge mix, 1/4 package	2
Chocolate fudge, prepared, 1/2 cup	3
Chocolate mix, 1/4 package	2
Chocolate, prepared, 1/2 cup	3
Coconut cream mix, 1/4 package	2
Coconut cream, prepared, 1/2 cup	3
Flan, prepared, 1/2 cup	3
Lemon mix, 1 serving (1/6 package)	1
Milk chocolate mix, 1/4 package	2
Vanilla mix, 1/4 package	2

	POINTS VALUE
Jell-O Fat Free 100 Calorie Packs Pudding Snacks	
Caramel Vanilla, 1	2
Chocolate, 1	2
Chocolate/vanilla swirls, 1	2
Devil's food & chocolate, 1	2
Tapioca, 1	2
Vanilla, 1	2
Jell-O Fat Free Cook & Serve	
Rice mix, 1/4 package	2
Rice, prepared, 1/2 cup	3
Tapioca mix, 1/4 package	2
Tapioca, prepared, 1/2 cup	3
Jell-O Fat Free Sugar Free Cook & Serve	
Banana cream, prepared, 1/2 cup	1
Chocolate mix, 1 serving (1/6 package)	0
Chocolate, prepared, 1/2 cup	1
Vanilla mix, 1/4 package	0
Vanilla, prepared, 1/2 cup	1
Jell-O Fat Free Sugar Free Instant	
Banana cream mix, 1/4 package	1
Butterscotch mix, 1/4 package	1
Butterscotch, prepared, 1/2 cup	1
Cheesecake mix, 1/4 package	1
Cheesecake, prepared, 1/2 cup	1
Chocolate fudge mix, 1/4 serving (11 g)	1
Chocolate fudge, prepared, 1/2 cup	1

	POINTS VALUE
Chocolate mix, 1/4 package	1
Chocolate, prepared, 1/2 cup	1
Lemon mix, 1/4 package	1
Lemon, prepared, 1/2 cup	1
Pistachio mix, 1/4 package	1
Pistachio, prepared, 1/2 cup	1
Vanilla mix, 1/4 serving (8 g)	1
Vanilla, prepared, 1/2 cup	1
White chocolate mix, 1/4 package	1
White chocolate, prepared, 1/2 cup	1
Jell-O Instant	
Banana cream mix, 1 serving (1/6 package)	2
Banana cream mix, 1/4 package	2
Banana cream, prepared, 1/2 cup	3
Butterscotch mix, 1/4 package	2
Butterscotch, prepared, 1/2 cup	3
Cheesecake mix, 1/4 package	2
Cheesecake, prepared, 1/2 cup	3
Chocolate cherry mix, 1/4 package	2
Chocolate fudge mix, 1/4 package	2
Chocolate fudge, prepared, 1/2 cup	3
Chocolate mix, 1/4 package	2
Chocolate, prepared, 1/2 cup	3
Coconut cream mix, 1/4 package	2
Coconut cream, prepared, 1/2 cup	3

CANDY, COOKIES & DESSERTS

Puddings, Jell-O Instant (con't)	POINTS VALUE
Devil's food mix, 1/4 package	2
Devil's food, prepared, 1/2 cup	3
French vanilla mix, 1/4 package	2
French vanilla, prepared, 1/2 cup	3
Lemon mix, 1/4 package	2
Lemon, prepared, 1/2 cup	3
Oreo cookies 'n cream with cookie pieces mix, 1 serving (31 g)	2
Pistachio mix, 1/4 package	2
Pistachio, prepared, 1/2 cup	3
Pumpkin spice mix, 1/4 package	2
Pumpkin spice, prepared, 1/2 cup	3
Vanilla mix, 1/4 package	2
Vanilla, prepared, 1/2 cup	3
White chocolate mix, 1/4 package	2
White chocolate, prepared, 1/2 cup	3
Jell-O Pudding Snacks	
Chocolate, 1 (106 g)	2
Chocolate, 1 (113 g)	3
Chocolate/Vanilla Oreo parfait, 1	2
Chocolate/vanilla swirls, 1	2
Tapioca, 1	2
Vanilla, 1	2
Jell-O Sugar Free Pudding	
Chocolate, 1	1
Chocolate vanilla swirls, 1	1

	POINTS VALUE
Creamy caramel, 1	1
Double chocolate, 1	1
Vanilla, 1	1
Jell-O Sugar Free Pudding Snacks	
Banana fudge sundae, 1	1
Chocolate mint fudge sundae, 1	1
Dulce de leche sundae, 1	1
Mochaccino sundae, 1	1
Jell-O X-Treme Pudding Sticks	
Variety pak, 1	1
Kozy Shack	
Banana pudding, 1/2 cup	3
Banana pudding, prepared with 1% milk, 4 oz	1
Bananas foster pudding, 3 1/2 oz	3
Black forest pudding, 3 1/2 oz	2
Cherries jubilee pudding, 3 1/2 oz	3
Chocolate pudding, 1/2 cup	3
Chocolate pudding, prepared with 1% milk, 4 oz	1
Cinnamon raisin rice pudding, 1/2 cup	3
Crème caramel flan, 4 oz	3
European style rice pudding, 1/2 cup	3
No sugar added apple pie a la mode, 3 1/2 oz	1
No sugar added bananas foster, 3 1/2 oz	1
No sugar added black forest, 3 1/2 oz	1

	POINTS VALUE
No sugar added cherries jubilee, 3 1/2 oz	1
No sugar added chocolate pudding, 4 oz	1
No sugar added rice pudding, 4 oz	1
No sugar added tapioca pudding, 4 oz	1
Restaurant style flan-Dulce de Leche, 4 oz	4
Rice pudding, 1/2 cup	3
Tapioca pudding, 1/2 cup	3
Vanilla pudding, prepared with 1% milk, 4 oz	2

Kraft Handi-Snacks

Banana, 1	2
Butterscotch, 1	2
Chocolate, 1	2
Chocolate (fat free), 1	1
Chocolate fudge, 1	2
Doubles banana split, 1	2
Doubles chocolate chip cookie, 1	2
Doubles fudge rocky road, 1	2
Pudding doubles, chocolate vanilla, 1 cup	2
Rice pudding, 1 cup	2
Sugar free chocolate, 1	1
Sugar free creamy caramel, 1	1
Sugar free vanilla, 1	1
Tapioca, 1	2
Vanilla, 1	2
Vanilla (fat free), 1	2

Minute

	POINTS VALUE
Rice pudding, as packaged, 1 serving (25 g)	2
Tapioca, 1 Tbsp	0

Uncle Ben's

Rice pudding mix, smooth and creamy cinnamon & raisins, 1/2 cup (cooked)	3
Rice pudding mix, smooth and creamy French vanilla, 1/2 cup	2

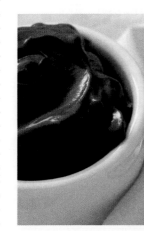

Asian Sauces

7 Paths

	POINTS VALUE
Dueling songbirds sweet & sour with guava stir fry sauce, 1/4 cup	2
Kama's crazy taxi Thai chili peanut stir fry sauce, 1/4 cup	2
Last boat to Luzon mango ginger stir fry sauce, 1/4 cup	1
Lost again pineapple sweet & sour stir fry sauce, 1/4 cup	2
Secret red door Thai peanut stir fry sauce, 1/4 cup	2
Shoulda turned left citrus teriyaki stir fry sauce, 1/4 cup	1
Somewhere near Shanghai sesame ginger stir fry sauce, 1/4 cup	2
Twice happiness black pepper stir fry sauce, 1/4 cup	1

A Taste of Thai

Garlic chili pepper sauce, 1 tsp	0
Pad Thai sauce, 2 Tbsp	2
Panang curry base, 1 tsp	1
Peanut sauce mix, 1/4 envelope	1
Red curry base, 1 tsp	1

Cherchies

Asian grilling & stir fry sauce with sherry, 2 Tbsp	2

Contadina

	POINTS VALUE
Sweet & sour sauce, 2 Tbsp	1

Eden

Wasabi powder, 1 tsp	0

Eden Organic

Genmai miso, organic - soybean & brown rice, 1 Tbsp	0
Hacho miso, organic - soybean, 1 Tbsp	1
Mugi miso, organic - soybean & barley, 1 Tbsp	0
Shiro miso, organic - rice & soybean, 1 Tbsp	1
Shoyu, 1 Tbsp	0
Shoyu, reduced sodium, 1 Tbsp	0
Tamari, 1 Tbsp	0

Eden Selected

Shoyu - imported, 1 Tbsp	0

House of Tsang

Bangkok padang sauce, 1 Tbsp	1
Classic stir fry sauce, 1 Tbsp	1
General Tsao sauce, 1 tsp	1
Ginger flavored soy sauce, 1 Tbsp	0
Hoisin sauce, 1 tsp	0
Hunan smokehut hibachi grill sauce, 1 Tbsp	1
Imperial citrus stir fry, 1 Tbsp	1
Kobe steak hibachi grill sauce, 1 Tbsp	1
Korean teriyaki sauce, 1 Tbsp	1

	POINTS VALUE
Low sodium ginger flavored soy sauce, 1 Tbsp	0
Low sodium soy sauce, 1 Tbsp	0
Oyster flavored stir fry, 1 Tbsp	1
Saigon sizzle sauce, 1 Tbsp	1
Spicy brown bean sauce, 1 tsp	0
Sweet & sour stir fry sauce, 1 Tbsp	1
Sweet ginger sesame hibachi grill sauce, 1 Tbsp	1
Szechuan spicy stir fry sauce, 1 Tbsp	1
Teriyaki hibachi grill sauce, 1 Tbsp	1
Thai peanut hibachi grill sauce, 1 Tbsp	1
Kraft	
Sweet 'n sour sauce, 1 dipping cup	1
San-J	
Asian bbq sauce, 2 Tbsp	1
Organic shoyu, 1 Tbsp	0
Organic wheat free tamari, 1 Tbsp	0
Organic wheat free tamari reduced sodium, 1 Tbsp	0
Reduced sodium tamari, 1 Tbsp	0
Sweet & tangy sauce, 2 Tbsp	1
Szechuan, 1 tsp	0
Tamari, 1 Tbsp	0
Teriyaki sauce, 1 Tbsp	0
Thai peanut, 2 Tbsp	1

	POINTS VALUE
Simply Asia	
General Tsao stir-fry sauce, 2 Tbsp	2
Ginger teriyaki stir-fry sauce, 2 Tbsp	1
Kung Pao stir-fry sauce, 2 Tbsp	1
Mandarin orange stir-fry sauce, 2 Tbsp	1
Szechwan stir-fry sauce, 2 Tbsp	2
Thai Kitchen	
10-minute simmer sauce, green curry, 1/2 cup	2
10-minute simmer sauce, Panang curry, 1/2 cup	2
10-minute simmer sauce, red curry, 1/2 cup	2
10-minute simmer sauce, yellow curry, 1/2 cup	2
Peanut satay sauce dipping & all-purpose sauce, 2 Tbsp	2
Premium fish sauce, 1 Tbsp	0
Premium fish sauce, less sodium, 1 Tbsp	0
Spicy Thai chili all-purpose sauce & marinade, 1 Tbsp	0
Tree of Life	
Organic shoyu soy sauce, 1 Tbsp	0
Organic wheat free tamari soy sauce, 1 Tbsp	0
Yoshida	
Cracked pepper & garlic, 1 Tbsp	1
Gourmet sauce, 1 Tbsp	1

Asian Sauces, Yoshida (con't)	POINTS VALUE
Hawaiian sweet & sour, 2 Tbsp	1
Spicy wing and rib sauce, 2 Tbsp	1
Traditional teriyaki, 1 Tbsp	0

Barbecue/Grilling Sauces

Annie's Naturals

Organic hot chipotle bbq sauce, 2 Tbsp	1
Organic original bbq sauce, 2 Tbsp	1
Organic smokey maple bbq sauce, 2 Tbsp	1

Boar's Head

Gourmet barbecue sauce - hot & spicy, 2 Tbsp	1
Gourmet barbecue sauce - sweet & mild, 2 Tbsp	1

Bull's Eye

Brewers best with guinness, 2 Tbsp	1
Honey garlic bonanza, 2 Tbsp	1
Honey smoke, 2 Tbsp	1
Honey teriyaki, 2 Tbsp	1
Original, 2 Tbsp	1
Premium select, 2 Tbsp	1
Ragin' buffalo bbq sauce, 2 Tbsp	1
Smokehouse hickory, 2 Tbsp	1
Smokin' chipotle barbecue sauce, 2 Tbsp	1
Spicy honey, 2 Tbsp	1
Spicy hot, 2 Tbsp	1
Steakhouse with A1 barbecue sauce, 2 Tbsp	1
Sweet & sticky barbecue sauce, 2 Tbsp	1
Sweet hickory smoke, 2 Tbsp	1

	POINTS VALUE
Sweet homestyle blend, 2 Tbsp	1
Texas style mesquite, 2 Tbsp	1

Consorzio

BBQ sauce, original, 2 Tbsp	1

Goldwater's

Bisbee barbeque sauce, 2 Tbsp	1
Grand Canyon cranberry grill sauce, 2 Tbsp	1

Heinz Thick & Rich

Cajun style barbecue sauce, 2 Tbsp	1
Chunky barbecue sauce, 2 Tbsp	1
Hawaiian barbecue sauce, 2 Tbsp	1
Honey mustard barbeque sauce, 2 Tbsp	1

Jack Daniel's

Hickory brown sugar, 2 Tbsp	1
Honey smokehouse, 2 Tbsp	1
Spicy original recipe, 2 Tbsp	1
Jack Daniel's No. 7	
Original recipe, 2 Tbsp	1

K.C. Masterpiece

Hickory barbecue sauce, 2 Tbsp	1
Hickory brown sugar barbecue sauce, 2 Tbsp	1
Honey barbecue sauce, 2 Tbsp	1
Honey steakhouse barbecue sauce, 2 Tbsp	1
Honey teriyaki barbecue sauce, 2 Tbsp	1
Mesquite barbecue sauce, 2 Tbsp	1
Original barbecue sauce, 2 Tbsp	1
Spicy original barbecue sauce, 2 Tbsp	1

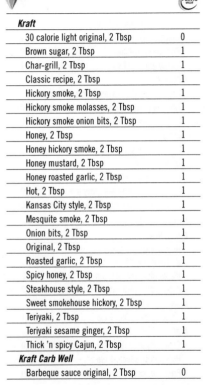

	POINTS VALUE
Kraft	
30 calorie light original, 2 Tbsp	0
Brown sugar, 2 Tbsp	1
Char-grill, 2 Tbsp	1
Classic recipe, 2 Tbsp	1
Hickory smoke, 2 Tbsp	1
Hickory smoke molasses, 2 Tbsp	1
Hickory smoke onion bits, 2 Tbsp	1
Honey, 2 Tbsp	1
Honey hickory smoke, 2 Tbsp	1
Honey mustard, 2 Tbsp	1
Honey roasted garlic, 2 Tbsp	1
Hot, 2 Tbsp	1
Kansas City style, 2 Tbsp	1
Mesquite smoke, 2 Tbsp	1
Onion bits, 2 Tbsp	1
Original, 2 Tbsp	1
Roasted garlic, 2 Tbsp	1
Spicy honey, 2 Tbsp	1
Steakhouse style, 2 Tbsp	1
Sweet smokehouse hickory, 2 Tbsp	1
Teriyaki, 2 Tbsp	1
Teriyaki sesame ginger, 2 Tbsp	1
Thick 'n spicy Cajun, 2 Tbsp	1
Kraft Carb Well	
Barbeque sauce original, 2 Tbsp	0

	POINTS VALUE
Kraft Thick 'N Spicy	
Hickory bacon, 2 Tbsp	1
Hickory smoke, 2 Tbsp	1
Honey, 2 Tbsp	1
Mesquite smoke, 2 Tbsp	1
Original, 2 Tbsp	1
Muirhead	
Barbeque sauce, 1 Tbsp	2
Naturally Fresh	
Bar-b-q sauce, 2 Tbsp	1
Open Pit	
Hot bbq sauce, 2 Tbsp	1
Original bbq sauce, 2 Tbsp	1
Original onion bbq sauce, 2 Tbsp	1
Thick & tangy chile lime bbq sauce, 2 Tbsp	1
Thick & tangy original bbq sauce, 2 Tbsp	1
Walden Farms	
Hickory smoked barbeque sauce, 2 Tbsp	0
Honey barbeque sauce, 2 Tbsp	0
Original barbecue sauce, 2 Tbsp	0
Gravies	
Boston Market	
Beef gravy, 1/4 cup	1
Chicken gravy, 1/4 cup	1
Turkey gravy, 1/4 cup	1

297

CONDIMENTS, SAUCES & GRAVIES

Gravies (con't)	POINTS VALUE
Durkee	
Au jus branded mix, 1 tsp	0
Brown gravy mix, 2 tsp	0
Chicken gravy mix, 1 Tbsp	1
Country gravy mix, 1 1/3 Tbsp	1
Mushroom in brown gravy mix, 2 tsp	0
Onion in brown gravy mix, 2 tsp	0
Pork gravy mix, 2 tsp	0
Turkey gravy mix, 2 tsp	0
French's	
Au jus branded mix, 1 tsp	0
Brown gravy mix, 2 tsp	0
Chicken gravy mix, 1 Tbsp	0
Pork gravy mix, 2 tsp	0
Sausage flavored country gravy mix, 1 1/3 Tbsp	1
Turkey gravy mix, 2 tsp	1
Heinz	
Fat free beef gravy, 1/4 cup	0
Fat free chicken gravy, 1/4 cup	0
Fat free turkey gravy, 1/4 cup	0
Heinz HomeStyle	
Beef gravy, 1/4 cup	1
Bistro style au jus, 1/4 cup	0
Chicken gravy, 1/4 cup	1
Country sausage, 1/4 cup	1
Cream of chicken gravy, 1/4 cup	1

	POINTS VALUE
Mushroom gravy, 1/4 cup	0
Onion gravy, 1/4 cup	1
Pork gravy, 1/4 cup	0
Turkey gravy, 1/4 cup	1
McCormick	
Brown gravy dry seasoning mix, 1 Tbsp	0
Chicken gravy dry seasoning mix, 2 tsp	0
Turkey gravy dry seasoning mix, 2 tsp	0
Tofurky	
Mushroom & giblet gravy, 2 Tbsp	1
Tony Chachere's	
Creole instant roux mix, 1 tsp	0
Southern pantry brown gravy mix, 1 1/2 tsp	0
Southern pantry white gravy mix, 2 tsp	0
Horseradish	
Boar's Head	
Horseradish and beets grated in vinegar, 1 tsp	0
Horseradish grated in vinegar, 1 tsp	0
Pub style horseradish sauce, 1 tsp	0
Heinz	
Horseradish sauce, 1 tsp	1
Kraft	
Cream style horseradish, 1 tsp	0
Horseradish sauce, 1 tsp	0
Prepared horseradish, 1 tsp	0

	POINTS VALUE
Manischewitz	
Creamy horseradish sauce - original, 1 tsp	0
Creamy horseradish sauce - wasabi, 1 tsp	0
Creamy horseradish sauce with dill, 1 tsp	1
Creamy horseradish sauce with lemon, 1 tsp	1

Hot & Latin Sauces

	POINTS VALUE
Boar's Head	
Jalapeño pepper sauce, 1 tsp	0
Bufalo	
Chipotle hot sauce, 1 tsp	0
Especial hot sauce, 1 tsp	0
Jalapeno hot sauce, 1 tsp	0
Picante clasica hot sauce, 1 tsp	0
Chi-Chi's	
Fiesta squeezable taco sauce, 1 Tbsp	0
Picante medium, 2 Tbsp	0
Picante mild, 2 Tbsp	0
Goldwater's	
Chipotle red hot sauce, 1 Tbsp	0
Habanero green hot sauce, 1 Tbsp	0
La Estrellita	
Enchilada sauce, mild, 1/2 cup	1
Old El Paso	
Enchilada sauce, hot, 1/4 cup	1
Enchilada sauce, medium, 1/4 cup	1
Enchilada sauce, mild, 1/4 cup	1

	POINTS VALUE
Green chilli enchilada sauce, 1/4 cup	1
Picante - hot, 2 Tbsp	0
Picante - medium, 2 Tbsp	0
Picante - mild, 2 Tbsp	0
Taco sauce, hot, 1 Tbsp	0
Taco sauce, medium, 1 Tbsp	0
Taco sauce, mild, 1 Tbsp	0
Taco toppers - mild taco sauce, 2 Tbsp	0
Thick 'n chunky picante - hot, 2 Tbsp	0
Thick 'n chunky picante - medium, 2 Tbsp	0
Thick 'n chunky picante - mild, 2 Tbsp	0
Ortega	
Green taco sauce, mild, 1 Tbsp	0
Sunsun	
Louisiana hot sauce, 1 tsp	1
Taco Bell Home Originals	
Hot restaurant sauce, 1 tsp	0
Medium taco sauce, 2 Tbsp	0
Mild taco sauce, 2 Tbsp	0
Tostitos	
All natural medium picante sauce, 2 Tbsp	0
Trappey's	
Bull Louisiana hot sauce, 1 tsp	0
Chef magic jalapeno sauce, 1 tsp	0
Indi-pep West Indian style hot sauce, 1 tsp	0
Louisiana hot sauce, 1 tsp	0
Mexi-pep hot sauce, 1 tsp	0

CONDIMENTS, SAUCES & GRAVIES

Hot & Latin Sauces, Trappey's (con't)	POINTS VALUE
Red devil cayenne pepper sauce, 1 tsp	0
Red devil cayenne pepper sauce, buffalo-style, 1 tsp	0
Zapata	
Hot sauce, 1 tsp	0

Ketchup
Annie's Naturals
Organic ketchup, 1 Tbsp	0

Del Monte
Ketchup, 1 Tbsp	0
Sauce, chili, 1 Tbsp	0

Estee
No salt added ketchup, 1 Tbsp	0

Heinz
Chili sauce, 1 Tbsp	0
Hot ketchup made with tabasco, 1 Tbsp	0
Kid's EZ squirt blastin' green, 1 Tbsp	0
Kid's ketchup with vitamin c, 1 Tbsp	0
Light harvest ketchup, 1 Tbsp	0
Organic tomato ketchup, 1 Tbsp	0
Reduced sugar tomato ketchup, 1 Tbsp	0
Tomato ketchup, 1 Tbsp	0
Tomato ketchup, no salt added, 1 Tbsp	0

Heinz Ketchup Kick'rs
Hot and spicy flavored tomato ketchup, 1 Tbsp	0

	POINTS VALUE
La Estrellita	
Green vegetarian chile, 1/2 cup	1
Green vegetarian chile, medium, 1/2 cup	1
Hot green vegetarian chile, 1/2 cup	1
Manischewitz	
Tomato ketchup, 1 Tbsp	0
Muir Glen Organic	
Tomato ketchup, 1 Tbsp	0
Tree of Life	
Organic ketchup, 1 Tbsp	0
Walden Farms	
Ketchup/cocktail, 1 Tbsp	0
Thick & spicy, 2 Tbsp	0

Mayonnaise
Best Foods
Canola mayonnaise, 1 Tbsp	3
Light mayonnaise, 1 Tbsp	1
Mayonnaise with olive oil, 1 Tbsp	1
Real mayonnaise, 1 Tbsp	3
Reduced fat mayonnaise, 1 Tbsp	1

Boar's Head
Real mayonnaise, 1 Tbsp	3
Savory remoulade Cajun style mayonnaise, 1 Tbsp	3
Sun dried tomato pesto mayonnaise, 1 Tbsp	1

	POINTS VALUE
Hain Pure Foods	
Canola mayonnaise dressing, 1 Tbsp	3
Lite safflower mayonnaise, 1 Tbsp	1
Safflower mayonnaise, 1 Tbsp	3
Hellmann's	
Canola mayonnaise, 1 Tbsp	3
Light mayonnaise, 1 Tbsp	1
Mayonnaise with olive oil, 1 Tbsp	1
Real mayonnaise, 1 Tbsp	3
Reduced fat mayonnaise, 1 Tbsp	1
Kraft	
Fat free mayonnaise dressing, 1 Tbsp	0
Light mayonnaise, 1 Tbsp	1
Real mayonnaise, 1 Tbsp	3
Real mayonnaise hot 'n spicy super easy squeeze, 1 Tbsp	3
Kraft Mayonesa	
Real mayonnaise with lime juice, 1 Tbsp	3
Smart Balance	
Omega plus light mayo, 1 Tbsp	1
Smart Beat	
Fat free mayonnaise, 1 Tbsp	0
Spectrum Naturals	
Canola mayonnaise, 1 Tbsp	3
Dijon mayonnaise, organic, 1 Tbsp	3
Eggless vegan mayonnaise, organic, 1 Tbsp	1
Light canola mayonnaise, eggless, vegan, 1 Tbsp	1

	POINTS VALUE
Mayonnaise, organic, 1 Tbsp	3
Naturals spread, 1 Tbsp	3
Olive oil mayonnaise, organic, 1 Tbsp	3
Roasted garlic mayonnaise, organic, 1 Tbsp	3
Soy mayonnaise, organic, omega 3 with flax oil, 1 Tbsp	3
Wasabi mayonnaise, organic, 1 Tbsp	3
Mustard	
Annie's Naturals	
Organic Dijon mustard, 1 tsp	1
Organic honey mustard, 1 tsp	0
Organic horseradish mustard, 1 tsp	0
Organic yellow mustard, 1 tsp	1
Boar's Head	
Delicatessen style mustard, 1 tsp	0
Honey mustard, 1 tsp	0
Cherchies	
Banana pepper mustard, 1 Tbsp	0
Champagne mustard, 1 tsp	0
Cranberry mustard, 1 tsp	0
Key lime mustard, 1 Tbsp	1
Eden Organic	
Organic brown mustard, 1 tsp	0
Organic yellow mustard, 1 tsp	0
Grey Poupon	
Country dijon mustard, 1 tsp	0
Deli mustard, 1 tsp	0

CONDIMENTS, SAUCES & GRAVIES

Mustard, Grey Poupon (con't)	POINTS VALUE
Dijon mustard, 1 tsp	0
Harvest course ground, 1 tsp	0
Hearty spicy brown mustard, 1 tsp	0
Mild & creamy, 1 tsp	0
Savory honey mustard, 1 tsp	0
Heinz	
Spicy brown mustard, 1 tsp	0
Yellow mustard, 1 tsp	0
Kraft	
Horseradish mustard, 1 tsp	0
Yellow mustard, 1 tsp	0
Muirhead	
Honey mustard, 1 Tbsp	2
Horseradish mustard, 1 Tbsp	2
Tree of Life	
Organic dijon mustard, 1 tsp	0
Organic stone ground mustard, 1 tsp	0
Organic yellow mustard, 1 tsp	0
Organic yellow squeeze mustard, 1 tsp	0
Westbrae Natural	
Dijon style mustard, 1 tsp	0
Zatarain's	
Creole mustard, 1 tsp	0
Olives	
Faraon	
Spanish olives, 7	1
Spanish pimiento stuffed olives, 5 olives	1

	POINTS VALUE
Sardo	
Cocktail olives, 6	1
Kalamata olives, 4	1
Manzanilla olives, 5	1
Plain green olives, 2	1
Sliced green olives, 1 Tbsp	1
Stuffed queen olives, 2	0
Other Sauces	
Annie's Naturals	
Organic Worcestershire sauce, 1 Tbsp	0
Austex American Originals	
Hot dog chili sauce with onion, 1 Tbsp	0
Hot dog chili sauce, classic, 1 Tbsp	0
Boar's Head	
Brown sugar & spice ham glaze cooking sauce, 2 Tbsp	2
Castleberry's American Originals	
Hot dog chili sauce with onion, 1 Tbsp	0
Hot dog chili sauce, classic, 1 Tbsp	0
Cherchies	
Apple butter cooking & dipping sauce, 2 Tbsp	1
Raspberry chipotle cooking & dipping sauce, 2 Tbsp	1
Seafood seasoning sauce, 1 Tbsp	0
Chincoteague	
Premium white clam sauce, 1/2 cup	3
Red clam sauce, 1/2 cup	2

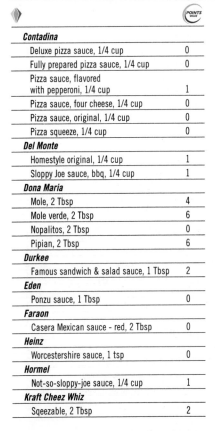

	POINTS VALUE
Contadina	
Deluxe pizza sauce, 1/4 cup	0
Fully prepared pizza sauce, 1/4 cup	0
Pizza sauce, flavored with pepperoni, 1/4 cup	1
Pizza sauce, four cheese, 1/4 cup	0
Pizza sauce, original, 1/4 cup	0
Pizza squeeze, 1/4 cup	0
Del Monte	
Homestyle original, 1/4 cup	1
Sloppy Joe sauce, bbq, 1/4 cup	1
Dona Maria	
Mole, 2 Tbsp	4
Mole verde, 2 Tbsp	6
Nopalitos, 2 Tbsp	0
Pipian, 2 Tbsp	6
Durkee	
Famous sandwich & salad sauce, 1 Tbsp	2
Eden	
Ponzu sauce, 1 Tbsp	0
Faraon	
Casera Mexican sauce - red, 2 Tbsp	0
Heinz	
Worcestershire sauce, 1 tsp	0
Hormel	
Not-so-sloppy-joe sauce, 1/4 cup	1
Kraft Cheez Whiz	
Sqeezable, 2 Tbsp	2

	POINTS VALUE
Lucky Leaf	
Lite strawberry fruit 'n sauce, no sugar added, 4 oz	1
Manischewitz	
Jellied cranberry sauce, 1/4 cup	2
Tomato & mushroom sauce, 1/4 cup	1
Muir Glen Organic	
Premium pizza sauce, 1/4 cup	1
Muirhead	
Apple cranberry chutney, 1 Tbsp	0
Apple pomegranate chutney, 1 Tbsp	0
Chocolate raspberry sauce, 1 Tbsp	1
Tangy cherry chutney, 1 Tbsp	1
Naturally Fresh	
Buffalo wing sauce, 2 Tbsp	2
Jackaroo meat sauce, 2 Tbsp	1
Seafood dipping sauce, 2 Tbsp	4
Ocean Spray	
Jellied cranberry sauce, 1/4 cup	2
Whole berry cranberry sauce, 1/4 cup	2
Ocean Spray Cran-Fruit	
For chicken, cranberry orange, 1/4 cup	2
For chicken, cranberry raspberry, 1/4 cup	2
Progresso	
Lobster, 1/2 cup	2
Red clam with tomato & basil, 1/2 cup	1
White clam (authentic), 1/2 cup	3
White clam with garlic & herbs, 1/2 cup	3

Other Sauces (con't)	POINTS VALUE

	POINTS VALUE
Ragu Old World Style	
Pizza sauce, 1/4 cup	0
Ragu Pizza Quick	
Traditional, 1/4 cup	1
Sabra	
Tahini, 1 serving (28 g)	2
Seneca	
Strawberry, 1 container	1
Snow's	
Red clam sauce, 1/2 cup	2
White clam sauce, 1/2 cup	2
T. Marzetti	
Homestyle cranberry sauce, 1/4 cup	2
Tree of Life	
Lime & chili chutney, 1 Tbsp	1
Major grey chutney, 1 Tbsp	1
Mango pomegranate chutney, 1 Tbsp	1
Mango raisin chutney, 1 Tbsp	1
Organic cranberry sauce, jellied, 1/4 cup	2
Organic sesame tahini, 2 Tbsp	4
Pineapple chutney, 1 Tbsp	1
Tree Top	
Apple pie a la mode naturally sweetened, 1 container	1
Mango peach naturally sweetened, 1 container	1
Pear naturally sweetened, 1 container	1

	POINTS VALUE
Walden Farms	
Scampi sauce, 2 Tbsp	0
Zapata	
Cheese sauce, mild, 1/4 cup	1
Cheese sauce, spicy, 1/4 cup	1

Pasta Sauces
Amy's

	POINTS VALUE
Family marinara pasta sauce, 1/2 cup	1
Garlic mushroom pasta sauce, 1/2 cup	2
Low sodium marinara sauce, 1/2 cup	1
Puttanesca sauce, 1/2 cup	1
Roasted garlic pasta sauce, 1/2 cup	3
Tomato basil pasta sauce, 1/2 cup	2
Aunt Millie's	
Italian sausage sauce, 1/2 cup	1
Marinara, 1/2 cup	1
Meat sauce, 1/2 cup	2
Traditional sauce, 1/2 cup	1
Barilla	
Marinara sauce, 1/2 cup	1
Tomato & basil sauce, 1/2 cup	1
Bertolli	
Alfredo with mushrooms, 1/4 cup	2
Creamy alfredo, 1/4 cup	3
Creamy garlic alfredo, 1/4 cup	3
Fire roasted tomato with cabernet, 1/2 cup	2

◆	POINTS VALUE
Five cheese, 1/2 cup	2
Italian sausage, romano & garlic, 1/2 cup	1
Marinara, 1/2 cup	1
Marinara with burgundy wine, 1 serving (126 g)	2
Mediterranean olive, 1/2 cup	2
Mushroom and garlic, 1 serving (127 g)	1
Olive oil & garlic, 1/2 cup	1
Organic olive oil garlic, 1/2 cup	1
Organic tomato & basil, 1/2 cup	2
Portobello mushroom with merlot, 1/2 cup	2
Tomato & basil, 1/2 cup	1
Vidalia onion & roasted garlic, 1/2 cup	1
Vodka sauce, 1/2 cup	3
CIBO Naturals	
Artichoke lemon pesto, 1/4 cup	6
Cilantro lime pesto, 1/4 cup	8
Classic basil pesto, 1/4 cup	9
Roasted red pepper pesto, 1/4 cup	2
Romesco sauce, 2 Tbsp	1
Sun dried tomato pesto (vegan), 1/4 cup	7
Classico	
Cabernet marinara, 1/2 cup	1
Caramelized onion and garlic, 1/2 cup	1
Creamy alfredo, 1/4 cup	3
Fire roasted tomato and garlic, 1/2 cup	1
Florentine spinach & cheese, 1/2 cup	2

◆	POINTS VALUE
Four cheese, 1/2 cup	1
Four cheese alfredo, 1/4 cup	2
Garden vegetable primavera, 1/2 cup	1
Italian sausage with green peppers & onions, 1/2 cup	2
Mushroom & ripe olives, 1/2 cup	1
Organic spinach & garlic, 1/2 cup	1
Organic tomato, herbs and spices, 1/2 cup	1
Roasted garlic, 1/2 cup	1
Roasted garlic alfredo, 1/4 cup	2
Roasted red pepper alfredo, 1/4 cup	2
Spicy red pepper, 1/2 cup	1
Spicy tomato & basil, 1/2 cup	1
Spicy tomato & pesto, 1/2 cup	2
Sun dried tomato pesto, 1/4 cup	2
Sun-dried tomato, 1/2 cup	1
Sun-dried tomato alfredo, 1/4 cup	2
Tomato & basil, 1/2 cup	1
Traditional sweet basil, 1/2 cup	1
Triple mushroom, 1/2 cup	1
Contadina	
Deluxe marinara sauce, 1/2 cup	1
Deluxe spaghetti sauce, 1/2 cup	1
◆ Italian paste - tomato paste product with Italian seasonings, 2 Tbsp	1
◆ Italian paste - tomato paste product with roasted garlic, 2 Tbsp	1

Pasta Sauces, Contadina (con't)	
◆ Italian paste - tomato paste product with tomato pesto, 2 Tbsp	1
◆ Italian style tomato sauce, 1/4 cup	0
Spaghetti sauce, 1/2 cup	1
◆ Tomato paste - 100% tomatoes, 2 Tbsp	0
◆ Tomato puree, 1/4 cup	0
◆ Tomato sauce, 1/4 cup	0
◆ Tomato sauce - extra thick & zesty, 1/4 cup	0
◆ Tomato sauce - garlic and onion, 1/4 cup	0
Del Monte	
Four cheese, 1/2 cup	1
◆ Organic tomato paste, 2 Tbsp	0
◆ Organic tomato sauce, 1/4 cup	0
◆ Sauce, tomato no salt added, 1/4 cup	0
Tomato & basil, 1/2 cup	1
Traditional, 1/2 cup	1
With garlic and onion, 1/2 cup	1
With green peppers and mushrooms, 1/2 cup	1
With meat, 1/2 cup	1
With mushrooms, 1/2 cup	1
Del Monte Chunky	
Garlic & herb, 1/2 cup	1
Italian herb, 1/2 cup	1
Eden Organic	
Pizza pasta sauce, 1/4 cup	0
Spaghetti sauce, 1/2 cup	1
Spaghetti sauce - no salt, 1/2 cup	1

Ellen Rose	
Artichoke & olive pesto, 2 Tbsp	2
Pesto sauce, 2 Tbsp	3
Sun dried tomato pesto, 2 Tbsp	5
Faraon	
◆ Tomato sauce, 1/4 cup	0
Lucini	
Hearty artichoke tomato pasta sauce, 1/2 cup	3
Rustic tomato basil pasta sauce, 1/2 cup	3
Sicilian eggplant & olive pasta sauce, 1/2 cup	2
Sicilian olive & wild caper sauce, 1/2 cup	3
Spicy Tuscan tomato sauce, 1/2 cup	3
Monterey Pasta Company	
Basil cream sauce with artichokes, 1/2 cup	5
Fresh herb alfredo sauce, 1/2 cup	5
Pesto sauce with garlic and basil, 1/4 cup	8
Sun dried tomato cream sauce, 1/2 cup	4
Sweet tomato basil sauce, 1/2 cup	1
Vodka cream sauce, 1/2 cup	4
Muir Glen Organic	
Cabernet marinara pasta sauce, 1/2 cup	1
Chunky tomato & herb pasta sauce, 1/2 cup	1
Fire roasted tomato pasta sauce, 1/2 cup	1
Four cheese pasta sauce, 1/2 cup	1
Garden vegetable pasta sauce, 1/2 cup	1
Garlic roasted garlic sauce, 1/2 cup	1

	POINTS VALUE
Italian herb pasta sauce, 1/2 cup	1
Portabello mushroom pasta sauce, 1/2 cup	1
◆ Premium chunky tomato sauce, 1/4 cup	0
◆ Premium tomato sauce, 1/4 cup	0
Spicy tomato pasta sauce, 1/2 cup	1
Sun dried tomato pasta sauce, 1/2 cup	1
Muirhead	
Tomato sauce, 1 Tbsp	0
Naturally Fresh	
Marinara, 2 Tbsp	0
Progresso	
Marinara (authentic), 1/2 cup	2
◆ Tomato puree, 1/4 cup	0
Ragu Cheese Creations	
Classic alfredo, 1/4 cup	3
Double cheddar, 1/4 cup	3
Lite parmesan alfredo, 1/4 cup	2
Roasted garlic parmesan, 1/4 cup	3
Ragu Chunky Gardenstyle	
Garden combination, 1/2 cup	2
Mama's special garden sauce, 1/2 cup	2
Mushrooms & green pepper, 1/2 cup	2
Roasted red pepper & onion, 1/2 cup	2
Sundried tomato & sweet basil, 1/2 cup	2
Super chunky mushroom, 1/2 cup	2
Super vegetable primavera, 1/2 cup	2
Tomato, basil & Italian cheese, 1/2 cup	2
Tomato, garlic & onion, 1/2 cup	2
Ragu Light	
No sugar added tomato & basil, 1/2 cup	1
Tomato & basil, fat free, 1/2 cup	1
Ragu Old World Style	
Flavored with meat, 1/2 cup	1
Marinara, 1/2 cup	2
Mushroom, 1/2 cup	1
Traditional, 1/2 cup	1
Ragu Organic	
Cheese, 1/2 cup	2
Garden veggie, 1/2 cup	1
Traditional, 1/2 cup	1
Ragu Rich & Meaty	
Classic Italian meat, 1/2 cup	3
Ragu Robusto	
Chopped tomato olive oil & garlic, 1/2 cup	2
Parmesan & romano, 1/2 cup	2
Roasted garlic, 1/2 cup	1
Sauteed beef, onions & garlic, 1/2 cup	2
Sauteed onion & garlic, 1/2 cup	2
Sauteed onion & mushroom, 1/2 cup	2
Seven-herb tomato, 1/2 cup	1
Six cheese, 1/2 cup	2
Sweet Italian sausage & cheese, 1/2 cup	2
Seeds of Change	
Arrabiatta di roma, 1/2 cup	2
Garden vegetable piemonte, 1/2 cup	1
Marinara di venezia, 1/2 cup	1

CONDIMENTS, SAUCES & GRAVIES

Pasta Sauces, Ragu Robusto (con't)	POINTS VALUE
Modena balsamic onion, 1/2 cup	2
Porcini mushroom di appenine, 1/2 cup	1
Puttanesca napoletana, 1/2 cup	2
Romagna three cheese, 1/2 cup	2
Sicilian spicy eggplant, 1/2 cup	2
Tomato basil genovese, 1/2 cup	1
Tuscan tomato and garlic, 1/2 cup	1
Vodka Americano sauce, 1/2 cup	3
Walden Farms	
Alfredo sauce, 1/4 cup	0
Marinara sauce, 1/3 cup	0

Pickles

B&G	POINTS VALUE
Bread & butter chips, 1 oz	1
Bread & butter chips, unsalted, 5 pieces	1
Crunchy kosher dills, 1 oz	0
Deluxe kosher dill spears, 1 oz	0
Dill gherkins, 1 oz	0
Hamburger dill chips, 1 oz	0
Kosher dill chips, 1 oz	0
Kosher dill spears, 1 oz	0
B&G Sandwich Toppers	
Bread & butter, 1 1/2 pieces	1
B&G Sugar Free	
Bread & butter chips, 1 oz	0
Sandwich toppers - bread and butter, 1 oz	0
Sweet gherkins, 1 oz	0

	POINTS VALUE
Boar's Head	
Kosher dill pickle - whole, 1/2	0
Sweet pickle chips with horseradish, 3	1
Cascadian Farm	
Baby dills, 1	0
Bread & butter chips, 5 slices	1
Kosher dills, 1	0
Kosher dills - reduced sodium, 1	0
Claussen	
Bread 'n butter chips, 4 slices	0
Burger slices, Kosher dill, 1 slice	0
Deli style hearty garlic wholes, 1/2	0
Deli style kosher dill halves, 1/2	0
Deli style kosher dill spears, 1	0
Kosher dill halves, 1/2	0
Kosher dill mini, 1	0
Kosher dill spears, 1	0
Kosher dill wholes, 1/2	0
New York deli style half sour wholes, 1/2	0
Sandwich slices deli style hearty garlic, 2 slices	0
Sandwich slices kosher dill, 2 slices	0
Sandwich slices, bread 'n butter, 2 slices	1
Hans Jurgen	
Cold pack pickles, 1 oz	0

	POINTS VALUE
Heinz	
Baby kosher dills, 1 oz	0
Bread & butter sandwich slices, 1 oz	1
Dill pickles, 1 oz	0
Genuine dill pickles, 1 oz	0
Hamburger dill chips, 1 oz	0
Kosher dill sandwich slices, 1 oz	0
Kosher dill spears, 1 oz	0
Kosher dills, 1 oz	0
Old fashioned bread and butter pickles, 1 oz	0
Polish dills, 1 oz	0
Sweet gherkins, 1 oz	1
Sweet pickles, 1 oz	1
Mrs. Fanning's	
Bread 'n butter pickles, 1 oz	1
Vlasic	
Bread & butter chips no sugar added, 3	0
Bread & butter sandwich stackers, 2	1
Bread & butter spears, 3/4	1
Bread & butter spears no sugar added, 1 serving (3/4 spear)	0
Kosher baby dills, 1	0
Kosher crunchy dills, 1 serving (1/2 pickle)	0
Kosher dill sandwich stackers, 2	0
Kosher dill snack'mms, 1 oz (2 pickles)	0
Kosher dill spears, 1 serving (3/4 spear)	0

	POINTS VALUE
Kosher midget dills, 3	0
Sweet bread & butter chips, 3	1
Sweet gherkins no sugar added, 3	0
Sweet relish no sugar added, 1 Tbsp	0
Zesty dill sandwich stackers, 2	0
Zesty garlic whole pickles, 1 serving (1/2 pickle)	0
Relish	
B&G	
Sweet relish, 1 Tbsp	1
B&G Sugar Free	
Sweet relish, 1 Tbsp	0
Cascadian Farm	
Sweet relish, 1 Tbsp	1
Claussen	
Premium sweet pickle relish, 1 Tbsp	0
Sweet pickle relish, 1 Tbsp	0
Del Monte	
Sweet pickle relish, 1 Tbsp	0
Heinz	
Hamburger relish, 1 Tbsp	0
Hot dog relish, 1 Tbsp	0
India relish, 1 Tbsp	0
Sweet relish, 1 Tbsp	0
Zesty relish, 1 Tbsp	0
Vlasic	
Dill relish, 1 Tbsp	0
Dill tabasco relish, 1 Tbsp	0

Seafood Sauces and Marinades

Cherchies

	POINTS VALUE
Seafood seasoning sauce, 1 Tbsp	0

Del Monte

Sauce, seafood cocktail, 1/4 cup	2

Heinz

Seafood cocktail sauce, 1/4 cup	1
Tartar sauce, 2 Tbsp	3
Zesty cocktail sauce, 1/4 cup	1

Kraft

Cocktail sauce, 1/4 cup	1
Lemon & herb flavor tartar sauce, 2 Tbsp	4
Nonfat tartar sauce, 2 Tbsp	1
Tartar sauce, 2 Tbsp	2

McCormick

Tartar sauce, 2 Tbsp	4

Naturally Fresh

Seafood cocktail, 2 Tbsp	0
Seafood cocktail sauce, 1 Tbsp	1
Seafood cocktail sauce, shelf stable, 2 Tbsp	0
Tartar sauce, 2 Tbsp	4
Tartar sauce, shelf stable, 2 Tbsp	4

Walden Farms

Cocktail sauce, 1 Tbsp	0

Weber Grill Creations

Mesquite, dry mix, 1 tsp	0

Steak, Meat Sauces and Marinades

A1

	POINTS VALUE
Bold & spicy, 1 Tbsp	0
Bold & spicy with Tabasco, 1 Tbsp	0
Carb well steak sauce, 1 Tbsp	0
Chicago steak house, 1 Tbsp	0
Cracked peppercorn, 1 Tbsp	0
Kobe sesame teriyaki, 1 Tbsp	1
New York steakhouse, 1 Tbsp	0
Original, 2 Tbsp	1
Roasted garlic, 1 Tbsp	0
Seafood marinade, ginger teriyaki with orange, 1 Tbsp	1
Seafood marinade, mango chipotle, 1 Tbsp	1
Seafood marinade, roasted garlic with lemon, 1 Tbsp	0
Smokey mesquite, 1 Tbsp	1
Steak house New Orleans Cajun, 1 Tbsp	1
Steak house teriyaki, 1 Tbsp	1
Steak sauce, 1 Tbsp	0
Steakhouse classic, 1 Tbsp	0
Steakhouse garlic & herb, 1 Tbsp	0
Steakhouse Jamaican jerk, 1 Tbsp	1
Steakhouse Texas mesquite, 1 Tbsp	0
Supreme garlic, 1 Tbsp	1
Teriyaki, 1 Tbsp	1
Thick & hearty, 1 Tbsp	1

	POINTS VALUE
Annie's Naturals	
Organic mango cilantro, 1 Tbsp	0
Organic smokey tomato marinade, 1 Tbsp	1
Organic spicy ginger marinade, 1 Tbsp	1
Organic steak marinade, 1 Tbsp	1
Organic teriyaki marinade, 1 Tbsp	1
Annie's Naturals All Natural	
Baja lime, 1 Tbsp	1
Consorzio	
Roasted garlic marinade, 1 Tbsp	1
Sesame orange, 1 Tbsp	1
Consorzio All Natural	
California teriyaki, 1 Tbsp	1
Roasted garlic and balsamic, 1 Tbsp	1
Durkee Grill Creations	
Chipotle marinade, dry mix, 1 tsp	0
Grill Mates	
Mesquite marinade, 2 tsp	0
Zesty herb marinade, 1 tsp	0
Heinz	
57 sauce, 1 Tbsp	0
Traditional steak sauce, 1 Tbsp	0
House of Tsang	
Mandarin marinade soy sauce, 1 Tbsp	1
House of Tsang Simply Tsang	
Ginger sesame marinade, 1 Tbsp	0
Jamaican jerk marinade, 1 Tbsp	1

	POINTS VALUE
Japanese steakhouse marinade, 1 Tbsp	1
Sweet & sour marinade, 1 Tbsp	1
Teriyaki marinade, 1 Tbsp	1
Jack Daniel's	
Ez marinader honey teriyaki, 1 Tbsp	1
Ez marinader mesquite, 1 Tbsp	1
Ez marinader slow roasted garlic and herb, 1 Tbsp	0
Original steak sauce, 1 Tbsp	0
Smokey steak sauce, 1 Tbsp	0
K.C. Masterpiece	
Garlic herb marinade, 1 Tbsp	1
Golden honey and dijon marinade, 1 Tbsp	1
Hickory and spice marinade, 1 Tbsp	1
Honey teriyaki with sesame marinade, 1 Tbsp	1
Spiced Caribbean jerk marinade, 1 Tbsp	0
Zesty lemon pepper marinade, 1 Tbsp	0
Mrs. Dash	
Garlic lime 10-minute marinade, 1 Tbsp	1
Lemon herb peppercorn 10-minute marinade, 1 Tbsp	1
Mesquite grille 10-minute marinade, 1 Tbsp	1
Southwestern chipotle 10-minute marinade, 1 Tbsp	1
Spicy teriyaki 10-minute marinade, 1 Tbsp	1
Zesty garlic herb 10-minute marinade, 1 Tbsp	1

Steak, Meat Sauces and Marinades (con't)

(POINTS VALUE)

Naturally Fresh

Lemon pepper, 2 Tbsp	3
Marinade, 2 Tbsp	0
Southwestern, 2 Tbsp	2

San-J

Japanese steak marinade, 1 Tbsp	0

Weber Grill Creations

Black peppercorn marinade, dry mix, 1 tsp	0
Italian herb, dry mix, 1 1/2 tsp	0
Tomato garlic pesto marinade, dry mix, 1 tsp	0
White wine & herb, dry mix, 1 tsp	0

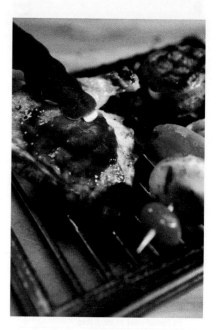

POINTS VALUE   POINTS VALUE

Butter & Butter Substitutes

Blue Bunny

Sweet cream butter, 1 Tbsp	3

Butter Buds

Powdered mix, 1 tsp	0
Sprinkles, 1 tsp	0

Land O Lakes

Butter sweet cream, salted stick, 1 Tbsp	3
Butter sweet cream, unsalted stick, 1 Tbsp	3
Country morning blend, soft, 1 Tbsp	3
Country morning blend, stick, 1 Tbsp	3
Honey butter, 1 Tbsp	2
Light butter with canola oil, 1 Tbsp	1
Light butter, stick, 1 Tbsp	2
Light butter, whipped, 1 Tbsp	1
Roasted garlic butter with oil, 1 Tbsp	3
Spreadable butter with canola oil, 1 Tbsp	3
Ultra creamy butter, salted, 1 Tbsp	3
Ultra creamy butter, unsalted, 1 Tbsp	3
Whipped butter, salted, 1 Tbsp	2
Whipped butter, unsalted, 1 Tbsp	2

Molly McButter

Natural butter, 1 tsp	0
Natural cheese, 1 tsp	0

Smart Balance

Butter blend stick, regular, 1 serving (14 g)	3
Butter blend stick, unsalted, 1 serving (14 g)	3
Butter blend stick, omega, 1 serving (14 g)	3

Cheese

4C

Grated Italian pecorino Romano sharp cheese, 1 serving (5 g)	1
Grated parmesan & Romano cheese, 1 serving (5 g)	1
Grated parmesan cheese, 1 serving (5 g)	1
Homestyle grated pecorino Romano cheese, 1 serving (5 g)	1

Alpine Lace

Reduced fat cheddar cheese, 1 oz	2
Reduced fat co-jack cheese, 1 oz	2
Reduced fat mozzarella cheese, 1 oz	2
Reduced fat reduced sodium lightly smoked provolone cheese, 1 oz	2
Reduced fat Swiss cheese, 1 oz	2
Reduced fat, American cheese, 1 oz	2
Reduced sodium muenster cheese, 1 oz	3

Athenos

Blue cheese crumbles, 1/4 cup	3
Blue cheese crumbles, 3 Tbsp	3
Feta cheese garlic & herb, 1 oz	2
Feta cheese traditional, 1 oz	2
Feta cheese traditional crumbles, 1/4 cup	2
Feta cheese with garlic & herb, 1/4 cup	2
Feta cheese with tomato & basil, 1 oz	2
Feta cheese with tomato basil crumbles, 1/4 cup	2

DAIRY & EGGS

Cheese, Athenos (con't)	POINTS VALUE
Gorgonzola cheese crumbles, 3 Tbsp	3
Reduced fat feta cheese slab, 1 oz	2
Blue Bunny	
1% lowfat cottage cheese, 1/2 cup	2
Homestyle large curd cottage cheese, 1/2 cup	3
Reduced fat 2% cottage cheese, 1/2 cup	2
Boar's Head	
25% lower sodium - 25% lower fat American cheese - yellow & white, 1 oz	2
28% lower sodium blue cheese crumbled, 1/4 cup	2
28% lower sodium creamy blue cheese, 1 oz	2
American cheese (loaf) - yellow or white, 1 oz	3
American cheese 120 sliced - yellow or white, 1 slice	2
American cheese 160, sliced - yellow or white, 2 slices	3
American sopressata & provolone slices, 1 serving (28 g)	3
Baby Swiss cheese, 1 oz	3
Butterkase cheese, 1 oz	3
Canadian cheddar cheese 3 yr. old, 1 oz	3
Cream cheese, 2 Tbsp	3
Cream havarti cheese, 1 oz	3
Cream havarti cheese plain with dill, 1 oz	3

	POINTS VALUE
Cream havarti cheese plain with jalapeño, 1 oz	3
Creamy gorgonzola cheese crumbled, 1/4 cup	3
Crumbled feta cheese, 1 oz	2
Double gloucester cheddar cheese, 1 oz	3
Edam cheese, 1 oz	2
Feta cheese, 1 oz	2
Fontina cheese, 1 oz	3
Gold label prem. imp Swiss, 1 oz	3
Gouda cheese, 1 oz	3
Grana padano cheese - pre-cut, 1 oz	3
Hickory smoked pasteurized process gruyere cheese, 1 oz	3
Horseradish cheddar cheese, 1 oz	3
Imported Italian grated pecorino romano cheese, 1 Tbsp	1
Imported Italian pecorino romano cheese - wedge, 1 Tbsp	1
Insalata panino, 1 oz	2
Lacey Swiss cheese, 1 oz	2
Longhorn colby cheese, 1 oz	3
Low sodium muenster cheese, 1 oz	3
Lower sodium provolone cheese, 1 oz	3
Monterey Jack cheese, 1 oz	3
Monterey Jack cheese with jalapeño, 1 oz	3
Mozzarella cheese, 1 oz	2

	POINTS VALUE
Muenster cheese, 1 oz	3
Natural Swiss cheese, 1 oz	3
Neufchatel cheese, 2 Tbsp	2
No salt added natural Swiss cheese, 1 oz	3
Parmigiano reggiano cheese - pre-cut, 1 oz	3
Picante/sharp provolone cheese, 1 oz	3
Pre-cut asiago cheese, 1 oz	4
Pre-cut creamy gorgonzola cheese, 1 oz	3
Pre-cut gruyere, 1 oz	3
Premium imported grated parmesan cheese, 1 Tbsp	0
Queso blanco cheese, 1 oz	2
Queso para freir cheese, 1 oz	2
Sharp cheddar cheese (white & yellow), 1 oz	3
Vermont cheddar cheese (white or yellow), 1 oz	3

Borden

	POINTS VALUE
Cheddar & Monterey Jack cheese (shredded), 1/4 cup	3
Cheddar cheese, extra sharp, 1 oz	3
Cheddar cheese, medium, 1 oz	3
Cheddar cheese, mild, 1 oz	3
Cheddar cheese, mild (shredded), 1/4 cup	3
Cheddar cheese, sharp, 1 oz	3
Cheddar cheese, sharp (shredded), 1/4 cup	3
Cheddar melt cheese (shredded), 1/4 cup	3

	POINTS VALUE
Colby & Monterey Jack cheese, 1 oz	3
Colby & Monterey Jack cheese (shredded), 1/4 cup	3
Colby & Monterey Jack slices, 2 slices	4
Colby cheese, 1 oz	3
Double twist string cheese, mozzarella, 1 stick	2
Four cheese Mexican cheese (shredded), 1/4 cup	3
Mild cheddar slices, 2 slices	4
Mozzarella cheese (shredded), 1/4 cup	2
Pizza cheese (shredded), 1/4 cup	3
Six cheese Italian cheese (shredded), 1/4 cup	2
String cheese, mozzarella, 1 serving (0.833 oz)	2
Swiss slices, 2 slices	3

Borden 2% Singles

	POINTS VALUE
American (white) reduced fat pasteurized prepared cheese product, 1 slice (3/4 oz)	1
American reduced fat pasteurized prepared cheese product, 1 slice (3/4 oz)	1
Sharp reduced fat pasteurized prepared cheese product, 1 slice (3/4 oz)	1

Borden Big!

	POINTS VALUE
American (white) pasteurized prepared cheese product, 1 slice	2
American pasteurized prepared cheese product, 1 slice	2

DAIRY & EGGS

Cheese (con't)	POINTS VALUE
Borden Deluxe	
American (white) pasteurized prepared cheese product, 1 slice (3/4 oz)	2
American pasteurized prepared cheese product, 1 slice (3/4 oz)	2
Borden Fat Free Singles	
♦ American (white) nonfat pasteurized prepared cheese product, 1 slice (3/4 oz)	1
♦ American nonfat pasteurized prepared cheese product, 1 slice (3/4 oz)	1
♦ Sharp nonfat pasteurized prepared cheese product, 1 slice (3/4 oz)	1
♦ Swiss nonfat pasteurized prepared cheese product, 1 slice (3/4 oz)	1
Borden Singles	
American (white) pasteurized prepared cheese product, 1 slice (3/4 oz)	2
American cheese pasteurized prepared cheese product, 1 slice (3/4 oz)	2
Swiss cheese, 1 slice (3/4 oz)	2
Boursin Light	
Garlic & fine herbs Gournay cheese, 1 2/3 Tbsp	1
Breakstone's	
Lowfat cottage cheese - 2% milkfat with added calcium & vitamin D, small curd, 1/2 cup	2
Ricotta cheese, 1/4 cup	3

	POINTS VALUE
Breakstone's 4-Pack	
2% milkfat, small curd (snack size), 4 oz	2
Breakstone's TempTee	
Whipped cream cheese, 2 Tbsp	2
Cabot	
Cheddar cheese, 1 oz (1" cube)	3
Fancy blend shredded cheese, 1/4 cup	3
Habanero cheddar, 1 oz (1" cube)	3
Jalapeno light cheddar cheese - 50% reduced fat, 1 oz (1" cube)	2
Light cheddar cheese - 50% reduced fat, 1 oz (1" cube)	2
Light cheddar cheese - 75% reduced fat, 1 oz (1" cube)	1
Light cheddar shredded cheese - 50% reduced fat, 1/4 cup (1 oz)	2
Pepper Jack, 1 oz (1" cube)	3
Reduced fat cheddar, 3/4 oz (1 bar)	1
Sharp cheddar, 3/4 oz (1 bar)	2
Sliced light cheddar cheese - 50% reduced fat, 1 slice	2
Swiss slices, 1 slice	3
Tomato basil cheddar, 1 oz (1" cube)	3
DiGiorno	
Asiago cheese wedge, grated, 2 tsp	1
Asiago cheese, wedge & cubes, 1 oz	3
Fior di latte fresh mozzarella cheese, 3 balls	2

	POINTS VALUE
Fresh twist parmesan cheese, grated, 2 Tbsp	1
Full moisture asiago cheese, shredded, 1/4 cup	3
Full moisture parmesan, shredded, 1/4 cup	3
Full moisture pecorino romano cheese, shredded, 1/4 cup	3
Full moisture romano cheese, shredded, 1/4 cup	3
Full moisture shaved parmesan cheese, shredded, 1/4 cup	3
Gourmet mozzarella cheese, 1 oz	2
Romano cheese wheels, grated, 2 tsp	1
Three cheese blend, shredded, 1/4 cup	3

DiGiorno Full-moisture Grated

Parmesan cheese, 2 tsp	1
Romano cheese, 2 tsp	1

Finlandia

Heavenly light imported Swiss cheese, 1 slice	1
Imported Swiss cheese, 1 oz	3
Sandwich naturals gouda cheese, 1 slice	2
Sandwich naturals havarti cheese, 1 slice	2
Sandwich naturals imported oltermanni cheese, 1 slice	2
Sandwich naturals muenster cheese, 1 slice	2
Sandwich naturals Swiss cheese, 1 slice	2

	POINTS VALUE
Follow Your Heart	
♦ Vegan gourmet cheese alternative, cheddar flavor, 1 oz	2
♦ Vegan gourmet cheese alternative, Monterey Jack flavor, 1 oz	2
♦ Vegan gourmet cheese alternative, mozzarella flavor, 1 oz	2
♦ Vegan gourmet cheese alternative, nacho flavor, 1 oz	2
Friendship	
All-natural California style cottage cheese with pineapple, 4% milkfat, 1/2 cup	3
All-natural California style cottage cheese, 4% milkfat, 1/2 cup	3
All-natural lowfat cottage cheese - no salt added, 1% milkfat, 1/2 cup	2
All-natural lowfat cottage cheese, 1% milkfat, 1/2 cup	2
All-natural lowfat whipped cottage cheese, 1% milkfat, 1/2 cup	2
All-natural pot style large curd cottage cheese, 2% milkfat, 1/2 cup	2
Farmer cheese, 2 Tbsp	1
Farmer cheese no salt added, 2 Tbsp	1
Lowfat cottage cheese with pineapple, 1% milkfat, 1/2 cup	2
♦ Nonfat cottage cheese, 1/2 cup	2
Nonfat cottage cheese with peaches, 1/2 cup	2
Nonfat cottage cheese with pineapple, 1/2 cup	2

Cheese (con't)	POINTS VALUE

Galaxy Foods

	POINTS VALUE
Rice cheddar flavor shreds, 1/3 cup	2
Rice cheddar flavored block, 1 oz	2
Rice mozzarella flavor shreds, 1/3 cup	2
Rice mozzarella flavored block, 1 oz	2
Rice parmesan flavored grated topping, 2 tsp	0
Rice slices American flavor, 1 slice	1
Rice slices cheddar flavor, 1 slice	1
Rice slices mozzarella flavor, 1 slice	1
Rice slices pepper Jack flavor, 1 slice	1
Rice slices Swiss flavor, 1 slice	1
Smoked provolone flavor alternative slices, 1 slice	1
Super stix mozzarella flavor snack sticks, 1 oz	2
Vegan cheddar flavor alternative slices, 1 slice	1
♦ Vegan cheddar flavor block, 1 oz	1
♦ Vegan mozzarella flavor, 1 slice	1
♦ Vegan mozzarella flavor block, 1 oz	1
♦ Vegan parmesan flavored grated topping, 2 tsp	0
Veggie American flavor alternative, 1 slice	1
Veggie cheddar flavor alternative, 1 slice	1
Veggie cheddar flavor alternative - shreds, 1/4 cup	2

	POINTS VALUE
Veggie cheddar flavor alternative-block, 1 oz	2
Veggie cheddar with jalapeño flavor, 1 slice	1
Veggie cheddar& pepper Jack cheese flavor alternative - shreds, 1/4 cup	2
Veggie chipotle flavor alternative - block, 1 oz	1
Veggie Monterey Jack & cheddar alternative - shreds, 1/4 cup	2
Veggie mozzarella flavor alternative, 1 slice	1
Veggie mozzarella flavor alternative - shreds, 1/4 cup	2
Veggie mozzarella flavor alternative-block, 1 oz	2
Veggie parmesan flavor topping-grated, 2 tsp	0
Veggie parmesan/mozzarella/romano flavor alternative - shreds (low fat), 1 oz	2
Veggie pepper Jack flavor alternative, 1 slice	1
Veggie pepper Jack flavor alternative - block, 1 oz	1
Veggie provolone smoked flavor alternative, 1 slice	1
Veggie Swiss flavor alternative, 1 slice	1

	POINTS VALUE
GG Golden Guernsey Dairy	
◆ Fat free cottage cheese, 1/2 cup	2
Low fat cottage cheese, 1/2 cup	2
Gourmet Goat	
Goat cream cheese log, 1 slice	2
Horizon Organic	
Lowfat cottage cheese, 1/2 cup	2
Reduced fat cream cheese, 2 Tbsp	2
Regular cottage cheese, 1/2 cup	3
Spreadable cream cheese, 2 Tbsp	3
Jarlsberg	
Lite sliced, 1 slice	1
Sliced, 1 slice	2
Knudsen	
Cottage cheese - 4% milkfat, large curd, 1/2 cup	3
Cottage cheese - 4% milkfat, small curd, 1/2 cup	3
Lowfat cottage cheese - 2% milkfat with added calcium & vitamin D, small curd, 1/2 cup	2
Knudsen Cottage Doubles	
Lowfat cottage cheese and blueberry topping, 1 container (5.5 oz)	3
Lowfat cottage cheese and peach topping with added calcium and vitamin D, 1 container (5.5 oz)	3

	POINTS VALUE
Lowfat cottage cheese and pineapple topping, 1 container (5.5 oz)	3
Lowfat cottage cheese and raspberry topping, 1 container (5.5 oz)	3
Lowfat cottage cheese and strawberry topping, 1 container (5.5 oz)	3
Knudsen Free	
◆ Free fat free cottage cheese, 1/2 cup	2
Knudsen LiveActive	
2% milkfat cottage cheese, small curd, 1 container	1
Kraft	
2% milk reduced fat sharp cheddar cheese, 4 slices	2
2% milk reduced-fat colby & 2% milk reduced-fat Monterey Jack cheese crumbles, 1/4 cup	2
2% reduced fat sharp cheddar cheese stick, 1	2
3-cheese blend crumbles (Monterey Jack, colby and cheddar cheeses), 1/4 cup	3
American pasteurized prepared cheese product, 1 slice	2
Bacon, spread, 2 Tbsp	2
Blue cheese crumbles, 3 Tbsp	3
Cheddar & Monterey Jack (shredded), 1/4 cup	3
Cheddar medium (shredded), 1/4 cup	3
Cheddar, mild (shredded), 1/4 cup	3

Cheese, Kraft (con't)	POINTS VALUE
Cheddar, sharp (shredded), 1/4 cup	3
Classic melts shredded American, mild cheddar & Monterey Jack cheeses, 1/4 cup	3
Colby & Monterey Jack (shredded), 1/4 cup	3
Colby & Monterey Jack cheese cubes, 4 pieces	3
Cracker cuts baby Swiss cheese slices, 3 slices	3
Cracker cuts extra sharp cheddar, 4 slices	3
Cracker cuts marbled colby & Monterey Jack cheese slices, 3 slices	3
Cracker cuts mild cheddar cheese slices, 3 slices	3
Cracker cuts sharp cheddar and marbled colby & high-moisture Monterey Jack, 4 slices	3
Cracker cuts sharp cheddar cheese slices, 3 slices	3
Easy cheese American, 1 serving (32 g)	2
Easy cheese cheddar, 1 serving (32 g)	2
Easy cheese cheddar 'n bacon, 1 serving (32 g)	2
Easy cheese pasteurized cheese snack, original cream cheese, 2 Tbsp	3
Easy cheese sharp cheddar, 1 serving (32 g)	2
Extra sharp cheddar cheese sticks, 1	3
Feta cheese crumbles, 1/4 cup	2

	POINTS VALUE
Grate it fresh parmesan cheese, 2 Tbsp	1
Grated parmesan & romano cheese blend, 2 tsp	1
Italian style five cheese - cheese shreds, 1 oz	2
Italian-style cheese crumbles (low-moisture part-skim mozzarella, provolone, asiago and romano), 1/4 cup	2
Low-moisture part-skim mozzarella (shredded), 1/4 cup	2
Low-moisture part-skim mozzarella cheese, 1 oz	2
Low-moisture part-skim mozzarella cheese crumbles, 1/4 cup	2
Macaroni & cheese topping, 2 tsp	1
Mediterranean-style cheese crumbles (provolone, feta & parmesan cheese), 1/4 cup	2
Mexican style cheese crumbles (sharp cheddar, asadero, and queso quesadilla cheeses, 1/4 cup	3
Mexican style natural shredded four cheese blend, 1/4 cup	3
Mexican style pasteurized prepared cheese product, 1 slice	2
Mexican style shredded queso quesadilla/asadero cheeses, 1/4 cup	2
Mild cheddar & Monterey Jack cheese cubes, 7 pieces	3
Mild cheddar cheese sticks, 1	3

	POINTS VALUE
Mild cheddar cheese, wax dipped, 1 oz	3
Mild marbled cheddar cheese, 1 oz	3
Olive and pimento, spread, 2 Tbsp	2
Organic pasteurized prepared cheese product, 1 slice	2
Organic shredded cheddar cheese, 1/4 cup	3
Organic shredded low-moisture part-skim mozzarella cheese, 1/4 cup	2
Organic string cheese, 1 stick	2
Parmesan cheese, grated, 2 tsp	1
Parmesan style topping, 2 tsp	1
Parmesan, shredded, 1/4 cup	3
Pasteurized process American cheese slices, 1 slice	2
Pasteurized process cheese food cheese n' onion, 1 oz	2
Pasteurized process cheese food with bacon & smoke flavor, 1 oz	2
Pasteurized process cheese food with garlic & natural flavor, 1 oz	3
Pasteurized process cheese food, garlic, 1 oz	2
Pimento, spread, 2 Tbsp	2
Pineapple, spread, 2 Tbsp	2
Reduced fat cheddar & Monterey Jack cheese cubes, 7 pieces	2
Reduced fat Italian style shredded cheese blend, 1/4 cup	2

	POINTS VALUE
Reduced fat Mexican style cheese crumbles, 1/4 cup	2
Reduced fat parmesan style grated topping, 2 tsp	0
Reduced-fat Monterey Jack pasteurized prepared cheese product with jalapeno pepper, 1 slice	1
Roka brand blue, spread, 2 Tbsp	2
Sharp cheddar cheese cubes, 7 pieces	3
Sharp cheese crumbles, 1/4 cup	3
Shredded 2% milk reduced fat sharp cheddar cheese with added calcium, 1/4 cup	2
Shredded queso asadero low-moisture part-skim cheese, 1/4 cup	2
Shredded queso quesadilla low-moisture whole milk cheese, 1/4 cup	2
Shredded sharp white cheddar cheese, 1/4 cup	3
Smoky Swiss & cheddar hickory smoked pasteurized process cheese food, 1 oz	2
String cheese reduced fat mozzarella cheese made with 2% milk, 1 stick	2
Swiss (shredded), 1/4 cup	3
Three cheese, shredded, 1/4 cup	3
Traditional feta cheese crumbles, 1/4 cup	2
Whole milk low-moisture mozzarella (shredded), 1/4 cup	2

Cheese (con't) — POINTS VALUE

Kraft 2%

Colby & Monterey Jack (shredded), 1/4 cup	2

Kraft 2% Milk Natural Cheese

Cheddar, mild, 1 oz	2
Cheddar, sharp, 1 oz	2
Colby, 1 oz	2
Mexican four cheese - cheese shreds, 1 oz	2
Monterey Jack, 1 oz	2

Kraft 2% Milk Reduced Fat Natural Shredded Cheese

Cheddar, mild (with calcium), 1/4 cup	2
Cheddar, sharp (with calcium), 1/4 cup	2
Mozzarella (with calcium), 1/4 cup	2

Kraft 2% Milk Singles

American, 2/3 oz	1
American, 3/4 oz	1
Mozzarella, 3/4 oz	1
Sharp cheddar, 3/4 oz	1
Swiss, 3/4 oz	1

Kraft Breakstone's TempTee

Pasteurized whipped cream cheese, 2 Tbsp	2

Kraft Classic Melts

Cheddar & American, 1 serving (28 g)	3
Four cheese, 1 serving (28 g)	3

Kraft Cracker Barrel

2% milk reduced fat extra sharp cheddar cheese sticks, 1	2

POINTS VALUE

Baby Swiss, 1 oz	3
Cheddar, aged reserve extra sharp, 1 oz	3
Cheddar, extra sharp, 1 oz	3
Cheddar, marbled sharp, 1 oz	3
Cheddar, sharp, 1 oz	3
Cheddar, Vermont sharp white, 1 oz	3
Cracker cuts 2% milk reduced fat extra sharp cheddar cheese slices, 3 slices	2
Cracker cuts extra sharp, 1 oz	3
Cracker cuts Vermont sharp white, 1 oz	3
Emmentaler cheese slices, 1 slice	2
Extra sharp cheddar cheese sticks, 1	3
Extra sharp cheddar cheese, colored, 1 oz	3
Extra sharp cheddar cheese, uncolored, 1 oz	3
Extra sharp cheddar spread, 2 Tbsp	3
Extra sharp white cheddar sticks, 1	3
Fontina cheese slices, 1 slice	2
Havarti cheese slices, 1 slice	2
Natural sharp cheddar slices, 1 slice	2
Sharp cheddar cheese sticks, 1	3
Sharp cheddar spread, 2 Tbsp	3
Shredded 2% milk reduced fat extra sharp cheddar cheese, 1/4 cup	2
Shredded 2% milk reduced fat sharp cheddar cheese, 1/4 cup	2
Shredded extra sharp cheddar cheese, 1/4 cup	3

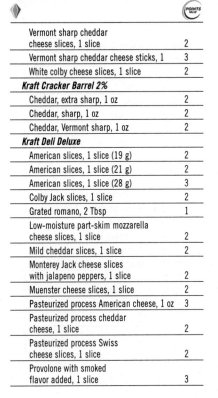

	POINTS VALUE
Vermont sharp cheddar cheese slices, 1 slice	2
Vermont sharp cheddar cheese sticks, 1	3
White colby cheese slices, 1 slice	2
Kraft Cracker Barrel 2%	
Cheddar, extra sharp, 1 oz	2
Cheddar, sharp, 1 oz	2
Cheddar, Vermont sharp, 1 oz	2
Kraft Deli Deluxe	
American slices, 1 slice (19 g)	2
American slices, 1 slice (21 g)	2
American slices, 1 slice (28 g)	3
Colby Jack slices, 1 slice	2
Grated romano, 2 Tbsp	1
Low-moisture part-skim mozzarella cheese slices, 1 slice	2
Mild cheddar slices, 1 slice	2
Monterey Jack cheese slices with jalapeno peppers, 1 slice	2
Muenster cheese slices, 1 slice	2
Pasteurized process American cheese, 1 oz	3
Pasteurized process cheddar cheese, 1 slice	2
Pasteurized process Swiss cheese slices, 1 slice	2
Provolone with smoked flavor added, 1 slice	3

	POINTS VALUE
Reduced fat 2% milk cheddar cheese slices, 1 slice	2
Reduced fat 2% milk pasteurized process American cheese with added calcium & vitamin d, 1 slice	2
Reduced fat 2% milk Swiss cheese, 1 slice	2
Sharp cheddar slices, 1 slice	2
Sharp pasteurized process cheddar cheese slices, 1 slice	3
Swiss, 1 slice (21 g)	2
Swiss slices, 1 slice (23 g)	2
Swiss slices, 1 slice (28 g)	3
Thin Swiss cheese slices, 2 slices	3
Kraft Deluxe Singles Pasteurized Process	
American, 1 oz	2
Pimento, 1 slice	2
Swiss, 1 slice	2
Kraft Free	
♦ Cheddar cheese (shredded), 1/4 cup	1
♦ Mozzarella cheese (shredded), 1/4 cup	1
Kraft Free Singles	
♦ American, 1 slice	1
♦ Mozzarella, 1 slice	1
♦ Sharp cheddar, 1 slice	1
♦ Swiss, 1 slice	1
Kraft Italian Style	
Mozzarella & parmesan (shredded), 1/4 cup	2

Cheese (con't)

	POINTS VALUE
Kraft Mexican Style	
Cheddar and Monterey Jack (shredded), 1/4 cup	3
Four cheese (shredded), 1/4 cup	3
Taco cheese (shredded), 1/4 cup	3
Kraft Natural Cheese	
Cheddar & Monterey Jack marbled, 1 oz	3
Cheddar, extra sharp, 1 oz	3
Cheddar, medium, 1 oz	3
Cheddar, mild, 1 oz	3
Cheddar, mild, 7 cubes	3
Cheddar, sharp, 1 oz	3
Colby, 1 oz	3
Colby & Monterey Jack, marbled, 7 cubes	3
Colby & Monterey Jack, marbled, 1 oz	3
Colby Monterey Jack, 1 oz	3
Low-moisture part-skim mozzarella, 1 oz	2
Monterey Jack, 1 oz	3
Monterey Jack with jalapeño peppers, 1 oz	3
Kraft Parm Plus!	
Garlic & herb, 2 tsp	0
Seasoning blend zesty red pepper, 2 tsp	0
Kraft Philadelphia	
Chive & onion (tub), 2 Tbsp	3
Chive, whipped, 2 Tbsp	2
Garden vegetable, 2 Tbsp	2

	POINTS VALUE
Honey nut flavor, 2 Tbsp	2
Neufchatel cheese (brick), 1 oz	2
Original (brick), 1 oz	3
Original (tub), 2 Tbsp	3
Original, whipped, 2 Tbsp	2
Pineapple, 2 Tbsp	2
Salmon (tub), 2 Tbsp	2
Strawberry, 2 Tbsp	2
Whipped cinnamon 'n brown sugar cream cheese, 2 Tbsp	2
Whipped garlic 'n herb cream cheese, 2 Tbsp	2
Whipped mixed berry cream cheese, 2 Tbsp	2
Whipped ranch cream cheese, 2 Tbsp	2
Kraft Philadelphia Free	
Fat free cream cheese, 1 oz	1
Strawberry, 2 Tbsp	1
Kraft Philadelphia Light	
Chive and onion, 2 Tbsp	2
Garden vegetable, 2 Tbsp	2
Garlic, 2 Tbsp	2
Jalapeño, 2 Tbsp	2
Original, 2 Tbsp	2
Strawberry, 2 Tbsp	2
Kraft Philly Flavors	
Cheesecake, 2 Tbsp	3

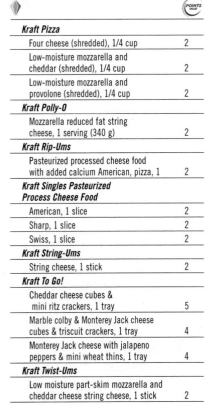

	POINTS VALUE
Kraft Pizza	
Four cheese (shredded), 1/4 cup	2
Low-moisture mozzarella and cheddar (shredded), 1/4 cup	2
Low-moisture mozzarella and provolone (shredded), 1/4 cup	2
Kraft Polly-O	
Mozzarella reduced fat string cheese, 1 serving (340 g)	2
Kraft Rip-Ums	
Pasteurized processed cheese food with added calcium American, pizza, 1	2
Kraft Singles Pasteurized Process Cheese Food	
American, 1 slice	2
Sharp, 1 slice	2
Swiss, 1 slice	2
Kraft String-Ums	
String cheese, 1 stick	2
Kraft To Go!	
Cheddar cheese cubes & mini ritz crackers, 1 tray	5
Marble colby & Monterey Jack cheese cubes & triscuit crackers, 1 tray	4
Monterey Jack cheese with jalapeno peppers & mini wheat thins, 1 tray	4
Kraft Twist-Ums	
Low moisture part-skim mozzarella and cheddar cheese string cheese, 1 stick	2

	POINTS VALUE
Low-moisture part-skim mozzarella string cheese, 1 stick	2
String cheese low moisture part-skim mozzarella and cheddar cheese, 1 stick	2
Kraft Velveeta	
Extra thick cheese slices, 1 serving (34 g)	2
Mild Mexican, 1 oz	2
Pasteurized prepared cheese product, 1 oz	2
Pasteurized prepared cheese product slices, 1 slice	1
Pepper Jack pasteurized prepared cheese product with jalapeno pepper, 1 oz	2
Plain, 1 oz	2
Shredded pasteurized process mild cheddar cheese, 1/4 cup	3
Shreds, 1/4 cup	2
Kraft Velveeta Light	
Reduced fat pasteurized process cheese product, 1 oz	1
Kraft Velveeta Singles	
American, 1 slice	2
Land O Lakes	
American cheese, slice, yellow or white, 2 slices (1 oz)	3
American cheese, slice, yellow or white, 1 slice (0.67 oz)	2
American cheese, slice, yellow or white, 3/4 oz	2

Cheese, Land O Lakes (con't)	POINTS VALUE
Chedarella cheese, 1 oz	3
Cheddar cheese, mild, medium, sharp, extra sharp, 1 oz	3
Co-Jack cheese, 1 oz	3
Colby cheese, 1 oz	3
Hot pepper cheese, 1 oz	3
Monterey Jack cheese, 1 oz	3
Mozzarella cheese, 1 oz	2
Pasteurized process American cheese, 1 oz (1" cube)	3
Pasteurized process cheese product with jalapeno peppers, 1 slice	2
Pasteurized process cheese product, individually wrapped slices, 1 slice	2
Provolone, 1 slice	3
Swiss cheese, 1 oz	3
White process cheese product - individually wrapped slices, 1 slice	2
Yellow process cheese product - individually wrapped slices, 1 slice	2
Land O Lakes Deli	
American cheese loaf, sharp, yellow or white, 1 oz	3
American cheese, less salt, 1 oz	3
Brick cheese, 1 oz	3
Cheddar cheese prints, medium & sharp, 1 oz	3
Co-Jack cheese, 1 oz	3

	POINTS VALUE
Extra sharp flavor process cheddar cheese, 1 oz	3
Italian mozzarella cheese, 1 oz	2
Italian provolone cheese, 1 oz	3
Jalapeno flavor process Jack cheese, 1 oz	3
Jalapeno flavor process cheese food, 1 slice	2
Longhorn colby cheese, 1 oz	3
Monterey Jack cheese prints, 1 oz	3
Muenster cheese naturals, 1 oz	3
Process American cheese yellow or white, 1 oz	3
Process light jalapeno cheese, 1 oz	2
Swiss & American cheese, 1 oz	3
Swiss cheese, 1 oz	3
Land O Lakes Naturally Slender	
Pasteurized process cheese product with jalapeno peppers, 1 slice	2
Reduced fat pasteurized process American cheese product with peppers, 1 oz	2
White American, 1 oz (1" cube)	2
Land O Lakes Pre-Sliced Naturally Slender	
Reduced fat white American cheese, 1 slice	2
Reduced fat yellow American cheese, 1 slice	2
Land O Lakes Reduced Fat Snack'N Cheese To-Go	
Co-Jack cheese portions, 1 piece	2
Mild cheddar cheese, 1 piece	2

	POINTS VALUE
Laughing Cow, The	
Gourmet cheese & baguettes, 1 serving (21 g)	1
Light creamy French onion cheese wedges, 1 wedge	1
Light creamy garlic & herb cheese wedges, 1 wedge	1
Light creamy Swiss original flavor cheese wedges, 1 wedge	1
Light gourmet cheese bites, 5 pieces	1
Mini babybel, bonbel, 1 piece	2
Mini babybel, gouda, 1 piece	2
Mini babybel, light original, 1 cheese	1
Mini babybel, mild cheddar, 1 piece	2
Mini babybel, original, 1 piece	2
Light N' Lively	
Lowfat cottage cheese with added calcium, 1/2 cup	2
Light N' Lively 4-Pack	
Lowfat cottage cheese with added calcium, 4 oz	2
Light N' Lively Free	
◆ Fat free cottage cheese with calcium, 1/2 cup	2
Litehouse	
Blue cheese crumbles, 1/4 cup	3

	POINTS VALUE
Madame Chevre Elite	
Cranberry with port in a cup, 2 Tbsp	1
Goat cream cheese log, 1 slice	2
Roasted red pepper in a cup, 2 Tbsp	1
Maple Street Creamery	
Garlic & herb spreadable cheese, 2 Tbsp	2
Horseradish & bacon spreadable cheese, 2 Tbsp	2
Jalapeno spreadable cheese, 2 Tbsp	2
Traditional Jack spreadable cheese, 2 Tbsp	2
Market Day	
American cheese, 1 slice	2
String cheese, 1 oz (about 1" cube)	2
Morning Glory	
◆ Fat free cottage cheese, 1/2 cup	2
Low fat cottage cheese, 1/2 cup	2
Naturally Fresh	
Strawberry cream cheese, 2 Tbsp	2
Philadelphia	
Blueberry, 2 Tbsp	2
Cream cheese spread, 1 pouch	2
Raspberry, 2 Tbsp	2
Swirls - brown sugar'n cinnamon, 2 Tbsp	2
Swirls - garlic 'n herb, 2 Tbsp	2
Swirls - triple berry, 2 Tbsp	2
Philadelphia Jammin' Swirls	
Blueberry, 2 Tbsp	2
Strawberry, 2 Tbsp	2

Cheese (con't) ⬥ | POINTS VALUE
| | POINTS VALUE

Polly-O

Asiago cheese, 1 oz	3
Caruso low-moisture mozzarella cheese, 1 oz	2
Caruso low-moisture part-skim mozzarella cheese, 1 oz	2
⬥ Fat free mozzarella cheese loaf, 1 oz	1
⬥ Fat free ricotta, 1/4 cup	1
Fior di latte fresh mozzarella cheese, 1 1/2 oz	3
Fresh mozzarella cheese, 1 oz	2
Fresh, fancy shredded parmesan cheese, 1/4 cup	3
Full moisture shredded parmesan cheese, 1/4 cup	3
Gourmet mozzarella cheese, 1 oz	2
Low-moisture part-skim mozzarella cheese, 1/4 cup	2
Low-moisture part-skim mozzarella cheese, 1 oz	2
Low-moisture whole-milk mozzarella cheese, 1 oz	2
Part skim ricotta cheese, 1/4 cup	2
Provolone cheese (not smoked), 1 oz	3
Reduced fat mozzarella cheese loaf, 1 oz	1
Ricotta cheese, 1/4 cup	3
Shredded, whole milk mozzarella, 1 oz	2
Smoked low-moisture whole milk mozzarella loaf, 1 slice (21 g)	2
Smoked low-moisture whole milk mozzarella loaf, 1 oz	2
String cheese reduced fat mozzarella cheese made with 2% milk, 1	2
Whole milk mozzarella, 1 serving (28 g)	2

Polly-O String-Ums

Low moisture part-skim mozzarella, 1 stick	2

Président

Brie light, 1 oz	2
⬥ Crumbled feta, fat free California tomato, 1 oz	1
⬥ Crumbled feta, fat free Mediterranean herbs, 1 oz	1
⬥ Crumbled feta, fat free plain, 1 oz	1
⬥ Fat free feta, 1 cube (1")	1
⬥ Fat free feta, California tomato & basil, 1 cube (approx. 1")	1
⬥ Fat free feta, Mediterranean herbs, 1 cube (approx. 1")	1

Rite

Cream cheese & lox spread, 2 Tbsp	2
Cream cheese & scallion spread, 2 Tbsp	2

Smart Balance

Cream cheese, 1 serving (30 g)	2
Creamy cheddar slices, 1 slice	1
Light cream cheese, 1 serving (30 g)	2
Part skim cheddar-style product, 1 oz	2
Part-skim mozzarella style product, 1 oz	2
Regular cream cheese, 1 serving (30 g)	2

	POINTS VALUE
Smart Beat	
◆ Fat free American, mellow cheddar, lactose free slices, 1 slice	1
◆ Fat free American, sharp cheddar slices, 1 slice	1
Sonoma Cheese Company	
Garlic & herb spreadable cheese, 2 Tbsp	2
Garlic Jack, 1 serving (1 oz)	3
Habanero Jack, 1 serving (1 oz)	3
Horseradish & bacon spreadable cheese, 2 Tbsp	2
Hot pepper Jack, 1 serving (1 oz)	3
Jalapeno spreadable cheese, 2 Tbsp	2
Mediterranean Jack, 1 serving (1 oz)	3
Pesto Jack, 1 serving (1 oz)	3
Traditional Jack, 1 serving (1 oz)	3
Traditional Jack spreadable cheese, 2 Tbsp	2
SoyaKaas	
Cream cheese style - garden vegetable, 1 slice	1
Cream cheese style - garlic & herb, 1 slice	1
Cream cheese style - plain, 1 oz	2
◆ Fat free jalapeno mexi-kaas, 1 oz	1
◆ Fat free mild cheddar style, 1 oz	1
◆ Fat free mozzarella style, 1 oz	1
◆ Garlic & herb, 1 oz	2

	POINTS VALUE
◆ Gouda style, 1 slice	2
◆ Grated parmesan style, 1 tsp	1
◆ Hickory smoked cheddar style, 1 oz	2
◆ Jalapeño Mexi-kaas, 1 oz	2
◆ Mild cheddar style, 1 oz	2
◆ Monterey Jack style, 1 oz	2
◆ Mozzarella style, 1 oz	2
◆ Sliced American cheddar style, 1 slice	1
◆ White cheddar horseradish style, 1 oz	2
◆ White cheddar style, 1 slice	1
Tofu Rella	
◆ Cheddar, 1 oz	2
◆ Garlic-herb, 1 oz	2
◆ Jalapeño, 1 oz	2
◆ Monterey, 1 oz	2
◆ Mozzarella, 1 oz	2
Tree of Life	
Natural cheese, mild cheddar, 1 serving (1 oz)	3
Natural cheese, mozzarella, 1 serving (1 oz)	2
Natural cheese, razor sharp cheddar, 1 serving (1 oz)	3
Natural cheese, sharp cheddar, 1 serving (1 oz)	3
Natural cheese, Swiss, 1 serving (1 oz)	3

Cheese, Tree of Life (con't)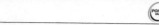

	POINTS VALUE
Organic cheese, 33% reduced fat cheddar, 1 serving (1 oz)	3
Organic cheese, jalapeno Jack, 1 serving (1 oz)	3
Organic cheese, mild cheddar, 1 serving (1 oz)	3
Organic cheese, Monterey Jack style, 1 serving (1 oz)	3
Organic cheese, mozzarella, 1 serving (1 oz)	2
Vegie Kaas	
Mild cheddar style, 1 oz	1
♦ Mozzarella style, 1 oz	1
Weight Watchers	
Light string cheese, 1 piece	1
Reduced fat cheddar cheese snacks, 1 piece	1
Reduced fat cream cheese spread, 1 container	1
Reduced fat shredded 4 cheese Mexican style blend, 1/3 cup	2
Reduced fat shredded cheddar cheese, 1 pouch	2
Reduced fat shredded mozzarella cheese, 1/3 cup	2
Reduced fat whipped cream cheese, 2 Tbsp	1
Singles, 1 slice	1

	POINTS VALUE
Wholesome Valley Organic	
American flavor slice, 1 slice	1
Cheddar flavor slice, 1 slice	1
Mozzarella flavor slice, 1 slice	1
Woolwich Dairy	
Goat feta slice, 1 slice	3
Goat mozzarella, 1 slice	3
White goat cheddar, 1 slice	3

Cream/Creamers
Blue Bunny

	POINTS VALUE
Half & half, 2 Tbsp	1
Heavy whipping cream, 1 Tbsp	1
Sour cream, regular, 2 Tbsp	2
Breakstone's	
♦ Fat free sour cream, 2 Tbsp	1
Reduced fat sour cream, 2 Tbsp	1
Sour cream, 2 Tbsp	2
Carnation Coffee-Mate	
Amaretto, liquid, 1 Tbsp	1
Chocolate raspberry, liquid, 1 Tbsp	1
Cinnamon vanilla creme, liquid, 1 Tbsp	1
Cinnamon vanilla crème, powder, 4 tsp	1
Coconut crème, liquid, 1 Tbsp	1
Coconut crème, powder, 4 tsp	1
Creamy chocolate, powder, 4 tsp	1
Crème brulee, liquid, 1 Tbsp	1

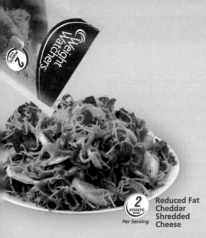

2 POINTS VALUE Per Serving — **Reduced Fat Cheddar Shredded Cheese**

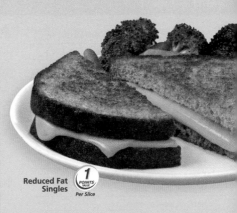

Reduced Fat Singles — 1 POINTS VALUE Per Slice

BRILLIANT
cheesiness.

1 POINTS VALUE Per Serving — **Reduced Fat Whipped Cream Cheese Spread**

Weight Watchers®shredded cheeses, cream cheeses, singles, and cheese snacks all provide a delicious, convenient option to high calorie, full-fat cheeses.

WeightWatchers·

Visit WeightWatchers.com/cheese for more information.

DAIRY & EGGS

 Cream/Creamers, Carnation Coffee-Mate (con't)

	POINTS VALUE
Crème brulee, powder, 4 tsp	1
Fat free cinnamon vanilla crème, liquid, 1 Tbsp	1
Fat free French vanilla, liquid, 1 Tbsp	1
Fat free French vanilla, powder, 4 tsp	1
Fat free hazelnut, liquid, 1 Tbsp	1
Fat free, liquid, 1 Tbsp	0
Fat free, powder, 1 tsp	0
French vanilla, liquid, 1 Tbsp	1
French vanilla, powder, 4 tsp	1
Hazelnut, liquid, 1 Tbsp	1
Hazelnut, powder, 4 tsp	1
Irish creme, liquid, 1 Tbsp	1
Lite, powder, 1 tsp	0
Low fat, liquid, 1 Tbsp	0
Regular, liquid, 1 Tbsp	0
Regular, powder, 1 tsp	0
Sugar free French vanilla, liquid, 1 Tbsp	0
Sugar free French vanilla, powder, 1 Tbsp	1
Sugar free hazelnut, liquid, 1 Tbsp	0
Sugar free hazelnut, powder, 1 Tbsp	1
Sugar free vanilla caramel, powder, 1 Tbsp	1
Toasted almond, liquid, 1 Tbsp	1
Toffee nut, liquid, 1 Tbsp	1
Toffee nut, powder, 4 tsp	1
Vanilla caramel, liquid, 1 Tbsp	1

	POINTS VALUE
Vanilla caramel, powder, 4 tsp	1
Vanilla chai spice, liquid, 1 Tbsp	1
Vanilla chai spice, powder, 4 tsp	1
Vanilla nut, liquid, 1 Tbsp	1
Flavia	
Latte creamer, 1 sachet	1
Friendship	
All-natural sour cream, 2 Tbsp	2
Light sour cream, 2 Tbsp	1
Nonfat sour cream, 2 Tbsp	1
GG Golden Guernsey Dairy	
Half & half, 1 fl oz	1
Reduced fat sour cream, 2 Tbsp	1
Sour cream, 2 Tbsp	2
International Delight	
Amaretto, 1 Tbsp	1
Amaretto, fat free, 1 Tbsp	1
Chocolate cream, 1 Tbsp	1
Cinnamon hazelnut, 1 Tbsp	1
Cinnamon hazelnut, fat free, 1 Tbsp	1
French vanilla, 1 Tbsp	1
French vanilla, fat free, 1 Tbsp	1
Hazelnut, 1 Tbsp	1
Irish cream, 1 Tbsp	1
Irish cream, fat free, 1 Tbsp	1
Reduced sugar French vanilla, 1 Tbsp	1

	POINTS VALUE
Reduced sugar hazelnut, 1 Tbsp	1
Southern butter pecan, 1 Tbsp	1
Vanilla hazelnut, 1 Tbsp	1
Vanilla toffee caramel, 1 Tbsp	1
Knudsen	
◆ Fat free sour cream, 2 Tbsp	1
Hampshire sour cream, 2 Tbsp	2
Light sour cream, 2 Tbsp	1
Land O Lakes	
Fat free half & half, 2 Tbsp	0
Morning Glory	
Half & half, 1 fl oz	1
Reduced fat sour cream, 2 Tbsp	1
Sour cream, 2 Tbsp	2
Silk	
French vanilla, 1 Tbsp	0
Hazelnut, 1 Tbsp	0
Plain, 1 Tbsp	0
Splenda	
Flavors for coffee, caramel, 1 packet	0
Flavors for coffee, cinnamon spice, 1 packet	0
Flavors for coffee, French vanilla, 1 packet	0
Flavors for coffee, hazelnut, 1 packet	0
Flavors for coffee, mocha, 1 packet	0
White Wave Silk	
French vanilla soy creamer, 1 Tbsp	0
Hazelnut soy creamer, 1 Tbsp	0
Original plain soy creamer, 1 Tbsp	0

Egg and Egg Substitutes

	POINTS VALUE
Egg Beaters	
Cheese & chive, 1/4 cup	1
◆ Egg white, refrigerated, 3 Tbsp	1 (5)
◆ Frozen, 1/4 cup	1 (5)
◆ Garden vegetable, refrigerated, 1/4 cup	1 (5)
◆ Refrigerated, 1/4 cup	1 (5)
◆ Southwestern, refrigerated, 1/4 cup	1
Eggland's Best	
◆ Brown egg, 1 large	2 (5)
◆ Cage free egg, 1 extra large	2 (5)
◆ Cage free egg, 1 large	2 (5)
◆ Egg, 1 jumbo	2 (5)
◆ Egg, 1 large	2 (5)
◆ Egg, 1 extra large	2 (5)
◆ Hard cooked and peeled eggs, 1	1 (5)
◆ Organic egg, 1 extra large	2 (5)
◆ Organic egg, 1 large	2 (5)
Gold Circle Farms	
◆ 98% pasteurized egg product, 1/4 cup	1 (5)
◆ DHA omega-3, grade A extra large egg, 1	2 (5)
◆ DHA Omega-3, grade A large egg, 1	2 (5)
◆ DHA omega-3, grade A medium egg, 1	2 (5)
Horizon Organic	
◆ 98% organic egg whites, 1/4 cup	1 (5)
◆ 100% organic egg whites, 3 Tbsp	1 (5)
◆ Extra large shell eggs, 1	2 (5)

DAIRY & EGGS

Egg and Egg Substitutes, Horizon Organic (con't)	POINTS VALUE
Jumbo shell eggs, 1	2 (5)
Large shell eggs, 1	2 (5)
Medium shell eggs, 1	2 (5)
Market Day	
Mini cheese omelets, 1	1
Morningstar Farms	
Scramblers, frozen, 1/4 cup	1
Nature's Harmony	
Grade A large eggs, 1	2 (5)
Nest Fresh	
Brown egg, 1 jumbo	2 (5)
Brown egg, 1 medium	2 (5)
Brown egg, 1 large	2 (5)
Brown egg, 1 extra large	2 (5)
Folic/vitamin b egg, 1 medium	2 (5)
Folic/vitamin b egg, 1 large	2 (5)
Folic/vitamin b egg, 1 extra large	2 (5)
Folic/vitamin b egg, 1 jumbo	2 (5)
Omega-3 egg, 1 jumbo	2 (5)
Omega-3 egg, 1 medium	2 (5)
Omega-3 egg, 1 extra large	2 (5)
Omega-3 egg, 1 large	2 (5)
Organic brown egg, 1 jumbo	2 (5)
Organic brown egg, 1 large	2 (5)
Organic brown egg, 1 extra large	2 (5)
Organic brown egg, 1 medium	2 (5)
White egg, 1 large	2 (5)
White egg, 1 extra large	2 (5)

	POINTS VALUE
White egg, 1 medium	2 (5)
White egg, 1 jumbo	2 (5)
Margarine	
Blue Bonnet	
Light soft spread, 1 Tbsp	1
Light Stick, 1 Tbsp	2
Original soft spread, 1 Tbsp	2
Stick, 1 Tbsp	3
Country Crock	
Light margarine plus omega, 1 Tbsp	1
Margarine with calcium, 1 Tbsp	1
Regular margarine plus omega, 1 Tbsp	2
Country Crock Shedd's Spread	
Light margarine, 1 Tbsp	1
Earth Balance	
All natural buttery spread, 1 Tbsp	3
Buttery stick, 1 serving (14 g)	3
Organic whipped buttery spread, 1 serving	2
Fleischmann's	
Light soft spread, 1 Tbsp	1
Made with olive oil soft spread, 1 Tbsp	2
Original soft spread, 1 Tbsp	2
Original stick, 1 Tbsp	3
Unsalted soft spread, 1 Tbsp	2
Unsalted stick, 1 Tbsp	3
I Can't Believe It's Not Butter!	
Mediterranean blend, 1 Tbsp	2
Mediterranean blend light, 1 Tbsp	1

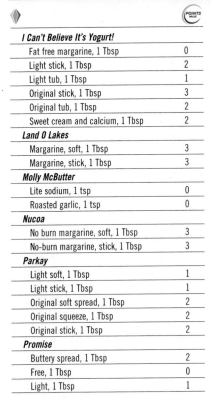

I Can't Believe It's Yogurt!	POINTS VALUE
Fat free margarine, 1 Tbsp	0
Light stick, 1 Tbsp	2
Light tub, 1 Tbsp	1
Original stick, 1 Tbsp	3
Original tub, 1 Tbsp	2
Sweet cream and calcium, 1 Tbsp	2
Land O Lakes	
Margarine, soft, 1 Tbsp	3
Margarine, stick, 1 Tbsp	3
Molly McButter	
Lite sodium, 1 tsp	0
Roasted garlic, 1 tsp	0
Nucoa	
No burn margarine, soft, 1 Tbsp	3
No-burn margarine, stick, 1 Tbsp	3
Parkay	
Light soft, 1 Tbsp	1
Light stick, 1 Tbsp	1
Original soft spread, 1 Tbsp	2
Original squeeze, 1 Tbsp	2
Original stick, 1 Tbsp	2
Promise	
Buttery spread, 1 Tbsp	2
Free, 1 Tbsp	0
Light, 1 Tbsp	1

Smart Balance	POINTS VALUE
37% light spread, 1 Tbsp	1
64% with flax oil margarine, 1 Tbsp	2
67% buttery spread, 1 Tbsp	2
Extra virgin olive oil spread, light, 1 serving (11 g)	1
Extra virgin olive oil spread, regular, 1 serving (11 g)	2
Light buttery spread with flax, 1 Tbsp	1
Low sodium buttery spread, 1 serving (11 g)	2
Omega spread, light, 1 serving (11 g)	1
Omega spread, regular, 1 serving (11 g)	2
Organic whipped buttery spread (margarine), 1 Tbsp	2
Smart Balance Omega Plus	
Buttery spread with phytosterols, 1 Tbsp	2
Smart Beat	
Fat free squeeze margarine, 1 Tbsp	0
Trans fat free super light margarine, 1 Tbsp	1
Soy Garden	
Natural buttery spread, 1 Tbsp	3

Milk and Milk Based Drinks
Blue Bunny

	POINTS VALUE
Egg nog, 1/2 cup	4
◆ Fat free buttermilk, 1 cup	2
◆ Fat free skim milk, 1 cup	2
Holly nog (egg nog flavored lowfat milk), 1 cup	6

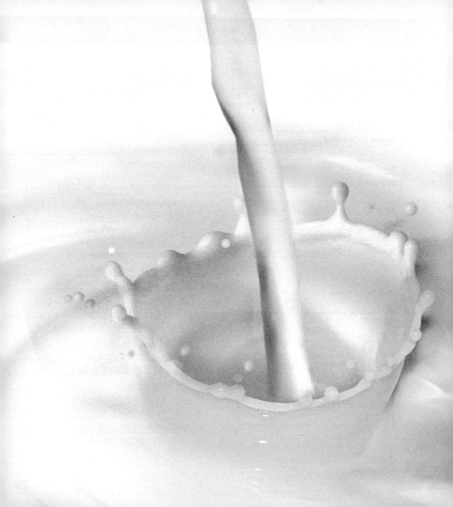

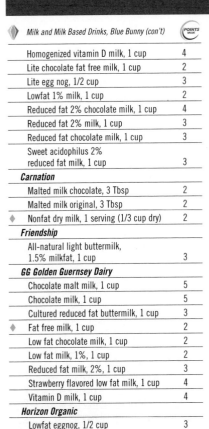

Milk and Milk Based Drinks, Blue Bunny (con't)	POINTS VALUE
Homogenized vitamin D milk, 1 cup	4
Lite chocolate fat free milk, 1 cup	2
Lite egg nog, 1/2 cup	3
Lowfat 1% milk, 1 cup	2
Reduced fat 2% chocolate milk, 1 cup	4
Reduced fat 2% milk, 1 cup	3
Reduced fat chocolate milk, 1 cup	3
Sweet acidophilus 2% reduced fat milk, 1 cup	3
Carnation	
Malted milk chocolate, 3 Tbsp	2
Malted milk original, 3 Tbsp	2
Nonfat dry milk, 1 serving (1/3 cup dry)	2
Friendship	
All-natural light buttermilk, 1.5% milkfat, 1 cup	3
GG Golden Guernsey Dairy	
Chocolate malt milk, 1 cup	5
Chocolate milk, 1 cup	5
Cultured reduced fat buttermilk, 1 cup	3
Fat free milk, 1 cup	2
Low fat chocolate milk, 1 cup	2
Low fat milk, 1%, 1 cup	2
Reduced fat milk, 2%, 1 cup	3
Strawberry flavored low fat milk, 1 cup	4
Vitamin D milk, 1 cup	4
Horizon Organic	
Lowfat eggnog, 1/2 cup	3

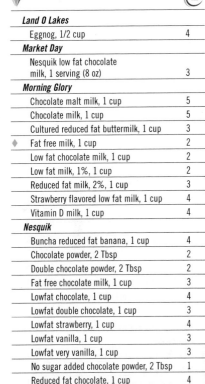

	POINTS VALUE
Land O Lakes	
Eggnog, 1/2 cup	4
Market Day	
Nesquik low fat chocolate milk, 1 serving (8 oz)	3
Morning Glory	
Chocolate malt milk, 1 cup	5
Chocolate milk, 1 cup	5
Cultured reduced fat buttermilk, 1 cup	3
Fat free milk, 1 cup	2
Low fat chocolate milk, 1 cup	2
Low fat milk, 1%, 1 cup	2
Reduced fat milk, 2%, 1 cup	3
Strawberry flavored low fat milk, 1 cup	4
Vitamin D milk, 1 cup	4
Nesquik	
Buncha reduced fat banana, 1 cup	4
Chocolate powder, 2 Tbsp	2
Double chocolate powder, 2 Tbsp	2
Fat free chocolate milk, 1 cup	3
Lowfat chocolate, 1 cup	4
Lowfat double chocolate, 1 cup	3
Lowfat strawberry, 1 cup	4
Lowfat vanilla, 1 cup	3
Lowfat very vanilla, 1 cup	3
No sugar added chocolate powder, 2 Tbsp	1
Reduced fat chocolate, 1 cup	4
Reduced fat double chocolate, 1 cup	4

DAIRY & EGGS

Milk and Milk Based Drinks, Nesquik (con't)	POINTS VALUE
Reduced fat strawberry, 1 cup	4
Reduced fat very vanilla, 1 cup	4
Strawberry powder, 2 Tbsp	2
Odwalla	
New super protein latte, 8 fl oz	4
Super protein chocolate, 8 fl oz	4
Super protein vanilla al'mondo, 8 fl oz	4
Quaker	
Milk chiller - chocolate, 8 fl oz	3
Milk chiller - strawberry, 8 fl oz	3
Smart Balance	
1% milk, 1 serving (8.75 fl oz)	3
Chocolate milk, 1 serving (8.75 fl oz)	3
Lactose free milk, 1 serving (8.75 fl oz)	2
Skim milk, 1 serving (8.75 fl oz)	2
Thai Kitchen	
Coconut milk, 2 fl oz	3
Coconut milk, unsweetened, premium, 2 fl oz	3
Lite coconut milk, 2 fl oz	1
Organic coconut milk, 2 fl oz	3
Organic lite coconut milk, 2 fl oz	1

Yogurt and Yogurt Drinks
Blue Bunny

	POINTS VALUE
♦ Fat free plain yogurt, 1 cup	2

Blue Bunny Light

	POINTS VALUE
Black cherry burst fat free yogurt, 4 oz	1
Black cherry burst fat free yogurt, 6 oz	2
Key lime pie fat free yogurt, 6 oz	2
Key lime pie fat free yogurt, 4 oz	1
Strawberry sensation fat free yogurt, 6 oz	2
Strawberry sensation fat free yogurt, 4 oz	1
Vanilla crème fat free yogurt, 6 oz	2
Vanilla crème fat free yogurt, 4 oz	1
Blue Bunny Light No Sugar Added Fat Free	
Black cherry burst yogurt, 6 oz	2
Black cherry burst yogurt, 4 oz	1
Blackberry crème yogurt, 6 oz	2
Blueberry bliss yogurt, 6 oz	2
Cherry vanilla supreme yogurt, 6 oz	2
Key lime pie yogurt, 6 oz	2
Peach passion yogurt, 4 oz	1
Peach passion yogurt, 6 oz	2
Raspberry rhapsody yogurt, 6 oz	2
Strawberry banana supreme yogurt, 6 oz	2
Strawberry sensation yogurt, 4 oz	1
Strawberry sensation yogurt, 6 oz	2
Vanilla crème yogurt, 4 oz	1
Vanilla crème yogurt, 6 oz	2
Blue Bunny Light Omega 3	
Black cherry orchard low fat yogurt, 4 oz	2
Blackberry crème low fat yogurt, 4 oz	2
Raspberry crème low fat yogurt, 4 oz	2
Strawberry patch low fat yogurt, 4 oz	2

| POINTS VALUE
 | POINTS VALUE

	POINTS VALUE
Blue Bunny Light Superfruit	
Black currant fat free yogurt, 6 oz	2
Black currant fat free yogurt, 4 oz	1
Blackberry lingonberry fat free yogurt, 4 oz	1
Blackberry lingonberry fat free yogurt, 6 oz	2
Mango pomegranate fat free yogurt, 4 oz	1
Mango pomegranate fat free yogurt, 6 oz	2
Pomegranate blueberry fat free yogurt, 6 oz	2
Pomegranate blueberry fat free yogurt, 4 oz	1
Pomegranate cherry fat free yogurt, 4 oz	1
Pomegranate cherry fat free yogurt, 6 oz	2
Raspberry acai fat free yogurt, 4 oz	1
Raspberry acai fat free yogurt, 6 oz	2
Raspberry cranberry fat free yogurt, 6 oz	2
White cranberry strawberry fat free yogurt, 6 oz	2
Blue Bunny Lite 85 Fat Free	
Peach yogurt, 6 oz	2
Peach yogurt, 8 oz	2
Colombo	
Plain (low fat), 8 oz	3
Colombo Classic	
Banana/strawberry, 8 oz	5
Black cherry parfait, 8 oz	5
Blackberry burst, 8 oz	5
Blueberry, 8 oz	5
Cherry, 8 oz	5
Fruit burst, 8 oz	5

	POINTS VALUE
Peach, 8 oz	5
Raspberry, 8 oz	5
Strawberry, 8 oz	5
Vanilla, 8 oz	5
White chocolate raspberry, 8 oz	5
Colombo Fat Free	
Plain, 8 oz	2
Vanilla, 8 oz	3
Colombo Light	
Blueberry, 8 oz	2
Boston cream pie, 8 oz	2
Cherry vanilla, 8 oz	2
Juicy peach, 8 oz	2
Key lime pie, 8 oz	2
Lemon meringue, 8 oz	2
Mixed berries, 8 oz	2
Orange crème, 8 oz	2
Raspberry, 8 oz	2
Strawberry, 8 oz	2
Strawberry/banana, 8 oz	2
White chocolate raspberry, 8 oz	2
Colombo Low Fat	
French vanilla, 8 oz	4
Greek Gods	
Fig, 6 oz	6
Honey, 6 oz	6
Honey, 4 oz	4

Yogurt and Yogurt Drinks, Greek Gods (con't)	POINTS VALUE
◆ Non fat, 4 oz	1
◆ Non fat, 6 oz	1
Pomegranate, 6 oz	6
Traditional, 4 oz	4
Traditional Greek yogurt, honey flavored, 6 oz	6
Vanilla, 6 oz	4
Horizon Organic	
Blueberry blended lowfat yogurt, 1 container (6 oz)	3
Lemon blended lowfat yogurt, 1 container (6 oz)	3
Mixed berry fat free yogurt, 1 container (6 oz)	3
Organic blueberry fat free yogurt, 1 container (6 oz)	3
Organic blueberry low fat yogurt, 1 container (6 oz)	3
Organic cherry fat free yogurt, 1 container (6 oz)	3
Organic lemon low fat yogurt, 1 container (6 oz)	3
Organic mixed berry fat free yogurt, 1 container (6 oz)	3
Organic peach fat free yogurt, 1 container (6 oz)	3
Organic peach low fat yogurt, 1 container (6 oz)	3
Organic raspberry fat free yogurt, 1 container (6 oz)	3

	POINTS VALUE
Organic raspberry low fat yogurt, 1 container (6 oz)	3
Organic strawberry banana low fat yogurt, 1 container (6 oz)	3
Organic strawberry fat free yogurt, 1 container (6 oz)	3
Organic strawberry low fat yogurt, 1 container (6 oz)	3
Organic vanilla fat free yogurt, 1 container (6 oz)	3
Peach blended lowfat yogurt, 1 container (6 oz)	3
Strawberry banana blended lowfat yogurt, 1 container (6 oz)	3
Strawberry blended lowfat yogurt, 1 container (6 oz)	3
Weight Watchers	
Amaretto cheesecake nonfat yogurt, 6 oz	1
Berries 'n cream nonfat yogurt, 6 oz	1
Black cherry fat free yogurt, 4 oz	1
Black cherry nonfat yogurt, 6 oz	1
Boston crème pie nonfat yogurt, 6 oz	1
Cherry cheesecake nonfat yogurt, 6 oz	1
Key lime pie nonfat yogurt, 6 oz	1
Lemon cream pie fat free yogurt, 4 oz	1
Lemon cream pie nonfat yogurt, 6 oz	1
Peach nonfat yogurt, 4 oz	1
Peach nonfat yogurt, 6 oz	1
Raspberry nonfat yogurt, 6 oz	1

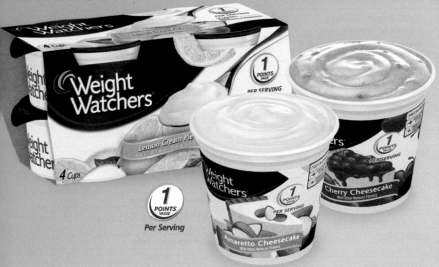

INDULGENT

creaminess.

Weight Watchers® yogurts bring unique and exciting
flavors with a *POINTS*® value of 1!

WeightWatchers®

Go to WeightWatchers.com/yogurt

DAIRY & EGGS

Yogurt and Yogurt Drinks, Weight Watchers (con't)	POINTS VALUE
Smooth & creamy strawberry shortcake fat free yogurt, 4 oz	1
Smooth & creamy white chocolate cheesecake fat free yogurt, 4 oz	1
Strawberry banana nonfat yogurt, 6 oz	1
Strawberry nonfat yogurt, 6 oz	1
Strawberry nonfat yogurt, 4 oz	1
Vanilla fat free yogurt, 4 oz	1
Vanilla nonfat yogurt, 6 oz	1
White chocolate raspberry nonfat yogurt, 6 oz	1
Yoplait Chocolate Whips!	
Chocolate, 4 oz	4
Chocolate cherry, 4 oz	4
Chocolate mint, 4 oz	4
Chocolate raspberry, 4 oz	4
Chocolate strawberry, 4 oz	4
Yoplait Go-Gurt	
Banana split, 1 tube	2
Berry blue, 1 tube	2
Berry bubblegum, 1 tube	2
Blue razzberry, 1 tube	2
Chill out cherry, 1 tube	2
Cool cotton candy, 1 tube	2
Crazy berry bolt, 1 tube	2
Melon berry, 1 tube	2
Paradise punch, 1 tube	2
Rad raspberry, 1 tube	2
Red rush, 1 tube	2

	POINTS VALUE
Shrek's donkeyberry blast, 1 tube	2
Shrek's ogreberry, 1 tube	2
Strawberry banana burst, 1 tube	2
Strawberry kiwi, 1 tube	2
Strawberry kiwi kick, 1 tube	2
Strawberry milkshake, 1 tube	2
Strawberry milkshake, 1 tube	2
Strawberry splash, 1 tube	2
Watermelon melt down, 1 tube	2
Yoplait Kids Yogurt	
Banana, 4 oz	2
Peach, 4 oz	2
Strawberry, 4 oz	2
Strawberry banana, 4 oz	2
Strawberry vanilla, 4 oz	2
Vanilla, 4 oz	2
Yoplait Kids Yogurt Drink	
Banana, 1 container	2
Mixed berry, 1 container	2
Strawberry, 1 container	2
Strawberry banana, 1 container	2
Yoplait Light	
Apple turnover, 6 oz	2
Apricot mango, 6 oz	2
Banana cream pie, 6 oz	2
Berries 'n cream, 6 oz	2
Blackberry, 6 oz	2
Blueberry, 4 oz	1

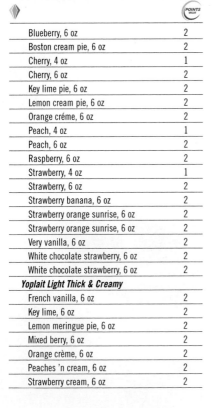

	POINTS VALUE
Blueberry, 6 oz	2
Boston cream pie, 6 oz	2
Cherry, 4 oz	1
Cherry, 6 oz	2
Key lime pie, 6 oz	2
Lemon cream pie, 6 oz	2
Orange créme, 6 oz	2
Peach, 4 oz	1
Peach, 6 oz	2
Raspberry, 6 oz	2
Strawberry, 4 oz	1
Strawberry, 6 oz	2
Strawberry banana, 6 oz	2
Strawberry orange sunrise, 6 oz	2
Strawberry orange sunrise, 6 oz	2
Very vanilla, 6 oz	2
White chocolate strawberry, 6 oz	2
White chocolate strawberry, 6 oz	2
Yoplait Light Thick & Creamy	
French vanilla, 6 oz	2
Key lime, 6 oz	2
Lemon meringue pie, 6 oz	2
Mixed berry, 6 oz	2
Orange crème, 6 oz	2
Peaches 'n cream, 6 oz	2
Strawberry cream, 6 oz	2

	POINTS VALUE
Yoplait Original	
Mango, 4 oz	2
Pina colada, 4 oz	2
Raspberry, 4 oz	2
Strawberry banana, 4 oz	2
Yoplait Original 99% Fat Free	
Banana crème, 6 oz	4
Berry banana, 6 oz	4
Blackberry harvest, 6 oz	4
Blueberry, 6 oz	4
Blueberry crumble, 6 oz	4
Boysenberry, 6 oz	4
Cherry, 6 oz	4
French vanilla, 6 oz	4
Guava, 6 oz	4
Harvest peach, 6 oz	4
Key lime pie, 6 oz	4
Lemon burst, 6 oz	4
Mandarin orange, 6 oz	4
Mango, 6 oz	4
Mixed berry, 6 oz	4
Orange créme, 6 oz	4
Original coconut cream pie, 6 oz	4
Passion fruit, 6 oz	4
Peach, 8 oz	5
Peach, 4 oz	2
Peach cobbler, 6 oz	4

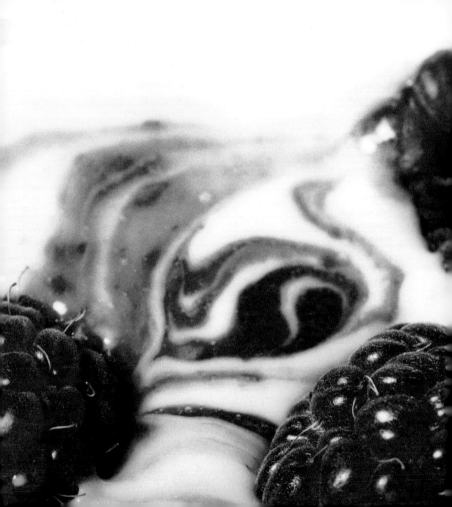

Yogurt and Yogurt Drinks, Yoplait Original 99% Fat Free (con't)	POINTS VALUE
Pina colada, 6 oz	4
Pineapple, 6 oz	4
♦ Plain fat free, 6 oz	2
♦ Plain fat free, 8 oz	3
Raspberry, 6 oz	4
Strawberry, 8 oz	5
Strawberry, 4 oz	2
Strawberry, 6 oz	4
Strawberry banana, 8 oz	5
Strawberry banana, 6 oz	4
Strawberry cheesecake, 6 oz	4
Strawberry kiwi, 6 oz	4
Strawberry mango, 6 oz	4
Tropical peach, 6 oz	4
Vanilla, 8 oz	5
White chocolate raspberry, 6 oz	4
Yoplait Thick & Creamy	
Banana, 6 oz	4
Blackberry harvest, 6 oz	4
Blueberries & cream, 6 oz	4
Crème caramel, 6 oz	4
Key lime pie, 6 oz	4
Lemon supreme, 6 oz	4
Orange crème, 6 oz	4
Peaches 'n cream, 6 oz	4
Raspberry cheesecake, 6 oz	4
Royal raspberry, 6 oz	4

	POINTS VALUE
Strawberries & cream, 6 oz	4
Strawberry, 6 oz	4
Strawberry banana, 6 oz	4
Vanilla, 6 oz	4
Yoplait Trix	
Berry bolt, 4 oz	2
Bubble gum, 4 oz	2
Cotton candy, 4 oz	2
Rainbow sherbet, 4 oz	2
Raspberry rainbow, 4 oz	2
Strawberry banana bash, 4 oz	2
Strawberry kiwi, 4 oz	2
Strawberry punch, 4 oz	2
Triple cherry, 4 oz	2
Very berry melon, 4 oz	2
Watermelon burst, 4 oz	2
Wild berry blue, 4 oz	2
Yoplait Whips!	
Creamy latte, 1 container	3
Dulce de leche, 1 container	3
Key lime pie, 1 container	3
Lemon meringue, 1 container	3
Orange crème, 1 container	3
Peaches n' cream, 1 container	3
Raspberry mousse, 1 container	3
Strawberry mist, 1 container	3

Seafood A-C

Acme

	POINTS VALUE
◆ Chubs, 2 oz	2

Bumble Bee

◆ Chopped clams, 1/4 cup	1 (5)
◆ Fancy whole baby clams, 2 oz	1 (5)
◆ Lump crabmeat, 1/4 cup (drained)	1 (5)
Seafood salad with crab and crackers, crackers only, 6	2
Seafood salad with crab and crackers, seafood salad only, 1 can	2
◆ White crabmeat, 2 oz (drained)	1 (5)

Chincoteague

Breaded fried clams, 3 oz	6
Chopped ocean clams, 1/2 cup	1 (5)
Eastern chopped sea clams, 1/2 cup	1
Eastern sea clam juice, 1/2 cup	0
Fried clams, 3 oz	6
◆ Ocean clam juice, 8 fl oz	0
Stuffed clams, frozen, 1 piece	3

Doxsee

◆ All natural clam juice, 1 Tbsp	0
◆ Chopped clams in clam juice, 1/4 cup	1 (5)
◆ Minced clams in clam juice, 1/4 cup	1 (5)

Eden

◆ Bonito flakes - cured, steamed & dried, 2 Tbsp	0

Gorton's

	POINTS VALUE
Premium fillets, cod, 1	6

Lascco

◆ Seafood & crab cocktail, 4 oz	2

Market Day

Crab cakes, 1	2
Krispy krunchy cod, 1 piece	5
◆ Pre-split king crab legs, 3 pieces	2

Phillips

Boardwalk crab cakes, 1	7
Crab & shrimp cake, 1	3
◆ Crab meat, 2 oz	1 (5)
Crab slammers, 2 pieces	4
Maryland style crab cake minis, 4	4
Maryland style crab cakes, 1	4
◆ Pasteurized king crab meat, 2 oz	1 (5)

Schwan's LiveSmart

◆ Catfish fillets, 1	2 (5)
◆ Alaskan cod fillets, 1 piece	2 (5)

Snow's

◆ All natural clam juice, 1 Tbsp	0
◆ Chopped clams in clam juice, 1/4 cup	1 (5)
◆ Minced clams in clam juice, 1/4 cup	1 (5)

Sol-Mex

◆ Baby clams, 1/2 cup	1 (5)
◆ Crab meat, 1/2 cup	2 (5)

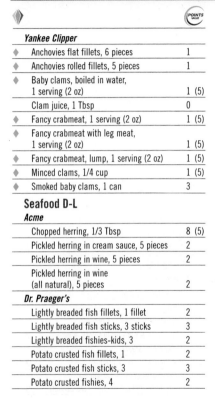

	POINTS VALUE
Yankee Clipper	
♦ Anchovies flat fillets, 6 pieces	1
♦ Anchovies rolled fillets, 5 pieces	1
♦ Baby clams, boiled in water, 1 serving (2 oz)	1 (5)
Clam juice, 1 Tbsp	0
♦ Fancy crabmeat, 1 serving (2 oz)	1 (5)
♦ Fancy crabmeat with leg meat, 1 serving (2 oz)	1 (5)
♦ Fancy crabmeat, lump, 1 serving (2 oz)	1 (5)
♦ Minced clams, 1/4 cup	1 (5)
♦ Smoked baby clams, 1 can	3

Seafood D-L

Acme

Chopped herring, 1/3 Tbsp	8 (5)
Pickled herring in cream sauce, 5 pieces	2
Pickled herring in wine, 5 pieces	2
Pickled herring in wine (all natural), 5 pieces	2

Dr. Praeger's

Lightly breaded fish fillets, 1 fillet	2
Lightly breaded fish sticks, 3 sticks	3
Lightly breaded fishies-kids, 3	2
Potato crusted fish fillets, 1	2
Potato crusted fish sticks, 3	3
Potato crusted fishies, 4	2

	POINTS VALUE
Gorton's	
Battered dipped fish portions, 1 serving (70 g)	5
Beer batter crispy battered fish fillets, 2 fillets	6
Beer batter tenders, 3 1/2 pieces	7
Crispy battered fish fillets, 2 fillets	6
Crispy battered popcorn fish, 1 serving (about 11 pieces)	7
Crunchy golden fish fillets, breaded, 2	6
Crunchy golden fish sticks, 6 sticks	6
Crunchy golden fish sticks breaded minced fish (30 pack), 6	6
Crunchy golden fish sticks breaded minced fish (44 pack), 6	6
Garlic and herb crunchy breaded fish fillets, 2 fillets	6
Garlic and herb crunchy breaded fish fillets, 2	6
Grilled tilapia fillets - roasted garlic butter, 1 fillet	2
Lemon herb crunchy breaded fish fillets, 2 fillets	6
Lemon pepper, battered, 2 fillets	7
Parmesan crunchy breaded fish fillets, 2 fillets	6
Potato crunch fish fillets, 2	5
Premium fillets, flounder, 1	6
Premium fillets, haddock, 1	6

FISH & SEAFOOD

Seafood D-L, Gorton's (con't)	POINTS VALUE
Ranch crunchy breaded fish fillets, 2 fillets	6
Southern fried country style crunchy breaded fish fillets, 2 fillets	6
Tenders, extra crunchy, 3 pieces	5
Tenders, original batter, 3 pieces	5
Gorton's Grilled Fillets	
Cajun blackened, 1 fillet	2
Classic char-grilled, 1 fillet	2
Garlic butter, 1 fillet	2
Italian herb, 1 fillet	2
Lemon butter, 1 fillet	2
Lemon pepper, 1 fillet	2
Ian's	
Fish portions, 1	5
Fish sticks, 5	4
Wheat free, gluten free battered fish, 1 serving (3.4 oz)	4
Wheat free, gluten free lightly breaded fish sticks, 5	4
Lascco	
Premium roll mop herring, 2 oz	2
Premium snack bit herring fillet, 2 oz	2
Premium sour cream herring fillet, 2 oz	3
Premium spiced cut herring, 2 oz	3
Premium wine snack herring fillet, 2 oz	2
Manischewitz	
Sweet gefilte fish, 1 piece (42 g)	1
Sweet gefilte fish, 1 piece (65 g)	1

	POINTS VALUE
Market Day	
Flounder del ray, 1 serving (6 oz)	4
Nathan's	
Herring in cream sauce, 1/4 cup	3
Herring in wine sauce, 1/4 cup	2
Herring tasti tidbits, 1/4 cup	2
Lunch herring, 1/4 cup	3
Old fashioned herring, 1/4 cup	3
Rite	
Chopped herring salad, 2 Tbsp	2
Creamy dill herring, 1/4 cup	3
Herring in cream, 1/4 cup	3
Herring in wine, 1/4 cup	2
Schwan's LiveSmart	
Haddock loins, 1 fillet (4 oz)	2 (5)
Pacific cod fillets, 1 serving (112 g)	2 (5)

Seafood M-P
Bumble Bee	
Whole oysters, 2 oz	2 (5)
Phillips	
Coconut mahi sticks, 3 pieces	7
White wine & herb mahi fillets, 4 oz	2
Schwan's LiveSmart	
Mahi mahi fillets, 1 fillet	2 (5)
Peachtree seasoning packet for mahi mahi filets, 1 serving (1/6 packet)	0

	POINTS VALUE
Yankee Clipper	
Smoked oysters, 1 can	3
Whole boiled oysters, 1/4 cup	1 (5)

Seafood Q-Z
Acme

	POINTS VALUE
Baked salmon salad, 4 Tbsp	5
Blue Hill Bay baked peppered salmon skin on portion, 2 oz	2
Blue Hill Bay baked salmon skin on portion, 2 oz	2
Blue Hill Bay whitefish salad, 4 Tbsp	4
Kippered salmon backs, 2 oz	3
Pre-sliced all natural smoked salmon, 2 oz	2 (5)
Pre-sliced all natural smoked salmon, 5 slices	2 (5)
Pre-sliced cold smoked salmon, 5 slices	2 (5)
Sliced nova, 3 slices	2 (5)
Whitefish, 2 oz	3 (5)
Whitefish salad, 4 Tbsp	4 (5)

Bumble Bee

	POINTS VALUE
Chunk light tuna in water, 1/4 cup (drained)	1 (5)
Chunk light tuna in water (3 oz can), 1 can	1 (5)
Chunk light tuna touch of lemon in water, 1/4 cup (drained)	1
Chunk white albacore in water, 1/4 cup (drained)	1 (5)

	POINTS VALUE
Chunk white albacore in water (3 oz can), 1 can (drained)	1 (5)
Deveined large shrimp, 1/4 cup (drained)	1 (5)
Deveined medium shrimp, 1/4 cup (drained)	1 (5)
Deveined small shrimp, 1/4 cup (drained)	1 (5)
Fat free tuna salad with crackers (crackers only), 6	2
Fat free tuna salad with crackers (tuna only), 1 cup	1
Pink salmon, 1 serving (2.2 oz)	2 (5)
Premium albacore tuna in water pouch, 1 pouch	2 (5)
Premium albacore tuna in water pouch, 2 oz	1 (5)
Prime fillet albacore steak entrees, ginger and soy, 4 oz	4
Prime fillet albacore steak entrees, lemon and cracked pepper, 4 oz	3
Prime fillet albacore steak entrees, mesquite grilled, 4 oz	3
Prime fillet solid white albacore in water, 2 oz (drained)	1 (5)
Red salmon, 1 serving (2.2 oz)	3 (5)
Regular broken shrimp, 1/4 cup (drained)	1 (5)
Regular jumbo shrimp, 1/4 cup (drained)	1 (5)
Regular large shrimp, 1/4 cup (drained)	1 (5)
Regular medium shrimp, 1/4 cup (drained)	1 (5)
Regular small shrimp, 1/4 cup (drained)	1 (5)

Seafood Q-Z, Bumble Bee (con't)	POINTS VALUE
◆ Sardines in hot sauce, 1 can	4
◆ Sardines in mustard, 1 can	3
Sardines in oil, 1 cup (drained)	3
◆ Sardines in water, 1 can (drained)	3 (5)
◆ Skinless and boneless pink salmon, 2 oz (drained)	1 (5)
Solid light tuna - tonno in olive oil, 2 oz (drained)	3
◆ Solid white albacore in water, 1 can (drained)	2 (5)
◆ Solid white albacore in water, 2 oz (drained)	1 (5)
◆ Tiny shrimp, 2 oz (drained)	1 (5)
Tuna salad original with crackers, crackers only, 6	2
Tuna salad original with crackers, tuna salad only, 1 can	5
Bumble Bee Easy Peel Sensations	
Lemon & cracked pepper, 1 can	3
Spicy Thai chili, 1 can	4
Sundried tomato & basil, 1 can	3
Bumble Bee Lunch on the Run	
Tuna salad - complete lunch kit, cookie only, 1	4
Tuna salad - complete lunch kit, crackers only, 6	2
Tuna salad - complete lunch kit, diced peaches only, 4 oz	1

	POINTS VALUE
Tuna salad - complete lunch kit, entire kit, 1	13
Tuna salad - complete lunch kit, tuna only, 1 serving (2.9 oz)	6
Bumble Bee Sensations	
Seasoned tuna medleys with crackers, crackers only, 6	2
Seasoned tuna medleys with crackers, lemon & pepper, tuna only, 3 oz	2
Seasoned tuna medleys with crackers, spicy Thai chili, tuna only, 3 oz	4
Seasoned tuna medleys with crackers, sundried tomato & basil, tuna only, 3 oz	3
Coral	
Chunk light tuna in oil, 1/4 cup	3
Chunk light tuna in oil (3 oz can), 1 can (drained)	3
◆ Chunk light tuna in water, 1/4 cup (drained)	1 (5)
Deming's	
◆ Pink salmon, 1/4 cup	2
◆ Red sockeye Alaska salmon, 1/4 cup	3
Double "Q"	
◆ Pink Alaska salmon, 1/4 cup	2
◆ Red sockeye salmon, 1/4 cup	3
Echo Falls	
◆ Cajun flavor smoked salmon, 2 oz	2
◆ Cracked pepper smoked salmon, 2 oz	2
◆ Scandinavian style grav lax, 2 oz	3

	POINTS VALUE
◆ Traditional smoked salmon, 2 oz	2 (5)
◆ Wild Alaskan sockeye smoked salmon, 2 oz	3 (5)
Fanci Food	
◆ Snails, very large, 6 pieces	1
Gorton's	
Popcorn shrimp, 22	6
Premium fillets, tilapia, 1	6
Gorton's Popcorn Shrimp	
Beer batter popcorn shrimp, 1 serving (about 18 shrimp)	7
Garlic & herb popcorn shrimp, 1 serving (about 22 shrimp)	6
Original popcorn shrimp, 1 serving (about 20 shrimp)	6
Gorton's Shrimp Temptations	
Beer batter, 5	6
Jumbo butterfly, 5	5
Lemon butter, 4 oz	3
Scampi, 4 oz	3
Lascco	
◆ Oven roasted salmon, 2 oz	2 (5)
◆ Premium nova sliced smoked salmon, 2 oz	1 (5)
◆ Shrimp cocktail, 4 oz	2
◆ Smoked salmon snack bits, 2 oz	1 (5)
Manischewitz	
Sweet whitefish & pike, 1 piece (69 g)	1
Sweet whitefish & pike, 1 piece (42 g)	0

	POINTS VALUE
Market Day	
◆ Classic salmon, 1 serving (2" wide piece)	7
Garlic & herb shrimp, 15	3
Jumbo party shrimp with sauce, 3 oz	1
◆ Large shrimp, 4 oz	1 (5)
Mediterranean salmon, 1 serving (12 oz)	10
Oven-ready butterfly shrimp, 4	5
Parmesan seasoned shrimp, 1 serving (42)	3
Popcorn shrimp, 21	5
Seasoned salmon, 4 oz (raw, about 2" wide piece)	7
Seasoned scallops, 1 serving (4 oz)	4
◆ Tilapia fillets, 1 serving (4 oz)	2 (5)
Tortilla crusted tilapia, 1 piece	6
◆ Wild Alaskan grilled salmon, 1 fl oz	2 (5)
Nathan's	
◆ Smoked salmon, 2 oz	1
Ocean Beauty	
Ahi tuna fajitas, 8 oz	2
Florentine salmon roulade, 4 oz	4
Honey-garlic salmon burger, 1 burger	2
Lemon dill salmon burger, 1 burger	1
Mediterranean salmon roulade, 4 oz	5
Salmon burger fillet, 1 burger	2
Salmon fajita, 8 oz	2
Southwest tuna burger, 1 burger	2
Tuna burger, 100% fat free, 1 burger	2
Tuna burger, 98% fat free, 1 burger	2

Seafood Q-Z (con't) POINTS VALUE

 POINTS VALUE

Oven Poppers

Stuffed tilapia in a ginger teriyaki sauce, 1 piece	6
Stuffed tilapia in a lemon, garlic, butter sauce, 1 piece	6

Phillips

Breaded shrimp, 5	5
Buffalo shrimp, 5 pieces (with 3/4 oz sauce)	6
Coconut shrimp, 5	8
Crispy garlic shrimp, 8	5
◆ Lemon peppercorn ahi tuna, 4 oz	3
Salmon cakes, 1 cake	4

Progresso

Light solid tuna in olive oil, 1 can	4
Solid white albacore tuna in olive oil, 1/4 cup	2

Rite

◆ Gravlax salmon, 2 oz	2 (5)
◆ Nova salmon bits, 1/4 cup	3 (5)
Nova salmon spread, 2 Tbsp	1
◆ Smoked Atlantic salmon, 2 oz	2 (5)
Smoked pastrami salmon, 2 oz	2
◆ Smoked premium salmon, 2 oz	2 (5)
Smoked whitefish salad, 2 Tbsp	2

 POINTS VALUE

Sabra

Tuna salad kit, crackers only, 1 serving (1 oz)	2
Tuna salad kit, tuna only, 1 oz	4

Schwan's LiveSmart

Alaskan salmon, 1 serving (4 oz)	2 (5)
◆ Alaskan salmon, spice packet only, 1/4 tsp	0
◆ Fully cooked Alaskan salmon, 1 piece	3 (5)
◆ Jumbo cooked tail-off shrimp, 9	2 (5)

Season Brand

◆ Albacore tuna in water, 1 pouch	2 (5)
◆ Bristling sardines in water, 1 can	5 (5)
◆ Light tuna in water, 1 pouch	2 (5)
◆ Medium red salmon, 1/4 cup	2 (5)
◆ No salt added Norway sardines in water, 1 can	4 (5)
◆ No salt added pink salmon, 1/4 cup	2 (5)
◆ No salt added, skinless & boneless sardines in water, 1 can	3 (5)
◆ Pink salmon, 1/4 cup	2 (5)
Sardine fillets in lemon garlic sauce, 1 can	9
Sardine fillets in sweet & tangy Spanish style sauce, 1 can	10
◆ Sardines in water, 1 can	3 (5)
◆ Skinless & boneless sardines in water, 1 can	4 (5)

	POINTS VALUE
SnackMasters Natural Gourmet Jerky	
Ahi tuna - original, 1 oz	2
Salmon - original, 1 oz	2
Sol-Mex	
◆ Sardines in tomato sauce - hot, 1/4 cup	2
StarKist	
Albacore lunch to go - from Thailand, 1 kit	6
Chunk light tuna in oil, 1 serving (2.8 oz, drained)	3
Chunk light tuna in sunflower oil - pouch, 2 oz (drained)	3
◆ Chunk light tuna in water, 2 oz (drained)	1 (5)
◆ Chunk light tuna in water (pouch), 1 pouch	2 (5)
◆ Chunk light tuna in water (pouch), 2 oz	1 (5)
Chunk light water lunch to go - from Ecuador, 1 kit	6
Chunk light water lunch to go - from Thailand, 1 kit	6
◆ Chunk white tuna in water, 2 oz (drained)	2 (5)
◆ Chunk white tuna in water (low sodium/low fat), 2 oz (drained)	1 (5)
◆ Chunk white tuna in water - pouch, 2 oz	1 (5)
Hickory smoked tuna creations lunch to go, 1 kit	6
Solid light tuna fillets in olive oil, 2 oz (drained)	3
◆ Solid light tuna fillets in water, 2 oz (drained)	1

	POINTS VALUE
◆ Solid light tuna in water, 2 oz (drained)	1 (5)
Solid white tuna in oil, 2 oz (drained)	2
◆ Solid white tuna in water, 2 oz (drained)	2 (5)
Zesty lemon pepper tuna creations lunch to go, 1 kit	6
StarKist Lunch to Go	
Albacore, 1 kit	6
StarKist Select	
◆ Chunk light tuna in water, 2 oz (drained)	1 (5)
StarKist Tuna Creations	
Herb and garlic, 1 pouch	2
Hickory smoke, 2 oz	2
Sweet and spicy (Equador recipe), 2 oz	1
Zesty lemon pepper, 2 oz	1
Tree of Life	
◆ Wild chunk light Tongol tuna in spring water, 1/4 cup	1 (5)
◆ Wild chunk light Tongol tuna in spring water, no salt added, 1/4 cup	1 (5)
Underwood	
Brisling sardines in mustard sauce, 1 can	4
Brisling sardines in soybean oil, 1 can	6
Yankee Clipper	
Sardines in mustard sauce, 1/4 cup	2
Sardines in soybean oil, 1/4 cup	3
◆ Sardines in tomato sauce, 1/4 cup	2

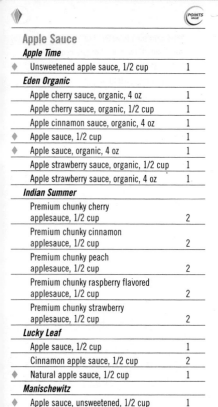

	POINTS VALUE
Apple Sauce	
Apple Time	
Unsweetened apple sauce, 1/2 cup	1
Eden Organic	
Apple cherry sauce, organic, 4 oz	1
Apple cherry sauce, organic, 1/2 cup	1
Apple cinnamon sauce, organic, 4 oz	1
Apple sauce, 1/2 cup	1
Apple sauce, organic, 4 oz	1
Apple strawberry sauce, organic, 1/2 cup	1
Apple strawberry sauce, organic, 4 oz	1
Indian Summer	
Premium chunky cherry applesauce, 1/2 cup	2
Premium chunky cinnamon applesauce, 1/2 cup	2
Premium chunky peach applesauce, 1/2 cup	2
Premium chunky raspberry flavored applesauce, 1/2 cup	2
Premium chunky strawberry applesauce, 1/2 cup	2
Lucky Leaf	
Apple sauce, 1/2 cup	1
Cinnamon apple sauce, 1/2 cup	2
Natural apple sauce, 1/2 cup	1
Manischewitz	
Apple sauce, unsweetened, 1/2 cup	1

	POINTS VALUE
Musselman's	
Apple sauce, 1/2 cup	1
Cinnamon apple sauce, 1/2 cup	2
Lite apple sauce, no sugar added, 1/2 cup	1
Lite cherry fruit 'n sauce, no sugar added, 1 container	1
Lite cinnamon apple sauce, no sugar added, 1/2 cup	1
Lite mixed berry fruit 'n sauce, no sugar added, 1 serving (113 g)	1
Lite orange mango fruit 'n sauce, no sugar added, 1 container	1
Lite peach fruit 'n sauce, no sugar added, 1 container	1
Lite raspberry fruit 'n sauce, no sugar added, 1 container	1
Lite strawberry fruit 'n sauce, no sugar added, 1 container	1
Natural apple sauce, 1/2 cup	1
Organic unsweetened apple sauce, 1 serving (113 g)	1
Sesame street cherry apple sauce (reduced sugar), 1 serving (113 g)	1
Sesame street grape apple sauce (reduced sugar), 1 serving (113 g)	1
Seneca	
Apricot flavored apple sauce, 1 container	1
Caramel apple, 1 container	1
Cinnamon, 1 container	1

	POINTS VALUE
Golden delicious, 1 container	1
♦ Natural, 1 container	1
Peach mango, 1 container	1
Pear flavored apple sauce, 1 container	1
Regular, 1 container	1
Wild berry, 1 container	1

Tree of Life

Organic apple sauce, cinnamon, 1/2 cup	2
♦ Organic apple sauce, unsweetened, 1/2 cup	1
Organic cinnamon apple sauce, 1	2
Organic cinnamon apple sauce, 1/2 cup	2
♦ Organic unsweetened apple sauce, 1	1
♦ Organic unsweetened apple sauce, 1/2 cup	1

Tree Top

Cinnamon naturally sweetened, 1 container	1
♦ Natural apple sauce, no sugar added, 1 container	1
Original naturally sweetened apple sauce, 1 container	1
Raspberry naturally sweetened, 1 container	1
Strawberry naturally sweetened, 1 container	1

Wilderness

♦ Applesauce, unsweetened, 1/2 cup	1
Chunky applesauce, 1/2 cup	1
Cinnamon applesauce, 1/2 cup	2
Mango flavored applesauce, 1/2 cup	2
♦ Natural applesauce, 1 container	1

	POINTS VALUE
Peach flavored applesauce, 1 container	2
Raspberry flavored applesauce, 1 container	2
Regular applesauce, 1/2 cup	1
Strawberry flavored applesauce, 1 container	2

Apples

Comstock

♦ Sliced apples in water, 2/3 cup	1 (2)

Lucky Leaf

Canned sliced apples, 1/2 cup	1 (2)

Musselman's

Canned sliced apples, 1/2 cup	1 (2)

Tree of Life

Apple rings, dried, 6 pieces	1

Apricots

Del Monte

Lite unpeeled apricot halves in extra lite syrup, 1/2 cup	1
Unpeeled apricot halves in heavy syrup, 1/2 cup	2

Del Monte Orchard Select

Unpeeled apricot halves in light syrup, 1/2 cup	1

Dole

♦ Apricots, 3 pieces	1 (2)

Sun-Maid

California apricots, 1/4 cup	2
Mediterranean apricots, 1/4 cup	1

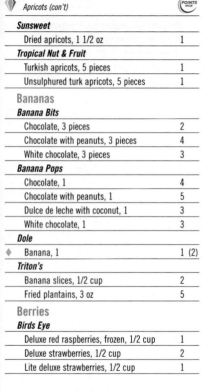

Apricots (con't)	POINTS VALUE
Sunsweet	
Dried apricots, 1 1/2 oz	1
Tropical Nut & Fruit	
Turkish apricots, 5 pieces	1
Unsulphured turk apricots, 5 pieces	1
Bananas	
Banana Bits	
Chocolate, 3 pieces	2
Chocolate with peanuts, 3 pieces	4
White chocolate, 3 pieces	3
Banana Pops	
Chocolate, 1	4
Chocolate with peanuts, 1	5
Dulce de leche with coconut, 1	3
White chocolate, 1	3
Dole	
Banana, 1	1 (2)
Triton's	
Banana slices, 1/2 cup	2
Fried plantains, 3 oz	5
Berries	
Birds Eye	
Deluxe red raspberries, frozen, 1/2 cup	1
Deluxe strawberries, 1/2 cup	2
Lite deluxe strawberries, 1/2 cup	1

	POINTS VALUE
Cascadian Farm	
Blackberries, 1 cup	1 (2)
Blueberries, 1 cup	1 (2)
Harvest berries, 1 cup	0
Premium strawberries, 1 cup	0 (2)
Red raspberries, 1/4 cup	0 (2)
Chocolate Bowl	
Dark chocolate cranberries, 12 pieces	3
Comstock	
Blueberries in heavy syrup, 1/2 cup	2
Dole	
Cranberries, 1/2 cup	0 (2)
Fresh frozen blackberries, 1 cup	1 (2)
Fresh frozen blueberries, 1 cup	1 (2)
Fresh frozen burst o berry, 1 cup	1
Fresh frozen red raspberries, 1 cup	1 (2)
Fresh frozen sliced strawberries with sugar, 1/2 cup	3
Fresh frozen whole strawberries, 1 cup	0 (2)
Fresh frozen wild blueberries, 1 cup	1 (2)
Raspberry, 1 cup	0 (2)
Strawberry, 8	0 (2)
Ocean Spray Craisins	
Sweetened dried cranberries, cherry flavor, 1/3 cup	2
Sweetened dried cranberries, orange flavor, 1/3 cup	2

◆		POINTS VALUE
	Sweetened dried cranberry, original flavor, 1/3 cup	2
Schwan's LiveSmart		
◆	Triple berry blend, 1 cup	1
◆	Whole blueberries, 3/4 cup	1 (2)
◆	Whole strawberries, 1 cup	0 (2)
Sun-Maid		
	Cape Cod cranberries, 1/3 cup	2
Sunsweet		
	Cranberry, 1 1/2 oz	2 (2)
	Cranberry, 1 bag	2 (2)
Traverse Bay Fruit Co.		
	Sweetened dried blueberries, 1/4 cup	2
Tree of Life		
	Blueberries, dried, 1/4 cup	2
	Cranberry concentrate, 8 tsp	2
	Dried cranberries, 1 serving (40 g)	2
◆	Organic blueberries, frozen, 1 cup	1 (2)
◆	Organic red raspberries, frozen, 2/3 cup	1 (2)
◆	Organic whole strawberries, frozen, 3/4 cup	1 (2)
Tropical Nut & Fruit		
	Dried blueberries, 1 serving (40 g)	2

Cherries

Cascadian Farm		
◆	Sweet cherries, 1 cup	1

◆		POINTS VALUE
Comstock		
	Dark sweet cherries pitted in heavy syrup, 1/2 cup	2
Del Monte		
	Dark, pitted cherries in heavy syrup, 1/2 cup	2
Dole		
◆	Cherries, 1 cup	1 (2)
◆	Fresh frozen dark sweet cherries, 1 cup	1
Eden		
	Dried Montmorency cherries, 1/4 cup	2
Futuro		
◆	Yellow cherries, 1 oz	0 (2)
Great Expectations		
	Maraschino cherries with stems, 1	0
Traverse Bay Fruit Co.		
	Sweetened dried cherries, 1/3 cup	2
Tree of Life		
	Dried cherries, 1 serving (28 g)	2
◆	Organic dark sweet cherries, frozen, 1/2 cup	2
Tropical Nut & Fruit		
	Bing cherries, 1/4 cup	2
	Dried cherries, 1/4 cup	2

Coconut

Tree of Life		
	Organic shredded coconut, 1 oz	4

Dried Fruit

Be Happy & Healthy

Sour wiggle giggle, 6 pieces	3

Betty Crocker Fruit Smoothie Blitz

All flavors and shapes, 1 regular pouch	1
All flavors and shapes, big pouch, 1 big pouch	3

Betty Crocker Sunkist with Calcium

All flavors and shapes, 1 regular pouch	2
All flavors and shapes, xxl, 10 pieces	2

Crispy Green

Crispy apples, 1 bag	1
Crispy apricots, 1 bag	1
Crispy peaches, 1 bag	1
Crispy pineapple, 1 bag	1

Dole

California seedless raisins, 1/4 cup	2
Chopped raisins, 1 oz	2
Cinnaraisins, 1/4 cup	3
Golden raisins, 1/4 cup	2
Pitted dates, 1/4 cup	2

Estee

Chocolatey covered raisins, 1/4 cup	4

Fruit by the Foot

All flavors, 1 roll	2

Fruit by the Foot Mini Feet

All flavors, 1 roll	1

Fruit Gushers

All flavors, 1 pouch	2

Fruit Roll-Ups

All flavors, 1 roll	1

Fruit Roll-Ups Mini Rolls

All flavors, 1 roll	1

Fruit Shapes

All flavors, 1 pouch	2

Kashi

Fruit leather - harvest grape, 1 pouch	1
Fruit leather - mango sunrise, 1 pouch	1
Fruit leather - orchard apple, 1 pouch	1
Fruit leather - orchard cherry, 1 pouch	1
Fruit leather - summer strawberry, 1 pouch	1
Fruit leather organic - organic grape, 1 pouch	1
Fruit leather organic - organic raspberry, 1 pouch	1
Fruit leather organic - organic strawberry, 1 pouch	1
Fruitabu organic smooshed apple twirl, 1	2
Fruitabu organic smooshed grape flavored twirl, 1	2
Fruitabu organic smooshed strawberry flavored twirl, 1	2
Fruitabu sploooshers - organic grape flavored tube, 1 tube	1

	POINTS VALUE
Fruitabu sploooshers - organic raspberry flavored tube, 1 tube	1
Fruitabu sploooshers - organic strawberry flavored tube, 1 tube	1
Kashi Stretch Island	
Fruit leather - abundant apricot, 1 pouch	1
Fruit leather - autumn apple, 1 pouch	1
Fruit leather organic - organic apricot, 1 pouch	1
Fruit leather, abundant apricot, 1 pouch	1
Fruit leather, bountiful blackberry, 1 pouch	1
Fruit leather, harvest grape, 1 pouch	1
Fruit leather, mango sunrise, 1 pouch	1
Fruit leather, orchard cherry, 1 pouch	1
Fruit leather, ripened raspberry, 1 pouch	1
Fruit leather, summer strawberry, 1 pouch	1
Kellogg's	
Fruit flavored snacks (all inclusive), 1 pouch	2
Fruit leather - ripened raspberry, 1 pouch	1
Yogos crazy berries, 1 pouch	2
Yogos island explosion, 1 pouch	2
Yogos rollers - yogurty striped- chacha cherry, 1 roll	2
Yogos rollers - yogurty striped- punch-a-licious, 1 roll	2
Yogos rollers - yogurty striped- strawberry splits, 1 roll	2
Yogos strawberry slam, 1 pouch	2

	POINTS VALUE
Market Day	
Fruit snacks variety pack, 1 serving (22.7 g)	2
Nature Valley Fruit Crisps	
Cinnamon apple fruit ripples, 1 pouch	1
Strawberry apple fruit ripples, 1 pouch	1
Ocean Spray	
Craisins 100 calorie pack original flavor, 1 oz	2
Sunbelt	
Fruit jammers, 13 pieces	2
Sun-Maid	
Calimyrna figs, 1/4 cup	2
Fruit bits, 1/4 cup	2
Golden raisins and cherries, 1/4 cup	2
Mission figs, 1/4 cup	2
Mixed fruit, 1/4 cup	1
Pitted dates, 1/4 cup	2
Raisins, 1/4 cup	2
Tart cherries, 1/4 cup	2
Tropical pineapples, 1/4 cup	3
Tropical trio, 1/4 cup	3
Washington apple, 1/4 cup	2
Yogurt raisins, 1/4 cup (30)	3
Sunsweet	
Berry blend, 1/4 cup	2
Blueberries, 1/4 cup	2
Cherries, sweet & tart, 1/4 cup	2

FRUITS

Dried Fruit, Sunsweet (con't)	POINTS VALUE
Cherry essence dried plums, 6	1
Cherry essence dried plums, 1 bag	1
Chocolate plum sweets, 14 pieces	2
Chopped dates, 1 1/2 oz	2
Mango, 6 pieces	2
Lemon essence prunes, 1 1/2 oz	1
Orange essence prunes, 1 1/2 oz	1
Orchard mix, 1/4 cup	1
Pitted dates, 1 1/2 oz	2
Pitted dried prunes, 1 1/2 oz	1
Tropical mix, 1/3 cup	3
Sunsweet Ones	
Super select California prunes, 4	1
Sunsweet Smart 60 Calorie Packs	
Cherry essence prunes, 1 bag	1
Prunes, 1 bag	1
Sunsweet Smart 70 Calorie Packs	
Mediterranean apricots, 1 bag	1
Premium Thailand mango, 1 bag	1
Tree of Life	
Banana chips, sweetened, 1/2 cup	5
Carob raisins, 1 serving (40 g)	4
Date sugar, 1 tsp	0
Deglate noor pitted dates, 5 pieces	2
Mixed fruit, unsulphured, 1/3 cup	1
Organic Medjool dates, dried, 5 pieces	2

	POINTS VALUE
Organic raisins, 1/4 cup	2
Organic raisins, 1 box	2
Organic raisins mini snack pack, 1 box	1
Thompson raisins, 1/4 cup	2
Yogurt raisins, 1 serving (40 g)	4
Tropical Nut & Fruit	
Banana chips, 1 oz	3
Black mission fig, 1/4 cup	1
Calimyrna figs, 1/4 cup	1
Currants, 1/4 cup	2
Dark raisins, 1/4 cup	2
Fruit medley, 1 serving (40 g)	2
Glazed red cherries, 1 piece	0
Imperial mixed fruit, 1/4 cup	1
Natural apple rings, 1 serving (40 g)	2
Natural apples, diced, 1 serving (40 g)	2
Pitted prunes, 1/4 cup	2
Sulphured apple dices, 1 serving (40 g)	2
Sulphured apple rings, 1 serving (40 g)	2
Sulphured gold raisins, 1/4 cup	2
Unsulfured unsweetened banana chip, 25 pieces	2
Welch's	
Berry medley, 1 serving (25.5 g)	2
Cherries, 1/4 cup	3
Mixed fruit, 1 serving (25.5 g)	2
Tropical sensation, 1 serving (25.5 g)	2

Fruit Cocktail/Salad

Del Monte

Cherry mixed fruit (plastic cup), 1/2 cup	1
Chunky mixed fruits in heavy syrup, 1/2 cup	2
Citrus salad in extra light syrup, 1/2 cup	2
Fruit cocktail in heavy syrup, 1/2 cup	2
♦ Fruit cocktail in water, artificially sweetened, 1/2 cup	1
♦ Fruit naturals chunky mixed fruits in fruit juice, 1/2 cup	1
♦ Fruit naturals fruit cocktail in fruit juices, 1/2 cup	1
Lite chunky mixed fruits in extra light syrup, 1/2 cup	1
Lite fruit cocktail in extra light syrup, 1/2 cup	1
♦ Mixed fruit - artificially sweetened, 1 container	0
Mixed fruit in cherry flavored gel, 1 cup	2
Tropical fruit in extra light syrup, 1/2 cup	1
♦ Tropical fruit salad in pineapple & passion fruit juices, 1/2 cup	1
Very cherry mixed fruit, 1/2 cup	2

Del Monte Fruit Cups

♦ Fruit naturals mixed fruit in fruit juices, 1 (4 oz cup)	1
Lite mixed fruit in extra light syrup, 1 (4 oz cup)	1
Mixed fruit in heavy syrup, 1 (4 oz cup)	1

Del Monte Fruit Rageous

Crazy cherry mixed fruit in cherry-flavored light syrup, 1 (4 oz cup)	2

Del Monte Fruit To-Go

Banana berry peaches in natural flavored light syrup, 1 (4 oz cup)	1
Fruity combo - mixed fruit with pineapple in light syrup, 1 (4 oz cup)	1

Del Monte Orchard Select

Mixed fruit in light syrup, 1/2 cup	2

Dole

Cherry mixed fruit in light syrup, 1	1
Diced pears in light syrup, 1	1
♦ Fresh frozen deluxe mixed fruits, 3/4 cup	1
Mixed fruit in peach gel, 1	2
Tropical fruit in light syrup, 1/2 cup	1
Tropical fruit salad in light syrup, canned, 1/2 cup	1

Dole Fruit Bowls

Cherry mixed fruit in light syrup, 1 container	1
Mixed fruit in light syrup, 1 container	1
Tropical fruit in lightly sweetened juice, 1 container	1

Dole Fruit in Gel

Mixed fruit in black cherry gel, 1 container	2

Market Day

Fruit singles, 1 serving (4 oz)	1
Spectrum blend fruit cup, 1 serving (6 oz)	2

Fruit Cocktail/Salad (con't) | POINTS VALUE

Schwan's LiveSmart

Fruit to go cups, 1	1
Golden fruit blend, 3/4 cup	1

Sunfresh

Citrus salad sections in light syrup, 1/2 cup	1
Tropical fruit mixed in light syrup w/ passion fruit juice, 1/2 cup	1
Tropical salad in extra light syrup, 1/2 cup	2

Tree of Life

Organic mixed berries, frozen, 3/4 cup	1

Fruit parfait

Dole

Apples & caramel crème parfait, 1 container	2
Fruit flurry - pineapple, 1 cup	2
Fruit flurry - pineapple mango, 1 cup	2
Fruit flurry - strawberry pineapple banana, 1 cup	3
Peaches & crème parfait, 1 container	3
Pineapple & crème parfait, 1 container	3

Grapefruit

Del Monte

Red grapefruit in extra light syrup, 1/2 cup	1
Red grapefruit in extra light syrup (color added), 1/2 cup	1

POINTS VALUE

Sunfresh

Red grapefruit in slightly sweetened grapefruit juice, 1/2 cup	1
Red grapefruit sections in light syrup, 1/2 cup	2
White grapefruit sections in light syrup, 1/2 cup	2

Grapes

Dole

Grapes, 1 1/2 cups	2 (2)

Kiwi

Dole

Kiwi, 2	1 (2)

Mangoes

Dole

Mango, 1/2	1 (2)

Herdez

Sliced mangos, 2 pieces	3

Sunfresh

Mango slices in light syrup, 1/2 cup	2

Tree of Life

Dried mango slices, unsulphured, 1 serving (40 g)	0

Triton's

Mango chunks, 1 cup	1

Tropical Nut & Fruit

Mango slices, 3 slices	3

Melons

Dole
- Cantaloupe, 1/4 — 1 (2)
- Honeydew melon, 1 serving (1/10) — 1 (2)

Fanci Food
Sweet pickled watermelon rind, 2 Tbsp — 1

Oranges

Del Monte
Mandarin oranges in
extra light syrup, 1/2 cup — 1

Del Monte Fruit Cups
Mandarin oranges in
light syrup, 1 (4 oz cup) — 1

Dole
Mandarin and crème, 1 — 2

Mandarin oranges in light syrup,
canned, 1/2 cup — 1

Dole Fruit Bowls
Mandarin oranges in light syrup,
1 container — 1

Mandarin oranges in light syrup, 1 cup — 2

Dole Fruit in Gel
Mandarins in orange gel, 1 container — 2

Sunfresh
Mandarin oranges in light syrup, 1/2 cup — 1

Orange sections in light syrup, 1/2 cup — 2

Tree of Life
Mandarin oranges in light syrup, 2/3 cup — 1

Papayas

Brooks
- Caribbean red papaya, 1 cup (cubes) — 1 (2)
- Caribbean sunrise papaya, 1 cup — 1 (2)

Dole
- Papaya, 1/2 — 1 (2)

Sunfresh
Papaya chunks in extra light syrup, 1/2 cup — 1

Tree of Life
Dried papaya spears, unsulphured,
1 serving (100 g) — 0

Triton's
- Papaya chunks, 1 cup — 1 (2)

Tropical Nut & Fruit
Papaya chunks, 1 serving (40 g) — 3

Peaches and Nectarines

Cascadian Farm
- Sliced peaches, 1 cup — 1 (2)

Del Monte
- Diced peaches - artificially
  sweetened, 1 container — 0 (2)
- Diced peaches - artificially
  sweetened, 1 can — 0 (2)

Halves, lite peaches in extra light syrup
(yellow cling), 1/2 cup — 1

Halves, peaches in heavy syrup
(yellow cling), 1/2 cup — 2

Peaches and Nectarines, Del Monte (con't)	POINTS VALUE

	POINTS VALUE
Halves, peaches in heavy syrup (yellow freestone), 1/2 cup	2
Peach chunks in extra light syrup, 1/2 cup	1
Peaches in peach flavored gel, 1 cup	2
Peaches in raspberry lemonade flavored gel, 1 cup	2
Peaches in strawberry banana flavored gel - lite, 1 cup	1
◆ Sliced, fruit nat. peaches in pear & peach juices (yellow cling), 1/2 cup	1 (2)
Sliced, peaches in natural raspberry flavored light syrup (yellow cling), 1/2 cup	1
Sliced, spiced peaches in light syrup (yellow cling), 1/2 cup	1
Sweet cinnamon chunky-cut peaches in light syrup (yellow cling), 1/2 cup	1
Whole, spiced peaches in heavy syrup (yellow cling), 1/2 cup	2
◆ Yellow cling peaches in water, artificially sweetened, 1/2 cup	0 (2)

Del Monte Fruit Cups

Diced peaches in heavy syrup, 1 (4 oz cup)	1
Fruit naturals diced peaches in pear and peach juices, 1 (4 oz cup)	1 (2)
Lite diced peaches in extra light syrup, 1 (4 oz cup)	1

Del Monte Fruit Rageous

Wild raspberry flavored peaches in light syrup, 1 (4 oz cup)	1

Del Monte Fruit To-Go

Peachy peaches in peach-flavored light syrup, 1 (4 oz cup)	1

Del Monte Orchard Select

Sliced, yellow cling peaches in light syrup, 1/2 cup	2

Dole

◆ Fresh frozen sliced peaches with flavor, 3/4 cup	1
◆ Nectarine, 1	1 (2)
◆ Peach, 1	0 (2)
Sliced peaches in light syrup, 1/2 cup	2

Dole Fruit Bowls

Yellow cling diced peaches in light syrup, 1 container	1
Yellow cling diced peaches in light syrup, 1 cup	1

Dole Fruit in Gel

Diced peaches in strawberry gel, 1 container	2

Pears
Del Monte

Diced pears in light syrup, 1 cup	1
◆ Halves, fruit naturals pears in pear juice, 1/2 cup	1 (2)
Halves, lite pears in extra light syrup, 1/2 cup	1
Halves, pear in heavy syrup, 1/2 cup	2
◆ Pears in water, artificially sweetened, 1/2 cup	1 (2)

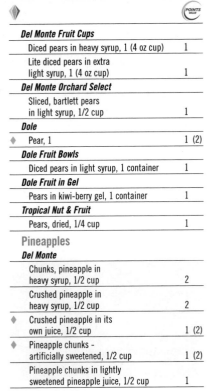

	POINTS VALUE
Del Monte Fruit Cups	
Diced pears in heavy syrup, 1 (4 oz cup)	1
Lite diced pears in extra light syrup, 1 (4 oz cup)	1
Del Monte Orchard Select	
Sliced, bartlett pears in light syrup, 1/2 cup	1
Dole	
Pear, 1	1 (2)
Dole Fruit Bowls	
Diced pears in light syrup, 1 container	1
Dole Fruit in Gel	
Pears in kiwi-berry gel, 1 container	1
Tropical Nut & Fruit	
Pears, dried, 1/4 cup	1

Pineapples

	POINTS VALUE
Del Monte	
Chunks, pineapple in heavy syrup, 1/2 cup	2
Crushed pineapple in heavy syrup, 1/2 cup	2
Crushed pineapple in its own juice, 1/2 cup	1 (2)
Pineapple chunks - artificially sweetened, 1/2 cup	1 (2)
Pineapple chunks in lightly sweetened pineapple juice, 1/2 cup	1
Pineapple chunks in pineapple juice, 1/2 cup	1
Pineapple crushed - artificially sweetened, 1/2 cup	1 (2)
Pineapple sliced - artificially sweetened, 1/2 cup	1 (2)
Pineapple tidbits - artificially sweetened, 1/2 cup	1 (2)
Sliced, pineapple in heavy syrup, 2 slices	2
Sliced, pineapple in its own juice, 2 slices	1 (2)
Del Monte Fruit Cups	
Pineapple tidbits in pineapple juice, 1 (4 oz cup)	1 (2)
Dole	
Fresh frozen pineapple chunks, 3/4 cup	2 (2)
Pineapple, 2 slices	1 (2)
Pineapple chunks in juice, 1/2 cup	1 (2)
Pineapple chunks in syrup, 1/2 cup	2
Pineapple crushed in juice, canned, 1/2 cup	1 (2)
Pineapple crushed in syrup, canned, 1/2 cup	2
Pineapple slices in juice, canned, 2 slices	1 (2)
Pineapple slices in syrup, canned, 2 slices	2
Pineapple tidbits in juice, canned, 1/2 cup	1 (2)
Pineapple tidbits in syrup, canned, 1/2 cup	2
Dole Fruit Bowls	
Pineapple tidbits in pineapple juice, 1 container	1 (2)

Pineapples (con't)

POINTS VALUE

Dole Fruit in Gel

Pineapple tidbits in lime gel, 1 container — 2

Dole Snack Jars

Pineapple chunks in light syrup, 1/2 cup — 1

Manischewitz

Crushed pineapple, 1/2 cup — 1

Sliced pineapple, 2 slices — 1

Sunfresh

Pineapple chunks in lightly sweetened pineapple juice, 1/2 cup — 1

Tree of Life

Pineapple rings, unsulphured, 1 Tbsp — 4

Triton's

Pineapple chunks, 1 cup — 1

Tropical Nut & Fruit

Natural pineapple, 2 pieces — 2

Pineapple wedge, 10 pieces — 2

Plums

Comstock

Purple plums sweet whole unpitted in heavy syrup, 1/2 cup — 2

Dole

Plum, 2 — 1 (2)

Sun-Maid

Pitted plums, 1/4 cup — 2

Specialty Fruits

Brooks

Star fruit - carambola, 1 cup — 1 (2)

Dole

Fresh frozen rhubarb chunks, 1 cup — 0

Persimmons, 1 medium — 1 (2)

Futuro

Pacaya date palm, 1 oz — 0

Herdez

Whole guavas, 4 pieces — 3

Triton's

Guava chunks, 1 cup — 0

Tangerines

Dole

Tangerine, 1 medium — 0 (2)

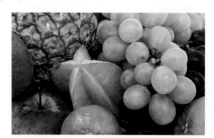

	POINTS VALUE
Dips	
Athenos	
Feta spread basil and tomato, 2 Tbsp	2
Feta spread original, 2 Tbsp	2
Blue Bunny	
Bacon & horseradish sour cream snack dip, 2 Tbsp	2
French onion sour cream snack dip, 2 Tbsp	2
Ranch dill sour cream snack dip, 2 Tbsp	2
Toasted onion sour cream snack dip, 2 Tbsp	2
CIBO Naturals	
Chipotle cheese dip, 2 Tbsp	3
Chipotle lime dip, 2 Tbsp	3
Cipollini onion dip, 2 Tbsp	3
Kalamata olive dip, 2 Tbsp	3
EatSmart	
◆ Three bean dip, 2 Tbsp	0
Emerald Valley Kitchen	
Organic black bean dip, 2 Tbsp	1
Organic classic 3 bean dip, 2 Tbsp	0
Frito-Lay	
French onion dip, 2 Tbsp	2
Fritos	
Bean dip, original flavor, 2 Tbsp	1
Chili cheese, 2 Tbsp	1

	POINTS VALUE
Hot bean dip, 2 Tbsp	1
Jalapeno cheddar flavor cheese dip, 2 Tbsp	1
Mild cheddar flavor cheese dip, 2 Tbsp	2
GG Golden Guernsey Dairy	
French onion dip, 2 Tbsp	1
Guiltless Gourmet	
◆ Mild black bean dip, 2 Tbsp	0
◆ Spicy black bean dip, 2 Tbsp	0
Hidden Valley	
Fat free original ranch party dip, prepared from mix, 2 Tbsp	1
Fiesta ranch party dip, prepared from mix, 2 Tbsp	2
French onion party dip, prepared from mix, 2 Tbsp	2
Original ranch party dip, prepared from mix, 2 Tbsp	2
K.C. Masterpiece Dip & Top Sauce	
Cool ranch bbq, 1 Tbsp	1
Honey dijon, 1 Tbsp	1
Kraft	
Bacon & cheddar, 2 Tbsp	2
Creamy ranch, 2 Tbsp	2
French onion, 2 Tbsp	2
Green onion, 2 Tbsp	2
Guacamole, 2 Tbsp	1
Jalapeño, 2 Tbsp	1

JAMS, SPREADS, SALSA & DIPS

Dips (con't)	POINTS VALUE
Kraft Cheez Whiz	
Light, 2 Tbsp	2
Plain, 2 Tbsp	2
Salsa con queso, 2 Tbsp	2
Lay's	
Creamy ranch dip, 2 Tbsp	1
French onion dip, 2 Tbsp	1
French onion flavored dry dip mix, 1 serving (1/16 of packet)	0
French onion flavored dry dip mix prepared with sour cream, 2 Tbsp	2
Green onion flavored dry dip mix, 1 serving (1/16 of packet)	0
Green onion flavored dry dip mix prepared with sour cream, 2 Tbsp	2
Ranch flavored dry dip mix, 1 serving (1/16 of packet)	0
Ranch flavored dry dip mix prepared with sour cream, 2 Tbsp	2
Litehouse	
Avocado dip, 2 Tbsp	4
Chocolate caramel dip, 2 Tbsp	3
Dilly dip, 2 Tbsp	4
Jalapeno ranch dip, 2 Tbsp	3
Lite ranch dip, 2 Tbsp	2
Low fat caramel dip, 2 Tbsp	2
Organic ranch dip, 2 Tbsp	4
Original caramel dip, 2 Tbsp	2

	POINTS VALUE
Ranch dip, 2 Tbsp	4
Reduced sugar caramel, 2 Tbsp	1
Toffee caramel dip, 1 serving (40 g)	2
Yogurt strawberry fruit dip, 2 Tbsp	1
Yogurt vanilla fruit dip, 2 Tbsp	2
Marzetti	
Cream cheese fruit dip - 100 calorie pack, 1	2
Light ranch veggie dip - 100 calorie pack, 1	3
Morning Glory	
French onion dip, 2 Tbsp	1
Naturally Fresh	
Bleu cheese dip, 2 Tbsp	4
Bleu cheese, shelf stable, 2 Tbsp	5
Caramel dip, 2 Tbsp	3
Chocolate dip, 2 Tbsp	1
Dijon honey mustard dip, 2 Tbsp	4
French onion dip, 2 Tbsp	3
French onion dip, refrigerated, 2 Tbsp	3
Honey mustard dip, 2 Tbsp	3
Hot sauce dip, 2 Tbsp	1
Ranch dip, 2 Tbsp	5
Ranch dip, shelf stable, 1 Tbsp	3
Ranch dressing, 2 Tbsp	3
Strawberry cream cheese dip, 2 Tbsp	2
Strawberry yogurt dip, 2 Tbsp	1

	POINTS VALUE
Sweet and sour sauce, 2 Tbsp	2
Vanilla yogurt dip, 2 Tbsp	1
Vegetable ranch dip, 2 Tbsp	4
Old El Paso	
Black bean, medium, 2 Tbsp	0
Cheese 'n salsa, low fat, medium, 2 Tbsp	1
Cheese 'n salsa, medium, 2 Tbsp	1
Cheese 'n salsa, mild, 2 Tbsp	1
Ortega	
Guacamole style dip, 2 Tbsp	1
Philadelphia	
Pourovers dip cream cheese spread & salsa, 2 Tbsp	2
Phillips	
Crab & spinach dip, 2 Tbsp	1
Maryland style crab dip, 2 Tbsp	2
Ruffles	
Rich & creamy smoky bacon & cheddar dip, 2 Tbsp	2
Rich & creamy sour cream & chive dip, 2 Tbsp	1
Sabra	
Moroccan matbucha dip, 1 serving (1 oz)	0
Turkish dip, 1 oz	1
T. Marzetti	
Blue cheese veggie dip, 2 Tbsp	4
Buffalo ranch veggie dip, 2 Tbsp	3

	POINTS VALUE
Celery and carrot dip, 1 1/2 oz	7
Chocolate fruit dip, 2 Tbsp	2
Cream cheese fruit dip, 2 Tbsp	2
Dill veggie dip, 2 Tbsp	3
Fat free caramel apple dip, 2 Tbsp	2
Fat free chocolate dip, 2 Tbsp	2
Fat free dill veggie dip, 2 Tbsp	1
Fat free ranch veggie dip, 2 Tbsp	1
Fat free southwestern veggie dip, 2 Tbsp	1
French onion veggie dip, 2 Tbsp	3
Guacamole dip, 2 Tbsp	4
Light caramel dip, 2 Tbsp	2
Light dill veggie dip, 2 Tbsp	2
Light ranch veggie dip, 2 Tbsp	2
Light vanilla yogurt fruit dip, 2 Tbsp	1
Natural strawberry flavored cream cheese fruit dip, 2 Tbsp	2
Organic ranch veggie dip, 2 Tbsp	4
Peanut butter caramel apple dip, 2 Tbsp	3
Ranch veggie dip, 2 Tbsp	3
Southwestern ranch veggie dip, 2 Tbsp	3
Spinach veggie dip, 2 Tbsp	4
T.G.I. Friday's	
Spinach, cheese & artichoke dip, 2 Tbsp	1
Taco Bell Home Originals	
Black bean con queso - mild, 2 Tbsp	1
Chili con queso, 2 Tbsp	1

JAMS, SPREADS, SALSA & DIPS

Dips (con't)	POINTS VALUE
Tostitos	
Creamy southwestern ranch dip, 2 Tbsp	1
Creamy spinach dip, 2 Tbsp	1
Monterey Jack queso, 2 Tbsp	1
Reduced fat zesty cheese dip, 2 Tbsp	1
Spicy queso supreme, 2 Tbsp	1
Walden Farms	
Bacon horseradish dip, 2 Tbsp	0
Bleu cheese dip, 2 Tbsp	0
Calorie free chocolate dip, 2 Tbsp	0
Calorie free marshmallow dip, 2 Tbsp	0
Caramel dip, 2 Tbsp	0
French onion dip, 2 Tbsp	0
Vegetable ranch dip, 2 Tbsp	0

Fruit spread

Polaner All Fruit	POINTS VALUE
Apricot, 1 Tbsp	1
Black cherry, 1 Tbsp	1
Blueberry, 1 Tbsp	1
Boysenberry, 1 Tbsp	1
Grape, 1 Tbsp	1
Orange marmalade, 1 Tbsp	1
Peach, 1 Tbsp	1
Pineapple, 1 Tbsp	1
Raspberry, 1 Tbsp	1
Seedless blackberry, 1 Tbsp	1

	POINTS VALUE
Seedless raspberry, 1 Tbsp	1
Seedless strawberry, 1 Tbsp	1
Strawberry, 1 Tbsp	1
Polaner Sugar Free	
Orange marmalade, 1 Tbsp	0
Smucker's Simply Fruit	
Apple butter, 1 Tbsp	1
Apricot, 1 Tbsp	1
Black cherry, 1 Tbsp	1
Black raspberry (seedless), 1 Tbsp	1
Blackberry (seedless), 2 Tbsp	1
Blueberry, 1 Tbsp	1
Grape, 1 Tbsp	1
Orange marmalade, 1 Tbsp	1
Peach, 1 Tbsp	1
Red raspberry, 1 Tbsp	1
Red raspberry (seedless), 1 Tbsp	1
Strawberry, 1 Tbsp	1
Strawberry (seedless), 1 Tbsp	1
Tree of Life	
Organic apricot fruit spread, 1 Tbsp	1
Organic blueberry fruit spread, 1 Tbsp	1
Organic cherry fruit spread, 1 Tbsp	1
Organic grape fruit spread, 1 Tbsp	1
Organic peach fruit spread, 1 Tbsp	1
Organic raspberry fruit spread, 1 Tbsp	1
Organic strawberry fruit spread, 1 Tbsp	1

	POINTS VALUE
Walden Farms No Carbs	
Apple butter fruit spread, 1 Tbsp	0
Apricot fruit spread, 1 Tbsp	0
Blueberry fruit spread, 1 Tbsp	0
Grape fruit spread, 1 Tbsp	0
Raspberry fruit spread, 1 Tbsp	0
Strawberry fruit spread, 1 Tbsp	0

Hummus

	POINTS VALUE
Athenos	
Artichoke and garlic, 2 Tbsp	1
Black olive, 2 Tbsp	1
Original, 2 Tbsp	1
Pesto, 2 Tbsp	1
Roasted eggplant, 2 Tbsp	1
Roasted garlic, 2 Tbsp	1
Roasted red pepper, 2 Tbsp	1
Three pepper, 2 Tbsp	1
Emerald Valley Kitchen	
Organic Greek olive hummus, 2 Tbsp	1
Organic hummus, 2 Tbsp	1
Organic red pepper hummus, 2 Tbsp	1
Organic smoked jalapeno & garlic hummus, 2 Tbsp	1
Organic spinach feta hummus, 2 Tbsp	1
Fantastic World Foods	
Original hummus, 2 Tbsp	1

	POINTS VALUE
Guiltless Gourmet	
Original hummus, 2 Tbsp	1
Roasted garlic hummus, 2 Tbsp	1
Marzetti	
Original hummus, 2 Tbsp	2
Roasted garlic hummus, 2 Tbsp	2
Roasted red pepper hummus, 2 Tbsp	2
Sabra	
Chunky (Marakesh) hummus, 1 oz	2
Classic hummus, 1 oz	2
Garlic hummus, 1 oz	2
Greek olive hummus, 1 oz	2
Hummus roasted red pepper, 1 oz	2
Luscious lemon hummus, 1 oz	2
Supremely spicy hummus, 1 oz	2
Swan Gardens	
Organic hummus, roasted garlic, 2 Tbsp	1
Organic hummus, roasted red peppers, 2 Tbsp	1
Organic hummus, traditional, 2 Tbsp	1
Tribe All Natural Hummus	
All natural hummus, 1 Tbsp	1
Calamata olive, 1 Tbsp	1
Chili pepper, 1 Tbsp	1
Chipotle, 1 Tbsp	1
Classic, 1 Tbsp	1

JAMS, SPREADS, SALSA & DIPS

Hummus, Tribe All Natural Hummus (con't)	POINTS VALUE
Eggplant (baba), 1 Tbsp	1
Forty spices, 1 Tbsp	1
French onion, 1 Tbsp	1
Garden vegetables, 1 Tbsp	1
Horseradish, 1 Tbsp	1
Jalapeno, 1 Tbsp	1
Organic chili pepper hummus, 1 Tbsp	1
Organic classic hummus, 1 Tbsp	1
Organic roasted red peppers hummus, 1 Tbsp	1
Roasted garlic, 1 Tbsp	1
Roasted red peppers, 1 Tbsp	1
Savory dill, 1 Tbsp	1
Scallion, 1 Tbsp	1
Sundried tomato basil, 1 Tbsp	1
Sundried tomato basil, 1 Tbsp	1
Zesty lemon, 1 Tbsp	1
Wholesome Valley Organic	
Classic hummus, 2 Tbsp	1
Garlic hummus, 2 Tbsp	1
Roasted red pepper hummus, 2 Tbsp	1
Spicy chipotle hummus, 2 Tbsp	1

Jams and Preserves
Cherchies

	POINTS VALUE
Cranberry preserves, 1 Tbsp	1
New England triple berry preserve with merlot, 1 Tbsp	1

	POINTS VALUE
White tea key lime raspberry preserve, 1 Tbsp	1
White tea pomegranate peach preserve, 1 Tbsp	1
Wild Maine blueberry preserve with burgundy, 1 Tbsp	1
Goldwater's	
Raspberry jam, 1 Tbsp	1
Polaner	
Concord grape jam, 1 Tbsp	1
Smucker's	
Black raspberry (seedless) jam, 1 Tbsp	1
Blackberry (seedless) jam, 1 Tbsp	1
Blackberry jam, 1 Tbsp	1
Boysenberry (seedless) jam, 1 Tbsp	1
Grape jam, 1 Tbsp	1
Red plum jam, 1 Tbsp	1
Red raspberry (seedless) jam, 1 Tbsp	1
Strawberry (seedless) jam, 1 Tbsp	1
Strawberry jam, 1 Tbsp	1
Sugar free blackberry jam, 1 Tbsp	0
Sugar free grape jam, 1 Tbsp	0

Jelly
Cherchies

	POINTS VALUE
Cherry hot pepper jelly, 1 Tbsp	1
Cranberry hot pepper jelly, 1 Tbsp	2
Lem'n hot pepper jelly, 1 Tbsp	2
Roasted garlic hot pepper jelly, 1 Tbsp	1

	POINTS VALUE
Goldwater's	
Jalapeno jelly, 1 Tbsp	1
Margarita jelly, 1 Tbsp	1
Prickly pear jelly, 1 Tbsp	1
Muirhead	
Apricot-jalapeno jelly, 1 Tbsp	1
Polaner	
Grape jelly, 1 Tbsp	1
Real currant jelly, 1 Tbsp	1
Real mint jelly, 1 Tbsp	1
Polaner Sugar Free	
Concord grape jelly, 1 Tbsp	0
Mint jelly, 1 Tbsp	0
Smucker's	
Apple jelly, 1 Tbsp	1
Black raspberry jelly, 1 Tbsp	1
Blackberry jelly, 1 Tbsp	1
Cherry jelly, 1 Tbsp	1
Cinnamon apple jelly, 1 Tbsp	1
Currant jelly, 1 Tbsp	1
Elderberry jelly, 1 Tbsp	1
Grape jelly, 1 Tbsp	1
Guava jelly, 1 Tbsp	1
Low sugar grape jelly, 1 Tbsp	1
Mint apple jelly, 1 Tbsp	1
Mixed fruit jelly, 1 Tbsp	1

	POINTS VALUE
Plum jelly, 1 Tbsp	1
Quince jelly, 1 Tbsp	1
Red raspberry jelly, 1 Tbsp	1
Strawberry jelly, 1 Tbsp	1

Marmalade
Muirhead

Tomato marmalade, 1 Tbsp	0

Polaner

California sweet orange marmalade, 1 Tbsp	1

Smucker's

Low sugar orange marmalade, 1 Tbsp	1
Sugar free orange marmalade, 1 Tbsp	0
Sweet orange marmalade, 1 Tbsp	1

Walden Farms No Carbs

Orange marmalade, 1 Tbsp	0

Other Spread and Dips
Apple Time

Apple butter, 1 Tbsp	1

CIBO Naturals

Fig & olive tapenade, 2 Tbsp	3
Kalamata olive Tuscan bean spread, 2 Tbsp	2
Lemon & garlic Tuscan bean spread, 2 Tbsp	1
Olive & garlic tapenade, 2 Tbsp	3
Olive trio bruschetta topping, 2 Tbsp	1

Other Spread and Dips, CIBO Naturals (con't)

	POINTS VALUE
Roasted garlic Tuscan bean spread, 2 Tbsp	1
Roasted red pepper Tuscan bean spread, 2 Tbsp	1
Tomato & artichoke bruschetta topping, 2 Tbsp	0
Tomato & basil bruschetta topping, 2 Tbsp	1
Classico	
Basil pesto, 1/4 cup	6
Bruschetta basil & tomato, 1 serving (15 g)	0
Bruschetta extra garlic, 1 serving (15 g)	0
Clearbrook Farms	
Apple butter, 1 Tbsp	1
Cherry butter, 1 Tbsp	1
Peach butter, 1 Tbsp	1
Pear butter, 1 Tbsp	1
Pumpkin butter, 1 Tbsp	1
Red raspberry butter, 1 Tbsp	1
Strawberry butter, 1 Tbsp	1
Triple berry butter, 1 Tbsp	1
Cure 81	
Deviled ham, 4 Tbsp	4
Eden Organic	
Apple butter, 1 serving (16 g)	0
Apple cherry butter, organic, 1 Tbsp	0
Cherry butter (Montmorency tart cherries), 1 Tbsp	1

	POINTS VALUE
Emerald Valley Kitchen	
Organic curry lime edamame spread, 2 Tbsp	1
Organic fiesta edamame spread, 2 Tbsp	1
Organic ginger wasabi edamame spread, 2 Tbsp	1
Kraft	
Sandwich spread, 1 Tbsp	1
Land O Lakes	
Fresh buttery taste spread, soft, 1 Tbsp	2
Fresh buttery taste spread, stick, 1 Tbsp	3
Lucky Leaf	
Apple butter, 1 Tbsp	1
Manischewitz	
Original apple butter spread, 1 Tbsp	0
MaraNatha Natural	
Creamy & raw almond butter, no salt added, 2 Tbsp	4
Creamy & raw sesame tahini, with salt, 2 Tbsp	5
Creamy & roasted almond butter, no salt added, 2 Tbsp	4
Creamy & roasted cashew butter, no salt added, 2 Tbsp	5
Creamy & roasted cashew macadamia butter, no salt added, 2 Tbsp	5
Creamy & roasted macadamia butter, no salt added, 2 Tbsp	6

	POINTS VALUE
Creamy & roasted sesame tahini, 2 Tbsp	5
Crunchy & roasted almond butter, no salt added, 2 Tbsp	4
Honey almond butter, 2 Tbsp	4
Honey peanut spread, 2 Tbsp	4
No stir creamy almond butter, 2 Tbsp	5
No stir crunchy almond butter, 2 Tbsp	5
MaraNatha Organic	
Creamy & raw almond butter, no salt added, 2 Tbsp	4
Creamy & raw sesame tahini, no salt added, 2 Tbsp	5
Creamy & roasted almond butter, no salt added, 2 Tbsp	4
Creamy & roasted sesame tahini, no salt added, 2 Tbsp	5
Crunchy & roasted almond butter, no salt added, 2 Tbsp	4
Muirhead	
Banana walnut butter, 1 Tbsp	0
Blueberry butter, 1 Tbsp	1
Cinnamon apple butter, 1 Tbsp	1
Ginger peachy butter, 1 Tbsp	0
Pear and port butter, 1 Tbsp	0
Pecan pumpkin butter, 1 Tbsp	0
Rutabaga butter, 1 Tbsp	0
Musselman's	
Apple butter, 1 Tbsp	1

	POINTS VALUE
Oscar Mayer	
Sandwich spread, 2 oz	3
Smucker's	
Cider apple butter, 1 Tbsp	1
Peach butter, 1 Tbsp	1
Spiced apple butter, 1 Tbsp	1
Soy Wonder	
Creamy, 2 Tbsp	4
Crunchy, 2 Tbsp	4
T. Marzetti	
Sugar free glaze for strawberries, 3 Tbsp	0
Tree of Life	
Natural creamy almond butter, 2 Tbsp	4
Natural creamy cashew butter, 2 Tbsp	5
Natural crunchy almond butter, 2 Tbsp	4
Organic cashew butter creamy, 2 Tbsp	5
Organic creamy almond butter, 2 Tbsp	4
Organic crunchy almond butter, 2 Tbsp	4
Organic or natural raw almond butter creamy, 2 Tbsp	4
Walden Farms	
Original bruschetta, 2 Tbsp	1

Peanut Butter
Better'n Peanut Butter

	POINTS VALUE
Low fat peanut spread, 2 Tbsp	2
Low fat peanut spread, low sodium, 2 Tbsp	2
Original, 2 Tbsp	2

JAMS, SPREADS, SALSA & DIPS

Peanut Butter (con't) POINTS VALUE

Fisher

Creamy peanut butter, 2 Tbsp	5
Crunchy peanut butter, 2 Tbsp	5

Laura Scudder's

Reduced fat peanut butter, 2 Tbsp	5

MaraNatha Natural

Creamy & roasted peanut butter with salt, 2 Tbsp	5
Creamy & roasted peanut butter, no salt added, 2 Tbsp	5
Crunchy & roasted peanut butter, no salt added, 2 Tbsp	5
Crunchy & roasted peanut butter, with salt, 2 Tbsp	5
No stir creamy & sweet peanut butter, 2 Tbsp	5
No stir crunchy & sweet peanut butter, 2 Tbsp	5

MaraNatha Organic

Creamy & roasted peanut butter, no salt added, 2 Tbsp	5
Creamy & roasted peanut butter, with salt, 2 Tbsp	5
Crunchy & roasted peanut butter, no salt added, 2 Tbsp	5
Crunchy & roasted peanut butter, with salt, 2 Tbsp	5
No stir creamy peanut butter, 2 Tbsp	5
No stir crunchy peanut butter, 2 Tbsp	5

Peanut Wonder

Low fat peanut spread, 2 Tbsp	2
Low fat peanut spread, low sodium, 2 Tbsp	2

Skippy

Carb options peanut spread, 2 Tbsp	5
Creamy peanut butter, 2 Tbsp	5
Creamy roasted honey nut peanut butter, 2 Tbsp	5
Natural super chunk, 2 Tbsp	5
Reduced fat creamy, 2 Tbsp	4
Reduced fat super chunk, 2 Tbsp	4
Super chunk peanut butter, 2 Tbsp	5
Super chunk roasted honey nut peanut butter, 2 Tbsp	5

Smart Balance

Omega natural peanut butter and omega-3 from flax oil, chunky, 2 Tbsp	5
Omega natural peanut butter and omega-3 from flax oil, creamy, 2 Tbsp	5

Smucker's

Reduced fat natural peanut butter, 2 Tbsp	5

Tree of Life

Blended organic creamy peanut butter, 2 Tbsp	5
Blended organic crunchy peanut butter, 2 Tbsp	5
Organic creamy peanut butter, 2 Tbsp	5

	POINTS VALUE
Organic creamy peanut butter, no salt added, 2 Tbsp	5
Organic crunchy peanut butter, 2 Tbsp	5
Organic crunchy peanut butter, no salt added, 2 Tbsp	5

Preserves
Clearbrook Farms

Bitter-sweet orange marmalade, 1 Tbsp	1
California apricot, 1 Tbsp	1
California peach, 1 Tbsp	1
Cranberry-orange, 1 Tbsp	1
Michigan black cherry, 1 Tbsp	1
Michigan damson plum, 1 Tbsp	1
Michigan red tart cherry, 1 Tbsp	1
Oregon black raspberry, 1 Tbsp	1
Oregon blackberry, 1 Tbsp	1
Oregon red raspberry, 1 Tbsp	1
Oregon strawberry, 1 Tbsp	1
Seedless Oregon red raspberry, 1 Tbsp	1
Wild Maine blueberry, 1 Tbsp	1

Polaner

Chunky apricot preserves, 1 Tbsp	1
Red raspberry preserves, 1 Tbsp	1
Strawberry preserves, 1 Tbsp	1

Polaner Sugar Free

Apricot, 1 Tbsp	0
Black cherry, 1 Tbsp	0

	POINTS VALUE
Blackberry, 1 Tbsp	0
Blueberry, 1 Tbsp	0
Peach, 1 Tbsp	0
Pineapple, 1 Tbsp	0
Raspberry, 1 Tbsp	0
Strawberry, 1 Tbsp	0

Smucker's

Apricot preserves, 1 Tbsp	1
Apricot-pineapple preserves, 1 Tbsp	1
Blueberry preserves, 1 Tbsp	1
Cherry preserves, 1 Tbsp	1
Low sugar apricot preserves, 1 Tbsp	1
Low sugar orange marmalade preserves, 1 Tbsp	1
Low sugar red raspberry preserves, 1 Tbsp	1
Low sugar strawberry preserves, 1 Tbsp	1
Peach preserves, 1 Tbsp	1
Pineapple preserves, 1 Tbsp	1
Plum preserves, 1 Tbsp	1
Red raspberry preserves, 1 Tbsp	1
Strawberry banana preserves, 1 Tbsp	1
Strawberry preserves, 1 Tbsp	1
Sugar free apricot preserves, 1 Tbsp	0
Sugar free boysenberry preserves, 1 Tbsp	0
Sugar free red raspberry preserves, 1 Tbsp	0
Sugar free strawberry preserves, 1 Tbsp	0

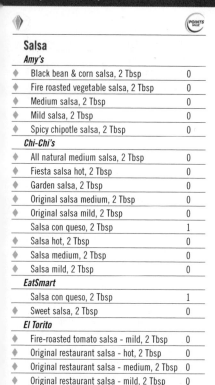

Salsa

Amy's

	POINTS VALUE
Black bean & corn salsa, 2 Tbsp	0
Fire roasted vegetable salsa, 2 Tbsp	0
Medium salsa, 2 Tbsp	0
Mild salsa, 2 Tbsp	0
Spicy chipotle salsa, 2 Tbsp	0

Chi-Chi's

All natural medium salsa, 2 Tbsp	0
Fiesta salsa hot, 2 Tbsp	0
Garden salsa, 2 Tbsp	0
Original salsa medium, 2 Tbsp	0
Original salsa mild, 2 Tbsp	0
Salsa con queso, 2 Tbsp	1
Salsa hot, 2 Tbsp	0
Salsa medium, 2 Tbsp	0
Salsa mild, 2 Tbsp	0

EatSmart

Salsa con queso, 2 Tbsp	1
Sweet salsa, 2 Tbsp	0

El Torito

Fire-roasted tomato salsa - mild, 2 Tbsp	0
Original restaurant salsa - hot, 2 Tbsp	0
Original restaurant salsa - medium, 2 Tbsp	0
Original restaurant salsa - mild, 2 Tbsp	0

Emerald Valley Kitchen

	POINTS VALUE
Organic fiesta salsa, 2 Tbsp	0
Organic green salsa, 2 Tbsp	0
Organic mango salsa, 2 Tbsp	0
Organic salsa - hot, 2 Tbsp	0
Organic salsa - medium, 2 Tbsp	0
Organic salsa - mild, 2 Tbsp	0

Goldwater's

Cochise corn & black bean salsa, 2 Tbsp	1
Mohave mango salsa, 2 Tbsp	0
Papago peach salsa, 2 Tbsp	0
Paradise pineapple salsa, 2 Tbsp	0
Rio verde tomatillo salsa, 2 Tbsp	0
Ruby raspberry salsa, 2 Tbsp	0
Sedona red hot salsa, 2 Tbsp	0
Sedona red salsa, 2 Tbsp	0
Smoky green salsa, 2 Tbsp	0
Smoky red salsa, 2 Tbsp	0

Green Mountain Gringo

Hot salsa, 2 Tbsp	0
Medium salsa, 2 Tbsp	0
Mild salsa, 2 Tbsp	0

Guiltless Gourmet

Roasted red pepper salsa, 2 Tbsp	0
Southwestern grill salsa, 2 Tbsp	0

	POINTS VALUE
Herdez	
Salsa casera, 2 tsp	0
Salsa casera medium, 2 tsp	0
Salsa casera mild, 2 tsp	0
Salsa hot, 2 Tbsp	0
Salsa medium, 2 tsp	0
Salsa ranchera, 2 Tbsp	0
Salsa taquera, 2 Tbsp	0
Salsa verde, 2 Tbsp	0
La Estrellita	
Green salsa, hot, 2 Tbsp	0
Kid's salsa, mild, 2 Tbsp	0
Red hot salsa, 2 Tbsp	0
Red salsa, medium, 2 Tbsp	0
Red salsa, mild, 2 Tbsp	0
Lance	
Don Pablo's hot salsa, 2 Tbsp	0
Don Pablo's medium salsa, 2 Tbsp	0
LaTortilla Factory	
Fire roasted roma tomato mild salsa, 2 Tbsp	0
Medium salsa, 2 Tbsp	0
Mild salsa, 2 Tbsp	0
Muir Glen Organic	
Black bean & corn, 2 Tbsp	0
Garlic cilantro salsa, 2 Tbsp	0
Hot salsa, 2 Tbsp	0

	POINTS VALUE
Medium chipotle salsa, 2 Tbsp	0
Medium salsa, 2 Tbsp	0
Mild salsa, 2 Tbsp	0
Naturally Fresh	
Salsa, medium, 2 Tbsp	0
Old El Paso	
Fiesta taco salsa, 2 Tbsp	0
Fresh Mexican salsa - smooth chipotle, 2 Tbsp	0
Fresh Mexican salsa - smooth pineapple chile, 2 Tbsp	0
Garden pepper salsa - medium, 2 Tbsp	0
Garden pepper salsa - mild, 2 Tbsp	0
Green chili salsa, 2 Tbsp	0
Salsa Mexicana - medium, 2 Tbsp	0
Salsa Mexicana - mild, 2 Tbsp	0
Taco toppers zesty ranch, 2 Tbsp	2
Thick 'n chunky salsa - hot, 2 Tbsp	0
Thick 'n chunky salsa - medium, 2 Tbsp	0
Thick 'n chunky salsa - mild, 2 Tbsp	0
Thick 'n chunky salsa - xtra mild, 2 Tbsp	0
Ortega	
Original salsa, mild, 2 Tbsp	0
Salsa verde, medium, 2 Tbsp	0
Preciosa	
Salsa picante, 1 Tbsp	0

JAMS, SPREADS, SALSA & DIPS

 Salsa (con't) POINTS VALUE

  POINTS VALUE

Santitas

Restaurant style salsa, 2 Tbsp	0

Seeds of Change

◆ Black bean & tomato medium salsa, 2 Tbsp	0
◆ Garlic & cilantro mild salsa, 2 Tbsp	0
◆ Garlic & cilantro spicy salsa, 2 Tbsp	0
◆ Traditional picante medium salsa, 2 Tbsp	0
◆ Traditional picante mild salsa, 2 Tbsp	0

Schwan's LiveSmart

Fruit and veggie salsa, 2/3 cup	1

Taco Bell Home Originals

Medium salsa con queso, 2 Tbsp	1
Mild salsa con queso, 2 Tbsp	1
◆ Thick 'n chunky medium salsa, 2 Tbsp	0
◆ Thick 'n chunky mild salsa, 2 Tbsp	0

Tostitos

◆ All natural chunky salsa mild, medium & hot, 2 Tbsp	0
◆ All natural salsa mild, medium or hot, 2 Tbsp	0
Black bean & corn salsa, 2 Tbsp	0
Pineapple and peach salsa, 2 Tbsp	0
◆ Restaurant style salsa, 2 Tbsp	0
Salsa con queso, 2 Tbsp	1

Zapata

◆ Fire roasted salsa roja, hot, 2 Tbsp	0
◆ Fire roasted salsa roja, medium, 2 Tbsp	0
◆ Fire roasted salsa roja, mild, 2 Tbsp	0
◆ Fire roasted salsa verde, medium, 2 Tbsp	0
◆ Fire roasted salsa verde, mild, 2 Tbsp	0

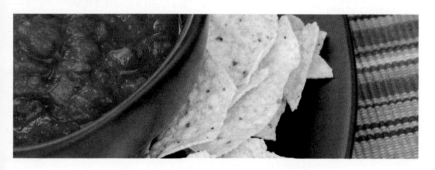

POINTS VALUE

POINTS VALUE

Bacon

Boar's Head

Canadian style bacon, 2 oz	2 (5)
Imported naturally smoked sliced bacon, 2 slices	2
Pancetta, 1/2 oz	1
Sliced bacon, 2 slices	2

Farmland

Butcher's cut extra thick sliced bacon, 1 slice	3
Cider house bacon, 2 slices	2
Fully cooked hickory bacon, 3 1/2 slices	2
Hickory smoked bacon, 2 slices	2
Hickory smoked bacon - center cut, 3 slices	2
Hickory smoked bacon - honey maple flavored, 2 slices	2
Lower sodium hickory smoked bacon, 2 slices	2
Thick sliced hickory smoked bacon - peppered, 1 slice	2

Hormel

Applewood smoked bacon, 2 slices	3
Bacon bits, 1 Tbsp	1
Bacon pieces, 1 Tbsp	1
Bacon, fully cooked, 2 1/2 slices	2
Bits, real crumbled bacon, 1 Tbsp	1
Bits, real crumbled bacon 30% less fat, 1 Tbsp	1
Canadian style bacon, 2 oz	2 (5)
Canadian style bacon, pizza, 1 package	3
Country sugar cured bacon, 2 slices	3
Crumbled bacon 30% less fat, maple, 1 Tbsp	1
Fully cooked bacon pieces, 1/2 oz	2
Lower sodium uncured bacon, 2 slices	2
Maple flavored bacon, 2 slices	2
Mesquite sliced bacon, 2 slices	2
Micro low salt bacon, 2 slices	2
Microwave bacon, cooked, 2 slices	2
Original uncured bacon, 2 slices	2
Real bacon pieces less fat, 1 Tbsp	1
Real crumbled bacon with picnic bacon 30% less fat, 1 Tbsp	1

Hormel Black Label

Bacon, cooked, 2 slices	2
Center cut bacon, cooked, 2 slices	2
Low salt bacon, cooked, 2 slices	2

Hormel Old Smokehouse

Bacon, 2 slices	3

Hormel Pillow Pack

Canadian bacon, 22 slices	2 (5)

Hormel Range Brand

Bacon, cooked, 2 slices	3

Bacon (con't) — POINTS VALUE

Jennie-O Turkey Store

Extra lean turkey bacon, 1 serving (15 g)	0
Full flavor turkey bacon, 1 serving (15 g)	1

Jones Dairy Farm

♦ Canadian bacon, 3 slices	2 (5)

Louis Rich

Bacon, turkey, 1 slice	1

Market Day

Fully cooked bacon slices, 3 pieces	2

Oscar Mayer

Bacon bits, real, 1 Tbsp	1
Bacon pieces, real, 1 Tbsp	1
Bacon, center cut, 2 slices	1
Canadian bacon with natural juices, 1 slice (8 oz.)	1 (5)
♦ Canadian style bacon made from pork sirloin hips with natural juices, 4 slices	1 (5)
♦ Canadian style bacon made from pork sirloin hips with natural juices, 97% fat free, 1 slice	1 (5)
Hickory country smoked bacon, 2 slices	2
Natural sliced bacon, 2 slices	2
Naturally hardwood smoked bacon, 2 slices	2
Ready to serve bacon, 3 slices	2
Ready-to-serve thick & hearty bacon, 2 slices	1

POINTS VALUE

Red Label

Canadian style bacon, 2 oz	2 (5)

Tyson

Fully cooked hickory bacon, 2 slices	2
Hickory bacon, 2 slices	2

Beef

Boar's Head

1st cut choice corned beef brisket - uncooked, 2.5 oz (cooked)	3
1st cut choice pastrami brisket, 2 oz	2
1st cut cooked choice corned beef brisket, 2 oz	2
All natural cap-off top round oven roasted beef, 2 oz	2
Cajun style seasoned eye rd oven roasted beef, 2 oz	2
Cooked cap-off choice corned beef top round, 2 oz	2
Cooked choice corned beef brisket, 2 oz	3
Custom cut cooked corned beef round, 2 oz	2
Deluxe low sodium - all natural cap-off choice top round, 2 oz	2
Italian style seasoned roasted beef with classic braciole seasoning, 2 oz	2
Londonport, top round seasoned roast beef, 2 oz	2
Natural flat cooked corned beef, 2 oz	2

	POINTS VALUE
No salt added choice cap off top round, 2 oz	2
Our deluxe oven roasted eye round, low sodium, 2 oz	2
Pepper seasoned eye round - low sodium, 2 oz	2
Red pastrami round, 2 oz	2
Seasoned filet of roast beef - cap off top round, 2 oz	2
USDA choice corned beef brisket - uncooked, 1 serving (2.4 oz)	5
Fast Classics	
Country fried steaks with gravy, 1 serving (1 steak & 2 Tbsp of gravy)	7
Fully cooked bacon cheeseburgers, 3 oz	5
Fully cooked beef burgers, 3 oz	5
Fast Fixin'	
Ribz for sandwiches, 1 patty	3
Sirloin beef Philly steak, 1	6
Hormel	
Corned beef, 2 oz	3
Roast beef w/ gravy, 1/2 cup	3
Sliced dried beef, 10 slices	1
Hormel Always Tender	
Beef strip steaks and garlic pepper, 4 oz	5
Beef strips and three pepper blend, 4 oz	5
Peppercorn beef fillet sirloin, 4 oz	3
Tequila lime beef fillet sirloin, 4 oz	3
Teriyaki beef fillet sirloin, 4 oz	3

	POINTS VALUE
Hormel Pillow Pack	
Dried beef, 10 slices	1
Market Day	
1/4 pound patties, 1 patty	7
Bacon wrapped ranch steaks, 1	8
Beef stew meat, 4 oz	6
Filet of sirloin steaks, 1 serving (6 oz)	10 (5)
French dip, 2/3 cup	2
Fully cooked pot roast, 3 oz	3
Ground beef, 4 oz (raw)	6
Home style gravy and beef tips, 2/3 cup	3
Marinated sirloin roast (garlic & herb), 4 oz	4
Meatloaf slices, 1 slice	7
Ranch steak, 5 oz (raw)	5
Teriyaki ranch steak, 1 steak	6
Teriyaki steak kabobs, 2 skewers	6
Mary Kitchen	
Corned beef hash, 1 cup	9
Roast beef hash, 1 cup	9
Schwan's LiveSmart	
Beef fajita meat, 3 oz	3
Tyson	
Beef pot roast in gravy, 5 oz	4
Beef steak tips in bourbon sauce, 1 serving (5 oz)	4
Beef tips in gravy, 5 oz	5
Country fried steak, 1 piece	8

Beef, Tyson (con't)

	POINTS VALUE
Roast beef in brown gravy, 5 oz	3
Seasoned beef strips (boxed), 3 oz	3
Seasoned steak strip (boxed), 3 oz	3
Steak fingers, 2 pieces	6

Chicken
Alexia

	POINTS VALUE
Chicken nuggets with broccoli and cheddar cheese, 6	5
Chicken nuggets with spinach and feta cheese, 6	5

Boar's Head

Golden classic oven roasted chicken breast, boneless, skinless, 2 oz	1
Hickory smoked chicken breast, 2 oz	1

Bumble Bee

Chicken salad with crackers, chicken salad only, 1 can	3
Chicken salad with crackers, crackers only, 6	2
◆ Prime fillet chicken breast lightly seasoned with garlic & herbs, 1 pouch	2
Prime fillet chicken breast with barbeque sauce, 1 pouch	4
◆ Prime fillet chicken breast with southwest seasonings, 1 pouch	2

Bumble Bee Lunch on the Run

Chicken salad - complete lunch kit, chicken salad only, 1 can	3

	POINTS VALUE
Chicken salad - complete lunch kit, crackers only, 6	2
Chicken salad - complete lunch kit, entire kit, 1	11
Chicken salad - complete lunch kit, mixed fruit cup only, 1 serving (4 oz)	1
Chicken salad, complete lunch kit, cookie only, 1	4

Fast Classics

Buffalo style chicken breast tenders, 3 oz	5
Buffalo style chicken chunks, 2 pieces	4
Buffalo style chicken wings, 3 oz	4
Chicken breast chunks, 2 pieces	4
Chicken breast tenders, 1 serving (3 oz)	4
Chicken fried chicken breasts, 1 serving (1 breast & 2 Tbsp gravy)	6
Crispy chicken breast strips, 1 serving (3 oz)	4
Flame roasted chicken breasts, 1	4
Honey bbq chicken wings, 3 oz	5
Tomato basil chicken breasts, 1 piece	3

Fast Fixin'

Chicken breast nuggets, 6	5
Chicken breast patties, 1 patty	5
Chicken breast strips, 3	5
Chicken cheese nuggets, 6	6
Dino bites, 4	6
Philly style chicken steaks, 1 piece	3
Popcorn chicken, 14 pieces	6

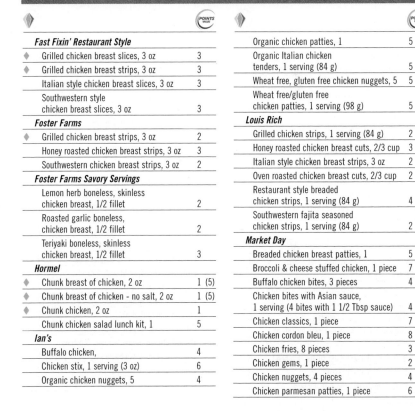

	POINTS VALUE
Fast Fixin' Restaurant Style	
Grilled chicken breast slices, 3 oz	3
Grilled chicken breast strips, 3 oz	3
Italian style chicken breast slices, 3 oz	3
Southwestern style chicken breast slices, 3 oz	3
Foster Farms	
Grilled chicken breast strips, 3 oz	2
Honey roasted chicken breast strips, 3 oz	3
Southwestern chicken breast strips, 3 oz	2
Foster Farms Savory Servings	
Lemon herb boneless, skinless chicken breast, 1/2 fillet	2
Roasted garlic boneless, chicken breast, 1/2 fillet	2
Teriyaki boneless, skinless chicken breast, 1/2 fillet	3
Hormel	
Chunk breast of chicken, 2 oz	1 (5)
Chunk breast of chicken - no salt, 2 oz	1 (5)
Chunk chicken, 2 oz	1
Chunk chicken salad lunch kit, 1	5
Ian's	
Buffalo chicken,	4
Chicken stix, 1 serving (3 oz)	6
Organic chicken nuggets, 5	4

	POINTS VALUE
Organic chicken patties, 1	5
Organic Italian chicken tenders, 1 serving (84 g)	5
Wheat free, gluten free chicken nuggets, 5	5
Wheat free/gluten free chicken patties, 1 serving (98 g)	5
Louis Rich	
Grilled chicken strips, 1 serving (84 g)	2
Honey roasted chicken breast cuts, 2/3 cup	3
Italian style chicken breast strips, 3 oz	2
Oven roasted chicken breast cuts, 2/3 cup	2
Restaurant style breaded chicken strips, 1 serving (84 g)	4
Southwestern fajita seasoned chicken strips, 1 serving (84 g)	2
Market Day	
Breaded chicken breast patties, 1	5
Broccoli & cheese stuffed chicken, 1 piece	7
Buffalo chicken bites, 3 pieces	4
Chicken bites with Asian sauce, 1 serving (4 bites with 1 1/2 Tbsp sauce)	4
Chicken classics, 1 piece	7
Chicken cordon bleu, 1 piece	8
Chicken fries, 8 pieces	3
Chicken gems, 1 piece	2
Chicken nuggets, 4 pieces	4
Chicken parmesan patties, 1 piece	6

Chicken, Market Day (con't) — POINTS VALUE

	POINTS VALUE
Chicken stir-fry kit, 1 1/3 cup	4
Chicken tenders, 1 piece	4
Chicnsteakes, 1 piece	2
Crispy chicnsteakes, 1 piece	5
Diced chicken tenderloin, 3/4 cup	2
Honey bbq chicken tenders, 1 piece	4
Popcorn chicken, 13 pieces	4
Seasoned chicken breast strips, 1 cup	3
Southwest chicnsteakes, 1 piece	3
Spicy buffalo wings, 4 pieces	6
Teriyaki chicnsteakes, 1 piece	4

Schwan's LiveSmart

	POINTS VALUE
Chicken breast meat for fajitas, 3 oz	3
Unbreaded chicken breast filets, 1 piece (4 oz)	2

Snow's

	POINTS VALUE
Premium chicken breast, 2 oz	1 (5)

T.G.I. Friday's

	POINTS VALUE
Bourbon glazed popcorn chicken, 3 pieces	4
Buffalo wings, 4 pieces	5
Honey bbq wings, 3 pieces	5
Spicy popcorn chicken, 1 serving (86 g)	4

Tyson

	POINTS VALUE
Breaded chicken breast fillets, 1 piece	6
Breast (all natural), 4 oz	3
Breast tenderloin (boxed), 1 piece	3

	POINTS VALUE
Buffalo boneless chicken wyngs, 3 pieces	3
Buffalo strips (bagged), 2 pieces	5
Buffalo style chicken strips, 2 pieces	5
Buffalo style hot wings (bone in), 4 pieces	6
Buffalo style popcorn chicken bites, 5 pieces	4
Chicken pattie-regular, 1 piece	4
Crispy chicken strips, 2 pieces	5
Crispy strips (bagged), 2 pieces	5
Diced chicken breast, 3 oz	2 (5)
Drumsticks (enhanced), 4 oz	4
Fajita chicken breast strips, 3 oz	3
Fresh or frozen boneless chicken breast with rib meat, 4 oz	2 (5)
Fresh or frozen chicken tender, 4 oz	2
Fresh or frozen drumsticks, 4 oz	4
Fresh or frozen skinless thighs, 4 oz	4 (5)
Fresh or frozen split breast, 4 oz	4
Fresh or frozen thighs, 4 oz	7
Fresh or frozen wings, 4 oz	7
Fresh whole bird, 4 oz	7
Grilled chicken breast strips, 3 oz	2
Honey battered breast tenders, 5 pieces	5
Honey bbq boneless chicken wyngs, 3 pieces	5
Honey bbq chicken strips, 1 piece	4
Honey bbq wings (bagged), 4 pieces	6

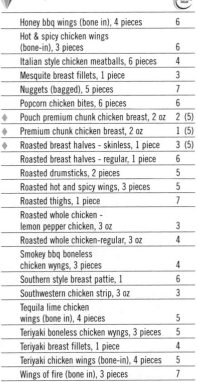

	POINTS VALUE
Honey bbq wings (bone in), 4 pieces	6
Hot & spicy chicken wings (bone-in), 3 pieces	6
Italian style chicken meatballs, 6 pieces	4
Mesquite breast fillets, 1 piece	3
Nuggets (bagged), 5 pieces	7
Popcorn chicken bites, 6 pieces	6
♦ Pouch premium chunk chicken breast, 2 oz	2 (5)
♦ Premium chunk chicken breast, 2 oz	1 (5)
♦ Roasted breast halves - skinless, 1 piece	3 (5)
Roasted breast halves - regular, 1 piece	6
Roasted drumsticks, 2 pieces	5
Roasted hot and spicy wings, 3 pieces	5
Roasted thighs, 1 piece	7
Roasted whole chicken - lemon pepper chicken, 3 oz	3
Roasted whole chicken-regular, 3 oz	4
Smokey bbq boneless chicken wyngs, 3 pieces	4
Southern style breast pattie, 1	6
Southwestern chicken strip, 3 oz	3
Tequila lime chicken wings (bone in), 4 pieces	5
Teriyaki boneless chicken wyngs, 3 pieces	5
Teriyaki breast fillets, 1 piece	4
Teriyaki chicken wings (bone-in), 4 pieces	5
Wings of fire (bone in), 3 pieces	7

Tyson Any'tizers

	POINTS VALUE
Barbeque style chicken wings, 3 pieces	5
Buffalo style boneless chicken wyngs, 3 pieces	4
Cheddar & bacon chicken bites, 4 pieces	6
Cheddar & jalapeno chicken bites, 4 pieces	4
Homestyle chicken fries, 7 pieces	5
Honey bbq boneless chicken wyngs, 3 pieces	5
Hot 'n spicy chicken wings, 3 pieces	6
Mini chicken bites, 13 pieces	7
Popcorn chicken, 6 pieces	5
Ranch flavored chicken fries, 7 pieces	5

Game Birds
Tyson

	POINTS VALUE
Cornish game hen, 4 oz	5

Ground Meat
Aidells

	POINTS VALUE
Buffalo style meatballs, 4	4
Chipotle meatballs, 4	3
Sun-dried tomato with parmesan & romano cheese meatballs, 3	4
Teriyaki meatballs, 4	4

Fast Fixin'

	POINTS VALUE
Beef meatballs, 3 oz	6
Italian style meatballs, 3 oz	7

Ground Meat (con't)	POINTS VALUE
Market Day	
Italian style meatballs, 4 pieces	4
Rosina	
Homestyle meatballs, 6	7
Italian-style meatballs, 3	6
Organic meatballs, 6	4
Swedish meatballs, 6	6
Turkey Italian style meatballs, 1 serving (85 g)	4
Turkey meatballs, 3	4
Rosina Presents Celentano	
Meatballs, Italian style, 3 (1 oz)	7
Meatballs, Italian-style, 6	7
Turkey meatballs, 3	4

Hot Dogs

	POINTS VALUE
Armour Healthy Ones	
Beef franks, 1	2
Ball Park Bun Size	
Beef franks, 1	5
Franks (made with beef, pork, turkey), 1	5
Smoked white turkey franks, 1	1
Ball Park Fat Free Franks	
Bun size smoked white turkey franks, 1	1
Fat free beef franks, 1	1
Fat free franks, 1	1
Lite beef franks, 1	3
Lite franks, 1	3

	POINTS VALUE
Ball Park Franks	
Beef franks, 1	5
Franks, made with beef, pork & turkey, 1	5
Ball Park GrillMaster	
Deli style beef, 1	7
Hearty beef, 1	7
Hot 'n spicy, 1	7
Smokehouse, 1	7
Ball Park Singles	
Beef franks, 1	4
Cheese franks, 1	4
Franks (made with beef, pork, turkey), 1	4
Boar's Head	
All natural salame with white wine, 1 oz	2
Beef frankfurter (natural casing) giants, 1	4
Beef frankfurters - skinless, 1	3
Cocktail beef frankfurters, natural casing, 5	5
Lite beef frankfurters, natural casing, 1	2
Lite beef frankfurters, skinless & natural casing, 1	2
Pork & beef frankfurter giants, natural casing, 1	4
Pork & beef frankfurter, skinless, 1	4
Farmland	
Hickory smoked hot dogs - original, 1	3
Premium beef franks, 1	5

	POINTS VALUE
Premium cheese franks, 1	3
Premium meat franks, 2 oz	5
Fluky's	
Fat free Chicago style hot dogs, 1 link	1
Foster Farms	
Chicken franks, 1	3
Turkey franks, 1	3
Hebrew National	
97% fat free beef franks, 1	1
Beef franks, 1	4
Jumbo beef franks, 1	7
Quarter pound beef franks, 1	9
Reduced fat beef franks, 1	4
Hormel	
Beef hot dog, 1	5
Cocktail smokies beef, 6	5
Smokies, 1	2
Smokies with cheese, 1	2
Ian's	
Wheat free, gluten free popcorn turkey corn dog, 1	8
Jennie-O Turkey Store	
Turkey wiener, 1	2
Louis Rich	
Bun-length brand turkey franks, 1 link	3
Turkey franks, 1 serving (45 g)	3

	POINTS VALUE
Oscar Mayer	
98% fat free wieners made with turkey, 1	1
Cheese hot dogs, made with pork, turkey & chicken, 1	4
Cheese turkey franks, 1	3
Deli style beef franks, 1	6
Fast franks beef frank with bun, 1	7
Fast franks wiener made with turkey, pork & chicken with bun, 1	7
Fat free wieners made with turkey & beef, 1	1
Franks, beef, 1	4
Franks, beef jumbo, 1	5
Franks, beef, bun-length, 1	5
Franks, beef, light, 1	2
Hot & spicy hot dogs, 1	6
Natural beef franks, 1	4
Premium beef franks, 1	6
Smoked hot dogs, 1	7
Smokies course ground wieners, 1	4
Turkey frank, 1	3
Wieners, bun-length, made with turkey & pork, 1	5
Wieners, jumbo, made with turkey & pork, 1	5
Wieners, light, made with turkey & pork, 1	2
Wieners, little, made with turkey & pork, 6	5
Wieners, made with turkey & pork, 1	4

Hot Dogs (con't)	POINTS VALUE
Wranglers	
Beef franks, 1	5
Cheese franks, 1	5
Smoked franks, 1	5

Luncheon/Deli Meat
Armour Healthy Ones

	POINTS VALUE
Baked ham, 1 serving (2 oz)	1
Browned chicken breast, 1 serving (2 oz)	1
Cooked ham, 1 serving (2 oz)	1
Honey ham, 1 serving (2 oz)	1
Honey maple ham, 1 serving (2 oz)	1
Honey roasted & smoked turkey breast, 1 serving (2 oz)	1
Meat franks, 1	2
Medium cooked roast beef, 1 serving (2 oz)	1
Medium rare roast beef, 1 serving (2 oz)	2
Mesquite smoked chicken breast, 1 serving (2 oz)	1
Mesquite smoked honey ham, 1 serving (2 oz)	1
Mesquite smoked turkey breast, 1 serving (2 oz)	1
Oven roasted chicken breast, 1 serving (2 oz)	1
Oven roasted turkey breast, 1 serving (2 oz)	1
Pastrami, 1 serving (2 oz)	1
Smoked ham, 1 serving (2 oz)	1

	POINTS VALUE
Smoked turkey breast, 1 serving (2 oz)	1
Southwest grill turkey breast, 1 serving (2 oz)	1
Virginia brand ham, 1 serving (2 oz)	1
Boar's Head	
Abruzzese, 1 oz	3
Abruzzese hot, 1 oz	3
All natural salame coated with course black pepper, 1 oz	2
All natural salame coated with herbs, 1 oz	2
Antipasto genoa salame & provolone slices, 1 serving (6 pieces meat/4 slices cheese)	3
Aroastica seasoned chicken breast, boneless/skinless, 2 oz	1
Bar B Q sauce basted breast of chicken, 2 oz	1
Beef bologna, 2 oz	4
Beef salami, 2 oz	3
Bianco d'oro Italian dry salame, 1 oz	3
Blazing buffalo-style roasted chicken breast, boneless/skinless, 2 oz	1
Bologna (pork & beef), 2 oz	4
Bologna, 28% lower sodium, 2 oz	4
Cap off top round pastrami, 2 oz	2
Choice pastrami brisket, 2 oz	4
Cooked salami, 2 oz	4
Dutch brand loaf, 2 oz	4
Garlic bologna, 2 oz	4

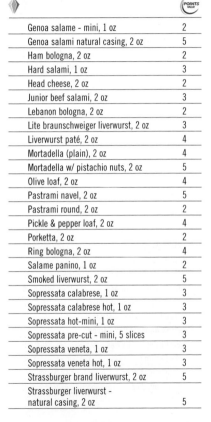

	POINTS VALUE
Genoa salame - mini, 1 oz	2
Genoa salami natural casing, 2 oz	5
Ham bologna, 2 oz	2
Hard salami, 1 oz	3
Head cheese, 2 oz	2
Junior beef salami, 2 oz	3
Lebanon bologna, 2 oz	2
Lite braunschweiger liverwurst, 2 oz	3
Liverwurst paté, 2 oz	4
Mortadella (plain), 2 oz	4
Mortadella w/ pistachio nuts, 2 oz	5
Olive loaf, 2 oz	4
Pastrami navel, 2 oz	5
Pastrami round, 2 oz	2
Pickle & pepper loaf, 2 oz	4
Porketta, 2 oz	2
Ring bologna, 2 oz	4
Salame panino, 1 oz	2
Smoked liverwurst, 2 oz	5
Sopressata calabrese, 1 oz	3
Sopressata calabrese hot, 1 oz	3
Sopressata hot-mini, 1 oz	3
Sopressata pre-cut - mini, 5 slices	3
Sopressata veneta, 1 oz	3
Sopressata veneta hot, 1 oz	3
Strassburger brand liverwurst, 2 oz	5
Strassburger liverwurst - natural casing, 2 oz	5

	POINTS VALUE
Carl Buddig	
Shaved brown sugar baked ham, 1 serving (56 g)	2
Carl Buddig Deli Cuts	
Shaved baked honey ham water added, 1 serving (56 g)	2
Shaved honey turkey breast, 1 serving (56 g)	2
Shaved oven-roasted turkey breast, 1 serving (56 g)	2
Shaved rotisserie chicken breast, 1 serving (56 g)	2
Shaved smoked ham, 1 serving (56 g)	2
Shaved smoked turkey breast, 1 serving (56 g)	2
Carl Buddig Original	
Beef, 2 oz	2
Beef, 1 package	2
Chicken, 1 package	2
Corned beef, 1 package	2
Corned beef, 2 oz	2
Ham with natural juices, 1 package	2
Ham with natural juices, 2 oz	2
Honey ham with natural juices, 2 oz	24
Honey ham with natural juices, 1 package	24
Honey turkey, 2 oz	2
Honey turkey, 1 package	2
Oven roasted turkey, 2 oz	2

MEAT & POULTRY

Luncheon/Deli Meat, Carl Buddig Original (con't)	POINTS VALUE
Oven roasted turkey, 1 package	2
Pastrami, 1 package	2
Pastrami, 2 oz	2
Turkey, 2 oz	2
Turkey, 1 package	2
Farmland	
Deli style - deli ham - 97% fat free, 1 oz	1
Deli style - smoked turkey breast - fat free, 1 slice	1
Deli style cooked ham & water product, 1 oz	1
Deli style honey ham, 97% fat free, 1 slice	1
Deli style honey turkey breast, 98% fat free, 1 oz	1
Deli style oven roasted turkey breast, 98% fat free, 1 oz	1
Foster Farms	
Breast variety pack, honey cured turkey breast, 3 slices	1
Breast variety pack, oven roasted chicken breast, 3 slices	1
Breast variety pack, smoked turkey breast, 3 slices	1
Club sandwich variety pack, oven roasted turkey breast, 4 slices	1
Club sandwich variety pack, smoked turkey breast, 4 slices	1
Club sandwich variety pack, turkey ham, 4 slices	1

	POINTS VALUE
Honey roasted & smoked turkey breast, 2 oz	2
Mesquite smoked turkey breast, 4 slices	1
Oven roasted chicken breast, 1 slice	1
Oven roasted turkey breast, 4 slices	1
Turkey variety pack, smoked turkey white meat, 1 slice	1
Turkey variety pack, turkey bologna, 1 slice	2
Turkey variety pack, turkey ham, 1 slice	1
Turkey variety pack, turkey pastrami, 1 slice	1
Value pack combo, chicken bologna, 2 slices	3
Value pack combo, oven roasted white turkey, 2 slices	1
Value pack combo, turkey pastrami, 2 slices	1
Hebrew National	
Beef bologna, 1 slice	2
Beef salami, 3 slices	4
Lean beef bologna, 4 slices	2
Lean beef salami, 4 slices	2
Hebrew National Deli Carved	
Beef bologna, 3 slices	5
Beef salami, 3 slices	4
Corned beef, 2 oz	2
Pastrami, 2 oz	2

Hormel	POINTS VALUE
Black forest ham, 2 oz	1
Black label chopped ham, 2 oz	4
Chicken Vienna sausage, 2 oz	3
Cooked corn beef, 2 oz	1
Cooked ham, 2 oz	1
Cooked pastrami, 2 oz	1
Double smoked ham, 2 oz	1
Homeland hard salami, 1 oz	2
Honey smoked turkey, 2 oz	1
Italian dry salami, 6 slices	3
Oven roasted turkey breast, 2 slices	1
Roasted turkey, 2 oz	1
San Remo genoa salami, 2 oz	6
Seasoned roast beef, 2 oz	1
Sliced honey ham, 2 oz	2
Smoked turkey breast, 2 oz	1
Spiced ham, 2 oz	4
Vienna sausage, 2 oz	4
Vienna sausage hot & spicy, 5 oz	4
Jennie-O Turkey Store	
Lunchmeat hickory smoked, 1 serving (56 g)	1
Lunchmeat honey smoked, 1 serving (56 g)	1
Lunchmeat pepper grilled, 1 serving (56 g)	1
Lunchmeat sun dried tomato, 1 serving (56 g)	1

Jones Dairy Farm	POINTS VALUE
Braunschweiger liverwurst chub, 2 oz	4
Braunschweiger liverwurst light chub, 2 oz	2
Braunschweiger liverwurst slices, 2 slices	4
Lance	
Beef & cheese, 1 package	4
Beef stick, 1 piece	1
Kippered beefsteak - original, 1 serving (25 g)	1
Kippered beefsteak - peppered, 1 serving (25 g)	1
Kippered beefsteak - teriyaki, 1 serving (25 g)	1
Original beef jerky, 1 piece	1
Peppered beef jerky, 1 piece	1
Spicy beef stick, 1 serving (12 g)	2
Teriyaki beef jerky, 1 piece	2
Louis Rich	
Chicken, white, oven roasted, 1 slice	1
Naturally smoked turkey breast & white turkey, 98% fat free, 1 slice	1
Oven roasted chicken breast, 3 slices	1
Turkey bologna, 1 slice	1
Turkey breast & white turkey, oven roasted 98% fat free, 1 slice	1
Turkey cotto salami, 1 slice	1
Turkey ham, smoked, chopped, 1 slice	1

Luncheon/Deli Meat (con't)   POINTS VALUE POINTS VALUE

Louis Rich Carving Board	
Turkey breast hickory smoked, 3 slices	1
Oscar Mayer	
98% fat free bologna made with turkey, 1 slice	1
All-American variety pak, bologna, 2 slices	4
All-American variety pak, cotto salami, 2 slices	3
All-American variety pak, ham, 2 slices	2
Bologna, beef, 1 slice	2
Bologna, beef, light, 1 slice	2
Bologna, garlic, 1 slice	4
Bologna, light, made with chicken-pork, 1 slice	2
Bologna, made with chicken and pork, 1 slice	2
Braunschweiger, liver sausage, 2 oz	5
Brown sugar ham, 5 slices	2
Canadian-style bacon, made from pork sirloin hips, 3 slices	1
Chicken breast, 5 slices	1
Chicken breast, oven roasted, 3 slices	2
Chopped honey ham, 1 slice	1
Cooked ham, 2 slices	1
Cooked ham, water added, 96% fat free, 1 slice	1
Cured roast beef, 6 slices	1

Deli shaved beef salami, 4 slices	4
Deli shaved Virginia brand ham, 6 slices	1
Fun pack: beef tacos, 1 package	10
Fun pack: cheesy chip nachos with strawberry-kiwi drink, 1 package	12
Fun pack: nachos with wild cherry drink, 1 package	14
Ham chopped, 1 slice	1
Ham, baked cooked, 3 slices	1
Ham, boiled, 3 slices	1
Ham, honey, 3 slices	1
Ham, honey & water product, 96% fat free, 3 slices	2
Ham, low sodium, 3 slices	2
Ham, smoked, 3 slices	1
Ham, smoked & water product, 3 slices	1
Hearty thick cut bologna made with chicken & pork, 1 slice	4
Honey ham, water added, thin sliced, 96% fat free, 5 slices	1
Honey smoked turkey, 1 slice	1
Honey smoked turkey breast, 5 slices	1
Luncheon loaf, spiced, 1 slice	2
Mesquite turkey breast, 5 slices	1
Natural smoked ham, 3 slices	1
Olive loaf, 1 slice	2
Oven roasted turkey breast, 6 slices	1

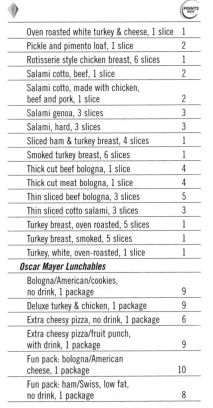

	POINTS VALUE
Oven roasted white turkey & cheese, 1 slice	1
Pickle and pimento loaf, 1 slice	2
Rotisserie style chicken breast, 6 slices	1
Salami cotto, beef, 1 slice	2
Salami cotto, made with chicken, beef and pork, 1 slice	2
Salami genoa, 3 slices	3
Salami, hard, 3 slices	3
Sliced ham & turkey breast, 4 slices	1
Smoked turkey breast, 6 slices	1
Thick cut beef bologna, 1 slice	4
Thick cut meat bologna, 1 slice	4
Thin sliced beef bologna, 3 slices	5
Thin sliced cotto salami, 3 slices	3
Turkey breast, oven roasted, 5 slices	1
Turkey breast, smoked, 5 slices	1
Turkey, white, oven-roasted, 1 slice	1

Oscar Mayer Lunchables

	POINTS VALUE
Bologna/American/cookies, no drink, 1 package	9
Deluxe turkey & chicken, 1 package	9
Extra cheesy pizza, no drink, 1 package	6
Extra cheesy pizza/fruit punch, with drink, 1 package	9
Fun pack: bologna/American cheese, 1 package	10
Fun pack: ham/Swiss, low fat, no drink, 1 package	8
Fun pack: turkey/cheddar, low fat, pudding, 1 package	8
Ham/American cheese/snicker/fruit punch, 1 package	9
Ham/cheddar, no drink, 1 package	8
Ham/cheddar/cookies, no drink, 1 package	9
Ham/Swiss, no drink, 1 package	8
Pepperoni pizza, no drink, 1 package	7
Pizza cracker stackers, 1 package	10
Turkey/American/cookies, no drink, 1 package	9
Turkey/cheddar, no drink, 1 package	8
White turkey/ham/no drink, 1 package	9

Oscar Mayer Lunchables Fun Pack

	POINTS VALUE
Bbq chicken shake up, 1 package	5
Breaded chicken nuggets, 1 package	7
Ham & turkey sub, 1 package	11
Low fat ham and cheddar, 1 package	9
Mini pizzas, 1 package	10
Mini's - cheeseburgers, 1 package	9
Mini's, hot dogs, 1 package	9
Nacho chicken shake up, 1 package	5
Pepperoni & cheese, 1 package	9
Pizza and treatza, 1 package	9
Turkey and American, 1 package	8
Turkey and cheddar, 1 package	8

Luncheon/Deli Meat (con't)

	POINTS VALUE
Oscar Mayer Lunchables Maxed Out	
Cheese pizza, 1 package	11
Chicken strips, 1 package	11
Double stacked tacos, 1 package	9
Ham and cheddar, 1 package	15
Nacho, 1 package	13
Pepperoni flavored sausage pizza, 1 package	12
Pizza stix, 1 package	14
Turkey and cheese, 1 package	16
Rustlers	
Beef jerky, 1 serving (9 g)	1
Spicy stick, 1 package	2
SnackMasters Natural Gourmet Jerky	
Beef jerky, hot & spicy, 1 oz	2
Beef jerky, original, 1 oz	2
Beef jerky, teriyaki, 1 oz	2
Turkey jerky, hot & spicy, 1 oz	1
Turkey jerky, original, 1 oz	2
Turkey jerky, teriyaki, 1 oz	2
Spam	
Classic, 2 oz	5
Classic single, 1 package	7
Garlic, 2 oz	4
Golden honey grail, 2 oz	5
Hot & spicy, 2 oz	5
Less salt, 2 oz	5

	POINTS VALUE
Lite, 2 oz	3
Oven roasted turkey, 2 oz	2
Smoked, 2 oz	5
Spread, 4 Tbsp	4
Turkey single, 1 package	3
With bacon, 2 oz	5
With cheese, 2 oz	5
Underwood	
Chicken spread, 1/4 cup	3
Deviled ham spread, 1/4 cup	4
Liverwurst spread, 1/4 cup	4
Roast beef spread, 1/4 cup	4

Pork/Ham

Black Label

	POINTS VALUE
Canned ham, 3 oz	2
Boar's Head	
42% lower sodium branded deluxe ham, 2 oz	1
All natural smoked uncured ham, 2 oz	1
All natural uncured ham, 2 oz	1
Baby black forest brand boneless smoked ham, 3 oz	2
Baby maple glazed honey coat ham, 3 oz	2
Black forest brand boneless smoked ham, 2 oz	1
Branded deluxe ham, 2 oz	1
Capocollo, 1 oz	2
Capocollo hot, 1 oz	2

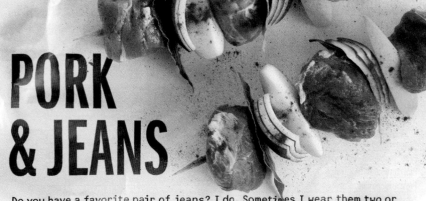

PORK
& JEANS

Do you have a favorite pair of jeans? I do. Sometimes I wear them two or three times a week because I like them so much. That's what I love about jeans. I can dress them up. I can dress them down. I can wear them to a dinner party or to do yard work.

Which brings me to The Other White Meat.® As with my jeans, I also enjoy pork two or three times a week and never get tired of it. I can dress it up—Apple-Pecan Tenderloin Medallions, or dress it down—kabobs. And because it's lean—one serving of pork tenderloin has less than 3 grams of fat—I can eat all I want and still look good in my skinny jeans. Suffice it to say pork and jeans fit me perfectly.

The Other White Meat®

Don't be blah.®

TheOtherWhiteMeat.com/PorkAnd

Pork/Ham, Boar's Head (con't)

	POINTS VALUE
Cooked capocollo sweet - natural casing, 2 oz	3
Gourmet pepper ham, 2 oz	1
Honey coat ham, 2 oz	1
Maple glazed honey coat ham, 2 oz	1
Maple glazed honey coat sweet slice ham, 3 oz	2
Pepper brand ham, 2 oz	2
Pesto parmesan oven roasted ham, 2 oz	2
Prosciutto di parma, 1 oz	1
Prosciutto panino, 1 oz	2
Prosciutto piccolo boneless, 1 oz	1
Prosciutto riserva stradolce boneless, 1 oz	1
Ready to eat ham, 3 oz	2
Rosemary & sundried tomato ham, 2 oz	2
Seasoned cooked fresh ham, 2 oz	2
Semi-boneless smoked ham, 3 oz	3
Skinless/shankless prosciutto, 1 oz	1
Smoked pork shoulder butt roast, 3 oz	4
Smoked Virginia ham, 2 oz	1
Spiced ham, 2 oz	3
St. Louis style pork spareribs in gourmet barbecue sauce, 3	11
Sweet slice boneless smoked ham, 3 oz	2
Tavern ham, 2 oz	1
Virginia brand ham, 2 oz	1

Casa Italia

	POINTS VALUE
Bellarrosto roasted prosciutto cotto, 1 oz	1
Grandoro prosciutto cotto, 1 oz	1

	POINTS VALUE
Porchetta (roasted pork loin), 1 oz	1
Rosemary roasted ham, 1 oz	1

Cure 81

	POINTS VALUE
Half ham, 3 oz	2
Ham with brown sugar, 3 oz	2
Quarter chunk, 3 oz	2
Quarter sliced, 3 oz	2

Curemaster

	POINTS VALUE
Ham, 3 oz	2

Farmland

	POINTS VALUE
Boneless smoked ham - classic cure, 3 oz	2
Boneless smoked ham - maple river, 3 oz	3
Boneless smoked ham - old fashioned pit ham, 3 oz	3
Boneless smoked ham - special select, 2 oz	1
Boneless smoked ham - tradition, 3 oz	3
Boneless smoked ham & water product, 3 oz	2
Cubed ham, 2 oz	1
Extra tender bone-in pork loin, 4 oz	3
Extra tender boneless pork loin - center cut, 4 oz	3
Extra tender boneless pork loin - center cut for chops, 4 oz	3
Extra tender boneless top round roast, 4 oz	3
Extra tender pork loin back ribs, 4 oz	8
Extra tender pork loin ribs, 4 oz	8
Extra tender pork spare ribs, 4 oz	8

	POINTS VALUE
Hickory smoked ham, 3 oz	3
Spiral sliced ham - bone-in half hickory smoked, 3 oz	4
Spiral sliced ham bone-in half - honey cured, 3 oz	3
Farmland - Special Select	
Boneless smoked ham - honey, 1 slice	1
Farmland Nutrition Wise	
Boneless center cut thick pork chops, 1/2	3
Boneless center cut thin pork chops, 1	3
Boneless pork sirloin tip roast, 4 oz	3
Extra tender boneless pork loin, 4 oz	3
Extra tender boneless pork tenderloin, 4 oz	3 (5)
Ground pork, 97% fat free fresh, 4 oz	3
Pork cubes, 4 oz	3
Pork strips, 4 oz	3
Hormel	
Chunk ham, 2 oz	2
Glazed ham with maple & brown sugar, 1 serving (5 oz)	4
Ham & cheese patties, 1	5
Ham patties, 1	5
Jalapeno pigs feet, 2 oz	2
Pickled pigs feet, 2 oz	2
Pickled pork hocks, 2 oz	3
Pickled pork tidbits, 2 oz	3
Hormel Always Tender	
Adobo pork cubes, 4 oz	3
Apple bourbon pork tenderloin, 4 oz	3

	POINTS VALUE
Babyback pork ribs with garlic, 4 oz	6
Babyback ribs, 4 oz	6
Babyback ribs with teriyaki, 4 oz	6
Boneless pork tenderloin, 4 oz	3
Boneless rib ends, 4 oz	4
Center cut boneless pork loin, 4 oz	4
Fajita pork strips, 4 oz	3
Fresh pork roast, 4 oz	4
Garlic pork tenderloin, 4 oz	3
Honey mustard pork loin fillet, 4 oz	3
Loin, 4 oz	5
Mesquite pork tenderloin, 4 oz	3
Mild Thai style, 4 oz	3
Mojo criollo loin filet, 4 oz	3
Onion garlic pork shoulder roast, 4 oz	5
Original pork loin, 4 oz	3
Peppercorn pork tenderloin, 4 oz	3
Picnic, 4 oz	6
Pork - citrus center cut loin fillet, 4 oz	3
Pork - onion garlic roast, 4 oz	5
Pork - original fillet, 4 oz	3
Pork - peppercorn chops, 1	4
Pork - roast flavored roast, 4 oz	4
Pork - sun dried tomato center cut loin fillet, 4 oz	3
Pork - teriyaki chops, 1	4
Pork boneless sirloin roast, 4 oz	3
Pork butts, 4 oz	7

Pork/Ham, Hormel Always Tender (con't)	POINTS VALUE
Pork crown roast, 4 oz	5
Pork medallions applewood smoked bacon, 6 oz	6
Pork medallions double smoked, 6 oz	6
Pork medallions peppered maple bacon, 6 oz	6
Pork shoulder roast, 4 oz	4
Raspberry chipotle tenderloin, 4 oz	3
Sesame ginger pork cubes, 4 oz	4
Spare ribs, 4 oz	8
Teriyaki tenderloin, 4 oz	3
Hormel Pillow Pack	
Diced ham, 2 oz	1
Hormel Spiral Cure 81	
Half ham, 3 oz	3
Jones Dairy Farm	
Dainty ham, 3 oz	2
Family ham, 2 oz	2
Ham slices, 2 slices	1
Ham steak, 3 oz	2
Market Day	
Baby back ribs, 4 oz	7
BBQ pulled pork, 1/2 cup	6
Bone-in pork chop, 1 chop	4
Boneless pork chops, 1 chop	4
Boneless pork riblets, 7 pieces	10
◆ Deluxe ham steaks, 1	4

	POINTS VALUE
◆ Pork tenderloins, 1 serving (4 oz)	3 (5)
Rack of pork roast, 1 piece	3
Spiral sliced ham, 3 oz	5
Stuffed pork chop, 1	10
Schwan's LiveSmart	
Fully cooked pork loin roast, 3 oz	3
Tyson	
Bbq seasoned pork mini ribs, 4 pieces	8
Maple & brown sugar glazed ham, 5 oz	4
Pork roast in gravy, 5 oz	3
Teriyaki pork strip, 3 oz	3

Sausage
Aidells

	POINTS VALUE
Artichoke & garlic sausage, 1 link	3
Cajun style andouille sausage, 1 link	4
Chicken & apple sausage, 1 link	4
Chorizo saussage, 1 link	4
Habanero & green chile sausage, 1 link	3
Mango sausage, 1 link	4
Pesto sausage, 1 links	4
Portobello mushroom sausage, 1 link	3
Roasted red pepper & corn sausage, 1 link	2
Spinach & feta sausage, 1 link	3
Sun-dried tomato with mozzarella cheese sausage, 1 link	3

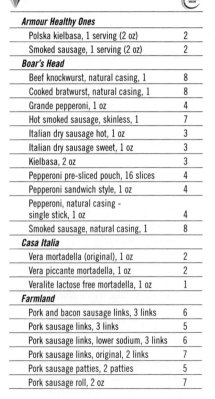

Armour Healthy Ones

	POINTS VALUE
Polska kielbasa, 1 serving (2 oz)	2
Smoked sausage, 1 serving (2 oz)	2

Boar's Head

Beef knockwurst, natural casing, 1	8
Cooked bratwurst, natural casing, 1	8
Grande pepperoni, 1 oz	4
Hot smoked sausage, skinless, 1	7
Italian dry sausage hot, 1 oz	3
Italian dry sausage sweet, 1 oz	3
Kielbasa, 2 oz	3
Pepperoni pre-sliced pouch, 16 slices	4
Pepperoni sandwich style, 1 oz	4
Pepperoni, natural casing - single stick, 1 oz	4
Smoked sausage, natural casing, 1	8

Casa Italia

Vera mortadella (original), 1 oz	2
Vera piccante mortadella, 1 oz	2
Veralite lactose free mortadella, 1 oz	1

Farmland

Pork and bacon sausage links, 3 links	6
Pork sausage links, 3 links	5
Pork sausage links, lower sodium, 3 links	6
Pork sausage links, original, 2 links	7
Pork sausage patties, 2 patties	5
Pork sausage roll, 2 oz	7

Fluky's

	POINTS VALUE
Fat free beef Polish sausage, 1 link	2

Hebrew National

Beef breakfast sausage, maple flavor, 2 links	4
Beef breakfast sausage, original flavor, 2 links	4
Beef breakfast sausage, reduced fat, 2 links	3
Beef knockwurst, 1 link	7
Beef polish sausage, 1 link	7

Hormel

Chunk pepperoni, 1 oz	4
Mild pepperoni, 15 slices	4
Pepperoni hot & spicy, 15 slices	4
Rosa grande pepperoni, 1 oz	4
Sliced pepperoni, 15 slices	4
Twin pepperoni, 1 oz	4

Hormel Little Sizzlers

Maple sausage, 3 links	6
Pork sausage hot & spicy, cooked, 3 links	6
Sausage link, cooked, 3 links	6
Sausage patties, cooked, 2 patties	6

Hormel Pillow Pack

Giant sliced pepperoni, 5 slices	4
Pepperoni, 14 slices	4
Pepperoni bite size, 1 oz	4
Pepperoni diced, 1 oz	4

Sausage, Hormel Pillow Pack (con't)	POINTS VALUE
Pepperoni hot & spicy, 14 slices	4
Thick slice pepperoni, 8 slices	4
Turkey pepperoni, 17 slices	2
Jennie-O Turkey Store
Beer brat, 1	6
Bratwurst, 1	4
Breakfast lovers sausage chubs, 1 serving (112 g)	4
Breakfast lovers sausage links, 1 serving (56 g)	4
Breakfast sausage link, mild, 1 serving (56 g)	4
Breakfast sausage pattie, 1 serving (64 g)	4
Cheddar brat, 1	6
Lean Italian sausage link, hot, 1 serving (109 g)	4
Lean Italian sausage link, sweet, 1 serving (109 g)	4
Smoked turkey sausage ring rope, 1 serving (56 g)	2
Sweet Italian dinner sausage, 1 serving (84 g)	4
Turkey kielbasa ring rope, 1 serving (56 g)	2
Jones Dairy Farm
All natural golden brown light sausage links, 3	4
All natural golden brown mild sausage links, 3	7
All natural golden brown mild sausage patties, 1	3

	POINTS VALUE
All natural light pork sausage & rice links, 2	3
All natural pork little sausages, 3	5
All natural pork sausage patties, 1	4
All natural roll sausage, 2 oz	6
Lance
Giant hot sausage, 1 serving (1.7 oz)	3
Hot sausage, 1 piece	2
Hot sausage, 1 piece	2
Louis Rich
Turkey polska kielbasa, 2 oz	2
Turkey sausage (original), 2.5 oz	3
Turkey smoked sausage, 2 oz	2
Market Day
Fully cooked turkey sausage links, 2 pieces	3
Old Smokehouse
Summer sausage, 2 oz	6
Oscar Mayer
Pepperoni, 14 slices	4
Pork sausage link, cooked, 2	4
Pork sausage patties, ready to serve, 2	5
Smokies sausage, little, made with pork & turkey, 6	5
Smokies, beef, 1	4
Summer sausage, 1 slice	2
Summer sausage, beef (thuringer cervelat), 2 slices	4
Rosina
Sausage meatballs, 6	7

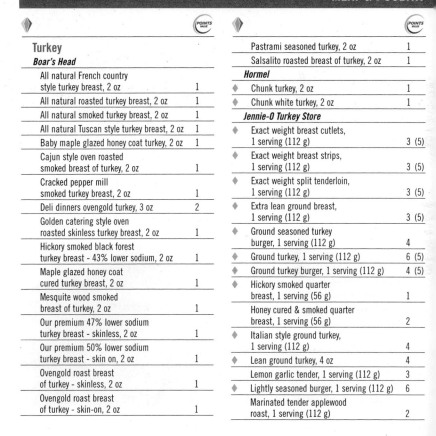

	POINTS VALUE
Turkey	
Boar's Head	
All natural French country style turkey breast, 2 oz	1
All natural roasted turkey breast, 2 oz	1
All natural smoked turkey breast, 2 oz	1
All natural Tuscan style turkey breast, 2 oz	1
Baby maple glazed honey coat turkey, 2 oz	1
Cajun style oven roasted smoked breast of turkey, 2 oz	1
Cracked pepper mill smoked turkey breast, 2 oz	1
Deli dinners ovengold turkey, 3 oz	2
Golden catering style oven roasted skinless turkey breast, 2 oz	1
Hickory smoked black forest turkey breast - 43% lower sodium, 2 oz	1
Maple glazed honey coat cured turkey breast, 2 oz	1
Mesquite wood smoked breast of turkey, 2 oz	1
Our premium 47% lower sodium turkey breast - skinless, 2 oz	1
Our premium 50% lower sodium turkey breast - skin on, 2 oz	1
Ovengold roast breast of turkey - skinless, 2 oz	1
Ovengold roast breast of turkey - skin-on, 2 oz	1

	POINTS VALUE
Pastrami seasoned turkey, 2 oz	1
Salsalito roasted breast of turkey, 2 oz	1
Hormel	
Chunk turkey, 2 oz	1
Chunk white turkey, 2 oz	1
Jennie-O Turkey Store	
Exact weight breast cutlets, 1 serving (112 g)	3 (5)
Exact weight breast strips, 1 serving (112 g)	3 (5)
Exact weight split tenderloin, 1 serving (112 g)	3 (5)
Extra lean ground breast, 1 serving (112 g)	3 (5)
Ground seasoned turkey burger, 1 serving (112 g)	4
Ground turkey, 1 serving (112 g)	6 (5)
Ground turkey burger, 1 serving (112 g)	4 (5)
Hickory smoked quarter breast, 1 serving (56 g)	1
Honey cured & smoked quarter breast, 1 serving (56 g)	2
Italian style ground turkey, 1 serving (112 g)	4
Lean ground turkey, 4 oz	4
Lemon garlic tender, 1 serving (112 g)	3
Lightly seasoned burger, 1 serving (112 g)	6
Marinated tender applewood roast, 1 serving (112 g)	2

Turkey, Jennie-O Turkey Store (con't)	POINTS VALUE
Marinated tender roast turkey, 1 serving (112 g)	2
◆ Oven ready bone in breast homestyle, 1 serving (112 g)	3 (5)
◆ Oven ready whole turkey homestyle, 1 serving (112 g)	4 (5)
◆ Oven roasted quarter breast, 1 serving (112 g)	2
◆ Premium 1/3 pound white turkey, 1 serving (149 g)	6
Savory seasoned turkey burger, 1 serving (112 g)	4
Seasoned pepper tender, 1 serving (112 g)	2
Tequila lime tender, 1 serving (112 g)	2
◆ Teriyaki tenderloin, 1 serving (112 g)	3
Turkey breakfast sausage links, 2	4
◆ Turkey breast tenderloins, 4 oz	2
◆ Turkey burger, 1 serving (112 g)	4
Turkey ham, 1 serving (56 g)	2
Turkey pastrami, 1 serving (56 g)	2

Jennie-O Turkey Store So Easy

Cheddar broccoli stuffed turkey breast, 1 serving (168 g)	5
◆ Slices - homestyle, 1 serving (140 g)	2
◆ So easy breast roast - homestyle, 1 serving (140 g)	2
Swiss cheese & ham stuffed turkey breast, 1 serving (168 g)	6

	POINTS VALUE
Traditional herb stuffing stuffed turkey breast, 1 serving (168 g)	6
White pepper & rice stuffed turkey breast, 1 serving (168 g)	6

Louis Rich

Oven roasted turkey breast, 3 slices	1
Turkey breast & white turkey, oven roasted, 2 slices	1
Turkey patties, white, 1	5

Market Day

Turkey breast roast, 4 oz	3

Oscar Mayer

Oven roasted turkey breast, 3 slices	1
Smoked turkey breast, 3 slices	1

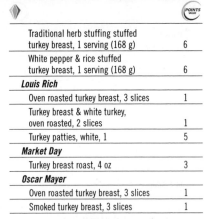

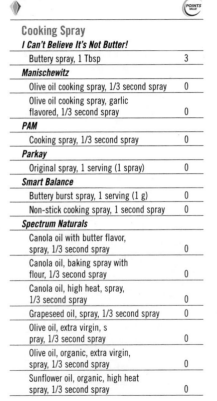

Cooking Spray

I Can't Believe It's Not Butter!

	POINTS VALUE
Buttery spray, 1 Tbsp	3

Manischewitz

Olive oil cooking spray, 1/3 second spray	0
Olive oil cooking spray, garlic flavored, 1/3 second spray	0

PAM

Cooking spray, 1/3 second spray	0

Parkay

Original spray, 1 serving (1 spray)	0

Smart Balance

Buttery burst spray, 1 serving (1 g)	0
Non-stick cooking spray, 1 second spray	0

Spectrum Naturals

Canola oil with butter flavor, spray, 1/3 second spray	0
Canola oil, baking spray with flour, 1/3 second spray	0
Canola oil, high heat, spray, 1/3 second spray	0
Grapeseed oil, spray, 1/3 second spray	0
Olive oil, extra virgin, s pray, 1/3 second spray	0
Olive oil, organic, extra virgin, spray, 1/3 second spray	0
Sunflower oil, organic, high heat spray, 1/3 second spray	0

Oils

Bertolli

	POINTS VALUE
Classico olive oil, 1 Tbsp	4
Extra light tasting olive oil, 1 Tbsp	4
Extra virgin olive oil, 1 Tbsp	4

Carapelli

Extra virgin olive oil, 1 Tbsp	4
Grapeseed oil, 1 Tbsp	4
Light olive oil, 1 Tbsp	4
Mild olive oil, 1 Tbsp	4
Premium extra virgin olive oil, 1 Tbsp	4

Consorzio All Natural

Basil flavored olive oil, 1 Tbsp	4
Dipping oil, herb flavored olive oil and balsamic vinegar, 1 Tbsp	3
Roasted garlic flavored extra virgin olive oil, 1 Tbsp	4
Roasted pepper flavored olive oil, 1 Tbsp	4

Eden Organic

Safflower oil, 1 Tbsp	4
Sesame oil, 1 Tbsp	4
Soybean oil, 1 Tbsp	4

Eden Selected

Extra virgin olive oil, 1 Tbsp	4
Hot pepper sesame oil, 1 Tbsp	4
Toasted sesame oil, 1 Tbsp	4

OILS, DRESSINGS & SEASONINGS

 Oils (con't)

	POINTS VALUE
Enova	
Cooking & salad oil, 1 Tbsp	4
Faraon	
Olive oil, 1 Tbsp	4
Filippo Berio	
Extra light olive oil, 1 Tbsp	4
Extra virgin olive oil, 1 Tbsp	4
Olive oil, 1 Tbsp	4
Hain Pure Foods	
Almond oil, 1 Tbsp	4
Avocado oil, 1 Tbsp	4
Canola oil, 1 Tbsp	4
Extra virgin olive oil, 1 Tbsp	4
Garlic oil, 1 Tbsp	4
Peanut oil, 1 Tbsp	4
Safflower oil, 1 Tbsp	4
Sesame oil, 1 Tbsp	4
Soybean oil, 1 Tbsp	3
Sunflower oil, 1 Tbsp	4
Walnut oil, 1 Tbsp	4
House of Tsang	
Hot chili sesame oil, 1 tsp	1
Mongolian fire oil, 1 tsp	1
Pure sesame oil, 1 tsp	1
Wok oil, 1 Tbsp	4

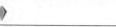

	POINTS VALUE
Lucini	
100% organic premium select extra virgin olive oil, 1 Tbsp	4
Premium select extra virgin olive oil, 1 Tbsp	4
Manischewitz	
Extra virgin olive oil, 1 Tbsp	4
Extra virgin olive oil - garlic & basil, 1 Tbsp	4
Extra virgin olive oil - hot roasted pepper, 1 Tbsp	4
Vegetable oil, 1 Tbsp	4
Milpas	
Corn oil, 2 tsp	3
Naturally Fresh	
Olive oil, 2 Tbsp	8
Planters	
Peanut oil, 1 Tbsp	4
PurOliva	
Puroliva, 2 tsp	2
Smart Balance	
Omega oil, 1 Tbsp	4
Spectrum Naturals	
Almond oil, refined, 1 Tbsp	4
Apricot kernel oil, refined, 1 Tbsp	4
Avocado oil, refined, 1 Tbsp	4
Canola oil, high heat, refined, 1 Tbsp	4

	POINTS VALUE
Canola oil, organic, refined, 1 Tbsp	4
Canola oil, refined, 1 Tbsp	4
Coconut oil, organic, refined, 1 Tbsp	4
Coconut oil, organic, unrefined, 1 Tbsp	4
Corn oil, unrefined, 1 Tbsp	4
Grapeseed oil, refined, 1 Tbsp	4
Olive oil, extra virgin, unrefined, 1 Tbsp	4
Olive oil, extra virgin, unrefined, Greek, 1 Tbsp	4
Olive oil, organic, extra virgin, Moroccan, wild harvest, 1 Tbsp	4
Olive oil, organic, extra virgin, unrefined, 1 Tbsp	4
Olive oil, organic, extra virgin, unrefined, California, 1 Tbsp	4
Olive oil, organic, extra virgin, unrefined, Italian, 1 Tbsp	4
Olive oil, organic, extra virgin, unrefined, Mediterranean, 1 Tbsp	4
Olive oil, organic, extra virgin, unrefined, Spanish Arbequina, 1 Tbsp	4
Peanut oil, unrefined, 1 Tbsp	4
Safflower oil, high heat, refined, 1 Tbsp	4
Safflower oil, organic, high heat, refined, 1 Tbsp	4
Sesame oil, organic, unrefined, 1 Tbsp	4
Sesame oil, refined, 1 Tbsp	4

	POINTS VALUE
Sesame oil, toasted, organic, unrefined, 1 Tbsp	4
Sesame oil, toasted, unrefined, 1 Tbsp	4
Sesame oil, unrefined, 1 Tbsp	4
Soy oil, organic, refined, 1 Tbsp	4
Sunflower oil, organic, high heat, refined, 1 Tbsp	4
Walnut oil, refined, 1 Tbsp	4

Tree of Life

	POINTS VALUE
Almond oil, 1 Tbsp	4
Avocado oil, 1 Tbsp	4
Macadamia nut oil, 1 Tbsp	4
Organic coconut oil, expeller pressed, 1 Tbsp	4
Organic extra virgin olive oil, 1 Tbsp	4
Sesame oil, 1 Tbsp	4
Walnut oil, 1 Tbsp	4

Salad Dressings
Annie's Naturals

	POINTS VALUE
Artichoke parmesan, 2 Tbsp	4
Balsamic vinaigrette, 2 Tbsp	3
Caesar dressing, 2 Tbsp	3
Cowgirl ranch, 2 Tbsp	3
Goddess dressing, 2 Tbsp	4
Lemon & chive dressing, 2 Tbsp	4
Light Italian dressing, 2 Tbsp	1

OILS, DRESSINGS & SEASONINGS

Salad Dressings, Annie's Naturals (con't)	POINTS VALUE
Low fat gingerly vinaigrette, 2 Tbsp	1
Low fat honey mustard vinaigrette, 2 Tbsp	1
Low fat raspberry vinaigrette, 2 Tbsp	1
Organic Asian sesame, 2 Tbsp	4
Organic balsamic vinaigrette, 2 Tbsp	3
Organic bbq sweet and spicy, 2 Tbsp	1
Organic buttermilk, 2 Tbsp	2
Organic Caesar dressing, 2 Tbsp	3
Organic cowgirl ranch, 2 Tbsp	3
Organic creamy asiago cheese dressing, 2 Tbsp	3
Organic cucumber yogurt dressing, 2 Tbsp	2
Organic French dressing, 2 Tbsp	3
Organic goddess dressing, 2 Tbsp	4
Organic green garlic dressing, 2 Tbsp	3
Organic green goddess, 2 Tbsp	4
Organic oil & vinegar, 2 Tbsp	4
Organic papaya poppyseed, 2 Tbsp	4
Organic pomegranate vinaigrette, 2 Tbsp	2
Organic red wine & olive oil, 2 Tbsp	5
Organic roasted garlic vinaigrette, 2 Tbsp	3
Organic sesame ginger with chamomile, 2 Tbsp	3
Organic shiitake and sesame vinaigrette, 2 Tbsp	3
Organic shiitake and sesame vinaigrette, 2 Tbsp	3

	POINTS VALUE
Organic thousand island, 2 Tbsp	2
Roasted red pepper, 2 Tbsp	2
Tuscany Italian, 2 Tbsp	2
Woodstock dressing, 2 Tbsp	3
Consorzio	
Balsamic vinaigrette dressing, 2 Tbsp	2
Mango fat-free dressing & marinade, 1 Tbsp	0
Raspberry & balsamic fat-free dressing, 1 Tbsp	0
Strawberry & balsamic fat-free dressing, 1 Tbsp	0
El Torito	
Cilantro pepita Caesar salad dressing, 2 Tbsp	4
Serrano ranch salad dressing, 2 Tbsp	4
Ellen Rose	
Caesar dressing, 2 Tbsp	4
Herb vinaigrette, 2 Tbsp	6
Lowfat orange ginger dressing, 2 Tbsp	0
Oriental dressing, 2 Tbsp	5
Raspberry vinaigrette, 2 Tbsp	5
Follow Your Heart	
Low fat ranch dressing, 2 Tbsp	1
Original vegenaise, 1 Tbsp	3
Spicy Southwest Ranch Dressing, 2 Tbsp	1

	POINTS VALUE
Good Seasons	
Asian sesame mix, 1 serving (1/8 of envelope)	0
Asian sesame with ginger, 2 Tbsp	3
Asian sesame, prepared, 2 Tbsp	4
Basil vinaigrette mix, 1/8 envelope	0
Basil vinaigrette, prepared, 2 Tbsp	4
Cheese garlic dry mix, 1/8 envelope	0
Cheese garlic, prepared, 2 Tbsp	4
Classic balsamic vinaigrette with extra virgin olive oil, 2 Tbsp	2
Creamy Caesar with aged parmesan, 2 Tbsp	3
Fat free Italian dry mix, 1/8 envelope	0
Fat free Italian, prepared, 2 Tbsp	0
Garlic & herb, prepared, 2 Tbsp	4
Garlic and herb dry mix, 1/8 envelope	0
Gourmet Caesar dry mix, 1/8 envelope	0
Gourmet Caesar, prepared, 2 Tbsp	4
Gourmet parmesan Italian dry mix, 1/8 envelope	0
Gourmet parmesan Italian, prepared, 2 Tbsp	4
Italian dry mix, 1/8 envelope	0
Italian vinaigrette with extra virgin olive oil, 2 Tbsp	2
Italian, prepared, 2 Tbsp	4

	POINTS VALUE
Light Greek vinaigrette with oregano & athenos feta cheese, 2 Tbsp	1
Light honey dijon, 2 Tbsp	1
Light red raspberry vinaigrette with poppyseed, 2 Tbsp	2
Mild Italian dry mix, 1/8 envelope	0
Mild Italian, prepared, 2 Tbsp	4
Roasted garlic dry mix, 1/8 envelope	0
Roasted garlic, prepared, 2 Tbsp	4
Sun dried tomato vinaigrette with roasted red pepper, 2 Tbsp	2
Zesty Italian dry mix, 1/8 envelope	0
Zesty Italian, prepared, 2 Tbsp	4
Heinz	
Creamy Italian, 1 oz	3
Italian, 1 oz	3
Thousand island, 1 oz	4
Henri's	
Fat free French, 2 Tbsp	1
Fat free honey mustard, 2 Tbsp	1
Hidden Valley	
BLT ranch with bacon and tomato, 2 Tbsp	4
Buttermilk recipe original ranch, prepared from mix, 2 Tbsp	3
Caesar with crushed garlic, 2 Tbsp	3
Coleslaw, 2 Tbsp	4

OILS, DRESSINGS & SEASONINGS

Salad Dressings, Hidden Valley (con't)	POINTS VALUE
Fat free French with honey and bacon, 2 Tbsp	1
Fat free original ranch, 2 Tbsp	1
Fat free original ranch with bacon, 2 Tbsp	1
French with honey and bacon, 2 Tbsp	4
Light BLT ranch with bacon and tomato, 2 Tbsp	2
Light original ranch, 2 Tbsp	2
Light original ranch with sour cream, 2 Tbsp	2
Light original ranch with sun dried tomato and feta, 2 Tbsp	2
Milk recipe original ranch, prepared from mix, 2 Tbsp	3
Original ranch, 2 Tbsp	4
Original ranch with bacon, 2 Tbsp	4
Original ranch with garlic, 2 Tbsp	4
Original ranch with sun dried tomato and feta, 2 Tbsp	4
Reduced calorie original ranch, prepared from mix, 2 Tbsp	1
Jackaroo	
Jalapeno ranch dressing, 2 Tbsp	3
Kraft	
Asian toasted sesame, 2 Tbsp	2
Blue cheese ranch, 2 Tbsp	4
Buttermilk ranch dressing, 2 Tbsp	3

	POINTS VALUE
Caesar ranch, 2 Tbsp	3
Caesar with bacon, 2 Tbsp	3
Catalina, 2 Tbsp	3
Cilantro flavored pepper ranch, 2 Tbsp	3
Classic Caesar, 2 Tbsp	3
Coleslaw, 2 Tbsp	3
Coleslaw maker, 2 Tbsp	3
Creamy French, 2 Tbsp	4
Creamy garlic, 2 Tbsp	3
Creamy Italian, 2 Tbsp	3
Cucumber ranch, 2 Tbsp	3
French style fat free salad dressing, 1 serving (35 g)	1
Garlic ranch, 2 Tbsp	3
House Italian, 2 Tbsp	2
Peppercorn ranch, 2 Tbsp	3
Ranch, 2 Tbsp	3
Ranch with bacon, 2 Tbsp	3
Roasted red pepper Italian with parmesan, 2 Tbsp	1
Roka blue cheese, 2 Tbsp	3
Russian, 2 Tbsp	3
Sour cream & onion ranch, 2 Tbsp	3
Thousand island, 2 Tbsp	2
Thousand island with bacon, 2 Tbsp	3
Three cheese Italian, 2 Tbsp	4

	POINTS VALUE
Three cheese ranch, 2 Tbsp	3
Tuna salad maker super easy squeeze, 1 Tbsp	1
Zesty Italian, 2 Tbsp	2
Kraft Carb Well	
Classic Caesar, 2 Tbsp	3
Italian, 2 Tbsp	2
Ranch, 2 Tbsp	3
Roka blue cheese, 2 Tbsp	3
Kraft Free	
Blue cheese flavored, 2 Tbsp	1
Caesar Italian, 2 Tbsp	1
Catalina, 2 Tbsp	1
Classic Caesar, 2 Tbsp	1
Creamy Italian, 2 Tbsp	1
French style, 2 Tbsp	1
Honey dijon, 2 Tbsp	1
Italian, 2 Tbsp	0
Peppercorn ranch, 2 Tbsp	1
Ranch, 2 Tbsp	1
Sour cream & onion ranch, 2 Tbsp	1
Thousand island, 2 Tbsp	1
Zesty Italian, 2 Tbsp	0
Kraft Light Done Right	
Asian toasted sesame, 2 Tbsp	1
Balsamic vinaigrette, 2 Tbsp	1

	POINTS VALUE
Catalina, 2 Tbsp	1
Classic Caesar, 2 Tbsp	2
Creamy French, 2 Tbsp	2
Cucumber ranch, 2 Tbsp	1
Golden Caesar, 2 Tbsp	2
House Italian, 2 Tbsp	1
Ranch, 2 Tbsp	2
Raspberry vinaigrette, 2 Tbsp	2
Red wine vinaigrette, 2 Tbsp	1
Roka bleu cheese salad dressing, 1 serving (29 g)	2
Thousand island, 2 Tbsp	1
Three cheese ranch, 2 Tbsp	2
Zesty Italian, 2 Tbsp	1
Kraft Miracle Whip	
Dressing, 1 Tbsp	1
Dressing, hot & spicy, 1 serving (15 g)	1
Fat free dressing, 1 Tbsp	0
Light dressing, 1 Tbsp	1
Kraft Special Collection	
Caesar Italian with oregano, 2 Tbsp	3
Caesar vinaigrette with parmesan, 2 Tbsp	2
Classic Italian vinaigrette, 2 Tbsp	1
Creamy poppyseed, 2 Tbsp	3
Italian pesto vinaigrette, 2 Tbsp	2
Parmesan Italian with basil, 2 Tbsp	3

OILS, DRESSINGS & SEASONINGS

Salad Dressings, Kraft Special Collection (con't)	POINTS VALUE
Roasted garlic vinaigrette, 1 serving (32 g)	1
Sweet honey catalina, 2 Tbsp	4
Tangy tomato bacon, 2 Tbsp	3
Kraft Special Collections	
Greek vinaigrette, 2 Tbsp	3
Parmesan romano, 2 Tbsp	4
Sun dried tomato, 2 Tbsp	2
Litehouse	
Bacon bleu cheese, 2 Tbsp	4
Balsamic vinaigrette, 2 Tbsp	2
Big bleu, 2 Tbsp	5
Bleu cheese lite, 2 Tbsp	2
Bleu cheese vinaigrette, 2 Tbsp	4
Bleu cheese, 2 Tbsp	4
Caesar, 2 Tbsp	2
Chunky bleu cheese, 2 Tbsp	4
Chunky garlic caesar, 2 tsp	4
Coleslaw, 2 Tbsp	3
Cranberry vinaigrette, 2 Tbsp	1
Creamy cilantro, 2 Tbsp	3
Creamy sesame ginger, 2 Tbsp	3
Feta Greek, 2 Tbsp	4
Garlic vinaigrette, 2 Tbsp	3
Hail Caesar, 2 Tbsp	4
Honey mustard dressing, 2 Tbsp	4
Huckleberry vinaigrette, 2 Tbsp	0

	POINTS VALUE
Jalapeno ranch, 2 Tbsp	3
Lite 1000, 2 Tbsp	2
Lite honey dijon, 2 Tbsp	2
Pomegranate blueberry vinaigrette, 2 Tbsp	0
Poppyseed pourable, 2 Tbsp	4
Ranch homestyle, 2 Tbsp	3
Ranch salsa dressing, 2 Tbsp	2
Ranch, 2 Tbsp	3
Raspberry walnut vinaigrette, 2 Tbsp	4
Red wine oil vinaigrette, 2 Tbsp	3
Red wine olive oil, 2 Tbsp	3
Roquefort, 2 Tbsp	2
Sesame ginger, 2 Tbsp	1
Soy ginger, 2 Tbsp	2
Spinach dressing, 2 Tbsp	1
Sweet French, 2 Tbsp	3
Thousand island, 2 Tbsp	4
Zesty Italian, 2 Tbsp	3
Zesty Italian vinaigrette, 2 Tbsp	3
Litehouse Organic	
Balsamic, 2 Tbsp	4
Caesar, 2 Tbsp	3
Ranch pourable, 2 Tbsp	4
Raspberry lime, 2 Tbsp	1
Maple Grove	
Fat free balsamic vinaigrette, 2 Tbsp	0
Fat free Caesar dressing, 2 Tbsp	0

	POINTS VALUE
Fat free cranberry balsamic vinaigrette, 2 Tbsp	1
Fat free Greek dressing, 2 Tbsp	1
Fat free honey dijon dressing, 2 Tbsp	1
Fat free lime basil vinaigrette, 2 Tbsp	1
Fat free poppyseed dressing, 2 Tbsp	1
Fat free raspberry vinaigrette, 2 Tbsp	1
Fat free vidalia dressing, 2 Tbsp	1
Fat free wasabi dijon dressing, 2 Tbsp	1
Lite Caesar dressing, 2 Tbsp	2
Lite honey mustard dressing, 2 Tbsp	2
Maple fig vinaigrette all natural, 2 Tbsp	1
Sesame ginger all natural, 2 Tbsp	1
Strawberry balsamic all natural, 2 Tbsp	1
Sugar free bacon vinaigrette dressing, 2 Tbsp	3
Sugar free balsamic vinaigrette dressing, 2 Tbsp	0
Sugar free dijon dressing, 2 Tbsp	2
Sugar free Italian with white balsamic dressing, 2 Tbsp	3
Sugar free raspberry vinaigrette, 2 Tbsp	0

Marzetti

	POINTS VALUE
Asiago peppercorn dressing, 2 Tbsp	5
Asian ginger dressing, 2 Tbsp	3
Baja ranch dressing, 2 Tbsp	4

	POINTS VALUE
Bistro blue cheese dressing, 2 Tbsp	5
Buffalo blue cheese dressing, 2 Tbsp	4
Chunky blue cheese dressing, 2 Tbsp	4
Classic ranch dressing, 2 Tbsp	5
Ginger mango vinaigrette, 2 Tbsp	3
Honey balsamic dressing, 2 Tbsp	3
Honey French blue cheese dressing, 2 Tbsp	4
Honey French dressing, 2 Tbsp	5
Honey mustard dip & dressing, 2 Tbsp	4
House balsamic vinaigrette dressing, 2 Tbsp	2
Italian with blue cheese vinaigrette, 2 Tbsp	3
Light balsamic vinaigrette dressing, 2 Tbsp	1
Light blue cheese dressing, 2 Tbsp	2
Light Caesar dressing, 2 Tbsp	2
Light honey dijon dressing, 2 Tbsp	2
Light honey French dressing, 2 Tbsp	2
Light raspberry cabernet vinaigrette, 2 Tbsp	2
Light slaw dressing, 2 Tbsp	3
Lite Caesar dressing, 2 Tbsp	2
Lite ranch dressing, 2 Tbsp	2
Organic balsamic vinaigrette, 2 Tbsp	3
Organic blue cheese dressing, 2 Tbsp	4

OILS, DRESSINGS & SEASONINGS

Salad Dressings, Marzetti (con't)	POINTS VALUE
Organic Caesar dressing, 2 Tbsp	4
Organic parmesan ranch dressing, 2 Tbsp	4
Poppyseed dressing, 2 Tbsp	4
Roasted garlic Italian vinaigrette dressing (house), 2 Tbsp	4
Slaw dressing, 2 Tbsp	4
Spinach salad dressing, 2 Tbsp	2
Strawberry chardonnay vinaigrette, 2 Tbsp	3
Supreme Caesar dressing, 2 Tbsp	4
Sweet Italian dressing, 2 Tbsp	4
Thousand island dressing, 2 Tbsp	4
Three cheese Italian dressing, 2 Tbsp	4
Ultimate blue cheese dressing, 2 Tbsp	5
White balsamic vinaigrette, 2 Tbsp	3
Muirhead	
Balsamic vinaigrette, 1 Tbsp	3
Hazel's sweet and sour dressing, 1 Tbsp	1
Herbes de provence vinaigrette, 1 Tbsp	3
Pomegranate vinaigrette, 1 Tbsp	3
Nasoya	
Dijon style nayonaise, 1 Tbsp	1
Fat free nayonaise, 1 Tbsp	0
Nayonaise, 1 Tbsp	1
Vegi-dressing, creamy dill, 2 Tbsp	2
Vegi-dressing, creamy Italian, 2 Tbsp	2
Vegi-dressing, garden herb, 2 Tbsp	2

	POINTS VALUE
Vegi-dressing, sesame garlic, 2 Tbsp	2
Vegi-dressing, thousand island, 2 Tbsp	2
Naturally Fresh	
Apple cranberry walnut, 2 Tbsp	1
Bacon bleu cheese, 1 Tbsp	5
Bleu cheese dressing, all natural, 2 Tbsp	5
Bleu cheese vinaigrette, 2 Tbsp	2
Buffalo ranch dressing, 2 Tbsp	3
Caesar dressing, 2 Tbsp	3
Classic bleu cheese dressing, 2 Tbsp	4
Classic Caesar dressing, 2 Tbsp	5
Classic oriental dressing, 2 Tbsp	4
Classic ranch dressing, 2 Tbsp	4
Cranberry orange dressing, 2 Tbsp	1
Cranberry walnut dressing, refrigerated, 2 Tbsp	3
Creamy cilantro dressing, 2 Tbsp	4
Fat-free balsamic vinaigrette, 2 Tbsp	0
Fat-free raspberry vinaigrette, 2 Tbsp	1
Ginger dressing, 2 Tbsp	2
Honey French dressing, 2 Tbsp	3
Honey mustard dressing, 2 Tbsp	4
Lite bleu cheese dressing, 2 Tbsp	3
Lite peppercorn ranch dressing, 2 Tbsp	2
Lite ranch dressing (with msg), 2 Tbsp	2
Mandarin ginger, 2 Tbsp	0

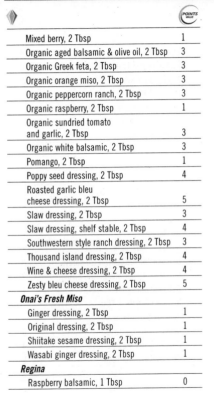

	POINTS VALUE
Mixed berry, 2 Tbsp	1
Organic aged balsamic & olive oil, 2 Tbsp	3
Organic Greek feta, 2 Tbsp	3
Organic orange miso, 2 Tbsp	3
Organic peppercorn ranch, 2 Tbsp	3
Organic raspberry, 2 Tbsp	1
Organic sundried tomato and garlic, 2 Tbsp	3
Organic white balsamic, 2 Tbsp	3
Pomango, 2 Tbsp	1
Poppy seed dressing, 2 Tbsp	4
Roasted garlic bleu cheese dressing, 2 Tbsp	5
Slaw dressing, 2 Tbsp	3
Slaw dressing, shelf stable, 2 Tbsp	4
Southwestern style ranch dressing, 2 Tbsp	3
Thousand island dressing, 2 Tbsp	4
Wine & cheese dressing, 2 Tbsp	4
Zesty bleu cheese dressing, 2 Tbsp	5
Onai's Fresh Miso	
Ginger dressing, 2 Tbsp	1
Original dressing, 2 Tbsp	1
Shiitake sesame dressing, 2 Tbsp	1
Wasabi ginger dressing, 2 Tbsp	1
Regina	
Raspberry balsamic, 1 Tbsp	0

	POINTS VALUE
San-J	
Tamari ginger dressing, 2 Tbsp	1
Tamari mustard, 2 Tbsp	1
Tamari peanut, 2 Tbsp	1
Tamari sesame, 2 Tbsp	1
Seeds of Change	
Balsamic vinaigrette, 2 Tbsp	2
French tomato salad dressing, 2 Tbsp	1
Greek feta vinaigrette, 2 Tbsp	2
Italian herb vinaigrette, 2 Tbsp	2
Roasted garlic vinaigrette, 2 Tbsp	2
Roasted red pepper vinaigrette, 2 Tbsp	1
Sweet basil vinaigrette, 2 Tbsp	2
Sweet dijon vinaigrette, 2 Tbsp	2
Seven Seas	
Creamy Italian, 2 Tbsp	3
Green goddess, 2 Tbsp	4
Red wine vinaigrette, 2 Tbsp	3
Viva Italian, 2 Tbsp	3
Viva robust Italian, 2 Tbsp	3
Seven Seas Free	
Red wine vinaigrette, 2 Tbsp	0
Viva Italian, 2 Tbsp	0

OILS, DRESSINGS & SEASONINGS

Salad Dressings (con't)	POINTS VALUE

Seven Seas Reduced Fat	
Red wine vinaigrette & oil, 2 Tbsp	1
Viva Italian, 2 Tbsp	1
Spectrum Naturals	
Omega-3 Asian ginger, organic, 2 Tbsp	4
Omega-3 creamy garlic ranch, organic, 2 Tbsp	3
Omega-3 golden balsamic, organic, 2 Tbsp	3
Omega-3 lemon sesame, organic, 2 Tbsp	4
Omega-3 pomegranate chipotle, organic, 2 Tbsp	4
Omega-3 shiitake sesame, organic, 2 Tbsp	3
Omega-3 vegan Caesar, organic, 2 Tbsp	3
Spin Blend	
Classic, 1 Tbsp	1
Light, 1 Tbsp	1
Walden Farms	
Asian, 2 Tbsp	0
Bacon ranch, 2 Tbsp	0
Balsamic vinaigrette, 2 Tbsp	0
Bleu cheese, 2 Tbsp	0
Caesar, 2 Tbsp	0
Classic French, 2 Tbsp	0
Coleslaw, 2 Tbsp	0
Creamy bacon, 1 packet	0
Creamy bacon, 2 Tbsp	0

	POINTS VALUE
Creamy Italian, 2 Tbsp	0
Honey dijon, 1 packet	0
Honey dijon, 2 Tbsp	0
Italian, 1 packet	0
Italian, 2 Tbsp	0
Italian with sun dried tomatoes, 2 Tbsp	0
Jersey sweet onion, 2 Tbsp	0
Ranch, 1 packet	0
Ranch, 2 Tbsp	0
Raspberry vinaigrette, 2 Tbsp	0
Russian, 2 Tbsp	0
Thousand island, 1 packet	0
Thousand island, 2 Tbsp	0
Zesty Italian, 2 Tbsp	0
Wish-Bone	
Balsamic basil light, 2 Tbsp	2
Balsamic breeze spritzer, 10 sprays	0
Balsamic Italian vinaigrette, 2 Tbsp	2
Balsamic vinaigrette, 2 Tbsp	1
Berry vinaigrette, 2 Tbsp	1
Blue cheese, 2 Tbsp	4
Cheese Italian, 2 Tbsp	3
Chunky blue cheese, 2 Tbsp	4
Creamy Caesar, 2 Tbsp	5
Creamy Italian, 2 Tbsp	3
Deluxe French, 2 Tbsp	3

	POINTS VALUE
Garlic ranch, 2 Tbsp	4
Honey dijon vinaigrette, 2 Tbsp	2
House Italian, 2 Tbsp	3
Italian, 2 Tbsp	2
Italian vinaigrette spritzer, 10 sprays	0
Lemon garlic herb, 2 Tbsp	2
Olive oil vinaigrette, 2 Tbsp	2
Ranch, 2 Tbsp	3
Raspberry hazelnut vinaigrette, 2 Tbsp	2
Raspberry walnut light, 2 Tbsp	2
Red wine mist spritzer, 10 sprays	0
Red wine vinaigrette, 2 Tbsp	2
Robusto Italian, 2 Tbsp	2
Romano basil vinaigrette, 2 Tbsp	2
Russian, 2 Tbsp	2
Sesame ginger light, 2 Tbsp	2
Skippy natural, 2 Tbsp	5
Spring onion ranch, 2 Tbsp	4
Sweet and spicy French, 2 Tbsp	4
Thousand island, 2 Tbsp	4
Western creamy French, 2 Tbsp	4
Western original, 2 Tbsp	4
Western with bacon, 2 Tbsp	4
Western with blue cheese, 2 Tbsp	4
Wish-Bone Fat Free	
Blue cheese, 2 Tbsp	1
Italian, 2 Tbsp	0

	POINTS VALUE
Ranch, 2 Tbsp	0
Red wine vinaigrette, 2 Tbsp	1
Western, 2 Tbsp	1
Wish-Bone Just 2 Good!	
1000 island, 2 Tbsp	1
Blue cheese, 2 Tbsp	1
Country Italian, 2 Tbsp	1
Creamy Caesar, 2 Tbsp	1
Deluxe French, 2 Tbsp	1
Honey dijon, 2 Tbsp	1
Italian, 2 Tbsp	1
Light blue cheese, 2 Tbsp	1
Parmesan/peppercorn ranch, 2 Tbsp	1
Ranch, 2 Tbsp	1
Sweet and spicy French, 2 Tbsp	1
Western, 2 Tbsp	2

Seasonings
4C

	POINTS VALUE
Seasoned coating mix for chicken, 1 serving (10 g)	1
Seasoned coating mix for pork, 1 serving (11 g)	1
A Taste of Thai	
Chicken & rice dinner seasoning, 1/4 envelope	0
Spicy Thai peanut bake, 1/4 envelope	1

417

OILS, DRESSINGS & SEASONINGS

Seasonings (con't)	(POINTS VALUE)
A1	
Barbecue, 1/4 tsp	0
Classic, 1/4 tsp	0
Garlic & herb, 1/4 tsp	0
Savory pepper, 1/4 tsp	0
Ac'cent	
Flavor enhancer, 1/8 tsp	0
Chef Paul Prudhomme's Magic Seasoning Blends	
Blackened redfish magic, 1/4 tsp	0
Blackened steak magic, 1/4 tsp	0
Fajita magic, 1/4 tsp	0
Herbal pizza & pasta magic, 1/4 tsp	0
Hot & sweet pizza & pasta magic, 1/4 tsp	0
Magic barbecue seasoning, 1/4 tsp	0
Magic salt free seasoning, 1/4 tsp	0
Magic seasoning salt, 1/4 tsp	0
Meat magic, 1/4 tsp	0
Pork & veal magic, 1/4 tsp	0
Poultry magic, 1/4 tsp	0
Salmon magic, 1/4 tsp	0
Seafood magic, 1/4 tsp	0
Vegetable magic, 1/4 tsp	0
Cherchies	
Garlic 'n herbs seasoning, 1/4 tsp	0
Garlic seasoning, 1/4 tsp	0
Lem'n dill seasoning, 1 tsp	0
Lem'n dill seasoning, no salt, 1 tsp	0

	(POINTS VALUE)
Lem'n pepper spicy blend, 1 tsp	0
Pepper pizzazz seasoning, 1/4 tsp	0
Pepper'n lime seasoning, 1 tsp	0
Salsa seasoning with lime, 1 tsp	0
Chi-Chi's	
Fajita seasoning mix, 1/4 package	1
Fiesta restaurante seasoning mix, 1 tsp	0
Fiesta taco seasoning mix, 1 serving (1/5 package)	0
Durkee	
BBQ buffalo wing, mix, 1 Tbsp	1
Chili seasoning dry mix, 1 Tbsp	0
Meatloaf dry mix, 2 tsp	0
Pot roast dry mix, 2 tsp	0
Sloppy Joe seasoning, 2 tsp	0
Spaghetti dry mix, 1 Tbsp	0
Taco dry mix, 2 tsp	0
Eden	
Dulse flakes - organic, 1 tsp	0
Eden shake (furikake) - sesame & sea vegetable seasoning, 1/2 tsp	0
Sea salt - French coast, light grey, fine grind, 1/4 tsp	0
Sea salt - Portuguese coast, white, fine grind, 1/4 tsp	0
Shiso leaf powder (pickled beefsteak leaf), 1 tsp	0
Tekka, 1 tsp	0

	POINTS VALUE
Eden Organic	
Garlic gomasio (sesame salt), 1/2 tsp	0
Gomasio (sesame salt), 1/2 tsp	0
Kuzu root starch, 1 serving (9 g)	1
Seaweed gomasio (sesame salt), 1 serving (1.5 g)	0
Fanci Food	
Popcorn salt, finely ground, 1/4 tsp	0
Popcorn seasoning, butter flavor, 1/2 tsp	0
Popcorn seasoning, cheddar flavor, 1/2 tsp	0
Pop'n topper, all natural butter flavor seasoning, 3/4 tsp	0
Fisher Salad Buddies	
Pecan pieces, 1/4 cup	5
Slivered almonds, 1/4 cup	4
Sunflower kernels, 3 Tbsp	4
Walnut pieces, 1/4 cup	5
French's	
Beef stew branded, 2 tsp	0
Beef stew dry mix, 1 Tbsp	1
Buffalo wings, hot, mix, 1 tsp	0
Buffalo wings, mild, mix, 1 1/3 Tbsp	0
Buffalo wings, screaming hot, mix, 1 1/2 Tbsp	0
Cajun wings, dry mix, 1 Tbsp	0
Chili seasoning dry mix, 1 Tbsp	0
Enchilada seasoning, mix, 2 tsp	0
Meatloaf dry mix, 2 tsp	0

	POINTS VALUE
Onion chili-o mix, 1 1/3 Tbsp	0
Pot roast dry mix, 2 tsp	0
Roasting bag, pot roast, mix, 2 tsp	0
Sloppy Joe seasoning, 2 tsp	0
Spaghetti dry mix, 1 Tbsp	0
Taco dry mix, 2 tsp	0
Grill Mates	
BBQ seasoning blend, 3/4 tsp	0
Montreal chicken seasoning, 3/4 tsp	0
Montreal steak seasoning, 1/4 tsp	0
Teriyaki dry seasoning mix, 1 tsp	0
Kitchen Bouquet	
Kitchen bouquet, 1 tsp	0
Manischewitz	
Brisket & steak seasoning, 1/4 tsp	0
Fish seasoning, 1/4 tsp	0
Poultry seasoning, 1/4 tsp	0
McCormick	
Celery salt, 1/4 tsp	0
Chili dry seasoning mix, 1 1/3 Tbsp	0
Guacamole dry seasoning mix, 1 tsp	0
Lemon & pepper seasoning, 1 1/2 tsp	0
Poultry seasoning, 1/4 tsp	0
Salad supreme seasoning, 2 tsp	0
Season-all, 1/4 tsp	0
Seasoned meat tenderizer, 1/4 tsp	0
Taco dry seasoning mix, 2 tsp	0

Seasonings (con't) **POINTS** VALUE

 POINTS VALUE

Mrs. Dash

Classic Italiano, 1/4 tsp	0
Extra spicy, 1/4 tsp	0
Garlic & herb, 1/4 tsp	0
Hamburger grilling blend, 1/4 tsp	0
Lemon pepper, 1/4 tsp	0
Onion & herb, 1/4 tsp	0
Original blend, 1/4 tsp	0
Southwest chipotle, 1/4 tsp	0
Table blend, 1/4 tsp	0
Tomato basil garlic, 1/4 tsp	0

Mrs. Dash Grilling Blends

Mesquite, 1/4 tsp	0
Original chicken blend, 1/4 tsp	0
Original steak blend, 1/4 tsp	0

Old Bay

Old bay seasoning, 1/4 tsp	0

Old El Paso

Burrito seasoning mix, 2 tsp	0
Cheesy taco seasoning mix, 2 tsp	0
Chili seasoning mix, 1 Tbsp	0
Enchilada sauce mix, 2 tsp	0
Fajita seasoning mix, 2 tsp	0
Taco seasoning mix, 2 tsp	0
Taco seasoning mix, 40% less sodium, 2 tsp	0
Taco seasoning mix, hot and spicy, 2 tsp	0
Taco seasoning mix, mild, 2 tsp	0

Ortega

Taco seasoning, 1 Tbsp (1/6 envelope)	0

Oven Fry

Extra crispy chicken, 1/8 packet	1

Oven Fry Seasoned Coating

Extra crispy for chicken, 1 serving (15 g)	1
Extra crispy for pork, 1 serving (15 g)	1
Fish fry for fish, 1 serving (12 g)	1
Home style flour for chicken recipe, 1 serving (11 g)	1

Season Brand

Capers, 2 Tbsp	0

Shake 'N Bake

Barbecue chicken or pork, as packaged, 1 serving (1/8 packet)	1
Buffalo wing glazes for chicken, as packaged, 1 serving (1/10 packet)	1
Country mild recipe, as packaged, 1 serving (1/8 packet)	1
Extra crispy recipe for chicken, as packaged, 1 serving (1/8 packet)	1
Honey mustard chicken or pork, as packaged, 1 serving (1/8 packet)	1
Hot & spicy chicken or pork, as packaged, 1 serving (1/8 packet)	1
Italian chicken or pork, as packaged, 1 serving (1/8 packet)	1
Lemon pepper for chicken or pork, as packaged, 1 serving (1/8 packet)	1

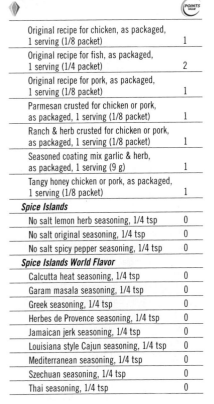

	POINTS VALUE
Original recipe for chicken, as packaged, 1 serving (1/8 packet)	1
Original recipe for fish, as packaged, 1 serving (1/4 packet)	2
Original recipe for pork, as packaged, 1 serving (1/8 packet)	1
Parmesan crusted for chicken or pork, as packaged, 1 serving (1/8 packet)	1
Ranch & herb crusted for chicken or pork, as packaged, 1 serving (1/8 packet)	1
Seasoned coating mix garlic & herb, as packaged, 1 serving (9 g)	1
Tangy honey chicken or pork, as packaged, 1 serving (1/8 packet)	1
Spice Islands	
No salt lemon herb seasoning, 1/4 tsp	0
No salt original seasoning, 1/4 tsp	0
No salt spicy pepper seasoning, 1/4 tsp	0
Spice Islands World Flavor	
Calcutta heat seasoning, 1/4 tsp	0
Garam masala seasoning, 1/4 tsp	0
Greek seasoning, 1/4 tsp	0
Herbes de Provence seasoning, 1/4 tsp	0
Jamaican jerk seasoning, 1/4 tsp	0
Louisiana style Cajun seasoning, 1/4 tsp	0
Mediterranean seasoning, 1/4 tsp	0
Szechuan seasoning, 1/4 tsp	0
Thai seasoning, 1/4 tsp	0

	POINTS VALUE
T. Marzetti	
Asian sesame salad topper, 1 Tbsp	1
Bac'n almond crunch salad toppings, 1 Tbsp	1
Fruit and nut salad topper, 1 Tbsp	1
Taco Bell Home Originals	
Fajita seasoning mix, 1 Tbsp	1
Taco seasoning mix, 2 tsp	0
Taco seasoning mix, chipotle flavor, 2 tsp	0
Taco seasoning mix, Santa Fe style flavor, 2 tsp	0
Weber	
Chicago steak, dry mix, 1/4 tsp	0
Gourmet burger, dry mix, 1/4 tsp	0
Kidk'n chicken, dry mix, 1/4 tsp	0
N'Orleans Cajun, dry mix, 1/4 tsp	0
Smokey mesquite, dry mix, 1/4 tsp	0
Sweet & tangy bbq, dry mix, 1/4 tsp	0
Zesty lemon seasoning for seafood & chicken, dry mix, 1/4 tsp	0
Zatarain's	
Creole seasoning, 1/8 tsp	0

Vinegars
Carapelli
Balsamic vinegar, 1 Tbsp	0

Eden Organic
Apple cider vinegar, 1 Tbsp	0
Brown rice vinegar, 1 Tbsp	0

OILS, DRESSINGS & SEASONINGS

 Vinegars (con't)

Eden Selected

Red wine vinegar, 1 Tbsp	0
Ume plum vinegar, 1 tsp	0

Fanci Food

Malt vinegar, 1 Tbsp	0
Red wine vinegar, 1 Tbsp	0
White wine vinegar, 1 Tbsp	0
White wine vinegar, raspberry, 1 Tbsp	0
White wine vinegar, tarragon, 1 Tbsp	0

Heinz

Apple cider vinegar, 1 Tbsp	0
Balsamic vinegar, 1 Tbsp	0
Distilled white vinegar, 1 Tbsp	0
Gourmet garlic wine vinegar, 1 Tbsp	0
Gourmet malt vinegar, 1 Tbsp	0
Premium tarragon vinegar, 1 Tbsp	0
Red wine vinegar, 1 Tbsp	0
Salad vinegar, 1 Tbsp	0

Lucini

Gran riserva balsamico vinegar, 1 Tbsp	0
Pinot grigio Italian wine vinegar, 1 Tbsp	0

Manischewitz

Balsamic vinegar, 1 Tbsp	0

Naturally Fresh

Red wine vinegar, 2 Tbsp	0
White wine vinegar, 2 Tbsp	0

Progresso

Balsamic vinegar, 1 Tbsp	0
Garlic flavored vinegar, 1 Tbsp	0
Red wine vinegar, 1 Tbsp	0

Regina

Balsamic vinegar, 1 Tbsp	0
Red wine vinegar, 1 Tbsp	0
Red wine vinegar with garlic, 1 Tbsp	0
White wine vinegar, 1 Tbsp	0

Spectrum Naturals

Apple cider vinegar, organic filtered, 1 Tbsp	0
Apple cider vinegar, organic unfiltered, 1 Tbsp	0
Balsamic vinegar, 1 Tbsp	0
Balsamic vinegar, organic, 1 Tbsp	0
Brown rice vinegar, organic, 1 Tbsp	0
Brown rice vinegar, organic, seasoned, 1 Tbsp	0
Distilled white vinegar, organic, 1 Tbsp	0
Golden balsamic vinegar, organic, 1 Tbsp	0
Red wine vinegar, organic, 1 Tbsp	0
White wine vinegar, organic, 1 Tbsp	0

Tree of Life

Apple cider vinegar, 1 Tbsp	0

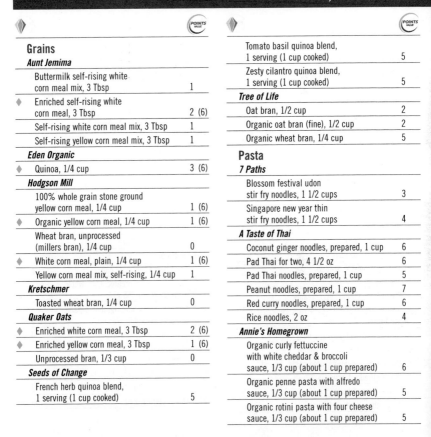

	POINTS VALUE
Grains	
Aunt Jemima	
Buttermilk self-rising white corn meal mix, 3 Tbsp	1
Enriched self-rising white corn meal, 3 Tbsp	2 (6)
Self-rising white corn meal mix, 3 Tbsp	1
Self-rising yellow corn meal mix, 3 Tbsp	1
Eden Organic	
Quinoa, 1/4 cup	3 (6)
Hodgson Mill	
100% whole grain stone ground yellow corn meal, 1/4 cup	1 (6)
Organic yellow corn meal, 1/4 cup	1 (6)
Wheat bran, unprocessed (millers bran), 1/4 cup	0
White corn meal, plain, 1/4 cup	1 (6)
Yellow corn meal mix, self-rising, 1/4 cup	1
Kretschmer	
Toasted wheat bran, 1/4 cup	0
Quaker Oats	
Enriched white corn meal, 3 Tbsp	2 (6)
Enriched yellow corn meal, 3 Tbsp	1 (6)
Unprocessed bran, 1/3 cup	0
Seeds of Change	
French herb quinoa blend, 1 serving (1 cup cooked)	5

	POINTS VALUE
Tomato basil quinoa blend, 1 serving (1 cup cooked)	5
Zesty cilantro quinoa blend, 1 serving (1 cup cooked)	5
Tree of Life	
Oat bran, 1/2 cup	2
Organic oat bran (fine), 1/2 cup	2
Organic wheat bran, 1/4 cup	5
Pasta	
7 Paths	
Blossom festival udon stir fry noodles, 1 1/2 cups	3
Singapore new year thin stir fry noodles, 1 1/2 cups	4
A Taste of Thai	
Coconut ginger noodles, prepared, 1 cup	6
Pad Thai for two, 4 1/2 oz	6
Pad Thai noodles, prepared, 1 cup	5
Peanut noodles, prepared, 1 cup	7
Red curry noodles, prepared, 1 cup	6
Rice noodles, 2 oz	4
Annie's Homegrown	
Organic curly fettuccine with white cheddar & broccoli sauce, 1/3 cup (about 1 cup prepared)	6
Organic penne pasta with alfredo sauce, 1/3 cup (about 1 cup prepared)	5
Organic rotini pasta with four cheese sauce, 1/3 cup (about 1 cup prepared)	5

Pasta (con't)

Asian Rhythms

Pad Thai noodles, 1 cup	7

Azumaya

Thin cut noodles, 1 cup	4
Wide-cut noodles, 1 cup	4

Barilla Plus

Angel hair, 2 oz (dry)	4
Elbows, 2 oz (dry)	4
Penne, 2 oz (dry)	4
Rotini, 2 oz (dry)	4
Spaghetti, 2 oz (dry)	4
Thin spaghetti, 2 oz (dry)	4

Barilla Whole Grain

Penne, 2 oz (dry)	3
Rotini, 2 oz (dry)	3
Spaghetti, 2 oz (dry)	3
Thin spaghetti, 2 oz (dry)	3

Birds Eye

Pasta & vegetables in a creamy cheese sauce, frozen, 1 cup	4

Bowl Appetit!

Cheddar broccoli pasta, 1 bowl	7
Garlic parmesan pasta, 1 bowl	7
Homestyle chicken flavored pasta, 1 bowl	5
Pasta alfredo, 1 bowl	8
Teriyaki rice, 1 bowl	5
Three-cheese rotini, 1 bowl	8

Carapelli

Creamy alfredo with penne, 1 cup	4
Four cheese with cavatappi, 1 cup	4
Roasted garlic & fusilli, 1 cup	4
Roasted red pepper radiatore, 1 cup	4
Tomato & basil gemelli, 1 cup	4
Tomato with spiral, 1 cup	4

Celentano Light

Broccoli stuffed shells, 1	6

Eden

Japanese brown rice udon, 2 oz	3
Lotus root soba, 2 oz	3
Mugwort soba, 2 oz	3
Soba, 2 oz	3
Wild yam soba, 2 oz	3

Eden Organic

Artichoke ribbons, 1/2 cup	4
Flax rice spirals, organic, 60% whole grain, 1 serving (55 g)	3
◆ Kamut & buckwheat rigatoni, organic, 100% whole grain, 1/2 cup	3 (6)
◆ Kamut ditalini, 1/2 cup	4 (6)
◆ Kamut elbows, organic 100% whole grain, 1/2 cup	4 (6)
◆ Kamut soba, organic, 1/2 cup	3 (6)
◆ Kamut spaghetti, 2 oz	3 (6)
◆ Kamut spirals, 2 oz	3 (6)

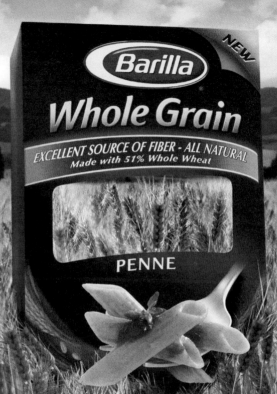

NEW

Barilla

Whole Grain

EXCELLENT SOURCE OF FIBER - ALL NATURAL
Made with 51% Whole Wheat

PENNE

We harvest the great-tasting Whole Grain.
You gather the compliments.

Introducing Barilla Whole Grain.
Taste you love. Nutrition you need. Whole grain pasta you've been waiting for.

PASTA, RICE & GRAINS

Pasta, Eden Organic (con't)	POINTS VALUE
Kamut udon, 1/2 cup	4 (6)
Kamut vegetable spirals, 1/2 cup	4 (6)
Parsley garlic ribbons, 1/2 cup	4
Parsley garlic spaghetti, 1/2 cup	3
Rye spirals, 1/2 cup	3
Saffron ribbons, 1/2 cup	4
Small vegetable shells, 1/2 cup	4
Soba, 1/2 cup	4
Spaghetti, 2 oz	3
Spelt & buckwheat gemelli, organic, 100% whole grain, 1/2 cup	4 (6)
Spelt ribbons, 1/2 cup	4 (6)
Spelt soba, 1/2 cup	4
Spelt spaghetti, 1/2 cup	4 (6)
Spelt udon, organic, 1/2 cup	4 (6)
Spelt ziti rigati, 1/2 cup	4 (6)
Spinach ribbons, 1/2 cup	3
Spinach spirals, 1/2 cup	3
Twisted pair gemelli, 1/2 cup	4 (6)
Udon, wheat and rice, organic, 1/2 cup	4
Vegetable alphabets, organic, 60% whole grain, 1/2 cup	4
Vegetable alphabets, whole grain, 1/2 cup	4
Vegetable ribbons, 1/2 cup	4
Vegetable shells, 1/2 cup	3
Vegetable spirals, 1/2 cup	3
Whole grain udon, 1/2 cup	3

	POINTS VALUE
Eden Selected	
Bifun (rice) pasta, 2 oz	4
Harusame (mung bean) pasta, 2 oz	4
Kuzu pasta, 2 oz	4
Soba - 100% buckwheat, 2 oz	3 (6)
Faraon	
Pasta - alphabet, 1/3 cup	4
Pasta - elbow, 1/4 cup	5
Pasta - fettucini, 1 cup	5
Pasta - fideo fine cut, 1 cup	5
Pasta - macaroni, 1 cup	5
Pasta - ojo perdiz, 1/3 cup	4
Pasta - pens, 1 cup	5
Pasta - rings, 1/3 cup	3
Pasta - shells, 1 cup	5
Pasta - small elbow, 1 cup	5
Pasta - small shells, 1/3 cup	5
Pasta - stars, 1/3 cup	3
Pasta - vermicelli, 1/2 cup	4
Pasta - wheel, 1 cup	5
Food for Life	
Ezekiel 4:9, fettuccini, 2 oz	4
Ezekiel 4:9, linguine, 2 oz	4
Ezekiel 4:9, penne, 2 oz	4
Ezekiel 4:9, spaghetti, 2 oz	4

	POINTS VALUE
Hodgson Mill	
Organic lasagna with milled flax seed, 2 oz	4
Organic whole wheat angel hair with milled flax seed, 2 oz	3
Organic whole wheat fettuccine with milled flax seed, 2 oz	3
Organic whole wheat penne with milled flax seed, 2 oz	3
Organic whole wheat spaghetti with milled flax seed, 2 oz	3
Organic whole wheat spirals with milled flax seed, 2 oz	3
Veggie rotini spirals, 2 oz	4
◆ Whole wheat angel hair pasta, 2 oz	3 (6)
◆ Whole wheat bow tie pasta, 2 oz	3 (6)
◆ Whole wheat egg noodles, 2 oz	3 (6)
◆ Whole wheat elbows, 2 oz	3 (6)
◆ Whole wheat fettuccine, 2 oz	3 (6)
◆ Whole wheat lasagna, 2 oz	3 (6)
◆ Whole wheat medium shells, 2 oz	3 (6)
◆ Whole wheat penne, 2 oz	3 (6)
◆ Whole wheat radiatores, 2 oz	3 (6)
◆ Whole wheat spaghetti, 2 oz	3 (6)
◆ Whole wheat spinach spaghetti, 2 oz	3 (6)
◆ Whole wheat spirals, 2 oz	3 (6)
◆ Whole wheat thin spaghetti, 2 oz	3 (6)
◆ Whole wheat veggie bows, 2 oz (dry)	3 (6)
◆ Whole wheat veggie radiatore, 2 oz	3 (6)

	POINTS VALUE
◆ Whole wheat veggie rotini spirals, 2 oz (dry)	3 (6)
◆ Whole wheat veggie wagon wheels, 2 oz (dry)	3 (6)
◆ Whole wheat yolkless pasta ribbons, 2 oz	3 (6)
Italian Village	
Cavatelli, 1 cup	5
Kraft	
Spaghetti with meat sauce, as packaged, 5 1/2 oz	6
Kraft Noodle Classics	
Savory chicken, prepared, 1 cup	7
Kraft Spaghetti Classics	
Tangy Italian, prepared, 1 cup	4
Manischewitz	
Egg noodle flakes and alphabets, 1/3 cup	4
Egg noodles - fine, medium, wide and bows, 1 1/2 cups	4
Kluski egg noodles, 1 1/4 cups	4
Noodle pudding mix, 1 serving (36 g)	3
◆ Whole grain noodle style pasta, yolk free extra wide, 1 1/4 cups	3
◆ Whole grain noodle style pasta, yolk free medium, 1 1/4 cup	3
Yolk free noodles, extra wide, 1 3/4 cups	4
Yolk free noodles, fine, 1 1/2 cups	4
Yolk free noodles, medium, 1 1/4 cups	4
Yolk free noodles, wide, 1 3/4 cups	4

PASTA, RICE & GRAINS

Pasta (con't)

	POINTS VALUE
Manischewitz Passover Gold	
Egg noodles, extra fine, 2 oz	4
Egg noodles, medium, 2 oz	4
Egg noodles, wide, 2 oz	4
Yolk free, 2 oz	4
Market Day	
Chicken fettuccini alfredo, 1 tray	9
Monterey Pasta Company	
Egg fettuccine, 1 1/4 cups	5
Egg linguine, 1 1/4 cups	5
Organic fettuccine, 1 1/4 cups	5
Organic linguine, 1 1/4 cups	5
Whole wheat fettuccine with flaxseed, 1 1/4 cups	4
Whole wheat linguine with flaxseed, 1 1/4 cups	4
Monterey Pasta Company Whole Wheat Borsellini	
Whole wheat five cheese borsellini, 1 cup	6
Nasoya	
Chinese style noodles, 1 cup	4
Japanese style noodles, 1 cup	4
Near East	
Angel hair pasta with spicy tomato, prepared, 1 serving	5
Couscous Moroccan pasta, prepared, 1 1/4 cups	5
Fusilli pasta with parmesan & romano, prepared, 1 serving	6

	POINTS VALUE
Gemelli pasta with tomato parmesan, prepared, 1 serving	7
Radiatore pasta basil & herb, prepared, 1 serving	5
Vermicelli pasta with roasted garlic & olive oil, prepared, 1 serving	6
Pasta Roni	
Angel hair pasta with herbs, prepared, 1 cup	7
Angel hair pasta with lemon & butter, prepared, 1 cup	8
Angel hair pasta with parmesan cheese, prepared, 1 cup	7
Broccoli au gratin, prepared, 1 cup	6
Broccoli, prepared, 1 cup	8
Chicken & garlic low fat, prepared, 1 cup	4
Chicken, prepared, 1 cup	7
Creamy garlic sauce with corkscrew pasta, prepared, 1 cup	8
Fettuccine alfredo, prepared, 1 cup	11
Fettuccine alfredo, reduced fat, prepared, 1 cup	6
Four cheese sauce with corkscrew pasta, prepared, 1 cup	8
Garlic alfredo, prepared, 1 cup	8
Herb & butter, prepared, 1 cup	7
Homestyle chicken, prepared, 1 cup	5
Linguine with chicken & broccoli, prepared, 1 cup	8

	POINTS VALUE
Linguine with creamy chicken parmesan, prepared, 1 cup	9
Mild cheddar, prepared, 1 cup	6
Parmesano, prepared, 1 cup	5
Romanoff, prepared, 1 cup	9
Shells & white cheddar, prepared, 1 cup	6
Stroganoff, prepared, 1 cup	8
Vermicelli with roasted garlic & olive oil, prepared, 1 cup	8
White cheddar & broccoli sauce with rigatoni, prepared, 1 cup	7
Rosetto	
Cheese stuffed shells, 2 pieces	6
Rosina Presents Celentano	
Cavatelli, 1 cup	5
Schwan's LiveSmart	
Sweet and savory roasted apple orzo, 1 cup	5
Thai Kitchen	
Original pad Thai stir-fry rice noodles mix, 1/2 package	5
Pad Thai with chili stir-fry rice noodles mix, 1/2 package	5
Savory garlic stir-fry rice noodles mix, 1/2 package	5
Stir-fry rice noodles, 2 oz	3
Thai peanut stir-fry rice noodles mix, 1/2 package	5
Thin rice noodles, 1/2 package	8

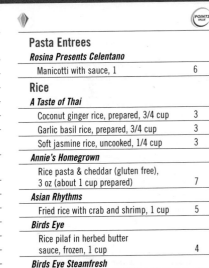

	POINTS VALUE
Pasta Entrees	
Rosina Presents Celentano	
Manicotti with sauce, 1	6
Rice	
A Taste of Thai	
Coconut ginger rice, prepared, 3/4 cup	3
Garlic basil rice, prepared, 3/4 cup	3
Soft jasmine rice, uncooked, 1/4 cup	3
Annie's Homegrown	
Rice pasta & cheddar (gluten free), 3 oz (about 1 cup prepared)	7
Asian Rhythms	
Fried rice with crab and shrimp, 1 cup	5
Birds Eye	
Rice pilaf in herbed butter sauce, frozen, 1 cup	4
Birds Eye Steamfresh	
Long grain white rice, 3/4 cup	3
Long grain white rice with mixed vegetables, 1 cup	3
♦ Whole grain brown rice, 1 cup	3 (6)
Bowl Appetit!	
Cheddar broccoli rice, 1 bowl	6
Herb chicken vegetable rice, 1 bowl	5
Carolina	
♦ Brown long grain rice, uncooked, 1/4 cup	3 (6)
Chicken rice mix, 2 oz (about 1/3 cup rice mix and 1 Tbsp seasoning)	4

PASTA, RICE & GRAINS

Rice, Carolina (con't)

POINTS VALUE

Classic pilaf rice mix, 2 oz (about 1/3 cup rice mix and 3/4 tsp seasoning)	4
Long grain & wild rice mix, 2 oz (about 1/3 cup rice mix and 2 Tbsp seasoning)	3
Long grain rice, uncooked, 1/4 cup	3
Spanish rice mix, 2 oz (about 1/3 cup rice mix and 1 Tbsp seasoning)	3
Spicy saffron yellow, 2 oz (about 1/4 cup rice mix and 2 Tbsp seasoning)	3
Thai jasmine rice, uncooked, 1/4 cup	3
Yellow rice mix, 2 oz (about 1/3 cup rice and 2 tsp seasoning)	4

Carolina Gold

Parboiled long grain rice, uncooked, 1/4 cup	3

Casbah

Rice pilaf, 1 serving (45 g)	3
Spanish pilaf, 1 serving (45 g)	3

Fanci Food

◆ Wild rice, 1/4 cup (unprepared)	3 (6)

Fantastic World Foods

Arborio rice, 1/4 cup	3
Basmati rice, 1/4 cup	3
Jasmine rice, 1/4 cup	3

Faraon

E-Z cook long grain rice, uncooked, 1/4 cup	3
Long grain rice, uncooked, 1/4 cup	3

POINTS VALUE

Gourmet House

◆ Canadian lake & river wild rice, 1/4 cup (dry)	3 (6)
◆ Minnesota cultivated wild rice, 1/4 cup (dry)	3 (6)

Green Giant

Cheesy rice & broccoli, frozen, 1 package	5

Mahatma

Basmati, 1/4 cup (dry)	3
Beef rice mix, 2 oz (about 1/4 cup rice mix and 1.5 Tbsp seasoning)	4
Broccoli & cheese rice mix, 2 oz (about 1/3 cup rice mix and 1/4 cup seasoning)	4
◆ Brown long grain rice, uncooked, 1/4 cup	3 (6)
Chicken rice mix, 2 oz (about 1/3 cup rice mix and 1 Tbsp seasoning)	4
Classic pilaf rice mix, 2 oz (about 1/3 cup rice mix and 3/4 tsp seasoning)	4
Long grain & wild rice mix, 2 oz (about 1/3 cup rice mix and 2 Tbsp seasoning)	3
Long grain rice, uncooked, 1/4 cup	3
Nacho cheese rice mix, 2 1/2 oz (about 1/4 cup rice mix and 3 Tbsp seasoning)	5
Spanish rice mix, 2 oz (about 1/3 cup rice mix and 1 Tbsp seasoning)	3
Spicy saffron yellow, 2 oz (about 1/4 cup rice mix and 2 Tbsp seasoning)	3
Thai jasmine rice, uncooked, 1/4 cup	3
Yellow rice mix, 2 oz (about 1/3 cup rice mix and 2 tsp seasoning)	4

	POINTS VALUE
Mahatma Gold	
Parboiled long grain rice, uncooked, 1/4 cup	3
Manischewitz	
Lentil pilaf mix, 1/4 cup	2
Rice pilaf mix, 1/4 cup	3
Spanish pilaf mix, 1/4 cup	3
Market Day	
Vegetable fried rice, 1 cup	2
Wild rice blend, 3/4 cup	2
Marrakesh Express	
Parmesan cheese, 1 cup	4
Roasted red pepper, 1 cup	4
Sun dried tomato and herb, 1 cup	4
Wild mushroom, 1 cup	4
Minute	
Enriched pre-cooked boil-in-bag long grain white rice, prepared, 1 cup	4
Enriched pre-cooked boil-in-bag long grain white rice, 1/2 bag (dry, 1 cup cooked)	4
Instant enriched long grain white rice, prepared, 1 cup	3
Instant enriched premium long grain white rice, prepared, 1 cup	3
♦ Instant whole grain brown rice, prepared, 2/3 cup	3 (6)
Instant, enriched, long grain premium rice, 1/2 cup (dry, 1 cup cooked)	4

	POINTS VALUE
Instant, enriched, long grain white rice, 1/2 cup (dry, 1 cup cooked)	4
♦ Instant, whole grain brown rice, 1/2 cup (dry, 2/3 cup cooked)	3 (6)
Minute Ready to Serve	
Chicken rice mix, 1 container (approx. 1 cup)	4
Long grain & wild rice mix, 1 container (approx. 1 cup)	4
Long grain white rice, 1 container (approx. 1 cup)	4
Natural whole grain brown rice fully cooked, 1 container (approx. 1 cup)	3 (6)
Yellow rice mix with real saffron, 1 container (approx. 1 cup)	4
Near East	
Brown rice pilaf mix, prepared, 1 cup	4
Chicken rice pilaf mix, prepared, 1 cup	4
Curry rice pilaf mix, prepared, 1 cup	4
Garlic & herb pilaf mix, prepared, 1 cup	4
Lentil pilaf mix, prepared, 1 cup	3
Long grain and wild rice pilaf mix, prepared, 1 cup	4
Spanish rice pilaf mix, prepared, 1 cup	6
Toasted almond pilaf mix, prepared, 1 cup	5
Wheat pilaf mix, prepared, 1 cup	4
Wild mushroom & herb pilaf mix, prepared, 1 cup	4

Rice (con't)

	POINTS VALUE
Near East Creative Grains	
Chicken & herbs, prepared, 1 cup	5
Creamy parmesan, prepared, 1 cup	6
Roasted garlic, prepared, 1 cup	4
Roasted pecan & garlic, prepared, 1 cup	5
Old El Paso	
Cheesy Mexican rice, as packaged, 1/3 package	5
Cheesy Mexican rice, prepared, 1 serving (1/3 package)	6
Spanish rice, as packaged, 1/3 package	5
Spanish rice, prepared, 1 serving (1/3 package)	6
Rice-A-Roni	
Beef & mushroom, prepared, 1 cup	6
Beef flavor, 1/3 less salt, prepared, 1 cup	5
Beef flavor, prepared, 1 cup	7
Broccoli au gratin, 1/3 less salt, prepared, 1 cup	7
Broccoli, prepared, 1 cup	6
Chicken & broccoli, prepared, 1 cup	5
Chicken & garlic, prepared, 1 cup	6
Chicken & vegetables, prepared, 1 cup	6
Chicken flavor, 1/3 less salt, prepared, 1 cup	6
Chicken flavor, prepared, 1 cup	7
Chicken teriyaki, prepared, 1 cup	5

	POINTS VALUE
Chicken with mushrooms, prepared, 1 cup	8
Chicken, low fat, prepared, 1 cup	4
Fried rice, 1/3 less salt, prepared, 1 cup	5
Fried rice, prepared, 1 cup	7
Garden vegetable rice, prepared, 1 cup	6
Herb & butter, prepared, 1 cup	7
Herb roasted chicken, prepared, 1 cup	6
Lemon chicken rice, prepared, 1 cup	5
Long grain & wild chicken almonds, prepared, 1 cup	6
Long grain & wild rice original, prepared, 1 cup	5
Long grain & wild rice pilaf, prepared, 1 cup	5
Mexican style, prepared, 1 cup	5
Oriental stir fry, prepared, 1 cup	6
Rice pilaf, prepared, 1 cup	7
Savory chicken vegetable, low fat, prepared, 1 cup	4
Spanish rice, prepared, 1 cup	5
Stroganoff, prepared, 1 cup	8
White cheddar & herbs, prepared, 1 cup	8
Rice-A-Roni Cheesy Pleasers	
Country cheddar, prepared, 1 cup	8
Creamy 4 cheese, 1 cup	6
Parmesan chicken rice, prepared, 1 cup	8

	POINTS VALUE
Rice-A-Roni Savory Whole Grain	
Chicken & herbs rice, prepared, 1 cup	5
Roasted garlic rice, prepared, 1 cup	6
Spanish rice, prepared, 1 cup	5
Riceland	
Extra long grain rice, uncooked, 1/4 cup	3
Gold - perfected rice, cooked, 1 cup	3
Gold - perfected rice, uncooked, 1/4 cup	3
Long grain rice, cooked, 3/4 cup	3
Long grain rice, uncooked, 1/4 cup	3
Medium grain rice, cooked, 3/4 cup	3
Medium grain rice, uncooked, 1/4 cup	3
◆ Natural brown rice, cooked, 3/4 cup	3 (6)
◆ Natural brown rice, uncooked, 1/4 cup	3 (6)
Perfected rice, uncooked, 1/4 cup	3
Riceland Rice 'N Easy	
Broccoli & cheese, as packaged, 2 oz	4
Cajun, as packaged, 2 oz	3
Chicken, as packaged, 2 oz	4
Seeds of Change	
Moroccan lentil rice pilaf, 1 serving (1 cup cooked)	3
Seven grain pilaf blend, 1 serving (1 cup cooked)	5
Success 10 Minute	
Jasmine rice, 1/4 cup (dry)	3

	POINTS VALUE
Success Rice	
◆ Brown rice, 1/2 cup	3 (6)
Jasmine rice, boil-in-bag, 1/4 cup (3/4 cup prepared)	3
Natural long grain rice, 1/2 cup	4
Success Whole Grain Brown Rice Mix	
Creamy cheddar & broccoli, 1 serving (1/2 cup rice with 1 Tbsp seasoning, 1 cup prepared)	5
Herb roasted chicken, 1 serving (1/2 cup rice with 1 Tbsp seasoning, 1 cup prepared)	4
Multigrain pilaf, 1 serving (1/2 cup rice with 1 Tbsp seasoning, 1 cup prepared)	4
Portobello mushroom, 1 serving (1/2 cup rice with 1 Tbsp seasoning, 1 cup prepared)	4
Southwest chipotle, 1 serving (1/2 cup rice with 1 Tbsp seasoning, 1 cup prepared)	4
Sunsun	
Enriched long grain rice, uncooked, 1/4 cup	3
Thai Kitchen	
Jasmine rice mix, green chili & garlic, prepared, 1 cup (cooked)	5
Jasmine rice mix, lemongrass & ginger, prepared, 1 cup (prepared)	5

Rice, Thai Kitchen (con't)

	POINTS VALUE
Jasmine rice mix, roasted garlic & chili, prepared, 1 cup (cooked)	4
Jasmine rice mix, spicy Thai chili, prepared, 1 cup (cooked)	5
Jasmine rice mix, sweet chili & onion, prepared, 1 cup (cooked)	6
Jasmine rice mix, Thai yellow curry, prepared, 1 cup (cooked)	5
Jasmine rice select harvest, prepared, 1/2 cup (cooked)	3

Tony Chachere's

	POINTS VALUE
Creole dirty rice mix, 1/3 cup	3
Creole gumbo dinner mix, 2 Tbsp	1
Creole jambalaya dinner mix, 1/4 cup	3
Creole rice & gravy dinner mix, 1/4 cup	4

Uncle Ben's

	POINTS VALUE
Boil-in-bag rice, 1/3 cup	4
Enriched long grain instant rice, 1 cup	4
◆ Fast & natural instant whole grain, 1 cup	3
Long grain & wild rice fast cook, butter & herb, 2 oz (dry, or 1 cup cooked)	4
Long grain & wild rice, fast cook recipe, 2 oz (dry, or 1 cup cooked)	4
Long grain & wild rice, original recipe, 2 oz (dry, or 1 cup cooked)	4
Long grain & wild rice, roasted garlic & olive oil, 2 oz (dry, or 1 cup cooked)	3
Long grain & wild rice, vegetable pilaf, 2 oz (dry, or 1 cup cooked)	3

	POINTS VALUE
Long grain & wild sun-dried tomato florentine, 2 oz (dry, or 1 cup cooked)	3
◆ Natural whole grain brown rice, 1 cup	3
Original converted brand rice, 1 cup	3
Whole grain brown & wild rice, mushroom recipe, 2 oz (dry, or1 cup cooked)	4

Uncle Ben's Country Inn

	POINTS VALUE
Broccoli rice au gratin, 2 oz (dry, or 1 cup cooked)	4
Chicken, 2 oz (dry, or 1 cup cooked)	4
Chicken & broccoli, 2 oz (dry, or 1 cup cooked)	4
Chicken & vegetable, 2 oz (dry, or 1 cup cooked)	4
Chicken & wild, 2 oz (dry, or 1 cup cooked)	4
Mexican fiesta, 2 oz (dry, or 1 cup cooked)	4
Oriental fried rice, 2 oz (dry, or 1 cup cooked)	4
Rice pilaf, 2 oz (dry, or 1 cup cooked)	4

Uncle Ben's Ready Complete Meals

	POINTS VALUE
Asian style stir fried rice with chicken, 1 bowl	7
Long grain & wild rice with chicken, 1 bowl	7
Mexican style rice with beef, 1 bowl	7

Uncle Ben's Ready Rice Pouch

	POINTS VALUE
Butter & garlic flavored rice, 1 cup (cooked)	4
Cajun style with red beans & bell peppers, 1 cup (cooked)	4

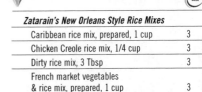

	POINTS VALUE
Chicken flavored whole grain brown, 1 cup (cooked)	4
Creamy four cheese flavored with vermicelli, 1 cup (cooked)	4
Garden vegetable with peas, carrots & corn, 1 cup (cooked)	4
Long grain & wild with 23 herbs & seasonings, 1 cup (cooked)	4
Original enriched long grain white rice, 1 cup (cooked)	4
Rice pilaf with orzo pasta, 1 cup (cooked)	4
Roasted chicken flavored with carrots & herbs, 1 cup (cooked)	4
Spanish style with tomatoes & peppers, 1 cup (cooked)	4
Teriyaki style with peas & carrots, 1 cup (cooked)	4
Whole grain brown rice, 1 cup (cooked)	5
Uncle Ben's Ready Whole Grain Medley Pouch	
Brown & wild rice, wild rice & red rice perfectly seasoned with herbs & spices, 1 cup (cooked)	4
Santa Fe brown rice, red & white wheat, black beans, corn, peppers, cilantro & seasonings, 1 cup (cooked)	4
Vegetable harvest, 1 cup (cooked)	4
Zapata	
Spanish rice, 2/3 cup	1

	POINTS VALUE
Zatarain's New Orleans Style Rice Mixes	
Caribbean rice mix, prepared, 1 cup	3
Chicken Creole rice mix, 1/4 cup	3
Dirty rice mix, 3 Tbsp	3
French market vegetables & rice mix, prepared, 1 cup	3
Garlic & herb rice mix, 1/4 cup	2
Gumbo mix, 2 Tbsp	1
Jambalaya mix, 3 Tbsp	3
Long grain & wild rice mix, 2 1/2 Tbsp	2
Spanish rice mix, 2 Tbsp	1
Yellow rice mix, 2 1/3 Tbsp	2

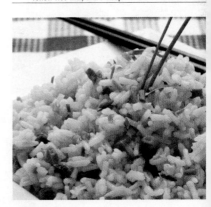

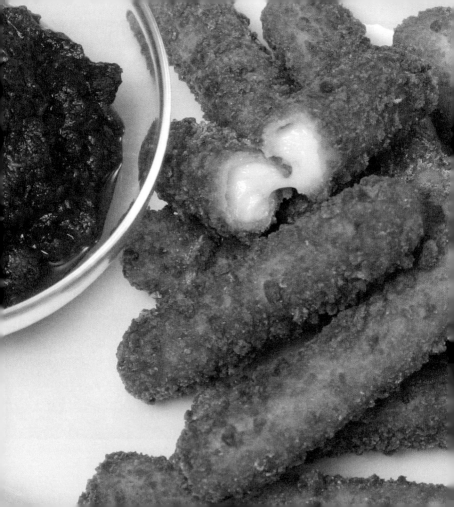

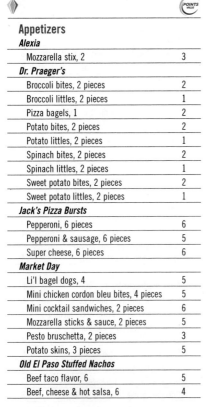

	POINTS VALUE
Appetizers	
Alexia	
Mozzarella stix, 2	3
Dr. Praeger's	
Broccoli bites, 2 pieces	2
Broccoli littles, 2 pieces	1
Pizza bagels, 1	2
Potato bites, 2 pieces	2
Potato littles, 2 pieces	1
Spinach bites, 2 pieces	2
Spinach littles, 2 pieces	1
Sweet potato bites, 2 pieces	2
Sweet potato littles, 2 pieces	1
Jack's Pizza Bursts	
Pepperoni, 6 pieces	6
Pepperoni & sausage, 6 pieces	5
Super cheese, 6 pieces	6
Market Day	
Li'l bagel dogs, 4	5
Mini chicken cordon bleu bites, 4 pieces	5
Mini cocktail sandwiches, 2 pieces	6
Mozzarella sticks & sauce, 2 pieces	5
Pesto bruschetta, 2 pieces	3
Potato skins, 3 pieces	5
Old El Paso Stuffed Nachos	
Beef taco flavor, 6	5
Beef, cheese & hot salsa, 6	4

	POINTS VALUE
Beef, cheese & mild salsa, 6	4
Chicken, cheese & salsa, 6	5
Nacho cheese, 6	4
Ore-Ida Bagel Bites	
Cheese & pepperoni, 4 pieces	4
Cheese, sausage & pepperoni, 4 pieces	4
Nacho cheese, 4 pieces	5
Supreme bagel bites, 4 pieces	4
Ultra five cheese, 4 pieces	5
Ore-Ida Stuffed Bagel Bites	
Pepperoni and cheese, 6 pieces	5
Three cheese, 4 pieces	4
Oscar Mayer Lunchables	
Cheese & salsa nacho lunch, 1 package	9
Phillips	
Crab & shrimp spring rolls, 3 (with 3/4 oz sauce)	4
Poppers	
Cheddar cheese stuffed jalapeños, 1 serving (76 g)	5
Cheddar cheese stuffed jalapeños, 1 serving (98 g)	7
Cream cheese stuffed jalapeños, 1 serving (77 g)	6
Cream cheese stuffed jalapeños, 1 serving (98 g)	7
Mozzarella nuggets, 3 pieces	2
Mozzarella sticks, 1 piece	2
Mozzarella sticks, 1 piece	2

PREPARED FOODS, SALADS & SIDES

Appetizers (con't)	POINTS VALUE

T.G.I. Friday's

Broccoli & cheddar potato skins, 3 pieces	4
Cheddar & bacon potato skins, 3 pieces	5
Cheddar & bacon potato skins, 2 pieces	3
Four cheese & pepperoni potato skins, 3 pieces	5
Mozzarella sticks with marinara sauce, 1 serving (1 mozzarella stick and 1 Tbsp sauce)	3

Thyme & Truffles Hors D'oeuvres

Cold canape assortment, 1 piece	2
Cranberry pecan spirals, 1 piece	2
Hors d'oeuvres party assortment, 1 piece	2
Mushroom leek crescent, 1 piece	2
Shrimp puff, 1 piece	2

Corn dog
Oscar Mayer

Corn dogs made with turkey, pork & chicken, 1	5

Dinner, refrigerated
Tyson

Carved turkey breast in gravy, 5 oz	4
Chicken breast medallions in marsala sauce, 4 oz	4
Chicken breast medallions in sesame teriyaki sauce, 4 oz	4
Chicken breast medallions in sweet roasted garlic sauce, 5 oz	4
Chicken breast medallions in Szechwan sauce, 5 oz	4
Pork roast with vegetables meal kit, 4 oz	8
Seasoned beef meatloaf, 5 oz	8

Egg Entrees
Market Day

Bacon quiche, 1 serving (1/8 quiche)	8
Breakfast casserole, 1/2 cup	4

Ethnic Entrees
7 Paths

Behind the temple mild curry noodle dinner for two, 1 cup (cooked)	4
Bye bye Bangkok spicy peanut noodle steamer, 1 bowl	6
Escape from Tokyo honey sesame noodle steamers, 1 bowl	4
Golden Gai sesame udon noodle dinner for two, 1 cup (cooked)	4

Amy's

Asian noodle stir-fry, 1	6
Black bean burrito, 1 package	5
Black bean tamale verde whole meal, 1	7
Black bean vegetable enchilada, 1 serving (4.75 oz)	4
Breakfast burrito, 1 package	5
Burrito - non dairy, 1 package	5
Burrito especial, 1 package	5
Cheddar cheese burrito, 1 package	6

	POINTS VALUE
Cheese enchilada, 1 serving (4.5 oz)	6
Cheese tamale verde whole meal, 1	8
Family size black bean vegetable enchilada, 1 serving (5 oz)	3
Family size cheese enchilada, 1 serving (4.8 oz)	5
Indian mattar paneer, 1 serving	6
Indian mattar tofu, 1 serving	5
Indian palak paneer, 1 serving (10 oz)	5
Indian paneer tikka, 1 serving	7
Indian samosa wrap, 1 serving	5
Indian spinach tofu wrap, 1 serving	7
Indian vegetable korma, 1 serving	6
Light in sodium black bean vegetable enchilada, 1/2	3
Light in sodium Indian mattar paneer, 1	6
Light in sodium Mexican casserole bowl, 1	8
Light in sodium refried black beans, 1/2 cup	2
Light in sodium traditional refried beans, 1/2 cup	2
Mexican quesadilla kids meal, 1	9
Mexican tamale pie, 1	2
Southwestern burrito, 1	6
Thai stir-fry, 1	6

Amy's Bowls

Mexican casserole bowl, 1 container	10
Santa Fe enchilada, 1 container	7
Teriyaki, 1 container	5

Amy's Whole Meals

	POINTS VALUE
Black bean enchilada, 1 serving (10 oz)	6
Cheese enchilada, 1 serving (9 oz)	7
Tortilla casserole & black beans bowl, 1	9

Asian Rhythms

Crab rangoon, 4 pieces	5
Crab rangoon, sweet chili sauce only, 2 Tbsp	1
Crispy dim sum, shrimp money bag, 4 pieces	4
Crispy dim sum, shrimp spring roll, 3 pieces	4
Crispy dim sum, shrimp wonton, 4 pieces	4
Crispy dim sum, sweet chili sauce only, 2 Tbsp	1
Ginger shrimp, sweet chili sauce only, 2 Tbsp	1
Steamed dim sum, seafood shumai, 4 pieces	2
Steamed dim sum, shrimp hagao, 4 pieces	3
Steamed dim sum, shrimp shumai, 4 pieces	2
Steamed dim sum, vinegar soy sauce only, 1 Tbsp	0
Thai green curry, 1 cup	6
Thai red curry sauce & jasmine rice, 1 cup	6

Betty Crocker Cookbook Favorites

Chipotle chicken with Mexican rice, prepared, 1 cup	8

Ethnic Entrees (con't)

	POINTS VALUE
Birds Eye Voila!	
Beef lo mein, 1 cup (cooked)	4
Chicken fajita, 1 serving (2 1/4 cups frozen, 1 cup cooked)	3
Chicken parmesan, 1 cup (cooked)	5
Birds Eye Voila! Family Skillets	
Alfredo chicken, 1 cup (cooked)	6
Cascadian Farm	
◆ Organic Chinese-style stir fry blend, 3/4 cup	0
◆ Organic Thai-style stir fry blend, 3/4 cup	0
Chicken Helper	
Cheesy chicken enchilada, prepared, 1 cup	7
Chicken fried rice, prepared, 1 cup	6
Eden Organic	
Refried black beans, 1/2 cup	2
Refried blacksoy & black beans, 1/2 cup	1
Refried kidney beans, 1/2 cup	1
Refried pinto beans, 1/2 cup	1
Spicy refried black beans, 1/2 cup	2
Spicy refried pinto beans, 1/2 cup	1
Ethnic Gourmet Taste of Greece	
Kotopoulo domato ke feta, 1 package	8
Ethnic Gourmet Taste of India	
Bean masala, 1 package	7
Chicken biryani over brown rice, 1 package	8
Chicken korma, 1 package	7

	POINTS VALUE
Chicken tandoori with spinach, 1 package	3
Chicken tikka masala, 1 package	4
Eggplant bharta, 1 package	6
Gujarati vegetable curry, 1 package	10
Palak paneer, 1 package	5
Shahi paneer, 1 package	13
Vegetable korma, 1 package	6
Ethnic Gourmet Taste of Italy	
Chicken arrabiata with penne, 1 package	7
Ethnic Gourmet Taste of Malaysia	
Malay chicken curry, 1 package	9
Ethnic Gourmet Taste of Santa Fe	
Chili relleno with mango salsa, 1 package	5
Ethnic Gourmet Taste of Thai	
Chicken pad Thai, 1 package	8
aeng kari kai, 1 package	9
Lemongrass & basil chicken, 1 package	8
Pad Thai with shrimp, 1 package	8
Pad Thai with tofu, 1 package	8
Fantastic World Foods	
Falafel, 1/4 cup	2
Instant refried beans, 1/4 cup	2
Green Giant Create A Meal!	
Stir fry sesame, prepared with chicken & oil, 1 cup	5
Stir fry teriyaki, as packaged, 1 1/2 cups	0
Stir-fry lo mein, as packaged, 2 cups	2

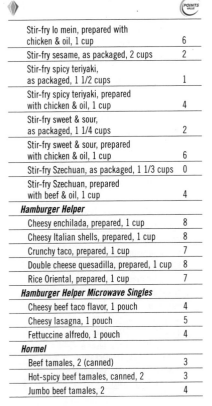

	POINTS VALUE
Stir-fry lo mein, prepared with chicken & oil, 1 cup	6
Stir-fry sesame, as packaged, 2 cups	2
Stir-fry spicy teriyaki, as packaged, 1 1/2 cups	1
Stir-fry spicy teriyaki, prepared with chicken & oil, 1 cup	4
Stir-fry sweet & sour, as packaged, 1 1/4 cups	2
Stir-fry sweet & sour, prepared with chicken & oil, 1 cup	6
Stir-fry Szechuan, as packaged, 1 1/3 cups	0
Stir-fry Szechuan, prepared with beef & oil, 1 cup	4
Hamburger Helper	
Cheesy enchilada, prepared, 1 cup	8
Cheesy Italian shells, prepared, 1 cup	8
Crunchy taco, prepared, 1 cup	7
Double cheese quesadilla, prepared, 1 cup	8
Rice Oriental, prepared, 1 cup	7
Hamburger Helper Microwave Singles	
Cheesy beef taco flavor, 1 pouch	4
Cheesy lasagna, 1 pouch	5
Fettuccine alfredo, 1 pouch	4
Hormel	
Beef tamales, 2 (canned)	3
Hot-spicy beef tamales, canned, 2	3
Jumbo beef tamales, 2	4

	POINTS VALUE
Hormel Individual Canned Servings	
Beef tamales, 1 can	4
Kashi	
Sweet & sour chicken, 1 package	6
Market Day	
Baked manicotti, 1	6
Carnitas enchiladas, 1 serving (12 oz)	12
Egg rolls with sauce, 3 pieces	7
Vegetable lasagna ratatouille, 1 serving (11.4 oz)	3
Monterey Pasta Company	
Artichoke & cheese borsellini, 1 cup	5
Garlic basil ravioli, 1 cup	6
Italian sausage borsellini, 1 cup	6
Made with organic spinach & cheese ravioli, 1 cup	5
Made with organic tomato basil mozzarella ravioli, 1 cup	6
Potato parmesan gnocchi, 1 cup	3
Snow crab ravioli with dill, 1 cup	5
Spinach mushroom tortelloni, 1 cup	5
Tri-color roasted chicken tortelloni, 1 cup	5
Mrs. T's	
4 cheese mini pierogies, 7	3
4 cheese pierogies, 3	5
American cheese pierogies, 3	5
Broccoli & cheese pierogies, 3	4

PREPARED FOODS, SALADS & SIDES

Ethnic Entrees, Mrs. T's (con't)	POINTS VALUE
Cheddar & bacon mini pierogies, 7	3
Cheddar & jalapeño pierogies, 3	4
Cheddar & real bacon mini pierogies, 7	3
Potato & cheddar mini pierogies, 7	3
Potato & cheddar pierogies, 3	4
Potato & onion pierogies, 3	3
Sauerkraut pierogies, 3	3
Sour cream & chive pierogies, 3	4

Near East

Falafel vegetarian patty mix, prepared, 5 patties	3

Old El Paso

Burrito dinner, prepared, 1	6
Fajita dinner no fuss, prepared, 2	7
◆ Refried beans, fat free, 1/2 cup	1 (5)
◆ Refried beans, spicy, fat free, 1/2 cup	1 (5)
Refried beans, traditional, 1/2 cup	1
◆ Refried beans, vegetarian, 1/2 cup	1
Soft taco dinner kit, prepared with chicken breast, 2	7
Soft taco dinner, prepared with ground beef, 2 tacos	8
Southwest style taco dinner, prepared with lean ground beef, 2 tacos	10
Southwest style taco dinner, ranch sauce & seasoning mix, prepared with chicken breast, 2	9
Stand 'n stuff taco dinner, prepared tacos with chicken breast, 2 tacos	7

	POINTS VALUE
Stand 'n stuff taco dinner, prepared tacos with lean ground beef, 2 tacos	8
Taco dinner, prepared tacos with chicken breast, 2 tacos	5
Taco dinner, prepared with ground beef, 2 tacos	6
Taco dinner, prepared, hard, 2 tacos	6
Taco dinner, prepared, soft, 2 tacos	7

Old El Paso Complete Skillet Meal

Crunchy enchilada style rice & chicken, as packaged, 1 serving (1/5 package)	4
Mexican style cheesy rice & beef, as packaged, 1 serving (1/5 package)	5

Schwan's LiveSmart

Chicken lo mein express bowl, 1 bowl	8
Oriental beef and broccoli with rice, 1 cup	6

Seeds of Change

Moroccan lentil tagine (with tomato sauce, pasta & vegetables), 1 tray	6
Spicy Thai peanut noodle, 1 tray	7
Spicy Yucatan frijoles & vegetables, 1 tray	6

Simply Asia

Ready in 10 minutes, chili garlic noodles, 1/3 package	6
Ready in 10 minutes, sesame teriyaki noodles, 1/3 package	6
Ready in 10 minutes, soy ginger noodles, 1/3 package	6

	POINTS VALUE
Ready in 10 minutes, spicy Kung Pao, 1/3 package	6
Ready in 10 minutes, spicy Szechwan noodles, 1/3 package	6
Ready in 10 minutes, toasted sesame garlic noodles, 1/3 package	7
Ready in 15 minutes, honey teriyaki stir-fry meal, 1/2 cup	5
Ready in 15 minutes, mandarin orange stir-fry meal, 1/2 cup	4
Ready in 15 minutes, spicy Kung Pao, 1/2 cup	4
Simply Asia Noodle Bowl	
Mandarin orange, 1 bowl	8
Roasted peanut, 1 bowl	11
Sesame teriyaki, 1 bowl	8
Soy ginger, 1 bowl	8
Spicy Kung Pao, 1 bowl	8
Spicy Mongolian, 1 bowl	9
Simply Asia Quick Noodles	
Honey teriyaki, 1 tray	8
Pad Thai, 1 tray	9
Sweet & sour chow mein, 1 tray	8
Szechwan garlic chow mein, 1 tray	9
Simply Asia Take Out	
Honey teriyaki, 1/2 box	5
Pad Thai, 1/2 box	5
Roasted peanut, 1/2 box	7

	POINTS VALUE
Spicy Kung Pao, 1/2 box	5
Sweet & sour chow mein, 1/2 box	5
Szechwan garlic chow mein, 1/2 box	5
T.G.I. Friday's	
Chicken quesadilla rolls, 2 pieces	6
Southwestern egg rolls, 1 piece	5
Steak quesadillas, 2 pieces	4
Taco Bell Home Originals	
Cheesy double decker taco dinner, prepared, 1	8
Fajita dinner, prepared, 2	8
♦ Fat free refried beans, 1/2 cup	1
♦ Fat free refried beans with mild green chilies, 1/2 cup	1
Refried beans, 1/2 cup	2
Soft taco dinner, prepared, 2	8
Taco dinner, prepared, 2	6
Ultimate nachos, prepared, 1/4 kit	6
Tamarind Tree	
Channa dal masala, 1 package	5
Dal makhani, 1 package	6
Thai Kitchen	
Garlic & roasted pepper rice noodles & sauce, 1/2 package	5
Ginger & sweet chili rice noodles & sauce, 1/2 package	5
Lemongrass & chili stir-fry rice noodles with seasoning, 1/2 package	6

PREPARED FOODS, SALADS & SIDES

Ethnic Entrees, Thai Kitchen (con't)

	POINTS VALUE
Original Pad Thai rice noodles & sauce, 1/2 package	5
Original pad Thai stir-fry rice noodles with sauce, 1/2 package	7
Stir-fry rice noodles with sauce, Thai curry, 1/2 package	6
Tangy sweet & sour rice noodles & sauce, 1/2 package	5
Thai basil & chili rice noodles & sauce, 1/2 package	5
Thai peanut rice noodles & sauce, 1/2 package	6
Thai peanut stir-fry rice noodles with seasoning, 1/2 packet	7
Toasted sesame stir-fry rice noodles with seasoning, 1/2 package	7

Thai Kitchen Noodle Cart

Pad Thai instant rice noodles & sauce, 1 package	5
Roasted garlic instant rice noodles & sauce, 1 package	5
Thai peanut instant rice noodles & sauce, 1 package	5
Toasted sesame instant rice noodles & sauce, 1 package	5

Thyme & Truffles Hors D'oeuvres

Mini quesadillas, 1 piece	1
Spanakopita, 1 piece	2

	POINTS VALUE
Tyson	
Beef steak fajita kit, 1 serving (1 fajita)	4
Beef steak quesadilla fresh meal kit, 1 serving (1 quesadilla)	6
Chicken enchilada meal kit, 1	5
Chicken fajita meal kit, 1	2
Chicken fried rice meal kit, 2 1/2 cups	9
Chicken quesadillas meal kit, 1	5
Chicken stir fry meal kit, 2 3/4 cups	8
Wanchai Ferry	
Cashew chicken, prepared, 1 serving (1/6 package)	7
Kung pao chicken, prepared, 1 serving (1/5 package)	7
Sweet & sour chicken, prepared, 1 serving (1/6 package)	6
Weight Watchers Smart Ones	
Chicken enchilada suiza, 1 package	6
Chicken oriental, 1 package	4
Szechuan style vegetables & chicken, 1 package	4
Traditional lasagna with meat sauce, 1 package	6
Weight Watchers Smart Ones Anytime Selections	
Calzone Italiano, 1 serving (283 g)	6
Chicken and cheese quesadilla, 1 serving (226 g)	4

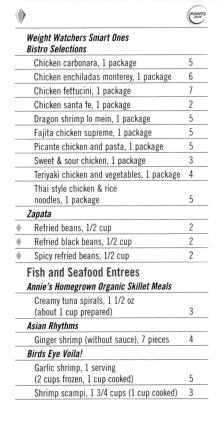

Weight Watchers Smart Ones Bistro Selections

	POINTS VALUE
Chicken carbonara, 1 package	5
Chicken enchiladas monterey, 1 package	6
Chicken fettucini, 1 package	7
Chicken santa fe, 1 package	2
Dragon shrimp lo mein, 1 package	5
Fajita chicken supreme, 1 package	5
Picante chicken and pasta, 1 package	5
Sweet & sour chicken, 1 package	3
Teriyaki chicken and vegetables, 1 package	4
Thai style chicken & rice noodles, 1 package	5

Zapata

Refried beans, 1/2 cup	2
Refried black beans, 1/2 cup	2
Spicy refried beans, 1/2 cup	2

Fish and Seafood Entrees
Annie's Homegrown Organic Skillet Meals

Creamy tuna spirals, 1 1/2 oz (about 1 cup prepared)	3

Asian Rhythms

Ginger shrimp (without sauce), 7 pieces	4

Birds Eye Voila!

Garlic shrimp, 1 serving (2 cups frozen, 1 cup cooked)	5
Shrimp scampi, 1 3/4 cups (1 cup cooked)	3

Gorton's Grilled Salmon

	POINTS VALUE
Classic grilled, 1 fillet	2
Lemon butter, 1 fillet	2

Gorton's Shrimp Bowl

Alfredo, 1 bowl	5
Fried rice, 1 bowl	7
Garlic butter, 1 bowl	5
Teriyaki, 1 bowl	6

Kashi

Lime cilantro shrimp, 1 package	5

Market Day

Fish & chips, 1 serving (2 fillets, 4 oz fries, 2 Tbsp tartar sauce)	13

Oven Poppers

Cod augratin, 1 piece	5
Cod stuffed with broccoli & cheese, 1 piece	3
Crab stuffed flounder, 1 piece	6
Crab stuffed sole, 1 piece	6
Flounder augratin, 1 piece	5
Flounder stuffed with broccoli & cheese, 1 piece	3
Flounder stuffed with garlic, shrimp & almonds, 1 piece	6
Salmon stuffed with spinach & cheese, 1 piece	7
Sole stuffed with garlic, shrimp & almonds, 1 piece	6
Sole stuffed with lump crabmeat, 1 piece	5

Fish and Seafood Entrees, Oven Poppers (con't)

	POINTS VALUE
Sole stuffed with shrimp & lobster in newburg sauce, 1 piece	4
Sole with spinach & cheese, 1/2 container	5
Tilapia stuffed with sun dried tomato, shrimp & lobster, 1 piece	4

Tuna Helper

Cheesy pasta, prepared, 1 cup	7
Cheesy pasta, reduced fat recipe, prepared, 1 cup	5
Creamy broccoli, prepared, 1 cup	7
Creamy broccoli, reduced fat recipe, prepared, 1 cup	5
Creamy parmesan, prepared, 1 cup	6
Creamy parmesan, reduced fat recipe, prepared, 1 cup	5
Creamy pasta, prepared, 1 cup	7
Creamy pasta, reduced fat recipe, prepared, 1 cup	6
Creamy roasted garlic, prepared, 1 cup	7
Creamy roasted garlic, reduced fat recipe, prepared, 1 cup	5
Fettuccine alfredo, prepared, 1 cup	7
Fettuccine alfredo, reduced fat recipe, prepared, 1 cup	5
Tetrazzini, prepared, 1 cup	7
Tetrazzini, reduced fat recipe, prepared, 1 cup	4
Tuna melt, prepared, 1 cup	6
Tuna melt, reduced fat recipe, prepared, 1 cup	5

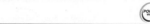

	POINTS VALUE

Weight Watchers Smart Ones

Shrimp marinara with linguini, 1 package	3
Tuna noodle gratin, 1 package	5

Meat and Poultry Entrees
Amy's Bowls

Teriyaki, 1 container	5

Amy's Whole Meals

Country dinner, 1	8

Annie's Homegrown Organic Skillet Meals

Cheddar chicken, 1 1/2 oz (about 1 cup prepared)	3
Cheeseburger macaroni, 1 serving (1.3 oz or about 1 cup prepared)	3

Betty Crocker Complete Meals

Chicken & buttermilk biscuits, 1 serving (1/5 package)	6
Homestyle dumplings & chicken, 1 serving (1/5 package)	5
Stroganoff, 1 serving (1/5 package)	4
Three cheese chicken, 1 serving (1/5 package)	5

Birds Eye

Garlic chicken, 1 serving (2 cups frozen, 1 cup cooked)	6

Birds Eye Viola!

Beef steak & garlic potato, 1 serving (1 2/3 cups frozen, 1 cup cooked)	4

	POINTS VALUE
Birds Eye Viola! Family Skillets	
Cheesy chicken, 1 serving (1 3/4 cup frozen, 1 cup cooked)	5
Birds Eye Voila!	
Alfredo chicken, 1 serving (1 1/2 cups frozen, 1 cup cooked)	7
Chicken & shrimp penne with vegetables, 1 serving (1 2/3 cups frozen, 1 cup cooked)	3
Chicken stir-fry, 1 serving (1 3/4 cups frozen, 1 cup cooked)	3
Chicken teriyaki & vegetables, prepared, 1 cup	2
Garden herb chicken, 1 serving (2 cups frozen, 1 cup cooked)	6
Garlic chicken, 1 serving (1 2/3 cups frozen, 1 cup cooked)	5
Pesto chicken primavera, 1 serving (2 cups frozen, 1 cup cooked)	4
Southwestern style chicken, 1 2/3 cups (1 cup cooked)	4
Teriyaki chicken, 1 serving (1 2/3 cups frozen, 1 cup cooked)	5
Three cheese chicken, 1 serving (1 2/3 cups frozen, 1 cup cooked)	4
Birds Eye Voila! Family Skillets	
Cheesy macaroni & beef, 1 cup (cooked)	8
Garlic chicken, 1 serving (1 2/3 cups frozen, 1 cup cooked)	5

	POINTS VALUE
Birds Eye World Market Blends	
Beef & broccoli stir-fry, 2 cups (frozen, 1 cup cooked)	3
Boston Market Home Style Meals	
Apple glazed pork with broccoli & rice au gratin, 1 package	7
Beef pot roast, 1 package	10
Chicken pot pie, 1 cup	14
Chicken primavera with penne pasta, 1 package	11
Chicken, broccoli & cheese pot pie, 1 cup	14
Country fried chicken with mashed potatoes & gravy and peas & carrots, 1 package	12
Glazed rotisserie white meat chicken with mashed potatoes & gravy and green beans & carrots, 1 package (383 g)	3
Glazed rotisserie white meat chicken with mashed potatoes & gravy and green beans & carrots, 1 package (453 g)	5
Home style chicken with noodles, 1 package	11
Honey roasted chicken with au gratin potatoes, 1 package	9
Meatloaf with mashed potatoes & gravy, 1 package (340 g)	13
Meatloaf with mashed potatoes & gravy, 1 package (453 g)	16
Roasted pork, 1 package	12

PREPARED FOODS, SALADS & SIDES

Meat and Poultry Entrees, Boston Market Home Style Meals (con't)	POINTS VALUE
Salisbury steak, 1 package	17
Swedish meatballs, 1 1/2 cups	20
Turkey breast medallions with mashed potatoes & gravy and green beans & carrots, 1 package	6
Turkey medallions, 1 package	9
Turkey pot pie, 1 cup	14
Chicken Helper	
Chicken teriyaki, prepared, 1 cup	6
Creamy chicken noodle, prepared, 1 cup	6
Four cheese, prepared, 1 cup	7
Jambalaya, prepared, 1 cup	5
Dinty Moore Hormel	
Roast beef & gravy with mashed potatoes, 1 bowl	4
Ethnic Gourmet Taste of Santa Fe	
Chipotle vegetarian chili lime sauce, 1 package	6
Lime chicken with ancho chile sauce, 10 oz	7
Zesty chicken with garlic mashed potatoes, 1 package	7
Fast Classics	
Steak fingers, gravy only, 1 serving (1/5 package)	2
Steak fingers, without gravy, 3 pieces	5
Green Giant Complete Skillet Meal	
Chicken teriyaki, 1/4 package	4
Creamy chicken parmesan, as packaged, 1/4 package	5

	POINTS VALUE
Creamy chicken parmesan, prepared, 1 cup	6
Garlic chicken pasta, as packaged, 1/4 package	4
Hamburger Helper	
Bacon cheeseburger, prepared, 1 cup	8
Cheddar cheese melt, prepared, 1 cup	7
Cheeseburger macaroni, prepared, 1 cup	7
Cheesy jambalaya, prepared, 1 cup	8
Cheesy nacho, prepared, 1 cup	8
Italian sausage, prepared, 1 cup	7
Philly cheesesteak, prepared, 1 cup	7
Potatoes stroganoff, prepared, 1 cup	7
Salisbury (homestyle), prepared, 1 cup	6
Hamburger Helper Complete Skillet Meal	
Pasta & beef with stroganoff sauce, as packaged, 1 serving (1/5 package)	7
Pasta & beef with stroganoff sauce, prepared, 1 cup	7
Hamburger Helper Microwave Singles	
Cheeseburger mac, 1 pouch	5
Stroganoff, 1 pouch	3
Hormel	
Beef roast, 5 oz	5
Beef roast family pack, 5 oz	5
Beef tips, 5 oz	4
Beef tips & gravy family pack, 5 oz	4
Chicken breast with gravy, 1	3
Family pack beef tips with gravy, 5 oz	4

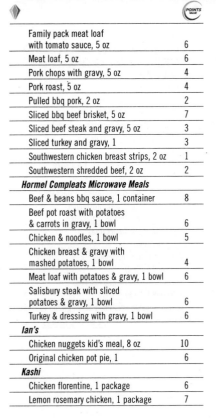

	POINTS VALUE
Family pack meat loaf with tomato sauce, 5 oz	6
Meat loaf, 5 oz	6
Pork chops with gravy, 5 oz	4
Pork roast, 5 oz	4
Pulled bbq pork, 2 oz	2
Sliced bbq beef brisket, 5 oz	7
Sliced beef steak and gravy, 5 oz	3
Sliced turkey and gravy, 1	3
Southwestern chicken breast strips, 2 oz	1
Southwestern shredded beef, 2 oz	2
Hormel Compleats Microwave Meals	
Beef & beans bbq sauce, 1 container	8
Beef pot roast with potatoes & carrots in gravy, 1 bowl	6
Chicken & noodles, 1 bowl	5
Chicken breast & gravy with mashed potatoes, 1 bowl	4
Meat loaf with potatoes & gravy, 1 bowl	6
Salisbury steak with sliced potatoes & gravy, 1 bowl	6
Turkey & dressing with gravy, 1 bowl	6
Ian's	
Chicken nuggets kid's meal, 8 oz	10
Original chicken pot pie, 1	6
Kashi	
Chicken florentine, 1 package	6
Lemon rosemary chicken, 1 package	7

	POINTS VALUE
Lemongrass coconut chicken, 1 package	6
Southwest style chicken, 1 package	4
Market Day	
Beef & broccoli with rice, 1 cup	5
Chicken and dumplings, 1 cup	5
Chicken breast Tuscan, 1 serving	8
Chicken pot pie, 1 cup	13
Individual chicken pot pies, 1 cup	16
Lemon caper chicken, 1 serving	7
Roast turkey with stuffing, 1 serving (12 oz)	6
Mary Kitchen	
50% less fat corned beef hash, 1 cup	6
Mary Kitchen Individual Canned Servings	
Corned beef hash, 1 cup	9
Schwan's LiveSmart	
Beef tips dinner, 1	6
Blackened chicken alfredo with vegetables dinner, 1 tray	6
Chicken fajita lean pouches, 1	5
Glazed chicken with rice and green bean medley, 1 tray	6
Ham & cheese lean pouches, 1	5
Roasted turkey & vegetables dinner, 1 tray	4
Salisbury steak dinner, 1	7
Sweet and sour chicken with rice, 1 cup	5
Turkey tenderloin & gravy, 5 oz	2

449

PREPARED FOODS, SALADS & SIDES

 Meat and Poultry Entrees (con't)

 POINTS VALUE   POINTS VALUE

Tyson

Chicken breast medallions in white wine and garlic sauce, 1 serving (5 oz)	3
Chicken broccoli and cheese, 1 piece	4
Chicken cordon bleu, 1 piece	9
Chicken kiev, 1 piece	12
Italian herb chicken, 1 serving (5 oz)	3

Wanchai Ferry

Spicy garlic chicken, prepared, 1 serving (1/6 package)	7

Weight Watchers Smart Ones

Chicken mirabella, 1 package	4
Honey dijon chicken, 1 package	4
Lemon herb chicken piccata, 1 package	4
Roast turkey medallions, 1 package	4
Salisbury steak with macaroni & cheese, 1 package	5
Santa fe style rice & beans, 1 package	6
Swedish meatballs, 1 package	5

Weight Watchers Smart Ones Bistro Selections

Beef pot roast, 1 package	3
Chicken marsala with broccoli, 1 package	4
Chicken parmesan, 1 package	5
Creamy parmesan chicken with garden vegetables, 1 package	4
Meatloaf with mashed potatoes, 1 package	5
Pepper steak, 1 package	5
Roast beef with gravy, 1 package	5
Roast beef with portabello gravy, 1 package	4
Roasted chicken with sour cream & chive mashed potatoes, 1 package	4
Salisbury steak and asparagus, 1 package	4
Sirloin beef and Asian style vegetables, 1 package	3
Slow-roasted turkey breast, 1 package	4
Stuffed turkey breast, 1 package	6
Teriyaki chicken & vegetables, 1 package	4
Turkey medallions with mushroom gravy and green beans, 1 package	4

Weight Watchers Smart Ones Fruit Inspirations

Cranbury turkey medallions, 1 serving (255 g)	7
Honey mango barbeque chicken, 1 serving (255 g)	5
Orange sesame chicken, 1 serving (255 g)	7
Pineapple beef teriyaki, 1 serving (255 g)	6

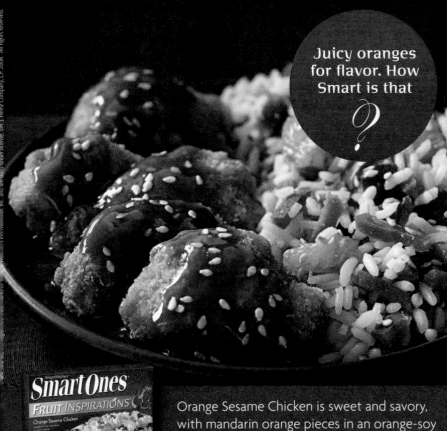

Juicy oranges for flavor. How Smart is that?

Smart Ones
FRUIT INSPIRATIONS
Orange Sesame Chicken

Orange Sesame Chicken is sweet and savory, with mandarin orange pieces in an orange-soy glaze. Just a *POINTS®* value of 7.

Special savings at eatyourbest.com

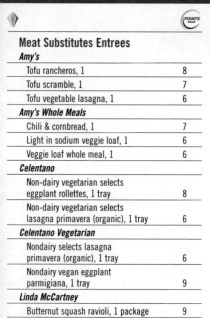

	POINTS VALUE

Meat Substitutes Entrees

Amy's

Tofu rancheros, 1	8
Tofu scramble, 1	7
Tofu vegetable lasagna, 1	6

Amy's Whole Meals

Chili & cornbread, 1	7
Light in sodium veggie loaf, 1	6
Veggie loaf whole meal, 1	6

Celentano

Non-dairy vegetarian selects eggplant rollettes, 1 tray	8
Non-dairy vegetarian selects lasagna primavera (organic), 1 tray	6

Celentano Vegetarian

Nondairy selects lasagna primavera (organic), 1 tray	6
Nondairy vegan eggplant parmigiana, 1 tray	9

Linda McCartney

Butternut squash ravioli, 1 package	9
Fire-grilled vegetarian chicken and vegetables, 1 package	6
Macaroni and cheese, 1 package	9
Spicy peanut pasta with vegetarian chicken, 1 package	8

Mon Cuisine

Vegan breaded chicken nuggets, 1 serving (0,85 g)	1
Vegan breaded chicken style cutlet in mushroom sauce, 10 oz	6
Vegan Italian stuffed shell pasta, 10 oz	4
Vegan Moroccan chicken, 10 oz	5
Vegan pot pie, 9 oz	15
Vegan veal style schnitzel in sauce, 10 oz	6
Vegetarian breaded chicken patties, 2 1/2 oz	2
Vegetarian grilled steak in mushroom gravy, 10 oz	5
Vegetarian salisbury steak in gravy, 10 oz	6
Vegetarian spaghetti & meatballs, 10 oz	7
Vegetarian stuffed cabbage in tomato sauce, 10 oz	4

Rosina

Non dairy vegetarian selects penne with roasted vegetables (made with organic ingredients), 1 tray	9
Non dairy vegetarian selects roasted vegetable lasagne, 10 oz	7
Non dairy vegetarian selects spinach & broccoli manicotti (organic), 1 tray	6
Non dairy vegetarian selects spinach & broccoli stuffed shells (organic), 1 tray	7

	POINTS VALUE
Tofurkey	
Roast & gravy (giblet & mushroom gravy only), 2 Tbsp	1
Roast & gravy (including stuffing), 4 oz	4
Wild rice & mushroom stuffing, 1/2 cup	2
Tofurky	
Vegetarian feast, cranberry-apple potato dumplings, 2 pieces	3
Vegetarian feast, giblet & mushroom gravy, 2 Tbsp	1
Vegetarian feast, roast with stuffing, 4 oz	4
Vegetarian feast, wishstix, 1/2 piece	0

Pasta and Vegetable Salads
Betty Crocker Suddenly Pasta Salad

	POINTS VALUE
Chipotle ranch, prepared, 2/3 cup	5

Betty Crocker Suddenly Salad

	POINTS VALUE
Caesar pasta, prepared, 1 cup	6
Classic pasta, prepared, 1 cup	5
Creamy Italian pasta, prepared, 3/4 cup	8
Creamy parmesan pasta, prepared, 1 cup	9
Ranch & bacon pasta, prepared, 3/4 cup	8

DiGiorno

	POINTS VALUE
Basil vinaigrette pasta salad, prepared, 3/4 cup	4
Three cheese Italian for club, as packaged, 1 serving (1/20 box)	5

	POINTS VALUE
DiLusso	
Chef salad (large), 1 container	8
Chef salad (small), 1 container	4
Chicken Caesar salad (large), 1 container	8
Chicken Caesar salad (small), 1 container	4
Chicken club salad (large), 1 container	8
Chicken club salad (small), 1 container	4
Chicken fajita salad (large), 1 container	6
Cobb salad (large), 1 container	11
Cobb salad (small), 1 container	6
Greek salad (large), 1 container	6
Ham & broccoli salad (large), 1 container	8
Southwest turkey salad (large), 1 container	6
Dole	
♦ Angel hair cole slaw, 3 oz	0
Dole Classic	
♦ Cole slaw, 3 oz	0
♦ Iceberg salad, 3 oz	0
Dole Complete Salads	
Bacon lettuce toss kit - bacon ranch dressing, 1 serving (0.69 fl oz)	2
Fall harvest kit - apple dijon vinaigrette dressing, 1 serving (0.8 fl oz)	2
Family Caesar kit - Caesar dressing, 1 serving (0.69 fl oz)	3
Garlic Caesar kit - garlic Caesar dressing, 1 serving (0.8 fl oz)	3

PREPARED FOODS, SALADS & SIDES

Pasta and Vegetable Salads, Dole Complete Salads (con't)	POINTS VALUE
Spring garden kit - raspberry vinaigrette dressing, 1 serving (0.7 fl oz)	2
Summer sun kit - tomato herb vinaigrette dressing, 1 serving (0.53 fl oz)	1
Taco toss kit - taco ranch dressing, 1 serving (0.66 fl oz)	2
Winter medley kit - cranberry vinaigrette dressing, 1 serving (0.83 fl oz)	3
Dole Complete Salads, with dressing	
Caesar, 1 serving (3.5 oz)	3
Light Caesar, 1 serving (3.5 oz)	2
Romano, 1 serving (3.5 oz)	2
Sunflower ranch, 1 serving (3.5 oz)	3
Dole Special Blends	
American blend, 3 oz	0
European blend, 3 oz	0
French blend, 3 oz	0
Italian blend, 3 oz	0
Romaine blend, 3 oz	0
Fortune of the East	
Thai peanut pasta salad, prepared, 2/3 cup	5
Green Giant	
Three bean salad, canned, 1/2 cup	1
Kraft	
Asian sesame, prepared, 1 cup	6
Basil vinaigrette, prepared, 3/4 cup	4
Caesar, prepared, 3/4 cup	9

	POINTS VALUE
Classic ranch with bacon, prepared, 3/4 cup	8
Garlic parmesan, prepared, 3/4 cup	9
Harvest ranch peppercorn, prepared, 1 cup	5
Italian, prepared, 3/4 cup	5
Santa Fe style ranch, prepared, 3/4 cup	4
Linsey	
Caesar salad kit, 1 serving (22 g)	3
Italian salad kit, 1 serving (22 g)	3
Light salad kit, 1 serving (22 g)	2
Oriental salad kit, 1 serving (22 g)	2
Spinach salad kit, 1 serving (22 g)	2
S&W	
Deli style bean salad, 1/2 cup	1
Dill garden salad, 1/2 cup	0
Marinated bean salad, 1/2 cup	1
Sabra To Go	
Red cabbage salad, 1 serving (1 oz)	2
Tyson	
Premium chunk chicken salad kit, 1 package	5
Westbrae Natural	
Country style marinated bean salad, 1/2 cup	1
Deli style marinated bean salad, 1/2 cup	1
Kashi	
Black bean mango, 1 package	7

	POINTS VALUE

Pasta/Rice Entrees
Amy's

Baked ziti kids meal, 1	7
Cheese lasagna, 1	8
Family size vegetable lasagna, 1 cup	5
Garden vegetable lasagna, 1 serving (10.3 oz)	6
Large size mac & cheese, 1 cup	8
Light in sodium vegetable lasagna, 1	6
Mac n' cheese kids meal, 1	8
Macaroni & cheese, 1	9
Macaroni & cheese, light in sodium, 1	9
Macaroni & soy cheeze, 1	8
Rice mac & cheese, 1 container	9
Vegetable lasagna, 1	6

Amy's Bowls

Baked ziti bowl, 1	8
Country cheddar bowl, 1 serving (9.5 g)	9
Pesto tortellini bowl, 1 serving (9.5 g)	10
Ravioli bowl, 1	8
Stuffed pasta shells, 1 container	6

Annie's Homegrown

Arthur mac & cheese, 2 1/2 oz (about 1 cup prepared)	6
Bunny shape pasta & yummy cheese, 2 1/2 oz (about 1 cup prepared)	6
Deluxe elbow & four cheese, 1 serving (3.6 oz or about 1 cup prepared)	7

	POINTS VALUE
Deluxe rotini & white cheddar, 1 serving (3.4 oz or about 1 cup prepared)	6
Deluxe shells & real age cheddar, 1 serving (3.6 oz or about 1 cup prepared)	7
Deluxe whole wheat shells & extra cheesy cheddar, 3 oz (about 1 cup prepared)	5
Macaroni & cheese, 1 cup (prepared)	6
Micro mac and real age cheese, 1/2 cup (packaged or 3/4 cup prepared)	5
Micro mac and white cheddar, 1/2 cup (packaged or 3/4 cup prepared)	5
Organic alfredo shells & cheddar, 2 1/2 oz (about 1 cup prepared)	5
Organic peace pasta with parmesan, 2 1/2 oz (about 1 cup prepared)	5
Organic shells & real age cheddar, 2 1/2 oz (about 1 cup prepared)	5
Organic shells with white cheddar, 2 1/2 oz (about 1 cup prepared)	5
Organic whole wheat shells & cheddar, 2 1/2 oz (about 1 cup prepared)	5
Shells & real age cheddar, 2 1/2 oz (about 1 cup prepared)	6
Shells & white cheddar, 2 1/2 oz (about 1 cup prepared)	6

Annie's Homegrown Organic Canned Meals

All stars, 1 cup	3
Arthur loops, 1 cup	3
BernieOs, 1 cup	3

PREPARED FOODS, SALADS & SIDES

Pasta/Rice Entrees, Annie's Homegrown Organic Canned Meals (con't)	POINTS VALUE
Cheesy ravioli, 1 cup	3
P'sghetti loops with soy meatballs, 1 cup	4
Annie's Homegrown Organic Skillet Meals	
Cheesy lasagna, 1 serving (1.3 oz or about 1 cup prepared)	2
Stroganoff, 1 serving (1.3 oz or about 1 cup prepared)	3
Annie's Homegrown Simply Organic Macaroni	
Macaroni & cheese, 2/3 cup (1 cup prepared)	5
Shells & cheese, 2/3 cup (1 cup prepared)	5
Back To Nature	
Back to nature cup, 1 package	4
Crazy bugs macaroni & cheese, as prepared, 1 cup	7
Harvest wheat & cheddar, as prepared, 1 cup	5
Organic macaroni & cheese, as prepared, 1 cup	7
Organic shells & cheese, as prepared, 1 cup	8
Organic white cheddar cheese & organic shells, as prepared, 1 cup	7
Original macaroni & cheese, as prepared, 1 cup	7
White cheddar & spirals, as prepared, 1 cup	7
White cheddar & whole wheat elbow, as prepared, 1 cup	6

	POINTS VALUE
Betty Crocker	
Chicken fettucine alfredo, prepared, 1 serving (1/5 package)	8
Chicken marsala with linguine, prepared, 1 serving (1/5 package)	7
Creamy basil parmesan chicken & pasta, prepared, 1 serving (1/5 package)	7
Garlic & herb chicken penne, prepared, 1 serving (1/6 package)	5
Betty Crocker Complete Meals	
Chicken fettuccini alfredo, 1 serving (1/5 package)	5
Lasagna pasta bake with meat sauce, 1 serving (1/5 package)	5
Birds Eye Voila!	
Pasta primavera with chicken, 2 cups (1 cup cooked)	5
Boca	
Lasagna - chunky tomato & herb sauce with meatless ground burger, 1 package	5
Boston Market Home Style Meals	
Lasagna with meat sauce layered with ricotta & meat sauce, 1 package	11
Macaroni & cheese, 1/2 cup	7
Celentano	
Organic ravioli, 1 cup	3
Celentano Light	
Cheese ravioli, blanched, 4	4
Manicotti florentine, 10 oz	6

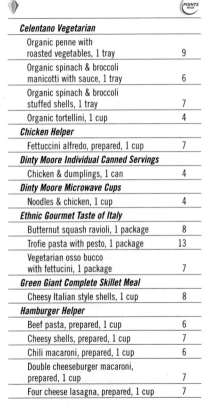

	POINTS VALUE
Celentano Vegetarian	
Organic penne with roasted vegetables, 1 tray	9
Organic spinach & broccoli manicotti with sauce, 1 tray	6
Organic spinach & broccoli stuffed shells, 1 tray	7
Organic tortellini, 1 cup	4
Chicken Helper	
Fettuccini alfredo, prepared, 1 cup	7
Dinty Moore Individual Canned Servings	
Chicken & dumplings, 1 can	4
Dinty Moore Microwave Cups	
Noodles & chicken, 1 cup	4
Ethnic Gourmet Taste of Italy	
Butternut squash ravioli, 1 package	8
Trofie pasta with pesto, 1 package	13
Vegetarian osso bucco with fettucini, 1 package	7
Green Giant Complete Skillet Meal	
Cheesy Italian style shells, 1 cup	8
Hamburger Helper	
Beef pasta, prepared, 1 cup	6
Cheesy shells, prepared, 1 cup	7
Chili macaroni, prepared, 1 cup	6
Double cheeseburger macaroni, prepared, 1 cup	7
Four cheese lasagna, prepared, 1 cup	7

	POINTS VALUE
Lasagna, prepared, 1 cup	6
Spaghetti, prepared, 1 cup	6
Three cheese, prepared, 1 cup	8
Tomato basil penne, prepared, 1 cup	7
Hamburger Helper Complete Skillet Meal	
Cheesy macaroni & beef, as packaged, 1 serving (1/5 package)	6
Cheesy macaroni & beef, prepared, 1 cup	7
Hodgson Mill	
Whole wheat macaroni & cheese, 2 oz (about 1/3 box)	4
Hormel Compleats Microwave Bowls	
Chicken & dumplings, 1 bowl	5
Chicken & rice, 1 bowl	6
Spaghetti with meat sauce, 1 bowl	5
Sweet & sour rice, 1 bowl	5
Teriyaki chicken with rice, 1 bowl	5
Hormel Compleats Microwave Meals	
Chicken alfredo chicken with penne pasta in alfredo sauce, 1 bowl	8
Lasagna/meat sauce, 1 bowl	6
Turkey & hearty vegetables, 1 bowl	4
Hormel Individual Canned Servings	
Beans and wieners, 1 can	6
Mac & cheese, 1 cup	6
Hormel Micro Cup Meals	
Lasagna with meat sauce, 1 cup	4
Spaghetti with meat sauce, 1 cup	4

PREPARED FOODS, SALADS & SIDES

Pasta/Rice Entrees (con't)	POINTS VALUE
Hormel Microcup Meals	
Southwest style rice, 1 cup	3
Teriyaki rice, 1 cup	4
Hormel Pasta Cups	
Cheese tortellini, 1 cup	4
Italian style, 1 cup	5
Lemon pepper, 1 cup	5
Ian's	
Mac & cheese - organic, 8 oz	7
Rotini & mini meatballs, 7 oz	6
Italian Village	
4-cheese large round ravioli, 4	5
Large round ravioli, 4	5
Mini round ravioli, 13	4
Square ravioli, 9	4
Italian Village Floresta	
Cheese tortellini, 1 cup (uncooked)	5
Meat tortellini, 1 cup (uncooked)	6
Kashi	
Chicken pasta pomodoro, 1 package	5
Pesto pasta primavera, 1 package	6
Kid's Kitchen	
Beans & wieners, 1 cup	7
Beefy macaroni, 1 cup	3
Cheezy mac 'n beef, 1 cup	6
Cheezy mac 'n franks, 1 cup	7
Cheezy mac 'n cheese, 1 cup	7
Mini beef ravioli, 1 cup	5

	POINTS VALUE
Noodle rings & chicken, 1 cup	3
Spaghetti & meatballs, 1 cup	5
Spaghetti rings & franks, 1 cup	6
Kraft	
All shapes, 1 cup	5
Deluxe sharp cheddar, as packaged, 1 serving (98 g)	7
Easy mac extreme cheese, 1 pouch	5
Easy mac macaroni & cheese, as packaged, 1 serving (61 g)	5
Homestyle macaroni, 3/4 cup	6
Macaroni & cheese spirals, as packaged, 1 serving (70 g)	5
Organic cheddar cheese & organic elbow pasta dinner, prepared, 1 cup	7
Organic white cheddar cheese & organic shells dinner, prepared, 1 cup	7
Original, 2 1/2 oz	5
Original, light, prepared, 1 cup	6
Original, prepared using classic recipe, 1 cup	10
Shapes - scooby doo, prepared using classic recipe, 1 cup	9
Spirals, prepared using classic recipe, 1 cup	9
Spirals, prepared using light recipe, 1 cup	6
Supermac original - pasta & sauce, prepared using classic recipe, 1 cup	7
Supermac original - pasta & sauce, prepared using light recipe, 1 cup	4

◇	POINTS VALUE
Three cheese, prepared using classic recipe, 1 cup	9
Three cheese, prepared using light recipe, 1 cup	6
Kraft Bistro Deluxe	
Classic cheddar, 1 cup	7
Creamy portobello mushroom, 1 cup	7
Sundried tomato parmesan, 1 cup	6
Three cheese italiano, 1 cup	7
Kraft Deluxe	
1/2 the fat made with 2% milk cheese, 3 1/2 oz	6
Four cheese blend, 1 cup	7
Original, as packaged, 3 1/2 oz	7
Kraft Easy Mac Cups	
Alfredo, 1 package	5
Bacon, 1 package	5
Original, 1 package	5
Triple cheese, 1 package	5
Kraft Premium	
Cheesy alfredo, 1 cup	5
Cheesy alfredo, prepared using classic recipe, 1 cup	8
Cheesy alfredo, prepared using light recipe, 1 cup	6
Mild white cheddar, prepared using classic recipe, 1 cup	8
Mild white cheddar, prepared using light recipe, 1 cup	6
Thick 'n creamy, 2 1/2 oz	5

◇	POINTS VALUE
Thick 'n creamy, prepared using classic recipe, 1 cup	8
Thick 'n creamy, prepared using light recipe, 1 cup	6
White cheddar, mild, 2 1/2 oz	5
Kraft Velveeta	
1/2 the fat, 4 oz	7
Bacon, prepared, 1 cup	8
Original, as packaged, 4 oz	8
Rotini and cheese with broccoli dinner, prepared, 1 cup	9
Market Day	
Cheese lasagna roll-up, 1 serving (3 oz)	3
Cheese ravioli, 7	4
Florentine lasagna roll-up, 1 serving (3 oz)	2
Mac & cheese singles, 1 pouch	7
Monterey Pasta Company	
Artichoke cheese ravioli with ripe olives, 1 cup	5
Atlantic lobster ravioli, 1 cup	5
Rainbow five cheese tortelloni, 1 cup	6
Roasted garlic chicken ravioli, 1 cup	5
Spinach ricotta ravioli, 1 cup	5
Whole wheat basil, tomato, & mozzarella ravioli, 1 cup	5
Whole wheat chicken and sundried tomato ravioli, 1 cup	4
Whole wheat classic Italian cheese tortellini, 1 cup	5

PREPARED FOODS, SALADS & SIDES

Pasta/Rice Entrees (con't)

POINTS VALUE

Monterey Pasta Company Whole Wheat Ravioli

Whole wheat spicy chicken pesto ravioli, 1 cup	5
Whole wheat Tuscan style roasted peppers ravioli, 1 cup	4

Monterey Pasta Company Whole Wheat Tortelloni

Whole wheat spinach & cheese tortelloni, 1 cup	5

Nutritious Living Hi-Lo

Chicken vegetable parmesan, 1 tray	3
Turkey chili Santa Fe, 1 tray	3

Old El Paso

Gordita dinner mix (with ranch sauce), prepared, 1 serving (1 tortilla, 2 Tbsp ranch sauce, 1 tsp seasoning mix)	8
Gordita dinner mix (with red sauce), prepared, 1 serving (1 tortilla, 2 Tbsp red sauce, 1 tsp seasoning mix)	8

Rosetto

All natural cheese ravioli, 9 pieces	4
All natural whole wheat & cheese ravioli, 9 pieces	4
Beef ravioli, 9 pieces	5
Beef ravioli made with organic durum wheat, 9 pieces	4
Cheese and broccoli ravioli, 4 pieces	5
Cheese manicotti, 2 pieces	6
Cheese ravioli, 9 pieces	5
Cheese tortellini, 1 cup	5
Chicken and herb ravioli, 9 pieces	4

	POINTS VALUE
Gourmet butternut squash ravioli, 9 pieces	4
Gourmet pesto ravioli with walnuts, 9 pieces	6
Italian style ravioli with sausage, 9 pieces	5
Large round cheese ravioli, 5 pieces	4
Small round cheese ravioli, 13 pieces	5

Rosina

Vegan organic ravioli, 1 cup	3
Vegan organic tortellini, 1 cup	4

Rosina Presents Celentano

Baked ziti with sauce, 8 oz	10
Cheese ravioli, 4	4
Cheese tortellini, 1 cup	5
Lasagna with sauce, 1 serving	9
Lasagna with sauce, 1/2 tray	6
Manicotti without sauce, 1/2 tray	8
Mini cheese ravioli, 12	4
Stuffed shells with sauce, 1/2 tray	6
Stuffed shells without sauce, 4	7

Rosina Presents Celentano Light

Light broccoli stuffed shells with sauce, 1 tray	6
Light lasagna with sauce, 1 tray	7
Light manicotti florentine with sauce, 1 tray	6
Light ravioli, 4	4
Light stuffed shells with sauce, 3 shells	7
Manicotti, 1 tray	7

	POINTS VALUE
Schwan's LiveSmart	
Six cheese tortellini, 1 cup	4
Seeds of Change	
Fettuccine alfredo di roma, 1	6
Hanalei vegetarian chicken teriyaki, 1 tray	5
Lasagna calabrese with eggplant & portobello mushroom, 1 tray	5
Spinach lasagna di parma, 1 tray	7
Venetian penne marinara, 1 tray	6
T.G.I. Friday's	
Four cheese toasted ravioli (toasted ravioli with sauce), 1 serving (98 g)	5
Weight Watchers Smart Ones	
Angel hair marinara, 1 package	3
Creamy rigatoni with broccoli & chicken, 1 package	6
Fettucini alfredo, 1 package	6
Lasagna Bolognese, 1 package	5
Lasagna florentine, 1 package	6
Macaroni & cheese, 1 package	5
Pasta primavera, 1 package	5
Ravioli florentine, 1 package	5
Spaghetti bolognese, 1 package	6
Three cheese macaroni, 1 package	6
Three cheese ziti marinara, 1 package	6
Weight Watchers Smart Ones Bistro Selections	
Penne pollo, 1 package	6

Pizza

	POINTS VALUE
A.C. LaRocco	
Cheese & garlic thin crust pizza, 1/3 pizza	5
Garden vegetarian, 1/3 pizza	5
Greek sesame thin crust pizza, 1/3 pizza	5
Quattro formaggio thin crust pizza, 1/3 pizza	4
Spinach & artichoke thin crust pizza, 1/3 pizza	4
Tomato & feta thin crust pizza, 1/3 pizza	5
Ultra thin bruschetta style pizza, 1/2 pizza	3
Ultra thin garlic chicken parmesan, 1/2 pizza	4
Ultra thin old world veggie pizza, 1/2 pizza	3
Alexia	
Pesto chicken with fresh mozzarella, 6 rolls	5
Sweet Italian sausage, roasted peppers & parmesan, 6 rolls	5
Amy's	
3 cheese pizza with cornmeal crust, 1/3 pizza	9
Cheese & pesto pizza with whole wheat crust, 1/3 pizza	8
Cheese pizza, 1 serving (4.33 oz)	7
Cheese pizza snacks, 1 serving (5-6 pieces)	4
Margherita pizza, 1/3 pizza	6
Mediterranean pizza with cornmeal crust, 1/3 pizza	8

Pizza, Amy's (con't) — POINTS VALUE

Mushroom and olive pizza, 1 serving (4.33 oz)	5
Pesto pizza, 1 serving (4.5 oz)	7
Rice crust cheese pizza, 1 serving (4 oz)	7
Rice crust spinach pizza, 1/3 pizza	8
Roasted vegetable pizza, 1 serving (4 oz)	6
Single serve cheese pizza, 1	9
Single serve margherita pizza, 1	8
Single serve mushroom & olive pizza, 1	10
Single serve non-dairy rice crust cheeze pizza, 1	11
Single serve pesto pizza, 1	10
Single serve roasted vegetable pizza, 1	9
Single serve spinach pizza, 1	10
Single serve spinach pizza, light in sodium, 1	10
Soy cheeze pizza, 1 serving (4.33 oz)	6
Spinach pizza, 1 serving (4.66 g)	7
Spinach pizza snack, 1 serving (5-6 pieces)	4
Veggie combo pizza, 1 serving (5.33 oz)	7

Boboli

100% whole wheat thin pizza crust, 1 serving (1/5 crust)	2
8" mini pizza crusts (2 pack), 1/2 crust	4
Original pizza crust, 12", 1/8 crust	3
Personal size pizza crust, 1/2 shell	4
Thin pizza crust, 1 serving (1/5 crust)	3

POINTS VALUE

Bravissimo

7" cheese pizza, 1/2	6
7" spinach pizza, 1/2	6
7" vegetable pizza, 1/2	5
9" cheese pizza, 1/3	6
9" pepperoni pizza, 1/3	6
9" roasted vegetable pizza, 1/3	4
9"·spinach mushroom pizza, 1/3	6

California Pizza Kitchen

Barbecue chicken, 1/3 pizza	6
Cajun recipe, 1/3 pizza	6
Five cheese and tomato, 1/3 pizza	7
Garlic chicken, 1/3 pizza	6
Hawaiian recipe, 1/3 pizza	6
Jamaican jerk chicken recipe pizza, 1/3 pizza	6
Sausage, pepperoni and mushroom, 1/3 pizza	6
Thai chicken, 1/3 pizza	6

California Pizza Kitchen Thin Crust

BBQ recipe chicken, 1/3	6
Cajun recipe, 1/3	6
Garlic chicken, 1/3	6
Margherita, 1/3	6
Sicilian recipe, 1/3	7
Sweet and spicy Italian, 1/3	6
White, 1/3	6

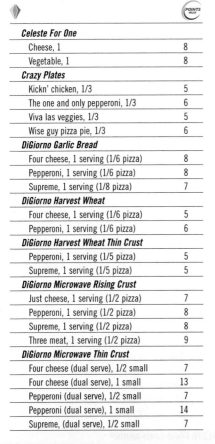

	POINTS VALUE
Celeste For One	
Cheese, 1	8
Vegetable, 1	8
Crazy Plates	
Kickn' chicken, 1/3	5
The one and only pepperoni, 1/3	6
Viva las veggies, 1/3	5
Wise guy pizza pie, 1/3	6
DiGiorno Garlic Bread	
Four cheese, 1 serving (1/6 pizza)	8
Pepperoni, 1 serving (1/6 pizza)	8
Supreme, 1 serving (1/8 pizza)	7
DiGiorno Harvest Wheat	
Four cheese, 1 serving (1/6 pizza)	5
Pepperoni, 1 serving (1/6 pizza)	6
DiGiorno Harvest Wheat Thin Crust	
Pepperoni, 1 serving (1/5 pizza)	5
Supreme, 1 serving (1/5 pizza)	5
DiGiorno Microwave Rising Crust	
Just cheese, 1 serving (1/2 pizza)	7
Pepperoni, 1 serving (1/2 pizza)	8
Supreme, 1 serving (1/2 pizza)	8
Three meat, 1 serving (1/2 pizza)	9
DiGiorno Microwave Thin Crust	
Four cheese (dual serve), 1/2 small	7
Four cheese (dual serve), 1 small	13
Pepperoni (dual serve), 1/2 small	7
Pepperoni (dual serve), 1 small	14
Supreme, (dual serve), 1/2 small	7

	POINTS VALUE
DiGiorno Rising Crust	
Four cheese, 12", 1 serving (1/6 pizza)	7
Four cheese, 8", 1/3 pizza	6
Italian sausage, 12", 1 serving (1/6 pizza)	8
Meatball marinara, 12", 1 serving (1/6 pizza)	7
Pepperoni, 12", 1 serving (1/6 pizza)	7
Pepperoni (2 or 3 pack), 1 serving (1/6 pizza)	8
Pepperoni, 8", 1/3 pizza	6
Sausage and pepperoni, 12", 1 serving (1/6 pizza)	8
Spicy chicken supreme, 12", 1 serving (1/6 pizza)	7
Spinach, mushroom, & garlic, 12", 1 serving (1/6 pizza)	6
Supreme, 12", 1 serving (1/6 pizza)	8
Supreme, 8", 1/3 pizza	7
Three meat, 12", 1 serving (1/6 pizza)	8
Three meat, 8", 1/3 pizza	7
DiGiorno Rising Crust Half & Half	
Cheese and pepperoni (cheese half), 1 serving (1/6 pizza)	7
Pepperoni/supreme (pepperoni half), 1 serving (1/6 pizza)	9
DiGiorno Rising Crust Microwave	
Cheese, 1	15
Pepperoni, 1	17
Supreme, 1	17
Three meat, 1	18

PREPARED FOODS, SALADS & SIDES

Pizza (con't)	POINTS VALUE
DiGiorno Stuffed Crust	
Four cheese, 1 serving (1/5 pizza)	8
Pepperoni, 1 serving (1/5 pizza)	8
Supreme, 1 serving (1/8 pizza)	8
Three meat, 1 serving (1/6 pizza)	8
DiGiorno Thin Crust	
Cheese, made with organic flour and cheese, 1 serving (1/4 of pizza)	7
Four cheese, 1 serving (1/5 of pizza)	7
Four meat, 1 serving (1/5 pizza)	7
Grilled chicken tomato & spinach, 1 serving (1/5 pizza)	6
Mushroom, pepperoni and bacon, 1 serving (1/5 pizza)	7
Pepperoni, 1 serving (1/5 pizza)	7
Spinach & garlic, made with organic flour, tomatoes and spinach, 1 serving (1/4 of pizza)	7
Spinach, mushroom, & garlic, 1 serving (1/5 pizza)	5
Supreme, 1 serving (1/5 pizza)	7
DiGiorno Ultimate	
Four cheese, 1 serving (1/5 pizza)	7
Four meat, 1 serving (1/5 pizza)	9
Pepperoni, 1 serving (1/5 pizza)	8
Supreme, 1 serving (1/5 pizza)	8
French Meadow Bakery	
Spelt pizza crust (alternative grain), 1 serving (1/3 of crust)	4

	POINTS VALUE
Ian's	
Organic French bread pizza, 1 serving (4 oz)	5
Pizza slices, 1 serving (2 oz)	2
Wheat free/gluten free French bread pizza, 1 serving (4 oz)	4
Jack's Naturally Rising Crust	
Cheese, 1 serving (1/6 pizza)	7
Combination, 1 serving (1/6 pizza)	7
Pepperoni, 1 serving (1/6 pizza)	7
Sausage, 1 serving (1/6 pizza)	7
The works, 1 serving (1/6 pizza)	7
Three meat, 1 serving (1/6 pizza)	7
Jack's Naturally Rising Pizza	
Bacon cheeseburger, 1 serving (1/6 pizza)	7
Jack's Original	
Bacon cheeseburger, 1/4 pizza	6
Canadian style bacon, 1/3 pizza	7
Cheese, 1/3 pizza	7
Hamburger, 1/4 pizza	6
Mexican, 1/4 pizza	6
Pepperoni, 1/3 pizza	9
Pepperoni & mushroom, 1/4 pizza	7
Pepperoni & sausage, 9", 1/2 pizza	8
Sausage, 1/4 pizza	6
Sausage & mushroom, 1/4 pizza	6
Sausage & pepperoni, 1/4 pizza	7
Spicy Italian sausage, 1/3 pizza	8
Supreme, 1/4 pizza	7

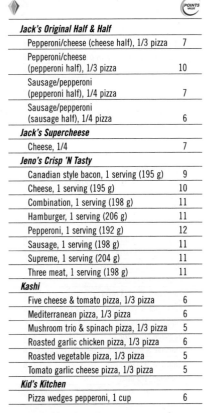

	POINTS VALUE
Jack's Original Half & Half	
Pepperoni/cheese (cheese half), 1/3 pizza	7
Pepperoni/cheese (pepperoni half), 1/3 pizza	10
Sausage/pepperoni (pepperoni half), 1/4 pizza	7
Sausage/pepperoni (sausage half), 1/4 pizza	6
Jack's Supercheese	
Cheese, 1/4	7
Jeno's Crisp 'N Tasty	
Canadian style bacon, 1 serving (195 g)	9
Cheese, 1 serving (195 g)	10
Combination, 1 serving (198 g)	11
Hamburger, 1 serving (206 g)	11
Pepperoni, 1 serving (192 g)	12
Sausage, 1 serving (198 g)	11
Supreme, 1 serving (204 g)	11
Three meat, 1 serving (198 g)	11
Kashi	
Five cheese & tomato pizza, 1/3 pizza	6
Mediterranean pizza, 1/3 pizza	6
Mushroom trio & spinach pizza, 1/3 pizza	5
Roasted garlic chicken pizza, 1/3 pizza	6
Roasted vegetable pizza, 1/3 pizza	5
Tomato garlic cheese pizza, 1/3 pizza	5
Kid's Kitchen	
Pizza wedges pepperoni, 1 cup	6

	POINTS VALUE
Linda McCartney	
Cheese pizza, 1/2	6
Mushroom and spinach pizza, 1/2	6
Market Day	
Breakfast pizzas, 1	11
Cheese pizza, 1/4	6
Cheese pizza eat-zzas, 1	8
Chicken club grilling pizzas, 1/2 pizza	12
Chicken pico de gallo pizzas, 1/2 pizza	9
Mediterranean pizzas, 1/2	9
Pepperoni pizza eat-zzas, 1	10
Taco pizza, 1/4	7
Palermo's Primo Thin Crust Pizza	
6 cheese, 1/3 pizza	7
BBQ recipe chicken, 1/3 pizza	7
Cheddar & tomato, 1/3 pizza	7
Greek, 1/3 pizza	7
Grilled chicken Caesar, 1/3 pizza	7
Ham & pineapple, 1/4 pizza	5
Margherita, 1/3 pizza	6
Sausage, 1/4 pizza	8
Special edition pepperoni, 1/3 pizza	9
Supreme, 1/3 pizza	8
Palermo's Primo Thin Pizza	
Primavera alfredo, 1/4 pizza	7
Vegetables & goat cheese, 1/3 pizza	6

Pizza (con't)	POINTS VALUE
Paraclete	
5" pizza shells, 1	1
7" pizza shells, 1	1
Pillsbury	
Classic pizza crust, refrigerated, 1 serving (1/5 loaf)	3
Schwan's LiveSmart	
BBQ recipe chicken pizza, 1	6
Fiesta chicken pizza, 1	5
Pepperoni pizza, 1	5
Roasted vegetable pizza, 1	4
Tomato basil margherita-style pizza, 1	4
SuperFoods	
Four cheese pizza, 1/3 pizza	5
Turkey and spinach pizza, 1/3 pizza	5
Veggie pizza, 1/3 pizza	5
Tombstone	
Brickoven style pepperoni, 1 serving (1/4 pizza)	7
Brickoven style sausage & pepperoni, 1 serving (1/4 pizza)	8
Brickoven style supreme, 1 serving (1/4 pizza)	7
Tombstone Brick Oven Style	
Cheese, 1/3	8
Classic sausage, 1/4	6
Deluxe, 1/4	6

	POINTS VALUE
Tombstone Garlic Bread	
Cheese, 1 serving (1/6 pizza)	8
Pepperoni, 1 serving (1/6 pizza)	8
Supreme, 1 serving (1/6 pizza)	8
Tombstone Light	
Vegetable pizza, 1 serving (1/5 pizza)	4
Tombstone Mini Deep Dish	
Cheese, 1 pizza	9
Pepperoni, 1 pizza	10
Supreme, 1 pizza	10
Tombstone Original	
Canadian style bacon, 1/4 pizza	7
Cheese, 1/4 pizza	7
Cheese, 9", 1/2 pizza	8
Deluxe, 1/5 pizza	6
Deluxe, 9", 1/3 pizza	6
Four meat,1/5 pizza	7
Hamburger, 1/5 pizza	7
Pepperoni, 1/4 pizza	9
Pepperoni, 9", 1/3 pizza	6
Pepperoni & sausage, 1 serving (1/4 pizza)	8
Pepperoni & sausage, 9", 1/3 pizza	6
Sausage,1/5 pizza	6
Sausage & mushroom, 1 serving (1/5 pizza)	6
Sausage, 9", 1/3 pizza	6
Supreme, 1/5 pizza	7

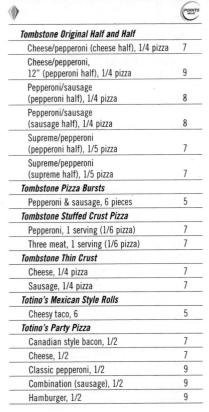

	POINTS VALUE
Tombstone Original Half and Half	
Cheese/pepperoni (cheese half), 1/4 pizza	7
Cheese/pepperoni, 12" (pepperoni half), 1/4 pizza	9
Pepperoni/sausage (pepperoni half), 1/4 pizza	8
Pepperoni/sausage (sausage half), 1/4 pizza	8
Supreme/pepperoni (pepperoni half), 1/5 pizza	7
Supreme/pepperoni (supreme half), 1/5 pizza	7
Tombstone Pizza Bursts	
Pepperoni & sausage, 6 pieces	5
Tombstone Stuffed Crust Pizza	
Pepperoni, 1 serving (1/6 pizza)	7
Three meat, 1 serving (1/6 pizza)	7
Tombstone Thin Crust	
Cheese, 1/4 pizza	7
Sausage, 1/4 pizza	7
Totino's Mexican Style Rolls	
Cheesy taco, 6	5
Totino's Party Pizza	
Canadian style bacon, 1/2	7
Cheese, 1/2	7
Classic pepperoni, 1/2	9
Combination (sausage), 1/2	9
Hamburger, 1/2	9

	POINTS VALUE
Mexican style taco beef, 1/2	9
Mini meatball, 1/2	8
Pepperoni, 1/2	9
Pepperoni trio, 1/2	9
Sausage, 1/2	9
Supreme (sausage & pepperoni), 1/2	9
Three cheese, 1/2	8
Three meat, 1/2	8
Totino's Pizza Rolls	
Cheese, 6 rolls	4
Combination (sausage & pepperoni), 6 rolls	5
Pepperoni, 6 rolls	5
Pepperoni trio, 6 rolls	5
Sausage, 6 rolls	5
Three meat, 6 rolls	5
Totino's Reduced Fat Pizza Rolls	
Pepperoni, 6	4
Totino's Ultimate Pizza Rolls	
Cheese, 3	4
Combination (sausage & reduced fat pepperoni), 3	4
Pepperoni & reduced fat pepperoni, 3	5
Weight Watchers Smart Ones Bistro Selections	
Four cheese pizza, 1 pizza	8
Pepperoni pizza, 1 pizza	8

	POINTS VALUE
Potato, Rice and Grain Sides	
Alexia	
Oven crinkles with onion & garlic, 1 serving (3 oz)	2
Oven crinkles with salt & pepper, 1 serving (3 oz)	2
Oven crinkles, classic, 1 serving (3 oz)	2
Oven fries - olive oil & sea salt, 1 serving (3 oz)	2
Oven fries - olive oil, rosemary & garlic, 1 serving (3 oz)	2
Oven reds - olive oil, parmesan & roasted garlic, 1 serving (3 oz)	2
Oven reds - olive oil, sun-dried tomatoes & pesto, 1 serving (3 oz)	2
Potato nuggets, 9 pieces	3
Red potatoes with garlic & parmesan, 1/2 cup	3
Sweet potato golden julienne fries, with sea salt, 1 serving (3 oz)	3
Waffle fries, 8 pieces	· 3
Yukon gold julienne fries with sea salt, 1 serving (3 oz)	2
Yukon gold potatoes & sea salt, 1/2 cup	3
Amy's	
Light in sodium brown rice & vegetable bowl, 1	5
Light in sodium shepherd's pie, 1	3

	POINTS VALUE
Amy's Bowls	
Brown rice & vegetables bowl, 1	5
Brown rice, black-eyed peas & veggies bowl, 1	6
Betty Crocker	
Russet harvest creamy butter mashed potatoes, prepared, 2/3 cup	3
Betty Crocker Deluxe Potatoes	
Cheesy cheddar au gratin, prepared, 1/2 cup	4
Cheesy cheddar au gratin, reduced-fat recipe, prepared, 1/2 cup	3
Creamy scalloped, prepared, 2/3 cup	3
Loaded au gratin, prepared, 1/2 cup	3
Mashed potato bake three cheese, prepared, 2/3 cup	4
Betty Crocker Mashed Potatoes	
Butter & herb mix, 2/3 cup	4
Four cheese mix, prepared, 1/2 cup	4
Four cheese mix, reduced-fat recipe, prepared, 1/2 cup	3
Homestyle creamy butter mashed potatoes, just add water, prepared, 2/3 cup	2
Homestyle recipe, prepared, 1/2 cup	4
Potato buds mix, prepared, 2/3 cup	4
Roasted garlic and cheddar, prepared, 1/2 cup	4
Roasted garlic and cheddar, reduced-fat recipe, prepared, 1/2 cup	3

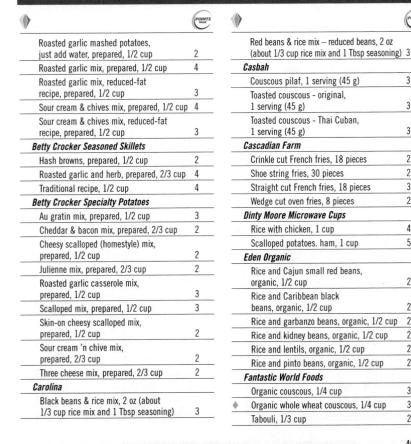

	POINTS VALUE
Roasted garlic mashed potatoes, just add water, prepared, 1/2 cup	2
Roasted garlic mix, prepared, 1/2 cup	4
Roasted garlic mix, reduced-fat recipe, prepared, 1/2 cup	3
Sour cream & chives mix, prepared, 1/2 cup	4
Sour cream & chives mix, reduced-fat recipe, prepared, 1/2 cup	3
Betty Crocker Seasoned Skillets	
Hash browns, prepared, 1/2 cup	2
Roasted garlic and herb, prepared, 2/3 cup	4
Traditional recipe, 1/2 cup	4
Betty Crocker Specialty Potatoes	
Au gratin mix, prepared, 1/2 cup	3
Cheddar & bacon mix, prepared, 2/3 cup	2
Cheesy scalloped (homestyle) mix, prepared, 1/2 cup	2
Julienne mix, prepared, 2/3 cup	2
Roasted garlic casserole mix, prepared, 1/2 cup	3
Scalloped mix, prepared, 1/2 cup	3
Skin-on cheesy scalloped mix, prepared, 1/2 cup	2
Sour cream 'n chive mix, prepared, 2/3 cup	2
Three cheese mix, prepared, 2/3 cup	2
Carolina	
Black beans & rice mix, 2 oz (about 1/3 cup rice mix and 1 Tbsp seasoning)	3

	POINTS VALUE
Red beans & rice mix – reduced beans, 2 oz (about 1/3 cup rice mix and 1 Tbsp seasoning)	3
Casbah	
Couscous pilaf, 1 serving (45 g)	3
Toasted couscous - original, 1 serving (45 g)	3
Toasted couscous - Thai Cuban, 1 serving (45 g)	3
Cascadian Farm	
Crinkle cut French fries, 18 pieces	2
Shoe string fries, 30 pieces	2
Straight cut French fries, 18 pieces	3
Wedge cut oven fries, 8 pieces	2
Dinty Moore Microwave Cups	
Rice with chicken, 1 cup	4
Scalloped potatoes. ham, 1 cup	5
Eden Organic	
Rice and Cajun small red beans, organic, 1/2 cup	2
Rice and Caribbean black beans, organic, 1/2 cup	2
Rice and garbanzo beans, organic, 1/2 cup	2
Rice and kidney beans, organic, 1/2 cup	2
Rice and lentils, organic, 1/2 cup	2
Rice and pinto beans, organic, 1/2 cup	2
Fantastic World Foods	
Organic couscous, 1/4 cup	3
♦ Organic whole wheat couscous, 1/4 cup	3 (6)
Tabouli, 1/3 cup	2

PREPARED FOODS, SALADS & SIDES

Potato, Rice and Grain Sides (con't) (POINTS VALUE)

Hamburger Helper

Cheesy baked potato, prepared, 1 cup	7
Cheesy hashbrowns, prepared, 1 cup	9

Hodgson Mill

◆ Whole wheat couscous, 1/3 cup	3 (6)
◆ Whole wheat couscous with milled flax seed & soy, 1/3 cup	4 (6)
Whole wheat garlic & basil couscous with milled flaxseed, 1/3 cup	4
Whole wheat parmesan cheese couscous with milled flaxseed, 1/3 cup	4

Ian's

Alphatots - alphabet shaped fun fries, 3 1/2 oz	4

Mahatma

Black beans & rice mix, 2 oz (about 1/3 cup rice mix and 1 Tbsp seasoning)	3
Red beans & rice mix - reduced beans, 2 oz (about 1/3 cup rice mix and 1 Tbsp seasoning)	3

Market Day

Quick 'n' crispy fries, 42	4

Marrakesh Express

Chicken with vegetables, 1 cup	3
Creamy pearls of pasta, 3 scoops	5
Curry, 1 cup	3
Mango salsa, 1 cup	4
Moroccan pasta, 1 cup	4
Parmesan cheese, 1 cup	4

(POINTS VALUE)

Plain, 1 cup	4
Sun dried tomato, 1 cup	3
Wild mushroom, 1 cup	4

Near East

Herbed chicken, prepared, 1 cup	4
Mediterranean curry, prepared, 1 cup	4
Parmesan, prepared, 1 cup	4
Roasted garlic and olive oil, prepared, 1 cup	4
Taboule wheat salad mix, prepared, 2/3 cup	2
Toasted pine nut, prepared, 1 cup	5
Tomato lentil, prepared, 1 cup	4

Ore-Ida

Cottage fries, 3 oz	3
Country style French fries, 3 oz	3
Country style steak fries, 3 oz	2
Crispers, 3 oz	5
Crispy crowns, 11 pieces	4
Crispy crunchies, 3 oz	4
Extra crispy fast food fries, 3 oz	3
Extra crispy golden crinkles, 3 oz	4
Extra crispy seasoned crinkles, 3 oz	3
Extra crispy steak fries, 3 oz	3
Fajita seasoned fries, 3 oz	3
Golden crinkles, 12 pieces	3
Golden fries, 14 pieces	2
Golden twirls, 1 1/3 cups	3

	POINTS VALUE
Oven chips, 3 oz	3
Pixie crinkles, 3 oz	3
Shoestrings, 32 pieces	3
Steak fries, 7 pieces	2
Texas crispers, 3 oz	3
Waffle fries, 3 oz	3
Zesties, 3 oz	3
Zesty twirls, 1 1/4 cups	3
Rice-A-Roni	
Red beans & rice, prepared, 1 cup	6
Schwan's LiveSmart	
Hash brown shreds, 3 oz	1
Quick bake French fries, 3 oz	3
Seeds of Change	
Athenian orzo, 1 tray	6
Risotto portobello di milano, 1 tray	6
Turkish seven grain pilaf, 1 tray	6
Tuscan style rice & beans, 1 serving (1 cup cooked)	3
Tony Chachere's	
Creole red beans and rice dinner mix, 1/4 cup	2
Old fashioned butter beans & rice mix, 1/4 cup	2
Southern white beans & rice mix, 1/4 cup	2
Weight Watchers Smart Ones	
Broccoli & cheddar roasted potatoes, 1 package	4

	POINTS VALUE
Zatarain's	
Blackened chicken alfredo, 1 package	13
Dirty rice with beef & pork, 1 package	9
Jambalaya seasoned with chicken, 1 package	8
Jambalaya seasoned with sausage, 1 package	8
Red beans & rice with sausage, 1 package	12
Sausage & chicken gumbo, 1 package	6
Zatarain's New Orleans Style Rice Mixes	
Black beans & rice, 3 Tbsp	2
Blackened chicken with yellow rice, 1 package	10
Red beans and rice, prepared, 1/2 cup	1
Rice	
Schwan's LiveSmart	
Microsteam brown rice, 1/2 pouch	6 (6)
Microsteam penne pasta, 1/2 pouch	4
Wild rice pilaf, 1 cup	3
Sandwiches	
Amy's	
Broccoli & cheese in a pocket sandwich, 1	6
Cheese pizza in a pocket sandwich, 1	6
Roasted vegetables in a pocket sandwich, 1	4
Soy cheeze pizza in a pocket sandwich, 1	6
Spinach feta in a pocket sandwich, 1	5

PREPARED FOODS, SALADS & SIDES

Sandwiches, Amy's (con't)	POINTS VALUE
Spinach pizza in a pocket sandwich, 1	6
Tofu scramble in a pocket sandwich, 1	4
Vegetable pie in a pocket sandwich, 1	6
Fast Fixin'	
On the go bbq rib sandwiches, 1	6
On the go cheeseburgers, 1	5
On the go chipotle chicken sandwiches, 1	7
Guiltless Gourmet	
Mediterranean spinach wrap, 1	5
Ian's	
Mini cheeseburgers, 1	5
Mini chicken patty sandwiches, 1	4
Jimmy Dean D-Lights	
Black forest ham, egg white and Swiss cheese on a muffin made with whole grain, 5	1
Canadian bacon, egg white and cheese on a honey wheat muffin, 1	5
Turkey sausage, egg white and cheese on a muffin made with whole grain, 1	5
Kangaroo	
Cheese omelet pita, 1	4
Santa Fe omelet pita, 1	4
Lightlife Smart Tortilla Wrap	
Breakfast scramble with smart bacon, 1	6
Market Day	
Breakfast bundles, 1 piece	4
Breakfast quesadilla, 1 serving (106 g)	7

	POINTS VALUE
Chop house cheeseburger, 1	10
Honey wheat pretzel turkey sandwich, 1	6
PB&J squarewiches, 1	6
Philly cheese steak kit, 1	15
Oscar Mayer	
Honey ham and Swiss melt, 1 package	9
Monterey turkey melt, 1 package	10
Oven baked ham and cheddar melt, 1 package	9
Smoked turkey breast/bacon/ mayonnaise, 1 package	5
Steakhouse cheddar melt, 1 package	10
Turkey cheddar dijon melt, 1 package	9
Oscar Mayer Deli Creations	
Smoked ham water added/natural mild cheddar cheese/mayonnaise, 1 package	6
Smoked ham water added/natural Swiss cheese/dijon mustard, 1 package	4
Smoked turkey breast/natural mild cheddar cheese/mayonnaise, 1 package	6
Pillsbury Frozen Sunrise Skillet Meal	
Sunrise skillet (potatoes, peppers, onions, sausage, biscuits), as packaged, 1 serving (1/8 package)	9
Sunrise skillet (potatoes, peppers, onions, sausage, biscuits), prepared with fat-free egg product including biscuit, 1 1/3 cups	11
Schwan's LiveSmart	
Toastwich ham & cheese, 1 piece	6

	POINTS VALUE
Weight Watchers Smart Ones Morning Express	
Breakfast quesadilla , 1 serving (113 g)	4
English muffin sandwich, 1 serving (113 g)	4
English muffin sandwich with Canadian bacon, 1 serving (113 g)	4
Stuffed breakfast sandwich, 1 serving (113 g)	4
Weight Watchers Smart Ones Bistro Selections	
Smartwich, pepperoni pizza, 1 serving (127 g)	6

Vegetable Sides

	POINTS VALUE
Alexia	
Onion rings, 6	5
Amy's	
Broccoli pot pie, 1	10
Country vegetable pie, 1	8
Non-dairy vegetable pot pie, 1	7
Shepherd's pie, 1	3
Vegetable pot pie, 1	9
Amy's Whole Meals	
Country dinner, 1	8
Southern meal with cornbread and beans, 1	7
Boar's Head	
◆ Sauerkraut, 2 Tbsp	0
Celentano Vegetarian	
Eggplant rollettes with sauce, 1 tray	8
Del Monte	
◆ Sauerkraut, 2 Tbsp	0

	POINTS VALUE
Dr. Praeger's	
Broccoli pancakes, 1	1
Potato pancakes, 1	2
Spinach pancakes, 1	2
Sweet potato pancakes, 1	1
Eden Organic	
◆ Sauerkraut, 1/2 cup	0
Ian's	
Onion rings, 6	3
Krrrrisp Kraut	
◆ Sauerkraut, 2 Tbsp	0
Ore-Ida	
Gourmet onion rings, 3 pieces	4
Rosina Presents Celentano	
Broccoli/spinach eggplant (rollette with sauce), 1 tray	8
Eggplant parmigiana, 1 cup	9
Eggplant parmigiana, 1/3 tray	9
Eggplant parmigiana, 1/2 small tray	8
Schwan's LiveSmart	
Herb garlic potato & vegetable blend, 1 cup	1
Mini bow tie pasta and vegetable blend, 1 cup	2
Roasted potatoes, broccoli and carrots with cheese sauce, 1 cup	2
Silver Floss	
◆ Sauerkraut, 2 Tbsp	0

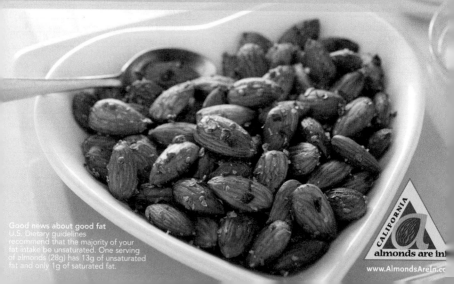

california almonds

How to show your sweet heart you care.

Step 1: Pick up some California Almonds from the snack, produce or baking aisle of the grocery store.

Step 2: Next time you or your sweetie is looking for snack, grab a handful of heart-healthy California Almo

Step 3: Feel satisfied knowing that just one ounce of almonds (about 23) can help you and your loved ones maintain a healthy cholesterol level.

Remember: Almonds are the snack that loves you back. They provide protein, fiber, vitamin E and more. Plus, they're low in saturated fat and always cholesterol-free. Now *that's* amore.

Good news about good fat
U.S. Dietary guidelines
recommend that the majority of your
fat intake be unsaturated. One serving
of almonds (28g) has 13g of unsaturated
fat and only 1g of saturated fat.

CALIFORNIA
almonds are in!
www.AlmondsAreIn.cc

Cheese Puffs

Cheetos

	POINTS VALUE
Chili limon flavored snacks, 21 pieces	4
Fantastix, chili cheese flavored baked corn & potato snack, 1 serving (28 g)	3

Garden of Eatin'

Cheddar puffs, 32 pieces	4
Crunchitos, 35	3

Little Bear

Crunchitos, 1 cup	3
Lite cheddar puffs, 2 cups	3
Original cheddar puffs, 2 cups	3

Market Day

Italian four cheese dipper, 1 slice	6

Cheese Snacks

Cheetos

Crunchy, 21 pieces	4

Snyder's of Hanover

Multigrain baked cheddar cheese crunchies, 1 cup	3
Multigrain white cheese puffs, 25	3
Multigrain yellow cheese puffs, 1 1/2 cups	3

Weight Watchers

Cheddar twists, 1 pouch	2

Corn Chips

Bachman

	POINTS VALUE
Corn chips, 1 oz	3
Corn chips, bbq flavored, 1 oz	3

Bugles

Chili cheese, 1 1/3 cups	4
Nacho cheese, 1 1/3 cups	4
Old El Paso salsa, 1 1/3 cups	4
Original, 1 1/3 cups	4
Original (single serving), 1 pouch	3
Smokin BBQ, 1 1/3 cups	4
Southwest ranch, 1 1/3 cups	4

Chester's

Flamin' hot flavored fries, 1 serving (24.8 g)	3

Corn Nuts

Barbecue, 1 package	4
Chile picante, 1 package	4
Crunchy toasted corn, 1/3 cup	3
Crunchy toasted corn, 1 package (22 g)	2
Crunchy toasted corn, 1 package (39 g)	4
Crunchy toasted corn, 1 package (48 g)	5
Crunchy toasted corn - chile, 1/3 cup	3
Crunchy toasted corn - chile, 1 package (22 g)	2
Crunchy toasted corn - chile, 1 package (39 g)	4

Corn Chips, Corn Nuts (con't)	POINTS VALUE
Crunchy toasted corn - chile, 1 package (48 g)	5
Crunchy toasted corn - nacho, 1/3 cup	3
Crunchy toasted corn - nacho, 1 package (22 g)	2
Crunchy toasted corn - nacho, 1 package (39 g)	4
Crunchy toasted corn - nacho, 1 package (48 g)	5
Crunchy toasted corn - original, 1/3 cup	3
Crunchy toasted corn - original, 1 package (39 g)	4
Crunchy toasted corn - original, 1 package (48 g)	5
Crunchy toasted corn - ranch, 1/3 cup	3
Crunchy toasted corn - ranch, 1 package (22 g)	2
Crunchy toasted corn - ranch, 1 package (39 g)	4
Crunchy toasted corn - ranch, 1 package (48 g)	5
Crunchy toasted corn - salsa, 1 package (22 g)	2
Crunchy toasted corn - salsa, 1 package (48 g)	5
Picante crunchy, 1 oz	3
Salsa jalisco, 1 oz	2
Salsa jalisco, 1 package	4

	POINTS VALUE
Fritos	
Bar-b-que, 29 pieces	4
Chili cheese, 31 pieces	4
Chips n' dip with chili cheese kit, 1 kit	6
Corn chips, 32 pieces	4
Flamin' hot flavor corn chips, 28 pieces	4
Flavor twists cheddar ranch flavored corn snacks, 23 pieces	4
Flavor twists honey bbq flavored, 23 pieces	4
Scoops!, 10 pieces	4
Garden of Eatin'	
Blue corn chips, 42 chips	4
Lance	
BBQ corn chips (blastin), 35	5
Hot fries, 1 oz	4
Solea Polenta Chips	
Guacamole chips, 1 oz	3
Mediterranean lime, 1 oz	3
Sea salt chips, 1 oz	3
Tuscan barbecue chips, 1 oz	3
Sun Chips	
Cinnamon flavor multigrain snacks, 15	3
French onion multigrain, 15	3
Garden salsa flavor multigrain snacks, 15 pieces	3
Harvest cheddar 100 calorie mini bites multigrain snacks, 1 package	2

	POINTS VALUE
Harvest cheddar multigrain, 15	3
Original multigrain, 16	3

Crackers

Annie's Homegrown

Cheddar bunnies, 50 pieces	3
Cheddar bunnies, 1 packet	3
Chocolate bunny grahams, 24 pieces	3
Chocolate chip bunny grahams, 24 pieces	3
Cinnamon bunny grahams, 24 pieces	3
Honey bunny grahams, 24 pieces	3
Sour cream & onion cheddar bunnies, 55 pieces	3
White cheddar blonde bunnies, 55 pieces	3
Whole wheat cheddar bunnies, 50 pieces	3

Austin

Animal crackers - sea animal, 1 package	3
Cheese crackers with cheddar cheese (sandwich), 1 package	5
Cheese crackers with cheddar Jack (sandwich), 1 package	5
Cheese crackers with megastuffed peanut butter (sandwich), 1 package	5
Cheese crackers with peanut butter (sandwich), 1 package	5
Chocolatey peanut butter, 1 package	5
Crispy crackers with cream cheese & chives (sandwich), 1 package	5
Dolphins & friends, 60	3

	POINTS VALUE
Grilled cheese flavored crackers (sandwich), 1 package	5
Super snack pack 8 ct cheese peanut butter, 1 package	3
Super snack pack 8 ct. toasty peanut butter, 1 package	3
Super snack pack cheese on cheese, 8 ct., 1 package	3
Super snack pack pb&j, 1 package	3
Toast and pb&J sandwich crackers, 1 package	4
Toasty crackers with peanut butter (sandwich), 1 package	5
Wheat crackers with cheddar cheese (sandwich), 1 package	5
Wheat crackers with cheddar cheese reduced fat (sandwich), 1 package	4
Zoo animal crackers, 1 package	3

Bachman

Jax baked cheese curls, 1 oz	3

Back to Nature

Classic rounds - flaky, buttery baked crackers, 5	2
Crispy wheats baked snack crackers, 1 pouch	3
Crispy wheats baked snack crackers, 17	3
Harvest whole wheats crackers, 6	2

Baked! Cheetos

Crunchy cheese flavored snacks, 34 pieces	3
Flamin' hot cheese flavored snacks, 1 package	3

Crackers (con't) (POINTS VALUE)

Baked! Cheetos Crunchy

Cheese flavored snacks (100 calorie mini bites), 1 package	2

Barbara's Bakery

Barbara's wheatines, all flavors, 1 large square	1
Cheese bites, 22	2
Cheese puffs, bakes, 1 1/2 cups	4
Cheese puffs, jalapeno, 3/4 cup	4
Cheese puffs, original, 3/4 cup	4
Cheese puffs, white cheddar, 1 1/2 cups	4
Original rite lite rounds, 5	1
Savory poppy rite lite rounds, 5	1
Tamari sesame rite lite rounds, 5	2

Barnum's Animals

Animal crackers, 1 serving (28 g)	2

Be Happy & Healthy

Reggae rice crackers, 1/2 cup	2

Carr's

Croissant crackers, 3 pieces	2
Poppy & sesame crackers, 4 pieces	2
Rosemary crackers, 7 pieces	3
Table water crackers, 5 pieces	1
Table water crackers baked with garlic & herbs, 4 pieces	1
Table water crackers with cracked pepper, 5 pieces	1

 (POINTS VALUE)

Table water crackers with sesame seeds, 5 pieces	1
Whole wheat crackers, 2 pieces	2

Cheetos

Asteroids crunchy cheese flavored snacks (100 calorie mini bites), 1 package	3
Asteroids flamin' hot cheese flavored snacks convenient cups, 1 cup	3
Bacon cheddar on cheese flavored crackers, 1 package	4
Cheddar cheese on golden toast crackers, 1 package	5
Cheddar jalapeno cheese flavored snacks, 21 pieces	4
Flamin' hot, 21 pieces	4
Flamin' hot jumbo puffs cheese flavored snacks, 13 pieces	4
Flamin' hot limon cheese flavored snacks, 28 pieces	4
Jumbo puffs cheese flavored snacks, 13	4
Mix & move cheese flavored snacks, 22	4
Natural white cheddar puffs cheese flavored snacks, 32 pieces	3
Puffs, 29 pieces	4
Reduced fat cheese flavored snacks, 35 pieces	3
Twisted cheese flavored snacks, 7 pieces	4

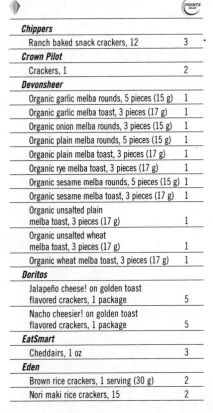

	POINTS VALUE
Chippers	
Ranch baked snack crackers, 12	3
Crown Pilot	
Crackers, 1	2
Devonsheer	
Organic garlic melba rounds, 5 pieces (15 g)	1
Organic garlic melba toast, 3 pieces (17 g)	1
Organic onion melba rounds, 3 pieces (15 g)	1
Organic plain melba rounds, 5 pieces (15 g)	1
Organic plain melba toast, 3 pieces (17 g)	1
Organic rye melba toast, 3 pieces (17 g)	1
Organic sesame melba rounds, 5 pieces (15 g)	1
Organic sesame melba toast, 3 pieces (17 g)	1
Organic unsalted plain melba toast, 3 pieces (17 g)	1
Organic unsalted wheat melba toast, 3 pieces (17 g)	1
Organic wheat melba toast, 3 pieces (17 g)	1
Doritos	
Jalapeño cheese! on golden toast flavored crackers, 1 package	5
Nacho cheesier! on golden toast flavored crackers, 1 package	5
EatSmart	
Cheddairs, 1 oz	3
Eden	
Brown rice crackers, 1 serving (30 g)	2
Nori maki rice crackers, 15	2

	POINTS VALUE
Finn Crisp	
Crispbread - fiber, 1 slice	0
Crispbread - multigrain, 1 slice	0
Crispbread - traditional, 1 slice	0
Rounds - multigrain, 1 slice	0
Rounds - sesame, 1 slice	1
Thin crisps - caraway, 2 slices	0
Thin crisps - multigrain, 2 slices	0
Thin crisps - original, 2 slices	0
Thin crisps - roast onion, 2 slices	0
Flat Earth	
Ranch carrot & green bean medley crunchy, 33 pieces	3
Frito-Lay	
Cream cheese & chive on toast flavored crackers, 1 package	5
Peanut butter on cheese crackers, 1 package	4
Peanut butter on toast crackers, 1 package	4
Gamesa	
Sabrosas crackers, 11	4
Saladitas saltine crackers, 9	3
GeniSoy Smart Hearts	
Garlic parmesan, 3/4 cup	2
Lightly salted, 3/4 cup	2
White cheddar, 3/4 cup	2
Good Health Guppies	
Cheddar crackers, 42	2

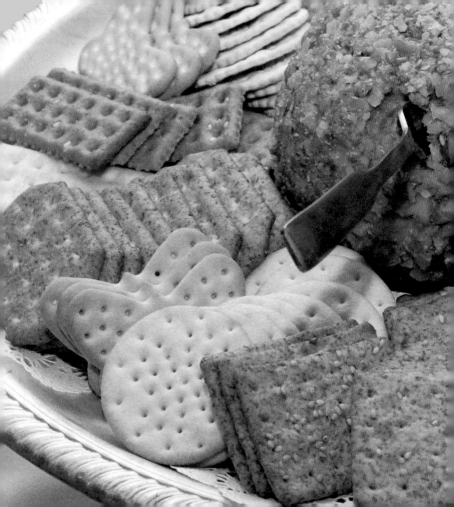

Crackers (con't)	POINTS VALUE
Good Health Quilts	
Dark rye crackers, 2	0
Light rye crackers, 2	1
Low sodium wheat crackers, 8	2
Original wheat crackers, 8	2
Health Valley	
Amaranth graham crackers, 6	2
Organic bruschetta vegetable crackers, 4	2
Organic cracked pepper crackers, 4	2
Organic garden herb crackers, 4	2
Organic sesame crackers, 4	1
Organic stoned wheat, 4	1
Organic whole wheat crackers, 4	1
Original rice bran graham crackers, 6	2
Jacoben's	
Blueberry, 1 slice	1
Cinnamon, 1 slice	1
Cinnamon-raisin, 1 slice	1
Honey maple, 1 slice	1
Original, 1 slice	1
Raspberry, 1 slice	1
Jax	
Cheddar cheese curls, 23 pieces	3
KA-ME	
Rice crunch cracker, black sesame & soy sauce, 17	2
Rice crunch cracker, seaweed, 19	2

	POINTS VALUE
Rice crunch crackers, cheese, 19	2
Rice crunch crackers, plain, 19	2
Rice crunch crackers, sesame, 19	2
Rice crunch crackers, wasabi, 19	3
Kashi TLC	
Country cheddar, 18	3
Entertained party cracker stoneground 7-grain, 4	2
Entertained party crackers Mediterranean bruschetta, 4	2
Entertained party crackers roasted garlic & thyme, 4	2
Fire roasted vegetable, 15	2
Honey sesame, 15	2
Natural ranch, 15	2
Original 7-grain, 15	2
Keebler	
Animal crackers dora the explorer, 9	3
Animal crackers hot wheels, 9	3
Cheese on club sandwich crackers, 1 package	4
Club cracker sticks butter herb, 12	3
Club cracker sticks, honey wheat, 12	3
Club cracker sticks, original, 12	3
Club crackers, multigrain, 4	1
Club crackers, multigrain puffed, 24	3
Club crackers, original, 4	1
Club crackers, puffed original, 24	3
Club crackers, reduced fat, 5	1

SNACKS

Crackers, Keebler (con't)	POINTS VALUE
Graham, cinnamon crisp, 8	3
Graham, cinnamon crisp, low fat, 8	2
Graham, honey, 8	3
Graham, honey, low fat, 8	2
Graham, original, 8	3
Sandwich crackers - cheese & peanut butter, 1 package	5
Sandwich crackers - toast & peanut butter, 1 package	5
Sandwich crackers - wheat & cheddar, 1 package	4
Scooby-doo cheddar crackers, 49	3
Special k snack bites, chocolatey, 1 pouch	2
Toasteds organic harvest wheat, 16	3
Toasteds, buttercrisp, 5	2
Toasteds, onion, 5	2
Toasteds, sesame, 5	2
Toasteds, wheat, 5	2
Town house bistro - corn bread, 2	2
Town house bistro - multigrain, 2	2
Town house flipsides, cheese pretzel, 5	1
Town house flipsides, original, 5	1
Town house toppers, garlic herb, 3	2
Town house toppers, original, 3	2
Town house, 50 % reduced fat, 6	1
Town house, original, 5	2
Town house, reduced sodium, 5	2

	POINTS VALUE
Town house, wheat, 5	2
Wheatables honey wheat snack crackers, 17	3
Wheatables multi grain snack crackers, 17	3
Wheatables original reduced fat, 19	3
Wheatables original snack crackers, 17	3
Zesta export sodas, 3	1
Zesta oyster crackers dot, 51	2
Zesta saltine crackers, original, 5	1
Zesta, saltine crackers, fat free, 5	1
Kellogg's	
All bran crackers garlic and herb, 18	2
All bran crackers multigrain, 18	2
All bran snack bites brown sugar cinnamon, 1 pouch	2
All bran snack bites honey oat & strawberry, 1 pouch	2
Special k snack bites strawberry, 1 pouch	2
Special k snack bites vanilla, 1 pouch	2
Kraft	
Cracker meal, 1/4 cup	2
Kraft Cheese Nips	
Baked snack crackers - cheddar, 1 package (35 g)	4
Baked snack crackers - cheddar, 1 package (47 g)	5
Baked snack crackers - spongebob squarepants, 25	3
Big crackers, 1 serving (31 g)	3

	POINTS VALUE
Cheddar, 29	3
Four cheese, 1 serving (30 g)	3
Mini, 1 package (21 g)	2
Peanut butter crackers, 1 package (39 g)	4
Real cheese crackers, 1 package (39 g)	5
Reduced fat cheddar, 31	3
Kraft Handi-Snacks	
Cheez'n breadsticks, 1	3
Cheez'n crackers, 1	2
Cheez'n pretzels, 1	2
Teddy graham bearwiches n' crème, 1	4
Lance	
Captain's wafers, 2 packages	2
Cheddar charged cheese ball, 27 pieces	4
Cheddar charged cheese puffs, 9 pieces	4
Cheese-on-wheat, 6	5
Cream cheese & chives on captain's wafers, 6	5
Crushed saltines, 1 oz	3
Gold-n-chees, 1 package	4
Graham crackers, 3	2
Nekot smores, 6	6
Nip chee, 6	5
Oblong melba toast, 4 slices	1
Oyster crackers, 1 package	1
Peanut butter wheat, 6	5
Peanut butter with honey on captain's wafers, 6	5

	POINTS VALUE
Reduced fat toastchee, 6	4
Saltines, 2 packages	1
Sesame twins, 2 packages	1
Smoked Swiss cheese on wheat, 6	5
Smokehouse cheddar on captain's. wafers, 6	4
Snack mix, gold-n-cheese, 1 package	5
Toastchee, 6	5
Toasty, 6	5
Triple cheese twisters cheese twists, 30 pieces	5
Wheat twins, 2 packages	1
Little Debbie	
Cheddar on cheese crackers, 1 serving (26 g)	3
Peanut butter cheese crackers, 4	3
Peanut butter toasty crackers, 4	3
Manischewitz	
Concord grape matzos, 1	2
Egg & onion matzo, 1	2
Egg matzo, 1	2
Egg matzo crackers, 1 oz	2
Everything matzo, 1	2
Matzo farfel, 1/4 cup	1
Matzo meal, 1/4 cup	2
Matzos, 1	2
Matzos, unsalted, 1	2
Saltine matzos, 1	2
Savory garlic matzos, 1	2
Thin matzo, unsalted, 1	2

Crackers, Manischewitz (con't)	POINTS VALUE
Thin matzos, salted, 1	2
Thin tea matzos, 1	2
White grape matzos, 1	2
Whole wheat matzos, 1	1
Yolk free egg matzos, 1	2
Market Day	
Cheddar cheese guppies, 1 pouch	2
Colby Jack cheese sticks, 1 stick	3
Giant cinnamon goldfish grahams, 1 pouch	3
Michael Season's	
Lite cheddar cheese curls, 1 cup	3
Mi-Del	
Honey grahams, 4	2
Nabisco	
Chicken in a biskit, 1 serving (31 g)	4
Grahams, 8 (2 full cracker sheets)	3
Sociables baked savory crackers, 1 serving (14 g)	2
Vegetable thins baked snack crackers, 1 serving (31 g)	4
Whole grain chips - apple, 16	2
Whole grain chips - banana, 16	2
Whole grain chips - tomato basil, 16	2
Nabisco Cheese Nips	
Crackers with real cheese, 1 package	3
Nabisco Honey Maid	
Chocolate grahams, 8	3
Chocolate sticks, 1 serving (31 g)	3

	POINTS VALUE
Cinnamon grahams, 8	3
Cinnamon grahams, lowfat, 8 (2 full cracker sheets)	2
Cinnamon sticks, 14	3
Cinnamon sticks, 1 package	4
Cinnamon sticks packs 2 go, 1 packet	2
Graham sticks - honey, 14	3
Honey grahams, 8	3
Honey grahams, lowfat, 8 (2 full cracker sheets)	2
Nabisco Kid Sense Fun Packs	
Teddy grahams cubs cinnamon, 1 serving (22 g)	2
Nabisco Premium	
Gold crackers, 1 serving (15 g)	2
Low sodium saltine, 5	1
Original saltine, 1 large packet (4 crackers)	1
Original saltine, 3 packets (2 crackers each)	1
Original saltine, 5	1
Soup & oyster crackers, 1 serving (15 g)	1
Unsalted tops saltine, 2 packages	1
Unsalted tops saltine, 5	1
Nabisco Ritz	
Baseball crackers, 1 serving (16 g)	2
Cheddar oven-toasted chips, 1 package	2
Cheddar oven-toasted chips, 1 serving (28 g)	3
Cracker sandwiches with real cheese, 1 package	5

	POINTS VALUE
Crackers, 1 serving (16 g)	2
Football shape crackers, 1 serving (16 g)	2
Garlic butter crackers, 1 serving (16 g)	2
Holiday crackers, 5	2
Low sodium crackers, 1 serving (16 g)	2
Mini original bite size, 1 serving (30 g)	4
Original chips, 1 serving (28 g)	3
Reduced fat crackers, 1 serving (15 g)	2
Toasted chips - sour cream & onion, 14	3
Toasted chips - sour cream & onion, 1 package	2
Toasted chips - sour cream & onion, 1 package	5
Whole grain chips - vegetable medley, 5	2
Whole wheat crackers, 1 serving (15 g)	1
Nabisco Ritz Bits	
Cheese cracker sandwiches, 1 package (35 g)	4
Cheese cracker sandwiches, 1 package (42 g)	5
Cheese cracker sandwiches go-pak, 1 serving (29 g)	4
Graham cracker s'mores cracker sandwiches, 1 package (35 g)	4
Graham cracker s'mores cracker sandwiches, 1 package (42 g)	5
Graham cracker s'mores cracker sandwiches, 2 packages (28 g)	3
Graham cracker s'mores cracker sandwiches, 9	3

	POINTS VALUE
Peanut butter cracker sandwiches, 1 package (35 g)	4
Peanut butter cracker sandwiches, 1 package (49 g)	6
Peanut butter cracker sandwiches, 1 serving (28 g)	3
Peanut butter cracker sandwiches, 1 serving (42 g)	5
Peanut butter cracker sandwiches go-pak, 1 serving (29 g)	3
Nabisco Royal Lunch	
Milk crackers, 1	1
Nabisco Teddy Cheddy	
Baked cheddar cheese crackers, 1 package	4
Baked cheddar cheese crackers, 31	3
Nabisco Teddy Grahams	
Chocolate graham snacks, 1 serving (30 g)	3
Chocolate graham snacks, 1 serving (35 g)	3
Chocolatey chip graham snacks, 1 serving (30 g)	3
Cinnamon graham snacks, 1 serving (30 g)	3
Cinnamon graham snacks, 1 serving (35 g)	3
Dora the explorer graham snacks, 1 serving (31 g)	3
Honey graham snacks, 1 serving (30 g)	3
Honey graham snacks, 1 serving (35 g)	3
Honey graham snacks go-pak, 1 serving (30 g)	3

Crackers, Nabisco Teddy Grahams (con't)

	POINTS VALUE
Honey graham snacks mini snak saks, 1 serving	3
Mini chocolatey chips graham snacks snak saks, 1 serving (30 g)	3

Nabisco Triscuit

Baked whole wheat crackers - low sodium, 6 crackers	2
Baked whole wheat crackers - original, 1 package	4
Baked whole wheat crackers - original, 6	2
Cheddar, 1 serving (28 g)	2
Deli-style rye, 1 serving (28 g)	2
Garden herb, 1 serving (28 g)	2
Reduced fat baked whole wheat crackers, 7	2
Roasted garlic, 1 serving (28 g)	2
Thin crisps, 1 serving (30 g)	2

Nabisco Uneeda

Biscuit, 2	1

Nabisco Wheat Thins

Baked snack crackers - big, 1 package (44 g)	4
Baked snack crackers - tomato and basil, 15	3
Baked snack crackers 100% whole grain, 16	3
Big, 1 serving (31 g)	3
Harvest crisps five grain baked snack crackers, 13	3
Honey, 1 serving (31 g)	3
Low sodium, 1 serving (31 g)	3
Multi-grain, 1 serving (30 g)	3

	POINTS VALUE
Original, 1 serving (35 g)	4
Original flavor baked snack crackers, 1 package (50 g)	5
Original flavor baked snack crackers, 16	3
Original packs 2 go, 1 packet	4
Ranch, 1 serving (29 g)	3
Reduced fat baked snack crackers, 16	3

Natural Nectar Cracklebred

Multigrain crackers, 3	1
Original crackers, 3	1
Sundried tomato & oregano crackers, 3	1

New Morning

Mini-bites, chocolate graham snacks, 1 packet	2
Mini-bites, honey graham snacks, 1 packet	2

Old London

Bacon flavor melba snacks, 5 pieces	1
Classic melba snacks, 5 pieces	1
Classic melba toast, 3 pieces	1
Garlic melba snacks, 5 pieces	1
Garlic melba toast, 3 pieces	1
Onion melba snacks, 5 pieces	1
Onion melba toast, 3 pieces	1
Rye melba snacks, 5 pieces	1
Rye melba toast, 3 pieces	1
Sesame melba snacks, 5 pieces	1
Sesame melba toast, 3 pieces	1
Unsalted sesame melba toast, 3 pieces	1

	POINTS VALUE
Unsalted whole grain melba toast, 3 pieces	1
Wheat melba toast, 3 pieces	1
Whole grain melba snacks, 5 pieces	1
Whole grain melba toast, 3 pieces	1
Pepperidge Farm	
Distinctive butter flavored thins, 4	2
Distinctive harvest wheat crackers, 3	2
Flavor blasted xtra cheddar goldfish, 51	3
Red Oval Farms	
Sesame and onion crackers, 2	1
Red Oval Farms Stoned Wheat Thins	
Crackers (oval shape) - seeds & grains, 4	2
Sabritones	
Lime & chili flavored wheat snacks, 23	4
Sesmark	
Rice thins - brown rice, 17	2
Rice thins - cheddar, 15	3
Rice thins - sesame, 16	3
Rice thins - teriyaki, 15	3
Savory minis - garlic, 40	3
Savory rice minis - lightly salted, 40	3
Savory thins - black sesame & garlic, 16	3
Savory thins - cracked wheat, 16	2
Savory thins - original, 15	3
Savory thins - teriyaki, 15	3
Savory thins - three cheese & tomato, 16	3
Savory thins - toasted onion & garlic, 16	2

	POINTS VALUE
Sunshine	
Krispy saltines with whole wheat, 5	1
Krispy, soup & oyster, 16	1
Krispy, unsalted tops, 5	1
Zesta saltines with whole wheat, 5	1
Sunshine Cheez-It	
Big, 13	4
Cheddar Jack, 25	4
Cheez-its, 27	4
Crisps cheddar, 36	3
Crisps four cheese, 36	3
Fiesta cheddar nacho, 25	4
Fiesta chili queso, 25	4
Gripz, 1 pouch	3
Gripz nacho micro, 1 pouch	3
Hot & spicy, 25	3
Parmesan garlic, 25	4
Pasteurized cheese snack aerosol - cheddar, 2 Tbsp	2
Pasteurized cheese snack aerosol - white cheddar, 2 Tbsp	2
Reduced fat, 29	3
Right bites 100 calories, 1 pouch	2
Shrek, 27	3
Sour cream & onion, 25	4
Sponge Bob, 30	3
Stix cheddar, 35	3
Stix white cheddar, 35	3

Crackers, Sunshine Cheez-It (con't)

	(POINTS VALUE)
Twisterz cheddar and cool ranch, 17	3
Twisterz cheddar and more cheddar, 17	3
Twisterz hot wings and cheesy blue, 17	3
White cheddar, 25	3

Tree of Life

Organic classic golden crackers, 6	2
Organic cracked pepper crackers, 10	2
Organic garden vegetable crackers, 10	2
Organic herb & garlic crackers, 10	2
Organic sesame & flax seed crackers, 10	3
Organic toasted onion crackers, 10	2
Organic water cracker cracked pepper, 4	1
Organic water cracker original, 4	1
Organic water cracker sesame, 4	2

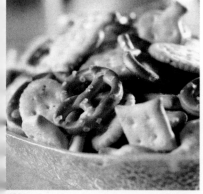

Glazed Fruit
Tropical Nut & Fruit

	(POINTS VALUE)
Diced orange peel glaze, 2 Tbsp	1
Glazed diced citron, 2 Tbsp	1
Glazed green cherries, 1 piece	0
Glazed pineapple slice, 1/2 piece	2
Mello mix, 1 Tbsp	1

Granola, Nutritional and Snack Bars
Gatorade

Chocolate chip bar, 1 bar	5

Quaker Oats Baked Muffin Bars

Banana, 1 bar	2
Blueberry, 1 bar	2

Quaker Oats Chewy Granola Bar

Dark chocolate cherry, 1 bar	2
Strawberry vanilla, 1 bar	2

Quaker Oats Simple Harvest

Chocolate chunk bar, 1 bar	3
Cinnamon brown sugar bar, 1 bar	3

Quaker Oats Simple Harvest Bar

Honey roasted nuts bar, 1 bar	3

Quaker Oats Sweet & Salty

Honey roasted peanut crunch bar, 2 bars	3
Oats, nuts & honey crunch bar, 2 bars	3
Toffee nut crunch bar, 2 bars	3

Quaker Oats Whole Grain Granola Bites

Chocolate, 1 bag	2
Cinnamon, 1 bag	2
Peanut butter, 1 bag	2

So decadent, if it weren't for the 90 calories, you might just blush.

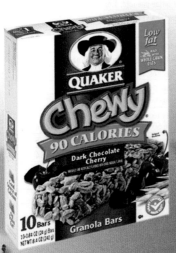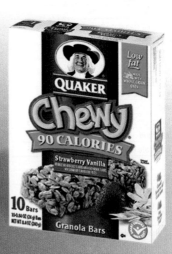

**Quaker 90 Calorie Chewy Granola Bars
in Decadent Flavors:
Dark Chocolate Cherry
& Strawberry Vanilla**

Nuts

Be Happy & Healthy

	POINTS VALUE
All about almonds, 23 pieces	4
Calypso cashews, 1/4 cup	4
Got nuts?, 1/4 cup	5

Blue Diamond

Oven roasted cinnamon brown sugar almonds, 1 oz	4
Oven roasted no salt almonds, 1 oz	4
Oven roasted sea salt almonds, 1 oz	4
Oven roasted vanilla bean almonds, 1 oz	4
Whole almonds, 1 bag	2

Brookside

Milk chocolate almonds, 9 pieces	5

Chocolate Bowl

Milk chocolate cashews, 12 pieces	5

DrSoy

Barbecue, 1 oz	3
Original, 1 oz	3
Ranch, 1 oz	3

Eden

Tamari almonds, dry roasted, 3 Tbsp	3

Estee

Candy coated peanuts, 1/4 cup	4

Everybody's Nuts

European roast pistachios, 1/4 cup	4
Roasted & salted pistachios, 1/4 cup	4
Roasted no salt pistachios, 1/4 cup	4
Salt & pepper pistachios, 1/4 cup	4

Fisher

Almonds, hickory smoked flavor, 1/4 cup	4
Almonds, roasted & salted, 1/4 cup	4
Butter toffee peanuts, 1 oz	3
Cashews, halves & pieces, 1 oz	4
Chopped pecans, 1 oz	5
Chopped walnuts, 1 oz	5
Deluxe mixed nuts, no peanuts, 1 oz	4
Fancy pecans, roasted & salted, 1 oz	6
Fancy pecans, roasted & salted, 1/4 cup	5
Honey roasted peanuts, dry roasted, 1 oz	4
Lightly salted mixed nuts, less than 50% peanuts, 1 oz	4
Macadamias, halves & pieces, 1 oz	5
Mixed nuts, less than 50% peanuts, 1 oz	4
Natural sliced almonds, 1 oz	4
Nature's nut mix, 1 oz	4
Peanuts, dry roasted, 1 package	2
Peanuts, honey roasted, 1 package	2
Peanuts, roasted salted, 1 package	2
Peanuts, salted in-shell, 1 oz (shelled peanuts)	4
Peanuts, unsalted in-shell, 1 oz (shelled peanuts)	4
Pecan halves, 1 oz	5
Pistachios, natural, 1 bag (1 bag shelled nuts)	4

GIVE YOUR HUNGER A TIME OUT.

NEW

No Added Oil

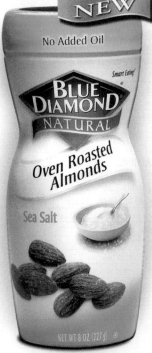

New Blue Diamond® Oven Roasted Almonds, baked to perfection, with no added oil, making each handful **MORE** flavorful and **MORE** satisfying... giving your hunger a time out, so you can make the most of your day. Need we say **MORE?**

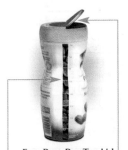

Easy Pour Pop-Top Lid
Portion Control Side Window

Sea Salt | Vanilla Bean | Cinnamon Brown Sugar | No Salt

MORE THAN A SNACK®

SNACKS

Nuts, Fisher (con't)	POINTS VALUE
Premium whole cashews, 1 oz	4
Raw peanuts, 1 oz	4
Slivered almonds, 1 oz	4
Spanish peanuts, redskin, 1 oz	4
Walnuts, 1 oz	5
Whole natural almonds, 1 oz	4
Fisher Chef's Naturals	
Chopped hazelnuts, 1 oz	4
Chopped macadamias, 1 oz	5
Pine nuts, 1 oz	5
Fisher Golden Roast	
Lightly salted peanuts, dry roasted, 1 oz	4
Peanuts, dry roasted, 1 oz	4
Unsalted peanuts, dry roasted, 1 oz	4
Frito-Lay	
Deluxe mixed nuts, 1/4 cup	4
Dry roasted peanuts, 1 serving (49.6 g)	7
Honey roasted cashews, 1 serving (42.5 g)	7
Honey roasted peanuts, 1 serving (30 g)	4
Hot peanuts, 1 serving (49.6 g)	7
Jumbo salted peanuts, 3 Tbsp	4
Nobby's nuts savory ranch crunchy coated peanuts, 2 oz	6
Nobby's nuts zesty salsa crunchy coated peanuts, 2 oz	6
Praline pecans, 1 serving (56.7 g)	8
Salted almonds, 1 serving (46.6 g)	7
Salted cashews, 3 Tbsp	6

	POINTS VALUE
Salted in-shell peanuts, 1 serving (28 g)	4
Salted in-shell pistachio nuts, 1 serving (25 g)	3
Salted peanuts, 1 package (49.6 g)	7
Smoked almonds, 1 serving (46.6 g)	7
GeniSoy	
BBQ, 1/4 cup	2
Chocolate soy nuts, 1/4 cup	5
Deep sea salted, 1/4 cup	2
Unsalted, 1/4 cup	2
Lance	
Cashews, 1 package	5
Honey toasted peanuts, 1 package	5
Hot & spicy peanuts, 1 package	7
Roasted peanuts (unsalted), 3/4 cup	4
Salted in shell roasted peanuts, 2/3 cup	4
Salted peanuts, 1 package	4
Nut Harvest	
Natural honey roasted peanuts, 2 Tbsp	4
Natural lightly roasted almonds, 2 Tbsp	5
Natural sea salted peanuts, 3 Tbsp	5
Natural sea salted whole cashews, 3 Tbsp	5
Planters	
Almonds, 1 oz	4
Black walnuts, 1 bag	9
Cashew halves & pieces lightly salted, 1 oz	4
Cashew halves with pieces, 1 oz	4
Cashew sesame mix with peanuts, 1 oz	4

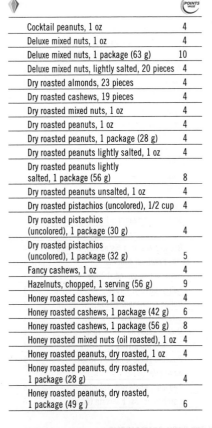

	POINTS VALUE
Cocktail peanuts, 1 oz	4
Deluxe mixed nuts, 1 oz	4
Deluxe mixed nuts, 1 package (63 g)	10
Deluxe mixed nuts, lightly salted, 20 pieces	4
Dry roasted almonds, 23 pieces	4
Dry roasted cashews, 19 pieces	4
Dry roasted mixed nuts, 1 oz	4
Dry roasted peanuts, 1 oz	4
Dry roasted peanuts, 1 package (28 g)	4
Dry roasted peanuts lightly salted, 1 oz	4
Dry roasted peanuts lightly salted, 1 package (56 g)	8
Dry roasted peanuts unsalted, 1 oz	4
Dry roasted pistachios (uncolored), 1/2 cup	4
Dry roasted pistachios (uncolored), 1 package (30 g)	4
Dry roasted pistachios (uncolored), 1 package (32 g)	5
Fancy cashews, 1 oz	4
Hazelnuts, chopped, 1 serving (56 g)	9
Honey roasted cashews, 1 oz	4
Honey roasted cashews, 1 package (42 g)	6
Honey roasted cashews, 1 package (56 g)	8
Honey roasted mixed nuts (oil roasted), 1 oz	4
Honey roasted peanuts, dry roasted, 1 oz	4
Honey roasted peanuts, dry roasted, 1 package (28 g)	4
Honey roasted peanuts, dry roasted, 1 package (49 g)	6

	POINTS VALUE
Honey roasted peanuts, dry roasted, 1 package (56 g)	7
Honey roasted peanuts, dry roasted, 1 package (70 g)	10
Lightly salted cocktail peanuts, 1 oz	4
Lightly salted mixed nuts, 1 oz	4
Lovers mix - cashew, 17 pieces	5
Lovers mix - macadamia, 22 pieces	5
Lovers mix - pecans, 24 pieces	5
Lovers mix - pistachio, 35 pieces	4
Macadamia nuts, 3 Tbsp	5
Macadamias, chopped, 1 bag (56 g)	11
Mix cashews with almonds and macadamias, 1 oz	5
Mix cashews with almonds and pecans, 1 oz	4
NUTrition energy mix, 1/4 cup	4
NUTrition lightly salted almonds, 1 serving (28 g)	4
NUTrition lightly salted smoked almonds, 1 serving (25 g)	4
NUTrition mixed nuts, lightly salted, 1 oz	4
NUTrition mixed nuts, roasted, lightly salted, 1 package (42 g)	6
NUTrition south beach diet mix, 21 pieces	4
Old fashioned peanuts (grandstand), 30 pieces	4
Pecan chips, 1 bag (56 g)	10
Pecan halves, 1 oz	5
Pecan pieces, 1 oz	5

SNACKS

Nuts, Planters (con't)	POINTS VALUE
Pecan pieces, 1 package (56 g)	10
Pine nuts, 1 bag (56 g)	9
Raw Spanish peanuts, 1 oz	3
Regular mixed nuts, 30 pieces	4
Salted peanuts, 1 package (28 g)	4
Salted peanuts, 1 package (56 g)	8
Salted peanuts, 35 pieces	4
Salted peanuts, 1 package (49 g)	7
Seasonuts bbq peanuts, 1 package (49 g)	7
Seasonuts bbq peanuts, 1 package (70 g)	10
Seasonuts honey mustard peanuts, 1 package (70 g)	10
Seasonuts honey mustard peanuts, 43 pieces	4
Select mix lightly salted cashews with almonds and pecans, 21 pieces	4
Select mix lightly salted cashews with almonds and pecans, 1 package (63 g)	10
Slivered almonds, 1/3 cup	5
Sliced almonds, 1 serving (33 g)	4
Slivered almonds, 1 serving (34 g)	5
Slivered almonds, 1 bag (56 g)	8
Smoked almonds, 1 package (42 g)	6
Spicy nuts & Cajun, 1 package (56 g)	7
Sweet 'n crunchy peanuts, 1 oz	3
Tavern nuts - coated redskin peanuts, 36 pieces	4
Unsalted cocktail peanuts, 1 oz	4
Unsalted mixed nuts, 1 oz	4
Walnut halves, 1 serving (30 g)	5

	POINTS VALUE
Walnut pieces, 1 serving (29 g)	5
Whole cashews, 1 package (63 g)	10
Whole cashews, 1 package (56 g)	3
Whole cashews, 1 oz	4
Whole lightly salted cashews, 1 oz	4
Planters Sweet Roasts	
Cinnamon (almonds, peanuts & pecans), 1 oz	4
Honey roasted (peanuts & cashews), 1 package	4
Vanilla (almonds, cashews & peanuts), 1 oz	4
Sabra	
Pine nuts, 1 oz	2
Sabritas	
Picante peanuts, 1 package	7
Salt & lime peanuts, 1 package	7
Sunkist	
Roasted & salted pistachios, 1/4 cup	4
Sunkist Almond Accents	
Butter toffee glazed, 1 Tbsp	1
Honey roasted, 1 Tbsp	1
Italian parmesan, 1 Tbsp	1
Original oven roasted, 1 Tbsp	1
Oven roasted no salt, 1 Tbsp	1
Ranch style, 1 Tbsp	1
Roasted garlic Caesar, 1 Tbsp	1
Tree of Life	
Almonds, whole raw, 1/4 cup	4
Carob almonds, 1 serving (40 g)	6

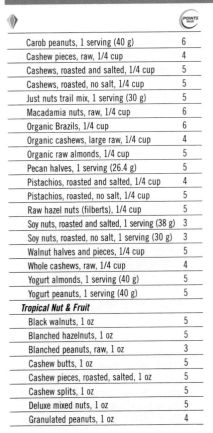

	POINTS VALUE
Carob peanuts, 1 serving (40 g)	6
Cashew pieces, raw, 1/4 cup	4
Cashews, roasted and salted, 1/4 cup	5
Cashews, roasted, no salt, 1/4 cup	5
Just nuts trail mix, 1 serving (30 g)	5
Macadamia nuts, raw, 1/4 cup	6
Organic Brazils, 1/4 cup	6
Organic cashews, large raw, 1/4 cup	4
Organic raw almonds, 1/4 cup	5
Pecan halves, 1 serving (26.4 g)	5
Pistachios, roasted and salted, 1/4 cup	4
Pistachios, roasted, no salt, 1/4 cup	5
Raw hazel nuts (filberts), 1/4 cup	5
Soy nuts, roasted and salted, 1 serving (38 g)	3
Soy nuts, roasted, no salt, 1 serving (30 g)	3
Walnut halves and pieces, 1/4 cup	5
Whole cashews, raw, 1/4 cup	4
Yogurt almonds, 1 serving (40 g)	5
Yogurt peanuts, 1 serving (40 g)	5
Tropical Nut & Fruit	
Black walnuts, 1 oz	5
Blanched hazelnuts, 1 oz	5
Blanched peanuts, raw, 1 oz	3
Cashew butts, 1 oz	5
Cashew pieces, roasted, salted, 1 oz	5
Cashew splits, 1 oz	5
Deluxe mixed nuts, 1 oz	5
Granulated peanuts, 1 oz	4

	POINTS VALUE
Honey roasted almonds, 1/4 cup	5
Honey roasted cashews, 1/4 cup	5
Honey roasted peanuts, 1/4 cup	4
In-shell peanuts, roasted, salted, 1 oz	4
Macadamia nuts, 1 oz	5
Mixed nuts and peanuts, 1/4 cup	5
Natural hazelnuts, 1 oz	5
Natural pistachios, 1/4 cup	4
Peanut butter stock, 1 oz	4
Pecan halves, 1 oz	5
Pecan halves, roasted & salted, 1 oz	6
Pecan pieces, 1 oz	5
Pine nuts (pignolias), 1/4 cup	4
Raw cashew butts, 1/4 cup	4
Raw cashew splits, 1/4 cup	4
Red pistachios, 1/4 cup	4
Redskin peanuts, 1 oz	5
Redskin peanuts, raw, 1 oz	4
Roasted pecan halves, 1 oz	6
Select mixed nuts, 1 serving (30 g)	5
Shelled raw pistachios, 1 oz	4
Sliced almonds, 1 oz	4
Slivered almonds, 1 oz	4
Smoked almonds, 1 oz	4
Soybeans roast/salt, 1 oz	2
Spanish peanuts, 1 oz	5
Walnut halves & pieces, 1/4 cup	5
Walnut pieces, 1/4 cup	5

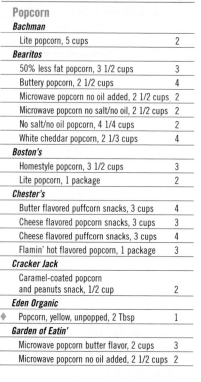

	POINTS VALUE

Popcorn
Bachman

Lite popcorn, 5 cups	2

Bearitos

50% less fat popcorn, 3 1/2 cups	3
Buttery popcorn, 2 1/2 cups	4
Microwave popcorn no oil added, 2 1/2 cups	2
Microwave popcorn no salt/no oil, 2 1/2 cups	2
No salt/no oil popcorn, 4 1/4 cups	2
White cheddar popcorn, 2 1/3 cups	4

Boston's

Homestyle popcorn, 3 1/2 cups	3
Lite popcorn, 1 package	2

Chester's

Butter flavored puffcorn snacks, 3 cups	4
Cheese flavored popcorn snacks, 3 cups	3
Cheese flavored puffcorn snacks, 3 cups	4
Flamin' hot flavored popcorn, 1 package	3

Cracker Jack

Caramel-coated popcorn and peanuts snack, 1/2 cup	2

Eden Organic

♦ Popcorn, yellow, unpopped, 2 Tbsp	1

Garden of Eatin'

Microwave popcorn butter flavor, 2 cups	3
Microwave popcorn no oil added, 2 1/2 cups	2

	POINTS VALUE

Good Health

Half naked popcorn, 3 1/2 cups	2
Organic popcorn, 3 1/2 cups	3

JOLLY TIME

♦ 100 calorie healthy pop butter 94% fat free, popped, 5 cups	1
♦ 100 calorie healthy pop kettle corn, 94% fat free, 4 cups	1
Better butter flavor microwave popcorn, popped, 4 cups	3
Mallow magic yummy marshmallow flavor microwave pop corn, popped, 2 1/2 cups	4
Sassy salsa kick'd up Southwest microwave popcorn, popped, 3 1/2 cups	3

JOLLY TIME American's Best

♦ 94% fat free butter flavor microwave pop corn, popped, 5 cups	1

JOLLY TIME Big Cheez

Ultimate cheddar microwave pop corn, popped, 3 1/2 cups	3

JOLLY TIME Blast O Butter

Light ultimate theatre style microwave pop corn, popped, 4 cups	2
Ultimate theatre style microwave pop corn, popped, 3 1/2 cups	3

JOLLY TIME Butter-Licious

Light butter flavor microwave pop corn, popped, 5 cups	2
Original butter flavor microwave pop corn, popped, 4 cups	3

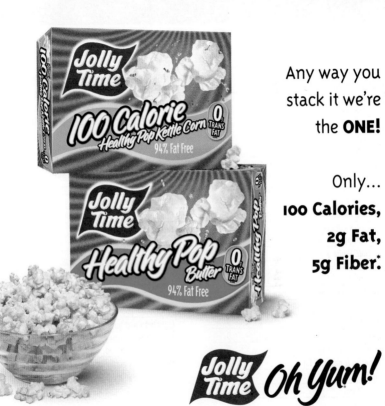

Any way you stack it we're the **ONE!**

Only...
**100 Calories,
2g Fat,
5g Fiber.***

Popcorn (con't) POINTS VALUE

JOLLY TIME Crispy 'N White

Light natural flavor white microwave pop corn, popped, 5 cups	2
Natural flavor white microwave pop corn, popped, 4 cups	3

JOLLY TIME Healthy Pop

♦ 94% fat free, butter flavor microwave pop corn, popped, 5 cups	1
94% fat free, caramel apple flavor microwave pop corn, popped, 5 cups	1
94% fat free, kettle corn microwave pop corn, popped, 4 cups	1

JOLLY TIME Kettle Mania

Kettle corn microwave pop corn, popped, 3 cups	3

JOLLY TIME White & Buttery

Butter, white microwave pop corn, popped, 4 cups	3

Kernel Season's Gourmet Popcorn Seasoning

Butter, 1/4 tsp	0
Caramel, 1/4 tsp	0
Kettle korn, 1/4 tsp	0
Nacho cheddar, 1 tsp	0
Parmesan & garlic, 1 tsp	0
Ranch, 1 tsp	0
Salt, 1/4 tsp	0
Sour cream & onion, 1 tsp	0
White cheddar, 1 tsp	0

  POINTS VALUE

Lance

White cheddar cheese popcorn, 1 package	4

Pop-Secret

100 calorie pop butter, popped, 1 bag	2
100 calorie pop kettle corn, popped, 1 bag	2
♦ 94% fat free butter (snack size), 1 bag	2
♦ 94% fat free butter, popped, 6 cups	2
94% fat free kettle corn, popped, 6 cups	2
94% fat free kettle corn, snack size, 1 bag	2
Butter popcorn, popped, 1 cup	1
Butter, popped, 1 cup	1
Cheddar, popped, 1 cup	1
Extra butter, popped, 1 cup	1
Homestyle (snack size), popped, 1 cup	1
Homestyle, popped, 1 cup	1
Jumbo pop butter, popped, 1 cup	1
Jumbo pop movie theater butter, popped, 1 cup	1
Kettle corn, popped, 1 cup	1
Light with real butter, popped, 1 cup	0
Movie theater butter (snack size), popped, 1 bag	1
Movie theater butter, popped, 1 cup	1
White cheddar popcorn, popped, 1 cup	1

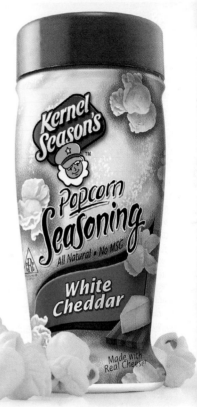

Popcorn (con't)

	POINTS VALUE
Robert's American Gourmet	
Chaos, 1 oz	3
Pirate's booty with golden caramel, 1 oz	2
Pirate's swords, 1 oz	3
Smart puffs, 1 oz	3
Tings, 1 oz	4
Veggie booty, 1 oz	3
Smart Balance	
Light butter, popped, 4 cups	2
Light popcorn (minibag), 1	3
Low fat, low sodium, 5 cups	2
Movie style, 3 1/2 cups	4
Smartfood	
Reduced fat white cheddar cheese flavored popcorn, 1 package	3
White cheddar cheese flavored popcorn, 1 3/4 cups	4
Tree of Life	
Organic butter flavored popcorn, popped, 4 cups	3
Organic lightly salted popcorn, popped, 4 cups	1

Potato Chips

	POINTS VALUE
Baked! Lay's	
Cheddar & sour cream flavored potato crisps, 14 pieces	2
Baken-ets	
Fried pork skins, 9 pieces	2

	POINTS VALUE
Hot n' spicy, fried, 9 pieces	2
Salt & vinegar fried pork skins, 9 pieces	2
Barbara's Bakery	
No salt added, 1 1/4 cups	4
Regular, 1 1/4 cups	4
Ripple, 1 1/4 cups	4
Yogurt & green onion, 1 1/4 cups	4
EatSmart	
French onion potato chips, 1 serving (1 oz)	3
Lightly salted potato chips, 1 serving (1 oz)	3
Sweet barbeque potato chips, 1 serving (1 oz)	3
El Isleno	
Plantains chips, 32 pieces	3
Good Health	
Au gratin bistro chips, 1 oz	1
Avocado oil potato chips with a pinch of sea salt, 1 oz	3
Avocado oil potato chips, Barcelona barbecue, 1 oz	3
Avocado oil potato chips, Chilean lime, 1 oz	3
Blue cheese bistro chips, 1 oz	3
Crème fraiche & green onion bistro chips, 1 oz	3
Sea salt bistro chips, 1 oz	3
Shoestring potato stix, 1 oz	4
Good Health Organic Chips	
Barbecue, 1 oz	3
Cracked pepper, 1 oz	3
Sea salt, 1 oz	3

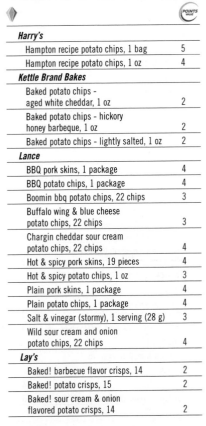

Harry's

	POINTS VALUE
Hampton recipe potato chips, 1 bag	5
Hampton recipe potato chips, 1 oz	4

Kettle Brand Bakes

	POINTS VALUE
Baked potato chips - aged white cheddar, 1 oz	2
Baked potato chips - hickory honey barbeque, 1 oz	2
Baked potato chips - lightly salted, 1 oz	2

Lance

	POINTS VALUE
BBQ pork skins, 1 package	4
BBQ potato chips, 1 package	4
Boomin bbq potato chips, 22 chips	3
Buffalo wing & blue cheese potato chips, 22 chips	3
Chargin cheddar sour cream potato chips, 22 chips	4
Hot & spicy pork skins, 19 pieces	4
Hot & spicy potato chips, 1 oz	3
Plain pork skins, 1 package	4
Plain potato chips, 1 package	4
Salt & vinegar (stormy), 1 serving (28 g)	3
Wild sour cream and onion potato chips, 22 chips	4

Lay's

	POINTS VALUE
Baked! barbecue flavor crisps, 14	2
Baked! potato crisps, 15	2
Baked! sour cream & onion flavored potato crisps, 14	2
Cheddar & sour cream artificially flavored potato chips, 15 pieces	4
Chili limon potato chips, 15 pieces	4
Classic, 15	4
Crab spice flavored potato chips, 15 pieces	4
Deli style original, 17	4
Dill pickle flavored potato chips, 17	4
Flamin' hot flavor potato chips, 17	4
Hot'n spicy barbecue flavored potato chips, 15	4
Jalapeno cheddar flavored potato chips, 15 pieces	4
Kettle cooked jalapeño potato chips, 15	3
Kettle cooked Maui onion potato chips, 15	3
Kettle cooked mesquite bbq, 18	3
Kettle cooked original, 16	3
Kettle cooked reduced fat original flavored potato chips, 18 pieces	3
Kettle cooked sea salt & malt vinegar potato chips, 18	3
Kettle cooked Southwestern ranch flavored potato chips, 18 pieces	3
Lightly salted potato chips, 20 pieces	4
Natural kettle cooked sea salt and vinegar, 16	4
Natural kettle cooked sea salted, 16	4
Salt & vinegar, 17	4
Sour cream & onion, 17	4
Stax cheddar flavored potato crisps, 12	4
Stax original flavor potato crisps, 13	4

Potato Chips (con't)

Lay's Light

Barbecue flavored potato chips, 20 pieces	1
Original potato chips, 20	1

Lay's Naturals

Country BBQ thick cut potato chips, 14	4
Sea salted thick cut potato chips, 17	4

Lay's Stax

Hot'n spicy barbecue flavored potato crisps, 12 pieces	4
Italian tomato basil flavor potato crisps, 12 pieces	4
Mesquite barbecue flavored potato crisps, 12 pieces	4
Ranch flavored potato crisps, 12 pieces	4
Salt & vinegar flavored potato crisps, 12 pieces	4
Spicy buffalo wings flavored potato crisps, 12 pieces	4
Sweet Thai chili flavor potato crisps, 12 pieces	4

Lay's Wavy Lay's

Au gratin flavored potato chips, 13	4
Hickory bbq flavored, 13	4
Potato chips, 11	4
Ranch flavored, 12	4

Manischewitz

Potato chips ripple, salted, 1 oz	4
Potato chips, unsalted, 1 oz	4
Potato stix, 1 bag	3

Maui

Maui style onion flavored potato chips, 14	4
Maui style potato chips, 14	4
Maui style salt & vinegar potato chips, 15	3

Michael Season's

Honey bbq reduced fat potato chips, 1 bag	2
Lightly salted reduced fat potato chips, 1 bag	2
Lite baked potato crisps, bbq, 19	2
Lite baked potato crisps, lightly salted, 21	2
Lite baked potato crisps, sour cream & onion, 19	2
Reduced fat kettle - lightly salted, 1 oz	3
Reduced fat kettle - sea salt & balsamic vinegar, 1 oz	3
Reduced fat kettle - sea salt & cracked pepper, 1 oz	3
Yogurt & green onion reduced fat potato chips, 1 bag	2

Miss Vickie's

Jalapeno, 15	3
Lime and black pepper flavored potato chips, 15	3
Mesquite BBQ flavored potato chips, 15	3
Original, 14	3
Sea salt & malt vinegar, 15	3

Munchos

Potato crisps, 16	4
Shrimp flavored potato crisps, 17	3

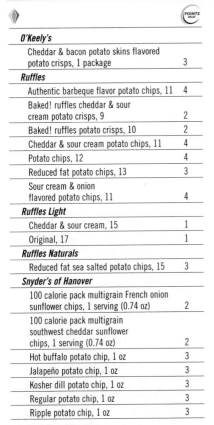

O'Keely's

Cheddar & bacon potato skins flavored potato crisps, 1 package	3

Ruffles

Authentic barbeque flavor potato chips, 11	4
Baked! ruffles cheddar & sour cream potato crisps, 9	2
Baked! ruffles potato crisps, 10	2
Cheddar & sour cream potato chips, 11	4
Potato chips, 12	4
Reduced fat potato chips, 13	3
Sour cream & onion flavored potato chips, 11	4

Ruffles Light

Cheddar & sour cream, 15	1
Original, 17	1

Ruffles Naturals

Reduced fat sea salted potato chips, 15	3

Snyder's of Hanover

100 calorie pack multigrain French onion sunflower chips, 1 serving (0.74 oz)	2
100 calorie pack multigrain southwest cheddar sunflower chips, 1 serving (0.74 oz)	2
Hot buffalo potato chip, 1 oz	3
Jalapeño potato chip, 1 oz	3
Kosher dill potato chip, 1 oz	3
Regular potato chip, 1 oz	3
Ripple potato chip, 1 oz	3

Salt & vinegar potato chip, 1 oz	3
Sour cream & onion potato chip, 1 oz	3

Solea Olive Oil Potato Chips

Cracked pepper and salt, 1 oz	3
Garlic, 1 oz	3
Parmesan, 1 oz	3
Rosemary, 1 oz	3
Sea salt, 1 oz	3
Sweet potato, 1 oz	3

Sun Chips

Apple 'n caramel flavored multigrain snacks, 15 pieces	3
Honey graham flavor multigrain snacks, 15 pieces	3

Terra

Blue potato chips, 15 chips	3
Crinkles blues jalapeno chili potato chips, 14	3
Crinkles candied sweet potato chips, 17	4
Crinkles red bliss potato chips bloody Mary, 12	3
Crinkles yukon golds garlic mashed potato chips, 17	3
Potpourri potato chips, 13 chips	3
Red bliss olive oil, 12 chips	3
Red bliss olive oil & fine herbs, 12 chips	3
Red bliss olive oil & roasted garlic parmesan, 12 chips	3
Red bliss olive oil & sun-dried tomatoes, 12 chips	3

Potato Chips, Terra (con't)

	POINTS VALUE
Spiced sweet potato chips, 17 chips	4
Spiced taro chips, 10 chips	3
Sweet potato chips, 1 bag (42 g)	4
Sweet potato chips, 17 chips	3
Unsalted potato chips au naturel, 18	3
Unsalted potato chips hickory bbq, 16	4
Unsalted potato chips lemon pepper, 16	4
Yukon gold onion & garlic potato chips, 9 chips	3
Yukon gold potato chips, original, 9 chips	3
Yukon gold salt & pepper potato chips, 9 chips	3
Yukon gold salt & vinegar potato chips, 9 chips	3

Terra Kettles

	POINTS VALUE
Chesapeake Bay & beer potato chips, 15	3
General Tso potato chips, 15	3
Pesto & smoked mozzarella, 15	3
Potato chips, Arrabiata, 15	3
Sea salt & pepper potato chips, 15	4
Sea salt & vinegar potato chips, 15	4
Sea salt with russets & blues potato chips, 15	4
Sea salt with russets and sweet potato chips, 15	4

Pretzels

Bachman

	POINTS VALUE
Butter twist, 5	2
Fat free thin pretzels, 11	2

	POINTS VALUE
Hard pretzel, 1	2
Honey wheat log splits, 9	2
Mini pretzels, 17	2
Nutzel, 1/2 cup	2
Nutzel, 19	2
Pita pretzel square, 11 pieces	2
Pretzel stix, 1 oz	2
Rods, 2	2
Sourdough bites, 10	2
Specials, 5	2
Thin 'n right pretzels, 12	2
Twist pretzel, 5	2

Combos

	POINTS VALUE
Cheddar cheese cracker, 1 bag (48.2 g)	6
Cheddar cheese cracker, 1 oz	3
Cheddar cheese pretzel, 1 bag (51 g)	5
Cheddar cheese pretzel, 1 oz	3
Nacho cheese pretzel, 1 bag (51 g)	5
Nacho cheese pretzel, 1 oz	3
Pepperoni pizza, 1 bag (48.2 g)	6
Pepperoni pizza, 1 oz	3
Pizzeria pretzel, 1 bag (51 g)	5
Pizzeria pretzel, 1 oz	3

Good Health

	POINTS VALUE
Salted peanut butter filled pretzels, 10	3
Unsalted peanut butter filled pretzels, 10 pieces	3

Hanover

	POINTS VALUE
Soft pretzels, 1	3

	POINTS VALUE
Harry's	
Everything sourdough, 1	2
Sourdough pretzels, 1	2
Unsalted sourdough pretzels, 1	2
Wheat honey pretzels, 1	2
Whole wheat honey, 1	2
Kettle Brand	
Baked pretzel chips - original, made with organic flour, 1 oz	2
Fully loaded, made with organic flour, 1 oz	2
Honey dijon, made with organic flour, 1 oz	2
Kidzels	
Kidzels, 1 bag (about 19 pieces)	2
Market Day	
Traditional pretzels with salt packets, 1	3
Otis Spunkmeyer	
Pretzel (with salt), 1	6
Rold Gold	
Baked cheddar flavored mini sticks pretzels, 18	3
Baked cinnamon flavored braided, 8	2
Baked garlic flavored braided twists pretzels, 8	2
Cheddar cheese flavor tiny twists pretzels, 20	2
Classic sticks, 48	2
Classic style braided twists pretzels, 8	2
Classic style rods, 3	2
Classic thins, 9	2

	POINTS VALUE
Classic tiny twists, 17	2
Dipped twists fudge coated pretzels, 6	3
Fat free tiny twists, 18	2
Hard sourdough, 1	2
Heartzels, 1 package	2
Holiday rings pretzels, 27	2
Holiday shapes pretzels, 17	2
Honey mustard, 20	2
Honey mustard & onion flavored mini sticks pretzels, 18	3
Honey wheat braided twists pretzels, 8	2
Schwan's LiveSmart	
Gourmet twist pretzels with salt, 1	4
Pretzel with cinnamon & sugar, 1	4
Soft stuffed pretzels with cheese, 2 sticks	3
Sweet cream cheese stuffed pretzels, 1	6
Snyder's of Hanover	
100 calorie pack minis, 1 package	2
100 calorie pack snaps, 1 package	2
100 calorie pack sticks, 1 package	2
12 multigrain sticks, 7	2
Butter sesame pretzel crackers, 1 serving (30 g)	2
Butter sesame sticks, 1 serving (1 oz)	2
Butter snaps pretzels, 1 oz	2
Buttermilk ranch pieces, 1 oz	3
Cheddar cheese filled pretzel sandwiches, 1 oz	3
Cheddar cheese pieces, 1 oz	3

505

Pretzels, Snyder's of Hanover (con't)	POINTS VALUE
Dipping sticks, 1 serving (1 oz)	2
Fudge covered peanut butter pretzel sandwiches, 1 serving (1 oz)	4
Fudge covered pretzel rods, 1 serving (19 g)	2
Garlic bread nibbler, 1 oz	3
Garlic bread pieces, 1 serving (1 oz)	3
Hard sourdough pretzel, 1 oz	2
Hershey's milk chocolate dips, 1 oz	3
Hershey's white chocolate dips, 1 oz	3
Homestyle pretzel, 1 oz	2
Honey mustard & onion nibbler, 1 oz	3
Honey mustard & onion pieces, 1 oz	3
Honey wheat pretzel sticks, 6 oz	2
Hot buffalo pretzel pieces, 1/3 cup	3
Jalapeño pieces, 1 oz	3
Mini pretzel, 1 oz	2
Multigrain honey mustard & onion nibblers, 13	3
Multigrain lightly salted pretzel sticks, 7	2
Multigrain olde tyme pretzels, 1 serving (30 g)	2
Nibbler pretzel, 1 oz	2
Old fashioned sticks, 1 oz	2
Olde tyme pretzel, 1 oz	2
Organic honey wheat pretzel, 1 oz	3
Organic oat bran pretzel, 1 oz	2
Organic pumpernickel and onion sticks, 1 oz	2
Original pretzel crackers, 1 serving (30 g)	2

	POINTS VALUE
Peanut butter filled pretzel sandwiches, 1 oz	3
Pretzel dips with hershey's special dark, 1 serving (1 oz)	3
Pretzel sticks, 1 oz	2
Pumpernickel & onion pretzel crackers, 1 serving (1 oz)	2
Pumpernickel and onion sticks, 7	2
Pumpernickel and onion with jalapeno cheese sandwiches, 8	3
Rod pretzel, 1 oz	2
Smokey barbeque potato chips, 1 serving (1.5 oz)	4
Snaps pretzels, 1 oz	2
Steakhouse onion pretzel pieces, 1/3 cup	3
Thin pretzel, 1 oz	2
Unsalted hard sourdough pretzel, 1 oz	2
Unsalted mini pretzel, 1 oz	2
Superpretzel	
Soft pretzel bites with 1/7 salt pak, 5	3
Soft pretzel bites without added salt, 5	3
Soft pretzel with 1/6 salt pak, 1	3
Soft pretzel without added salt, 1 (2 1/4 oz)	3
Superpretzel Pretzelfils	
Mozzarella, 2 sticks	3
Onion veggie cream cheese, 2 sticks	3
Pepperjack, 2 sticks	3
Pizza, 2 sticks	2
Superpretzel Softstix	
Cheese filled soft pretzel sticks, cheddar, 2	3

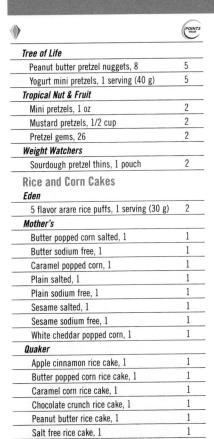

Tree of Life

	POINTS VALUE
Peanut butter pretzel nuggets, 8	5
Yogurt mini pretzels, 1 serving (40 g)	5

Tropical Nut & Fruit

Mini pretzels, 1 oz	2
Mustard pretzels, 1/2 cup	2
Pretzel gems, 26	2

Weight Watchers

Sourdough pretzel thins, 1 pouch	2

Rice and Corn Cakes

Eden

5 flavor arare rice puffs, 1 serving (30 g)	2

Mother's

Butter popped corn salted, 1	1
Butter sodium free, 1	1
Caramel popped corn, 1	1
Plain salted, 1	1
Plain sodium free, 1	1
Sesame salted, 1	1
Sesame sodium free, 1	1
White cheddar popped corn, 1	1

Quaker

Apple cinnamon rice cake, 1	1
Butter popped corn rice cake, 1	1
Caramel corn rice cake, 1	1
Chocolate crunch rice cake, 1	1
Peanut butter rice cake, 1	1
Salt free rice cake, 1	1
Salted rice cake, 1	1

Quaker Oats

	POINTS VALUE
White cheddar corn, 1	1

Quaker Oats Mini Delights

Buttered popcorn, 1 bag	2
Chocolatey drizzle, 1 bag	2

Quaker Oats Quakes

Apple cinnamon rice snacks, 8	1
BBQ rice snacks, 10	2
Caramel corn rice snacks, 7	1
Cheddar cheese rice snacks, 9	2
Chocolate crunch rice snacks, 7	1
Creamy ranch rice snacks, 10	2
Nacho rice snacks, 7	2
Sour cream & onion rice snacks, 10	2

Tree of Life

Oriental rice snacks, 1 serving (30 g)	2

Seeds, Snack and Trail Mixes

Be Happy & Healthy

Blueberry soft twisters, 4	2
Buzzworthy banana, 1/3 cup	3
Chocolate twisted bliss, 7 pieces	4
Debbie loves fruit, 1/4 cup	2
Green apple soft twisters, 4	2
Hit the road Jack, 3 Tbsp	3
Honey, I ate the peanuts, 35 pieces	4
Hot 'n healthy, 1/3 cup	2
Hot 'n sweet nuts, 1/4 cup	3
Nacho chips - they're mine, 33 pieces	3

507

SNACKS

Seeds, Snack and Trail Mixes, Be Happy & Healthy (con't)	POINTS VALUE
Power pistachios, 1/2 cup	3
Rockin raisins, 22 pieces	4
Rocky mountain munch, 1/4 cup	2
Sour wiggle giggle, 6 pieces	3
Soy glad you're healthy, 1/4 cup	3
Strawberry soft twisters, 4	2
Swinging sesame stix, 1/3 cup	5
Tammy's flax snacks, 1/4 cup	4
Whassup wasabi, 1/3 cup	3
Yogurt twisted bliss, 7 pieces	4
You've got trail!, 3 Tbsp	4
Yummy gummy in my tummy, 16 pieces	2
Zydeco Cajun mix, 1/3 cup	5
Boston's	
Snack mix, 1/2 cup	2
Chex	
Bold party blend, 1/2 cup	3
Bold party blend (single serve), 1 pouch	4
Cheddar cheese, 2/3 cup	3
Cheddar cheese, 1 pouch	4
Chocolate peanut butter, 2/3 cup	3
Chocolate turtle, 2/3 cup	3
Hot 'n spicy, 2/3 cup	3
Hot 'n spicy, 1 pouch	4
Peanut lovers, 1/2 cup	3
Peanut lovers, single serve, 1 pouch	5
Ranch, 2/3 cup	2
Simply chex cheddar, 2/3 cup	2

	POINTS VALUE
Sweet & salty caramel crunch, 1/2 cup	3
Sweet & salty caramel crunch, 1 pouch	4
Sweet & salty honey nut, 1/2 cup	3
Sweet & salty honey nut, 1 pouch	4
Traditional, 2/3 cup	3
Traditional, 1 pouch	4
Trail mix single serve snack mixes, 1 pouch	5
Trail mix snack mixes, 1/2 cup	3
Chex 100 Calorie Snack Mixes	
Cheddar, 1 pouch	2
Chocolate caramel, 1 pouch	2
Strawberry yogurt, 1 pouch	2
Chex Mix Select	
Apple cinnamon with walnuts, 2/3 cup	3
Tropical with almonds, 2/3 cup	3
Crunchies Food Company	
100% organic mixed fruit, 1/4 cup	0
Amaizing cornsnack, 1/3 cup	3
Banana crunchies, 3/4 cup	2
Blueberry crunchies, 1/4 cup	0
Mango crunchies, 1 cup	1
Organic mixed fruit, 1 cup	2
Organic strawberry crunchies, 1 1/3 cups	2
Organic sweet pea crunchies, 2/3 cup	1
Pineapple crunchies, 2/3 cup	2
Roasted mixed veggie crunchies, 1/4 cup	1
Strawberry crunchies, 1 1/4 cups	2
Tropical fruit crunchies, 3/4 cup	1
Very berry crunchies, 1 cup	2

	POINTS VALUE
DrSoy	
California blend trail mix, 1 oz	2
Tropical blend trail mix, 1 oz	2
Eden	
All mixed up, 3 Tbsp	3
Eden Organic	
Spicy pumpkin seeds, dry roasted with tamari, 1/4 cup	5
Estee	
Chocolatey covered fruit & nut mix, 1/4 cup	5
Fisher	
Sunflower kernels, dry roasted, 1 oz	4
Sunflower seeds, 1 oz (shelled)	4
Fisher Chef's Naturals	
Unsalted sunflower kernels, 1 oz	5
Flat Earth	
Apple cinnamon grove flavored baked fruit crisps, 14	3
Peach mango paradise flavored baked fruit crisps, 14	3
Wild berry patch flavored baked fruit crisps, 14	3
Frito-Lay	
BBQ flavored sunflower seeds, 1 serving (39 g)	7
Flamin' hot sunflower seeds, 1 serving (31 g)	5
Original trail mix, 3 Tbsp	4
Ranch! sunflower seeds, 1 serving (31 g)	5
Sunflower seed kernels, 1 serving (57 g)	10
Sunflower seeds, 1 serving (28 g)	4

	POINTS VALUE
Gardetto's	
Bruschetta bread crisp, 5	2
Deli-style mustard - single serve, 1 pouch	4
Deli-style mustard pretzel mix, 1/2 cup	3
Italian cheese blend, 1/2 cup	3
Original recipe, 1/2 cup	3
Original recipe, 1 pouch	5
Reduced fat original, 1/2 cup	3
Reduced fat original, 1 pouch	4
Special Italian recipe, 1/2 cup	3
Special Italian recipe, 1 pouch	5
Special request roasted garlic rye chips, 1/2 cup	4
Special request roasted garlic rye chips - single serve, 1 pouch	6
Special request rosemary & olive oil bread chips, 1/2 cup	3
GeniSoy Trail Mix	
Happy trails, 1/4 cup	3
Mountain medley, 1/4 cup	3
Tropical, 1/4 cup	2
Good Health	
Crispy cinnamon apple chips, 1 oz	3
Crispy original apple chips, 1 oz	3
Hodgson Mill	
Milled flax seed, 2 Tbsp	1
Organic golden milled flax seed, 2 Tbsp	1
Kids Chex	
Cheddar snack mixes, 2/3 cup	3

Seeds, Snack and Trail Mixes (con't) — *POINTS VALUE*

Lance

Sunflower seed kernels, 1 package	5
Sunflower seeds, in shell, 1/2 cup	3
Sunflower seeds, in shell, 2/3 cup	4
Sunflower seeds, in shell, 1 package	4

Lay's

Barbecue flavor, 15	4
Limon tangy lime, 17	4

Market Day

Munch packs, 1 pouch	5

Munchies

Cheese fix snack mix, 3/4 cup	3
Flamin' hot snack mix, 3/4 cup	3
Totally ranch snack mix, 3/4 cup	3

Nature's Path

Snack mix - bbq, 1 serving (30 g)	3
Snack mix - original, 1 serving (30 g)	3

Nut Harvest

Natural nut & fruit mix, 2 Tbsp	4

Ocean Spray Craisins

Trail mix, cranberry & chocolate, 3 Tbsp	3
Trail mix, cranberry, fruit & nuts, 3 Tbsp	3

Pepperidge Farm

Pumpernickel snack sticks, 15	2
Sesame snack sticks, 12	3

Philadelphia Snack Bites

Turtle snack bites, 1	3

Planters

Berry, nut and chocolate, 3 Tbsp	3
Dry roasted sunflower kernels, 1/4 cup	4
Honey nut medley, 4 Tbsp	4
Mixed nuts and raisins, 1 package	6
Mixed nuts and raisins, 3 Tbsp	4
Nut and chocolate mix, 1 package	6
Nut and chocolate mix, 3 Tbsp	4
Oil roasted sunflower kernels, 1/4 cup	4
Oil roasted sunflower kernels, 1 large package	9
Oil roasted sunflower kernels, 1 medium package	8
Oil roasted sunflower kernels, 1 small package	7
Pumpkin seeds, 1 package	5
Sesame nut mix, 1 oz	4
Spicy party mix with peanuts, 1/3 cup	4
Sunflower seeds, 3/4 cup	4
Sunflower seeds, 1 package (28 g)	4
Sunflower seeds, 1 package (43 g)	7
Trail mix golden nut crunch, 3 Tbsp	4
Trail mix sweet & nutty, 3 Tbsp	3

Planters Trail Mix

Fruit & nut mix, 3 Tbsp	3
Nut & chocolate mix, 1 large package	6
Nut & chocolate mix, 1 medium package	4
Nut & chocolate mix, 1 small package	3
Nuts, seeds & raisins, 3 Tbsp	4
Spicy nuts & Cajun sticks, 1 serving (29 g)	4

	POINTS VALUE
Quaker	
Baked cheddar snack mix, 3/4 cup	3
Cinnamon crunch snack mix, 1/2 cup	3
Honey graham snack mix, 1/2 cup	3
Kids snack mix, 1 cup	3
Traditional snack mix, 1/2 cup	3
Reese's	
Reese's really nuts trail mix, 1 package	7
Rold Gold	
Colossal cheddar flavor snack mix, 3/4 cup	4
Snyder's of Hanover	
Multigrain French onion sunflower chips, 16	3
Multigrain lightly salted sunflower chips, 16	3
Multigrain southwestern cheddar sunflower chips, 16	3
Spice Islands	
Sesame seed, whole, 1 serving (0.75 g)	0
Sunshine Cheez-It	
Party mix, 1/2 cup	3
Tree of Life	
Everyday trail mix, 1 serving (30 g)	3
Flax seed, 3 Tbsp	3
Nutty deluxe, trail mix, 1/4 cup	3
Organic golden flax seed, 3 Tbsp	3
Organic trail mix, 1/4 cup	3
Pumpkin seeds, roasted and salted, 1/4 cup	7
Sesame sticks, salted, 1/3 cup	4
Sunflower seed kernels, raw, 1/4 cup	5

	POINTS VALUE
Tropical Nut & Fruit	
After hours, 1 oz	4
Ah soy!, 1 oz	3
Banana split, 1 oz	3
Bartender's blend, 1 serving (30 g)	4
Bazaar mix, 1/3 cup	2
Berry good, 1 oz	3
Berry natural, 1 serving (30 g)	3
Blueberry thrill, 1 oz	3
Cajun harvest, 1 oz	4
California mix, 1 oz	3
California natural mix, 1 oz	2
Champion's choice, 1 oz	3
Checkmate, 1 oz	4
Cheese sesame sticks, 1 oz	4
Cinnamon splendor, 1 serving (30 g)	2
Convention mix, 1/3 cup	4
Corn nuts, 1 package	2
Country club, 1 oz	5
Diet delight, 1/4 cup	3
Festival mix, 1 oz	3
Firecracker hot & spicy, 1/2 cup	4
French quarter, 1 oz	4
Garlic sesame stick, 1 oz	4
Hawaiian mix, 1 oz	2
Hi-energy mix, 1 oz	2
Honey roasted sesame stix, 1 oz	4

Seeds, Snack and Trail Mixes, Tropical Nut & Fruit (con't)	POINTS VALUE
Hot Cajun corn sticks, 1 serving (28 g)	3
Hot rancheritos, 1/2 cup	2
Mexicali fire, 1 oz	4
Neptune's choice, 1 oz	4
Oat bran sticks, 1 oz	4
Oriental delight, 1 oz	4
Oriental delight natural, 1 oz	3
Poppy onion sticks, 1 oz	3
Rice snacks, natural, 2/3 cup	2
Rise 'n shine, 1/3 cup	3
Salty dog, 1 oz	4
Sesame nut mix, 1 oz	4
Sesame sticks, 1 oz	4
Sesame sticks hot & spicey, 1 oz	4
Sesame sticks roast pepper, 1 oz	4
Sesame sticks taco, 1 oz	4
Sienna cream crunch, 1 serving (30 g)	3
South of the border, 1 oz	4
Spicy rancheritos, 1/2 cup	2
Student mix, 1 oz	4
Sunburst, 1 oz	4
Sunflower seeds, raw, 1 oz	5
Sunflower seeds, roasted, 1 oz	5
Sweet & salty, 1 oz	4
Sweet caroline, 1 oz	4
Sweet tooth, 1 oz	3
Tahitian gold, 1/4 cup	3

	POINTS VALUE
The big cheese, 1 oz	3
Toasted sweet corn, 1 oz	3
Trail mix, 1 oz	3
Tropical's treasure, 1 oz	2
Whole flax seeds, 2 tsp	2
Yogurt ambrosia, 1/4 cup	2

Tortilla Chips
Amy's
Nacho snacks, 1 serving (5-6 pieces)	5

Bachman
Black bean tortilla chips, 8	3
Chipitos restaurant style tortilla chips, 6 pieces	3
Nacho tortilla chips, 12	3

Bearitos
Blue tortilla chips, 15	3
Blue tortilla chips, unsalted, 15	3
White tortilla chips, 15	3
White tortilla chips, unsalted, 15	3
Yellow tortilla chips, 15	3
Yellow tortilla chips, unsalted, 15	3

Chipitos
Black bean tortilla chips, 6	3
Nacho tortilla chips, 15	3
Restaurant style tortilla chips, 6 pieces	3
Sweet chile lime tortilla chips, 12 pieces	3
Thai barbecue tortilla chips, 12 pieces	3

Combos

	POINTS VALUE
Salsa tortilla, 1/3 cup	3
Salsa tortilla, 1 package	5

Doritos

Blazin' buffalo & ranch flavored tortilla chips, 12	3
Collisions, hot wings flavored tortilla chips, 11 pieces	3
Collisions, zesty taco flavored tortilla chips, 11 pieces	3
Cool ranch tortilla chips, 12 pieces	3
Fiery habanero flavored tortilla chips, 11 pieces	3
Jalapeno cheddar flavored tortilla chips, 11	3
Nacho cheese 100 calorie mini bites flavored tortilla chips, 1 package	2
Nacho cheese tortilla chips, 11 pieces	3
Natural nacho cheese tortilla chips, 11 pieces	3
Ranchero flavored tortilla chips, 12 pieces	3
Reduced fat cool ranch flavored tortilla chips, 11	3
Reduced fat nacho cheese flavored tortilla chips, 11 pieces	3
Salsa verde tortilla chips, 12 pieces	3
Sizzlin' picante flavored tortilla chips, 12 pieces	3
Smokin' cheddar bbq flavored tortilla chips, 12	3
Spicy nacho tortilla chips, 12 pieces	3

	POINTS VALUE
Taco tortilla chips, 12 pieces	3
Toasted corn tortilla chips, 13 pieces	3
X-13D flavored tortilla chips, 11 pieces	3

Doritos Baked!

Baked nacho cheese, 15 pieces	2

Doritos Light

Nacho cheese tortilla chips, 11 pieces	2

Garden of Eatin'

Baked blue tortilla chips, 19	2
Baked yellow tortilla chips, 19	2
Blue chips, salted, 15	3
Blue chips unsalted, 15 chips	3
Little soy blues, 13 chips	3
Mini white rounds, 18 chips	3
Mini white strips, 18 chips	3
Multigrain tortilla chips, everything, 16	3
Multigrain tortilla chips, sea salt, 16	3
Red hot blues, 15 chips	3
Red tortilla chips, 15	3
Salsa reds tortilla chips, 15 chips	3
Sesame blues, 9 chips	3
Sunny blues chips, 9 chips	3
Three pepper blue tortilla chips, 13	3
White tortilla chips, chili & lime, 10	3
White tortilla chips, guacamole, 10	3
White tortilla chips, key lime jalapeno, 15	3
White tortilla chips, pico de gallo, 7	3

Tortilla Chips, Garden of Eatin' (con't)

	POINTS VALUE
White tortilla chips, salted, 15	3
White tortilla chips, tamari, 9	3
Yellow corn chips, 42	4
Yellow tortilla chips, black bean, 13	3
Yellow tortilla chips, black bean chili, 13	3
Yellow tortilla chips, foccacia, 15	3
Yellow tortilla chips, Maui style, 15	3
Yellow tortilla chips, nacho cheese, 9	3
Yellow tortilla chips, salted, 13 chips	3

GeniSoy

Lightly salted, 1 serving (28 g)	2
Nacho, 1 serving (28 g)	2

Guiltless Gourmet Baked, Not Fried

Blue corn tortilla chips, 18	2
Chili lime tortilla chips, 18	2
Chili verde, 1 oz	2
Chili verde corn tortilla chips, 18	2
Chipotle, 1 oz	2
Chipotle corn tortilla chips, 18	2
Mucho nacho tortilla chips, 18	2
Spicy black bean tortilla chips, 18	2
Unsalted yellow corn tortilla chips, 18	2
Yellow corn tortilla chips, 18	2

Lance

Don Pablos bite size round white tortilla chips, 1 oz	3
Don Pablo's restaurant style white tortilla chips, 1 oz	3

	POINTS VALUE
LaTortilla Factory	
Bolsa grande tortillas, 2 (5.5")	2
King size yellow corn tortillas, 2 (7")	2
Restaurant style yellow corn chips, 12 chips	3
Safflower white corn, 1 serving (1 oz)	3
Super size white corn tortillas, 2 (7")	2
Traditional yellow corn, 1 serving (1 oz)	3
Little Bear	
Yellow corn chips, 42	4
Yellow tortilla chips, 15	3
Santitas	
100% white corn, 9	3
Tortilla chips, 9	3
Tortilla strips, 11	3
Snyder's of Hanover	
Multigrain golden flax tortilla strips, 11	3
Multigrain jalapeno red tortilla strips, 11	3
Multigrain lightly salted tortilla chips, 1 serving (28 g)	2
Multigrain savory blue tortilla strips, 11	3
Restaurant style tortilla chips, 8	2
White corn tortilla chip, 1 oz	3
Yellow corn tortilla chip, 1 oz	3
Terra	
Parsnips chips, 12	3
Stripes & blues gourmet bbq, 14	3
Stripes & blues sea salt, 14	3
Sweets and beets chips, 12	4

	POINTS VALUE
Tostitos	
100% white corn bite size tortilla chips, 24	3
100% white corn crispy rounds tortilla chips, 13	3
100% white corn restaurant style tortilla chips, 7	3
100% white corn restaurant style tortilla chips with a hint of jalapeno, 6 pieces	3
100% white corn restaurant style tortilla chips with a hint of lime flavor, 6	3
Bite size gold tortilla chips, 16 pieces	3
Chips n' dip with cheese kit, 1	5
Chips n' dip with salsa kit, 1	3
Flour tortilla chips, 14	3
Multigrain tortilla chips, 8	3
Natural blue corn restaurant style tortilla chips, 6	3
Natural yellow corn restaurant style tortilla chips, 6 pieces	3
Tostitos Baked!	
Scoops tortilla chips, 15	2
Tostitos Light	
Restaurant style tortilla chips, 6	2
Tostitos Scoops	
Tortilla chips, 13	3

Vegetable and Soy Chips

	POINTS VALUE
Amy's	
Spinach feta snacks, 1 serving (5-6 pieces)	4

	POINTS VALUE
Athenos	
Pita chips, garlic & herb, 11	3
Pita chips, original, 11	3
Pita chips, whole wheat, 11	2
EatSmart	
100 calorie pack veggie crisps, 1 serving (21.3 g)	2
Cheddar & jalapeno veggie crisps, 21	3
Garlic, parmesan & olive oil flavored soy crisps, 20	3
Sundried tomato and pesto veggie crisps, 1 oz	3
Tomato, romano & olive oil flavored soy crisps, 20 chips	3
Veggie crisps, 1 oz	3
Eden	
All mixed up too, 3 Tbsp	3
Brown rice chips, 1 serving (30 g)	4
Sea vegetable chips, 1 serving (30 g)	3
Vegetable chips, 1 serving (30 g)	3
Wasabi chips - hot'n spicy, 1 serving (30 g)	3
Flat Earth	
Farmland cheddar flavored baked veggie crisps, 12	3
Garlic & herb field flavored baked veggie crisps, 12	3
Tangy tomato ranch flavored baked veggie crisps, 12	3

Vegetable and Soy Chips (con't) | POINTS VALUE

Funyuns

Onion flavored rings, 13	3
Wasabi flavored rings, 13 pieces	3

Garden of Eatin'

Pita chips, Asian spice, 9 pieces	2
Pita chips, brown sugar & cinnamon, 8 pieces	2
Pita chips, Greek isle, 9 pieces	2
Pita chips, sea salt, 9	2

GeniSoy

Crispy dippers lightly salted, 1 oz	2
Soytato chips lightly salted, 26	2
Soytato chips, barbeque, 26	2
Soytato chips, sour cream & onion, 26	2
White cheddar, 1 oz	2

GeniSoy Crispy Dippers

Lightly salted, 1 oz	2
White cheddar, 1 oz	2

GeniSoy Potato Soy Crisps

Country style ranch, 17	2
Parmesan & garlic, 17	2
Sea salt & black pepper, 17	2
Texas roadhouse BBQ, 17	2

GeniSoy Smart Hearts

Garlic parmesan, 3/4 cup	2
Lightly salted, 3/4 cup	2
White cheddar, 3/4 cup	2

GeniSoy Soy Crisps

Apple cinnamon, 17	2
Creamy ranch, 17	2
Deep sea salt, 17	2
Nacho cheese, 17	2
Rich cheddar cheese, 17	2
Roasted garlic & onion, 17	2
Tangy salt 'n vinegar, 17	2
Zesty barbeque, 17	2

GeniSoy Soytato Chips

Barbeque, 26	2
Lightly salted, 26	2
Sour cream & onion, 26	2

Good Health

Veggie chips, 1 oz	3

Good Health Veggie Stix

Mixed vegetables, 1 oz	3

Kangaroo

Cinnamon sugar pita chips, 10	3
Garlic herb pita chips, 10	2
Sea salt pita chips, 10	2
Sea salt pita chips, 10	2
Whole grain French onion pita chips, 10	2

Kettle Brand

Baked pita chips, salt & pepper, made with organic flour, 1 oz	2
Baked pita chips, salt kissed, made with organic flour, 1 oz	2

	POINTS VALUE
Michael Season's	
Soy protein chips - original, 1 cup	2
Morningstar Farms	
Veggie bites broccoli cheddar, 3 pieces	4
Veggie bites egg florentine, 3 pieces	4
Veggie bites mushroom mozzarella, 3 pieces	4
Veggie bites spinach artichoke, 3 pieces	4
Old London	
Garlic bagel snacks, 5 pieces	1
Original bagel snacks, 5 pieces	1
Poppy seed bagel snacks, 5 pieces	1
Quaker Oats Soy Crisps	
BBQ, 26	3
White cheddar, 26	4
Robert's American Gourmet	
Veggie chips, 1 oz	3
Snyder's of Hanover	
Multigrain parmesan garlic & herb pita chips, 1 serving (1 oz)	3
Multigrain sea salt pita chips, 1 serving (1 oz)	3
Multigrain sundried tomato & herb pita chips, 1 serving (1 oz)	3
Stacy's	
Cinnamon sugar pita chips, 1 oz (8-10 chips)	3
Everything bagel chips, 12	3

	POINTS VALUE
Multigrain seasoned with sea salt pita chips, 7	3
Parmesan garlic & herb pita chips, 1 oz (8-10 chips)	3
Pesto & sundried tomato pita chips, 1 oz (8-10 chips)	3
Simply naked pita chips, 1 oz (8-10 chips)	3
Soy thin crisps simply cheese flavored baked, 18	3
Soy thin crisps sticky bun flavored baked soy crisps, 18	2
Soy thin crisps sweet bbq flavored baked soy crisps, 18	2
Texarkana hot pita chips, 1 oz (8-10 chips)	3
Toasted garlic flavored bagel chips, 13	2
Whole wheat bagel chips, 14	3
Terra	
Mediterranean exotic vegetable chips, 14 chips	3
Original exotic vegetable. chips, 14 chips	3
Stix, original, 1 oz	3
Taro chips, 10 chips	3
Zesty tomato exotic vegetable. chips, 14 chips	3

Bean and Chili

Amy's

	POINTS VALUE
Black bean chili, 1 cup	3
Light in sodium medium chili, 1 cup	5
Light in sodium spicy chili, 1 cup	5
Medium chili, 1 cup	5
Medium chili with vegetables, 1 cup	4
◆ Organic black bean vegetable soup, 1 cup	2
Organic Tuscan bean & rice soup, 1 cup	3
Spicy chili, 1 cup	5

Austex American Originals

Chili, no beans, 1 cup	9
Chili, with beans, 1 cup	8

Boca

Chili, 1 package (269 g)	2

Bush's

Homestyle chili, chunky with beans, 1 cup	5
Homestyle chili, hot with beans, 1 cup	5
Homestyle chili, no beans, 1 cup	5
Homestyle chili, original with beans, 1 cup	5

Castleberry's American Originals

Chili, no beans, 1 cup	9
Chili, with beans, 1 cup	8

Cattle Drive Gold

Chicken chili with beans, 1 cup	3
Chili with beans, 1 cup	6

Cherchies

	POINTS VALUE
9 spice red bean chili mix, 1 serving (56 g)	3
Black & navy bean soup mix, 1 serving (2 oz)	3
Cuban black beans soup mix, 1 serving (62 g)	3
Mixed bean soup mix, 1 serving (2 oz)	3
Spicy Southwest bean soup mix, 1 serving (2 oz)	3
White bean chili mix, 1 serving (1.77 oz)	3
White chili with red bell - jalapeno peppers, 1 serving (1/9 package)	3

Fantastic World Foods

◆ Baja black bean, 1 container	2
Blarney stone creamy potato soup, 1 oz (dry mix)	2
Buckaroo bean chili, 1 container	3
Cha cha chili bean simmer soup, 1 1/4 oz (dry mix)	2
Dutch split pea soup, 1 1/4 oz (dry mix)	2
New year hot and sour soup, 3/4 oz (dry mix)	1
Southwest tortilla bean, 1 container	3
◆ Vegetarian chili, 1/2 cup	3

Goldwater's

Senator's chili mix, 1 serving (1/4 oz)	0

Health Valley

◆ Black bean microwaveable bowl soup, 8 oz	2
◆ Fat-free black bean & vegetable, 8 oz	2
◆ Organic black bean soup, 8 oz	2

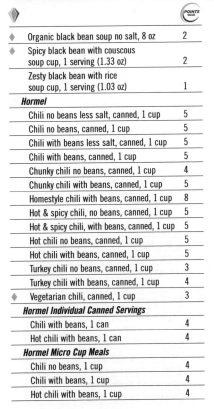

	POINTS VALUE
◆ Organic black bean soup no salt, 8 oz	2
◆ Spicy black bean with couscous soup cup, 1 serving (1.33 oz)	2
Zesty black bean with rice soup cup, 1 serving (1.03 oz)	1
Hormel	
Chili no beans less salt, canned, 1 cup	5
Chili no beans, canned, 1 cup	5
Chili with beans less salt, canned, 1 cup	5
Chili with beans, canned, 1 cup	5
Chunky chili no beans, canned, 1 cup	4
Chunky chili with beans, canned, 1 cup	5
Homestyle chili with beans, canned, 1 cup	8
Hot & spicy chili, no beans, canned, 1 cup	5
Hot & spicy chili, with beans, canned, 1 cup	5
Hot chili no beans, canned, 1 cup	5
Hot chili with beans, canned, 1 cup	5
Turkey chili no beans, canned, 1 cup	3
Turkey chili with beans, canned, 1 cup	4
◆ Vegetarian chili, canned, 1 cup	3
Hormel Individual Canned Servings	
Chili with beans, 1 can	4
Hot chili with beans, 1 can	4
Hormel Micro Cup Meals	
Chili no beans, 1 cup	4
Chili with beans, 1 cup	4
Hot chili with beans, 1 cup	4

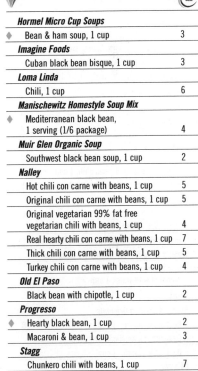

	POINTS VALUE
Hormel Micro Cup Soups	
◆ Bean & ham soup, 1 cup	3
Imagine Foods	
Cuban black bean bisque, 1 cup	3
Loma Linda	
Chili, 1 cup	6
Manischewitz Homestyle Soup Mix	
◆ Mediterranean black bean, 1 serving (1/6 package)	4
Muir Glen Organic Soup	
Southwest black bean soup, 1 cup	2
Nalley	
Hot chili con carne with beans, 1 cup	5
Original chili con carne with beans, 1 cup	5
Original vegetarian 99% fat free vegetarian chili with beans, 1 cup	4
Real hearty chili con carne with beans, 1 cup	7
Thick chili con carne with beans, 1 cup	5
Turkey chili con carne with beans, 1 cup	4
Old El Paso	
Black bean with chipotle, 1 cup	2
Progresso	
◆ Hearty black bean, 1 cup	2
Macaroni & bean, 1 cup	3
Stagg	
Chunkero chili with beans, 1 cup	7
Classic chili, 1 cup	7

SOUPS

Bean and Chili, Stagg (con't)

	POINTS VALUE
Country brand chili, with beans, 1 cup	7
Dynamite hot chili, with beans, 1 cup	7
Fiesta grille chili with beans, 1 cup	5
Laredo chili with beans, 1 cup	7
Quickdraw chili with beans, 1 bowl	5
Ranch house chicken chili, with beans, 1 cup	5
Santa Fe chicken chili with beans, 1 cup	4
Silverado beef 97% fat free chili, 1 cup	4
Silverado beef chili, with beans, 1 cup	5
Turkey ranchero chili, with beans, 1 cup	4
Vegetable garden 4-bean chili, 1 cup	3
White chicken chili with beans, 1 cup	5

Worthington

Chili, 1 cup	6

Wyler's Mrs. Grass

Homestyle three bean chili mix, 1/4 carton	2

Wyler's Soup Starter Homestyle Soup Mix

Hearty three bean chili, prepared with water, 1 cup	2

Beef

Austex American Originals

Beef stew, classic, 1 cup	8

Castleberry's American Originals

Beef stew, classic, 1 cup	8

Cherchies

Hearty beef & pasta soup mix, 1 serving (19 g)	1

Dinty Moore

	POINTS VALUE
Beef stew, 1 cup	4
Meatball stew, 1 cup	6

Dinty Moore Individual Canned Servings

Beef stew, 1 can	4

Dinty Moore Microwave Bowls

Beef stew, 1 bowl	6

Dinty Moore Microwave Cups

Beef stew, 1 cup	3

Hormel Micro Cup Meals

Beef stew, 1 cup	3

Hormel Micro Cup Soups

Beef vegetable, 1 cup	2

Market Day

Hearty beef stew, 2/3 cup	3

Muir Glen Organic Soup Chef Inspirations

Beef & vegetable soup, 1 cup	2

Progresso

Beef & baked potato, 1 cup	2
Beef & mushroom, 1 cup	2
Beef & vegetable, 1 cup	2
Beef barley, 1 cup	3
Beef barley 99% fat free, 1 cup	2
Chickarina with meatballs, 1 cup	2
Grilled steak with vegetable & penne, 1 cup	2

Progresso Carb Monitor Soups

Tuscan-style meatball, 1 cup	2

POINTS VALUE

Progresso Microwavable Soups

Beef & vegetable, 1 cup	2

Progresso Rich & Hearty Soups

Beef pot roast with country vegetables, 1 cup	2
Savory beef barley vegetable, 1 cup	2
Sirloin steak & vegetables, 1 cup	2
Steak & homestyle noodles, 1 cup	2
Steak & roasted russet potatoes, 1 cup	3
Steak & sauteed mushrooms, 1 cup	2
Vegetable beef slow cooked, 1 cup	2

Stagg

Steak house chili, no beans, 1 cup	8

Wyler's

Reduced sodium beef, 1 cube	0
Sodium free beef, 1 tsp	0
Zesty garlic beef, 1 cube	0

Wyler's Mrs. Grass

Homestyle beef stew mix, 1/4 carton	1
Homestyle beef vegetable mix, 1/4 carton	1

Wyler's Soup Starter Homestyle Soup Mix

Beef vegetable, prepared with water, 1 cup (1/7 package)	1
Hearty beef stew, prepared with water, 1 cup (1/8 package)	1

POINTS VALUE

Bouillon, Broth and Stocks

Cherchies

Gumbo with file seasoning soup mix, 1 serving (31 g)	2
Mexican tortilla soup mix, 1 serving (23 g)	1
Pasta e fagioli soup mix, 1 serving (2 oz)	3

Health Valley

Fat-free beef flavored broth, 8 oz	0
Fat-free beef flavored broth no salt, 8 oz	0
Fat-free chicken broth, 8 oz	1
Fat-free vegetable broth, 8 oz	0
Low fat chicken broth, 8 oz	1
Low fat chicken broth no salt, 8 oz	1

Herb-Ox

Beef bouillon cubes, 1	0
Beef instant bouillon powder, 1 tsp	0
Beef instant broth & seasoning, 1 packet	0
Beef instant broth & seasoning low sodium packet, 1	0
Chicken bouillon cubes, 1	0
Chicken instant bouillon powder, 1 tsp	0
Chicken instant broth & seasoning, 1 packet	0
Chicken instant broth & seasoning low sodium packet, 1	0
Garlic chicken bouillon cubes, 1	0
Vegetable bouillon cubes, 1	0

Bouillon, Broth and Stocks (con't)

Home Again

Beef base, 1 tsp	0
Chicken base, 1 tsp	0
Chicken base, no msg, 1 tsp	0
Chicken flavor stock, 1 tsp	0
Ham base, 3/4 tsp	0

Preciosa

Bacon bouillon, 1 tablet	0
Chicken bouillon, 1 tsp	0
Chicken/onion bouillon, 1 tsp	0

Progresso

Hearty penne in chicken broth, 1 cup	1
Southwestern style chicken chowder, 1 cup	2

San-J

White miso soup envelope, 1 package	1

Simply Asia Rice Noodle Soup Bowl

Garlic sesame, 1 (70 g)	5
Sesame chicken flavor, 1 (70 g)	5
Shiitake mushroom, 1 (70 g)	5
Spring vegetable, 1 (70 g)	5

Simply Asia Soup Bowl

Miso soup, 1 (178 g)	4
Sesame chicken soup, 1 (175 g)	8
Spring vegetable soup, 1 (172 g)	3
Szechwan hot & sour soup, 1 (178 g)	5

Thai Kitchen

Instant rice noodle soup, Bangkok curry, 1 package (45 g)	3
Instant rice noodle soup, garlic & vegetable, 1 package (45 g)	3
Instant rice noodle soup, lemongrass & chili, 1 package (68 g)	3
Instant rice noodle soup, spring onion, 1 package (45 g)	4
Instant rice noodle soup, Thai ginger, 1 package (68 g)	3
Rice noodle soup bowl, hot & sour, 1 (68 g)	5
Rice noodle soup bowl, lemongrass & chili, 1 (68 g)	5
Rice noodle soup bowl, mushroom, 1 (68 g)	5
Rice noodle soup bowl, roasted garlic, 1 (68 g)	5
Rice noodle soup bowl, spring onion, 1 (68 g)	5
Rice noodle soup bowl, Thai ginger, 1 (68 g)	5

Wyler's

Reduced sodium chicken, 1 cube	0

Chicken

4C

Noodle soup with real chicken broth, 1 serving (16 g)	1

Castleberry's American Originals

Brunswick stew, chicken & beef, 1 cup	6

Cherchies

Chicken pot pie soup mix, 1/4 cup	2

	POINTS VALUE
Dinty Moore	
Chicken & dumplings, 1 cup	5
Chicken & noodles, 1 cup	5
Chicken stew, 1 cup	5
Fantastic World Foods	
New England vegetarian chicken simmer soup, 1 oz (dry mix)	2
Vegetarian chicken noodle, 1/4 cup (dry mix)	2
Health Valley	
Chicken flavored noodles with vegetables soup cup, 1 serving (.99 oz)	2
Chicken noodle, 8 oz	2
Chicken rice, 8 oz	2
Organic cream of chicken, 8 oz	3
Hormel Micro Cup Soups	
Chicken & rice, 1 cup	2
Chicken noodle, 1 cup	2
Imagine Foods	
Creamy chicken, 1 cup	1
Manischewitz	
Original chicken noodle soup, 1 cup	1
Zesty chicken noodle soup, 1 cup	2
Market Day	
Chicken & dumpling soup, 1/2 cup	3
Chicken tortilla soup, 1 cup	5
Chicken with wild rice soup, 1 cup	2

	POINTS VALUE
Progresso	
Chicken & sausage gumbo soup, 1 cup	3
Chicken & wild rice, 1 cup	2
♦ Chicken barley, 1 cup	2
Chicken herb dumpling, 1 cup	2
Chicken noodle, 1 cup	2
Chicken noodle, 99% fat free, 1 cup	2
Chicken rice with vegetables, 1 cup	2
♦ Chicken vegetable, 1 cup	2
Grilled chicken Italiano with vegetables & penne, 1 cup	2
Hearty chicken & rotini, 1 cup	2
Homestyle chicken with vegetables & pasta, 1 cup	2
Minestrone with chicken, 1 cup	2
♦ Roasted chicken garden herb, 1 cup	1
Roasted chicken Italiano, 1 cup	1
Roasted chicken rotini, 1 cup	2
Progresso Carb Monitor Soups	
Chicken cheese enchilada flavor, 1 cup	4
♦ Chicken vegetable, 1 cup	1
Progresso Microwavable Soups	
Chicken noodle, 1 cup	2
Chicken wild rice, 1 cup	2
Progresso Reduced Sodium Soups	
Chicken & wild rice soup, 1 cup	2
Chicken gumbo, 1 cup	2
Chicken noodle, 1 cup	2

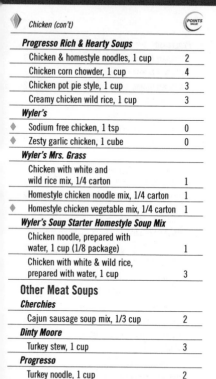

Chicken (con't)

POINTS VALUE

Progresso Rich & Hearty Soups

Chicken & homestyle noodles, 1 cup	2
Chicken corn chowder, 1 cup	4
Chicken pot pie style, 1 cup	3
Creamy chicken wild rice, 1 cup	3

Wyler's

Sodium free chicken, 1 tsp	0
Zesty garlic chicken, 1 cube	0

Wyler's Mrs. Grass

Chicken with white and wild rice mix, 1/4 carton	1
Homestyle chicken noodle mix, 1/4 carton	1
Homestyle chicken vegetable mix, 1/4 carton	1

Wyler's Soup Starter Homestyle Soup Mix

Chicken noodle, prepared with water, 1 cup (1/8 package)	1
Chicken with white & wild rice, prepared with water, 1 cup	3

Other Meat Soups

Cherchies

Cajun sausage soup mix, 1/3 cup	2

Dinty Moore

Turkey stew, 1 cup	3

Progresso

Turkey noodle, 1 cup	2

Seafood

POINTS VALUE

Asian Rhythms

Hot and spicy shrimp soup, 1 cup	4
Spicy coconut shrimp soup, 1 cup	5

Cape Cod

Premium New England style clam chowder, 1/2 cup	1

Chincoteague

Chesapeake Bay cream of crab soup, 1 cup	5
Crab & cheddar soup, 1/2 cup	2
Lobster and cheddar bisque, 1/2 cup	3
Manhattan clam chowder, 1/2 cup	2
New England clam chowder, 1/2 cup	2
Oyster stew, 1/2 cup	2
Premium clam bisque, 1/2 cup	2
Premium lobster bisque, 1/2 cup	2
Premium shrimp bisque, 1/2 cup	2
She crab soup, 1/2 cup	2
Vegetable red crab soup, 1 cup	2

Health Valley

Seafood Manhattan clam chowder, 8 oz	2
Seafood New England clam chowder, 8 oz	3

Hormel Micro Cup Soups

New England clam chowder, 1 cup	3

Market Day

Supreme lobster bisque, 1 cup	8

	POINTS VALUE
Phillips	
Clam chowder, 1 cup	4
Crab & corn chowder, 1 cup	8
Crab & shrimp chowder with garlic & tomato, 1 cup	3
Cream of crab soup, 1 cup	8
Lobster bisque, 1 cup	8
Shrimp bisque, 1 cup	7
Progresso	
◆ Manhattan clam chowder, 1 cup	2
New England clam chowder, 1 cup	4
New England clam chowder 99% fat free, 1 cup	2
Snow's	
Authentic New England clam chowder, 1 cup	5
New England clam chowder, 1/2 cup	2
New England corn chowder, 1/2 cup	2
Snow's 98% Fat Free	
Authentic New England clam chowder, 1 cup	2

Vegetables

4C
Recipe mix, onion, 1 serving (7 g)	0

Amy's
Butternut squash soup, 1 cup	2
Organic alphabet soup, 1 cup	1
Organic chunky tomato bisque, 1 cup	2

	POINTS VALUE
◆ Organic chunky vegetable soup, 1 cup	1
Organic corn chowder, 1 cup	4
Organic cream of mushroom soup, 3/4 cup	3
Organic cream of tomato soup, 1 cup	2
Organic fire roasted southwestern vegetable soup, 1 cup	2
◆ Organic lentil soup, 1 cup	3
◆ Organic lentil vegetable, 1 cup	3
Organic light in sodium butternut squash soup, 1 cup	2
Organic light in sodium chunky tomato bisque, 1 cup	2
Organic light in sodium cream of tomato soup, 1 cup	2
◆ Organic light in sodium lentil soup, 1 cup	3
◆ Organic light in sodium lentil vegetable soup, 1 cup	3
Organic light in sodium minestrone soup, 1 cup	1
◆ Organic light in sodium split pea soup, 1 cup	1
Organic minestrone soup, 1 cup	1
Organic no chicken noodle soup, 1 cup	2
Organic pasta & 3 bean, 1 cup	2
Organic potato leek soup, 1 cup	4
◆ Organic split pea soup, 1 cup	1
Organic Thai coconut soup (tom kha phak), 1/2 can	5
◆ Organic vegetable barley soup, 1 cup	1

SOUPS

 Vegetables (con't) POINTS VALUE

Cherchies

Barley & red lentil soup mix, 1 serving (2 oz)	0
Corn chowder, 1/3 cup (dry mix)	2
Corn chowder mix, 1 serving (29 g)	2
French country stew mix, 3 Tbsp	2
French potato soup, 1 serving (1/7 package)	1
French potato soup mix, 1 serving (12 g)	1
Gumbo mix with filé seasoning, 1 serving (1/9 package)	2
Italian wedding soup mix, 1/4 cup	1
Mexican tortilla soup, 1 serving (23 g)	1
Minestrone soup, 1/4 cup (dry mix)	2
Minestrone soup mix, 1/4 cup	2
Mushroom chowder mix, 1 serving (25 g)	1
Mushroom chowder with vegetables, 1/2 cup (dry mix)	1
Split pea & lentil soup mix, 1 serving (2 oz)	3
Vegetable chowder soup mix, 1 serving (1 oz)	2
Vegetable chowder with rice, 1 oz (dry mix)	2

Chi-Chi's

Fiesta tortilla soup mix, 1 serving (1/5 package)	2

Chincoteague

Premium corn chowder, 1/2 cup	2

Fantastic World Foods

Classic French onion, 1 container	2
Creamy potato, 1/4 cup (dry mix)	2
Creamy potato leek, 1 container	2

  POINTS VALUE

Green onion miso with tofu, 1 container	3
Hot & sour, 1 container	3
Mamma's minestrone, 1 container	3
Sesame miso, 1 container	3
Spicy Thai, 1 container	3
Split pea, 1/4 cup (dry mix)	2
Summer vegetable with rice, 1 container	1
Three-onion noodle, 1 container	3
Tuscan tomato & shells, 1 container	2
Vegetable barley, 1/4 cup (dry mix)	2
Vegetarian chicken noodle, 1 container	1

Health Valley

Cream potato with broccoli soup cup, 1 serving (0.83 oz)	1
Fat-free 14 garden vegetable soup, 8 oz	1
Fat-free 5 bean vegetable soup, 8 oz	2
Fat-free corn & vegetable soup, 8 oz	1
Fat-free lentil & carrots, 8 oz	1
Fat-free minestrone, 8 oz	1
Fat-free pasta Italiano soup cup, 1 serving (1.34 oz)	2
Fat-free pasta parmesan soup cup, 1 serving (.97 oz)	2
Fat-free split pea & carrots, 8 oz	1
Fat-free tomato vegetable, 8 oz	1
Fat-free vegetable barley, 8 oz	1
Lentil microwaveable bowl soup, 8 oz	2

	POINTS VALUE
Lentil with couscous soup cup, 1 serving (1.33 oz)	2
Minestrone microwaveable bowl soup, 8 oz	1
Organic cream of celery, 8 oz	2
Organic cream of mushroom, 8 oz	2
Organic lentil soup, 8 oz	1
Organic lentil soup no salt, 8 oz	1
Organic minestrone soup, 8 oz	1
Organic minestrone soup no salt, 8 oz	1
Organic mushroom barley, 8 oz	1
Organic mushroom barley no salt, 8 oz	1
Organic potato & leek soup, 8 oz	1
Organic potato & leek soup no salt, 8 oz	1
Organic split pea soup, 8 oz	1
Organic split pea soup no salt, 8 oz	1
Organic tomato soup, 8 oz	1
Organic tomato soup no salt, 8 oz	1
Organic vegetable soup, 8 oz	1
Organic vegetable soup no salt, 8 oz	1
Split pea microwaveable bowl soup, 8 oz	2
Tomato bisque microwaveable bowl soup, 8 oz	2
Vegetable, 1 cup	0
Vegetable microwaveable bowl soup, 8 oz	2

Imagine Foods

Acorn squash & mango soup, 1 cup	1
Corn chipotle bisque, 1 cup	2
Creamy broccoli, 1 cup	1
Creamy butternut squash, 1 cup	2
Creamy portobello mushroom soup, 1 cup	1
Creamy potato leek, 1 cup	2
Creamy sweet corn, 1 cup	2
Creamy tomato, 1 cup	1
Creamy tomato basil, 1 cup	2
Fire roasted tomato bisque, 1 cup	2
Sweet pea soup, 1 cup	1
Sweet potato, 1 cup	2

Lucini

Roman tomato cream soup, 1 cup	3
Rustic Italian minestrone soup, 1 cup	4

Manischewitz

Borscht with shredded beets, 1 cup	1
Clear borscht, 1 cup	1
Matzo ball & soup mix, 1 Tbsp (1 cup prepared)	1
Reduced sodium borscht, 1 cup	2
Schav, 1 cup	1

Market Day

Broccoli & cheese soup singles, 1 pouch	5
Italian wedding soup, 1/2 cup	3
Loaded baked potato soup, 1/2 cup	4
Minestrone soup, 1 cup	2

Muir Glen Organic Soup

Creamy tomato soup, 1 cup	4
Garden vegetable, 1 cup	1
Hearty tomato, 1 cup	2

Vegetables, Muir Glen Organic Soup (con't)

	POINTS VALUE
Lentil, 1 cup	2
Minestrone, 1 cup	2
Split pea, 1 cup	3
Nutritious Living Hi-Lo	
Home style beef stew, 1 tray	3
Phillips	
Vegetable crab soup, 1 cup	2
Progresso	
Creamy mushroom, 1 cup	3
Creamy tomato, 1 cup	4
French onion, 1 cup	1
Garden vegetable, 1 cup	1
Green split pea, 1 cup	3
Hearty tomato, 1 cup	2
Italian style wedding soup, 1 cup	3
Lentil, 1 cup	2
Lentil, 99% fat free, 1 cup	2
Minestrone, 1 cup	1
Minestrone, 99% fat free, 1 cup	1
Potato broccoli & cheese chowder, 1 cup	4
Split pea with ham, 1 cup	2
Tomato basil, 1 cup	3
Tomato rotini, 1 cup	2
Tomato vegetable Italiano, 1 cup	2
Vegetable, 1 cup	1
Vegetarian vegetable with barley, 1 cup	1

	POINTS VALUE
Progresso Light Soups	
Homestyle vegetable and rice soup, 1 cup	0
Italian-style vegetable soup, 1 cup	0
Savory vegetable barley soup, 1 cup	0
Southwestern-style vegetable soup, 1 cup	0
Vegetable and noodle soup, 1 cup	0
Progresso Microwavable Soups	
Italian-style wedding, 1 cup	3
Lentil, 1 cup	2
Minestrone, 1 cup	1
Vegetable, 1 cup	1
Progresso Reduced Sodium Soups	
Garden vegetable, 1 cup	1
Italian-style wedding soup with meatballs, 1 cup	2
Minestrone soup, 1 cup	2
San-J	
Vegan wakame soup envelope, 1 package	1
Uncle Ben's	
Broccoli cheese & rice, 1 cup (cooked)	2
Wyler's Mrs. Grass	
Cheddar broccoli mix, 1/4 carton	2
Potato, garlic and chives mix, 1/4 carton	2
Wyler's Soup Starter Homestyle Soup Mix	
Cheddar broccoli, prepared with water, 1 cup	2
Hearty chicken vegetable, prepared with water, 1 cup	1
Potato, garlic & chives, prepared with water, 1 cup	2

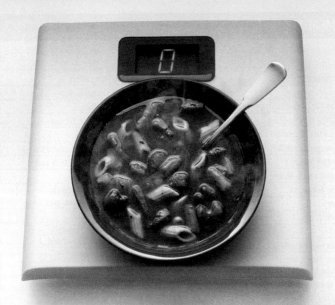

Progresso® Light Soup.

0 POINTS® value and **60 CALORIES** per serving on select varieties, endorsed by Weight Watchers.®

Try our Homestyle Vegetable and Rice,
Italian-Style Vegetable, Savory Vegetable Barley,
Southwestern-Style Vegetable, and Vegetable
and Noodle. See how the scale has been
tipped in your favor at ProgressoLight.com.

	POINTS VALUE
Meat Substitutes	
Amy's	
◆ All American veggie burger, 1	2
Bistro burger, 1 serving (2.5 oz)	2
Breakfast patties, 1 serving (1.33 oz)	2
◆ California veggie burger, 1	2 (5)
◆ Chicago veggie burger, 1	3 (5)
◆ Quarter pound veggie burger, 1	4
◆ Texas veggie burger, 1	2 (5)
Betty Crocker	
Bac Os chips or bits, 1 1/2 Tbsp	1
Boca	
◆ All American flame grilled burger, 1	1 (5)
◆ All-American classic burger (made with organic soy), 1	2 (5)
Bratwurst sausage, meatless, 1	3
Breakfast links, 2	1
Breakfast links (made with organic soy), 2	2
Breakfast patties, 1	1
Cheeseburger, 1	2
Cheeseburger (made with organic soy), 1	2
Chick'n hot & spicy buffalo wings, 1 serving (87 g)	3
◆ Garden burger, 1	2 (5)
◆ Grilled vegetable burger, 1	1 (5)
◆ Ground burger, 1/2 cup	1 (5)

	POINTS VALUE
Italian sausage, meatless, 1	3
Original chik'n nuggets, 4	4
Original chik'n patties, 1	3
◆ Original ground burger, 1/2 cup	1 (5)
◆ Original vegan burger, 1	1 (5)
◆ Original vegan burger (15 pound box), 1	2 (5)
◆ Original vegan burger (3 1/2 lb box), 1	1 (5)
◆ Roasted garlic burger, 1	1 (5)
◆ Roasted garlic burger (naturally flavored, made with organic soy), 1	2 (5)
◆ Roasted onion burger, 1	1 (5)
◆ Roasted onion burger (naturally flavored, made with organic soy), 1	2 (5)
Smoked sausage, meatless, 1	3
Spicy chik'n patties, 1	3
◆ Vegan burger, 1	1 (5)
Dr. Praeger's	
◆ Bombay veggie burgers, 1 burger	2 (5)
◆ California veggie burgers, 1 burger	2 (5)
California veggieballs, 2 pieces	1
◆ Italian veggie burgers, 1 burger	2 (5)
◆ Tex Mex veggie burgers, 1 burger	2 (5)
Fantastic World Foods	
◆ Nature's burger, 1/4 cup	3
Sloppy Joe mix, 1/4 cup	1
Taco filling, 1/4 cup	1

	POINTS VALUE
Lightlife	
Breakfast patties, 1 patty	1
♦ Burgers, 1 burger	1 (5)
Chicken patty, 1 patty	3
Chick'n nuggets, 4 nuggets	5
♦ Gimme lean, 2 oz	1
Gimme lean, sausage, 2 oz	1
♦ Lightburger 2 pack, 3 oz	2 (5)
Meatless meatballs, 5	3
Mushroom burgers, 5 oz	3 (5)
Smart dogs, 1 link	1
Smart pretzel dog, 1	7
Tofu pups, 1	1
♦ Veggie burger, 5 oz	2 (5)
Veggie dogs, 1 link	2
Lightlife Smart Bacon	
Smart bacon, 2 strips	1
Lightlife Smart BBQ	
Smart bbq, 1/4 cup	1
Lightlife Smart Chili	
Smart chili, 1 cup	3
Lightlife Smart Cutlets	
Chick'n fillet style veggie protein cutlets, 1	3
Lightlife Smart Deli	
Jumbos, 1	1

	POINTS VALUE
Lightlife Smart Franks	
Smart franks, 1 link	3
Lightlife Smart Ground	
♦ Original, 1/3 cup	1
♦ Taco, 1/3 cup	1
Lightlife Smart Links	
Breakfast, 2 links	1
Lightlife Smart Menu	
Chick 'n strips, 3 oz	1
Garlic teriyaki chick'n, 1 package	5
Orange sesame chick'n, 1 package	5
Steak strips, 3 oz	1
Veggie Bolognese, 1 package	4
Lightlife Smart Patties	
Mushroom burgers veggie protein patties, 1	2 (5
Lightlife Smart Sausages	
Chorizo veggie protein sausages, 1 link	3
Italian style veggie protein sausages, 1 links	3
Lightlife Smart Slice	
Bologna, 4 slices	1
Ham, 4 slices	2
Pepperoni, 1 oz	1
Turkey, 4 slices	1
Lightlife Smart Stuffer	
Chick'n broccoli melt, 1	4
Chick'n cordon melt, 1	4
Turk'y with cranberry stuffing, 1	4

Meat Substitutes (con't)

	POINTS VALUE
Lightlife Smart Tenders	
Lemon pepper chick'n veggie protein tenders, 3	3
Savory chick'n veggie protein tenders, 3	3
Lightlife Smart TexMex	
Smart Texmex, 1/4 cup	1
Lightlife Smart Tortilla Wrap	
Chick'n ranchero, 1	6
Mexican beef style, 1	7
Loma Linda	
Bolono slices, 3 slices	1
Chik-ketts, 2 slices (3/8" slices)	2
Choplets, 2 slices	1
Diced chik, 1/4 cup (drained)	1
Dinner roast, 1 slice (3/4" slice)	4
Frichik original, 2 pieces	3
Fripats, 1 pattie	3
Leanies, 1 link	2
Low fat frichiks, 2 pieces	2
Low fat veja-links, 1	1
Meatless chicken style roll, 1 slice (3/8" slice)	2
Meatless chicken style slices, 3 slices	2
Meatless corned beef (roll), 1 slice (3/8" slice)	3
Meatless corned beef (slices), 3 slices	4
Multigrain cutlets, 2 slices	1

	POINTS VALUE
Prime stakes, 1 piece	3
Prosage links, 2 links	1
Prosage roll, 1 slice (5/8" slice)	3
Saucettes, 1 link	2
Smoke turkey (roll), 1 slice (3/8" slice)	3
Smoked turkey (slices), 3 slices	4
Stakelets, 1 piece	3
Stripples, 2 strips	1
Super links, 1 link	3
Turkee slices, 3 slices	5
Vegetable skallops, 1/2 cup	1
Vegetable steaks, 2 slices	1
Vegetarian burger, 1/4 cup	1 (5)
Veja-links, 1 link	1
Wham (roll), 1 slice (3/8" slice)	3
Wham (slices), 3 slices	3
Morningstar Farms	
Asian veggie patties, 1	2 (5)
Breakfast pattie, with organic soy, frozen, 1 pattie	2
Breakfast starters with veggie sausage, 1/4 package	1
Burger - Philly cheese steak veggie, 1	2
Cheddar burger, 1	3
Chik patties, frozen, 1	3
Chik'n nuggets, frozen, 4	4
Chik'n tenders original, 2	4

	POINTS VALUE
Classic burger with organic soy, 1 pattie	3 (5)
Country scramble breakfast bites, 3 pieces	4
Garden veggie patties, frozen, 1	2 (5)
Ginger teriyaki veggie cakes, 1	2 (5)
Grillers burger style recipe crumbles, frozen, 2/3 cup	1 (5)
Grillers original, frozen, 1	3 (5)
Grillers prime, frozen, 1 pattie	4
Grillers vegan, 1	1 (5)
Meal starters chik'n, 12 strips	3
Meal starters steak strips, 12	3
Meatfree buffalo wings, frozen, 5	4
Meatfree corn dog, frozen, 1	3
Meatfree mini corn dogs, frozen, 4	4
Mushroom lover's burger, 1	3 (5)
Okara pattie, with organic soy, frozen, 1	2 (5)
Parmesan ranch chik patties, 1 pattie	4
Roasted herb chik'n, with organic soy, frozen, 1	2
Sausage style recipe crumbles, frozen, 2/3 cup	2
Southwest veggie cakes, 1	2 (5)
Spicy black bean burger, frozen, 1	2 (5)
TexMex burger with organic rice, beans and soy, frozen, 1 pattie	2 (5)
Thai burger, frozen, 1 pattie	2 (5)
Tomato basil pizza burger, frozen, 1 pattie	2

	POINTS VALUE
Vegan burger, with organic soy, frozen, 1 pattie	1 (5)
Veggie breakfast bacon strips, frozen, 2	1
Veggie breakfast sausage links, frozen, 2	1
Veggie breakfast sausage patties, 1 pattie	2
Veggie corn dog, frozen, 1	4
Veggie medley burger with organic soy, frozen, 1 pattie	2 (5)
Zesty tomato basil burger with organic soy, 1 pattie	2 (5)
Quorn	
Beef-style recipe grounds, 2/3 cup	1
Chick'n nuggets, 1 serving (65 g)	4
Chick'n recipe tenders, 1 cup	1
Chik'n patties, 1	3
Cranberry & goat cheese chik'n cutlet, 1	6
Garlic & herb chick'n cutlets, 1	4
Gruyere chick'n cutlets, 1	6
Meat-free meatballs, 4	2
Naked chick'n cutlets, 1	1
Southwestern chik'n wing, 1 serving (3-4 pieces)	4
Turk'y roast, 1 serving (1/5 roast)	1
Sabra	
Vegetarian liver, 1 oz	2
SuperBurgers	
Original, 1 patty	2
Texmex, 1 patty	2

◆ *Meat Substitutes (con't)* (POINTS VALUE)

Tofurky

Beer brats, 3 1/2 oz	6
Breakfast links, 1	2
Chipotle franks, 1	1
Cranberry & stuffing, 4 slices	2
Foot long veggie dog, 3 1/2 oz	3
Franks, 1	1
Hickory smoked, 5 slices	2
Italian deli, 5 slices	2
Italian sausage, 3 1/2 oz	6
Kielbasa, 3 1/2 oz	5
Oven roasted, 5 slices	2
Peppered, 5 slices	2
Philly-style steak, 5 slices	2
Vegetarian roast, 4 oz	4

Veggie Patch

Apple spice meatless sausage, 1 link	3
Artichokes & sundried tomato meatless sausage, 1 link	2
California veggie burgers, 1	1 (5)
Garlic portabella burgers, 1	2 (5)
◆ Garlic portabella burgers (club store size), 1	3 (5)
Jalapeno & cheddar meatless sausage, 1 link	2
Meatless buffalo wings, 4 wings	4
Meatless chick'n cutlets, 1	3
Meatless chick'n nuggets, 4 nuggets	4

◆ (POINTS VALUE)

Meatless garlic portabella meatballs, 4	3
Meatless meatballs, 4	2
Spinach nuggets, 4 nuggets	3
Veggie dog, 1	2

White Wave

◆ Chicken style seitan, 1 piece	2
Chicken style wheat meat, 1 serving (85 g)	2
◆ Traditional wheat gluten seitan, 1 serving (85 g)	3
Vegetarian stir fry strips, 1 serving (85 g)	2

Worthington

Bolono slices, 3 slices	1
Chic-ketts, 2 slices (3/8" slices)	2
Choplets, 2 slices	1
◆ Diced chik, 1/4 cup (drained)	1
Dinner roast, 1 slice (3/4" slice)	4
FriChik original, 2 pieces	3
FriPats, 1 pattie	3
Leanies, 1 links	2
Low fat frichik, 2 pieces	2
Low fat veja-links, 1 link	1
Meatless chicken style roll, 1 slice (3/8" slice)	2
Meatless chicken style slices, 3 slices	2
Meatless corned beef (roll), 1 slice (3/8" slice)	3
Meatless corned beef (slices), 3 slices	4

	POINTS VALUE
Multigrain cutlets, 2 slices	1
Prime stakes, 1 piece	3
Prosage links, 2	1
Prosage roll, 1 slice (5/8" slice)	3
Saucettes, 1 link	2
Smoke turkey (roll), 1 slice (3/8" slice)	3
Smoked turkey (slices), 3 slices	4
Stakelets, 1 piece	3
Stripples, 2 strips	1
Super links, 1	3
Turkee slices, 3 slices	5
Vegetable skallops, 1/2 cup	1
Vegetable steaks, 2 slices	1
Vegetarian burger, 1/4 cup	1 (5)
Veja-links, 1 link	1
Wham (roll), 1 slice (3/8" slice)	3
Wham (slices), 3 slices	3

Soy

Azumaya

	POINTS VALUE
Extra firm, 1 serving (79 g)	2 (5)
Firm, 1 serving (79 g)	2 (5)
Lite extra firm, 1 serving (79 g)	1 (5)
Lite silken, 1 serving (91 g)	1 (5)
Oriental spice tofu, 3 oz	2
Silken, 1 serving (1/5 block)	1
Zesty garlic tofu, 3 oz	2

Eden

	POINTS VALUE
Dried tofu, 1 serving (10 g)	1

House Foods

	POINTS VALUE
Organic tofu - extra firm, 3 oz	2 (5)
Organic tofu - firm, 3 oz (1" slice)	1 (5)
Organic tofu - medium firm (regular), 3 oz (1" slice)	1 (5)
Organic tofu - soft (silken), 3 oz (1" slice)	1 (5)
Premium tofu, extra firm, 1 slice	2 (5)
Premium tofu, extra soft, 3 oz	1 (5)
Premium tofu, firm, 1 slice	1 (5)
Premium tofu, medium firm, 1 slice	1 (5)
Premium tofu, soft, 1 slice	1 (5)
Tofu cutlet (Atsu-age), 2 1/2 oz	2
Tofu shirataki - angel hair, 4 oz	0
Tofu shirataki - fettuccine shape, 4 oz	0
Tofu shirataki - spaghetti shape, 4 oz	0
Tofu steak - Cajun, 1/4 package	2
Tofu steak - garlic & pepper, 1/4 package	2
Tofu steak - grilled, 1/4 package	2

Lightlife

	POINTS VALUE
Flax, 4 oz	5
Garden vegetable tempeh, 4 oz	5
Smoky tempeh strips, 3 slices	2
Soy, 4 oz	4
Three grain tempeh, 4 oz	5
Wild rice tempeh, 4 oz	6

SOY AND MEAT SUBSTITUTES

Soy (con't) — POINTS VALUE

Nasoya
Chinese spice tofu, 1 serving (1/4 package)	2
Extra firm tofu, 1 serving (1/5 package)	2 (5)
Firm tofu, 1 serving (1/5 package)	1 (5)
Garlic onion tofu, 1 serving (1/4 package)	2
Lite firm tofu, 1 serving (1/5 package)	1 (5)
Lite silken tofu, 1 serving (1/5 package)	0 (5)
Silken tofu, 1 serving (1/5 package)	1 (5)
Soft tofu, 1 serving (1/5 package)	1 (5)

Silk
Cultured soy - peach, 1 container	3
Cultured soy - raspberry, 1 container	3
Cultured soy - strawberry, 1 container	3

Silk Live!
Cultured soy - mango, 1 container	4

Toby's Tofu Paté
Classic, 2 Tbsp	1
Mild jalapeño, 2 Tbsp	1
Original, 2 Tbsp	2
Roasted garlic and red pepper, 2 Tbsp	1

Tofurky
Jurky - original, 4 pieces	2
Jurky - peppered, 4 pieces	2
Organic five grain tempeh, 3 oz	3
Organic soy tempeh, 3 oz	3
Spicy veggie tempeh, 3 oz	3

Tree of Life
Firm style, 1 serving (1/5 package)	3 (5)

POINTS VALUE

Organic tofu, 1 serving (1/5 package)	3 (5)
Reduced fat, 1 serving (1/5 package)	2 (5)
Smoked tofu, hot & spicy, 1 serving (85 g)	3
Smoked tofu, original, 1 serving (85 g)	3
Water pack, 1 serving (1/5 package)	2 (5)

White Wave
Baked tofu garlic herb Italian style, 1 piece	2
Baked tofu jalapeno Mexican style, 1 piece	2
Baked tofu lemon pepper style, 1 piece	2
Baked tofu sesame Thai style, 1 piece	2
Baked tofu teriyaki Oriental style, 1 piece	2
Baked tofu tomato basil style, 1 piece	2
Extra firm style tofu, 1 serving (1/4 block)	2 (5)
Five grain, 1 serving (1/3 block)	3
Organic extra firm, 1 serving (1/5 block)	2 (5)
Organic firm style tofu, 1 serving (1/5 block)	2 (5)
Organic soft style tofu, 1 serving (1/5 block)	2 (5)
Original soy, 1 serving (1/3 block)	3 (5)
Reduced fat tofu, 1 serving (1/5 block)	2 (5)
Soy rice, 1 serving (1/3 block)	3

White Wave Tofu Town
Grilled tofu tenders - Havana black bean, 1/2 package	4
Grilled tofu tenders - light tamari marinade, 1/3 package	3
Grilled tofu tenders - Mediterranean tahini sauce, 1/2 package	6
Grilled tofu tenders - sesame ginger teriyaki sauce, 1/2 package	5

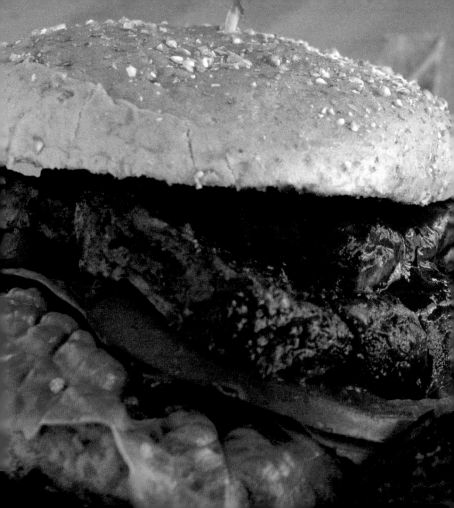

Artichokes

Birds Eye

Artichoke hearts, 12 pieces	0

Dole

Artichoke, 1 medium	0

Fanci Food

Artichoke bottoms, 3 pieces	0
Artichoke hearts quartered & marinated, 1 oz	0
Artichoke hearts, quarters, 3 pieces	0
Extra small artichoke hearts, 3 pieces	0
Hot artichoke hearts quartered & marinated, 1 oz	0
Marinated artichoke salad, 1 oz	0
Small artichoke hearts, 3 pieces	0

Progresso

Artichoke hearts (in brine), 2 pieces	0
Artichoke hearts (marinated), 2 pieces (with liquid)	2

Asparagus

Birds Eye

Asparagus cuts, 3/4 cup	0
Asparagus spears, 7	0

Cascadian Farm

Asparagus cuts, 2/3 cup	0

Del Monte

Green asparagus hand selected, 1/2 cup	0

Dole

Asparagus, 5 spears	0

Fanci Food

White asparagus spears, peeled, 1/2 cup	0

Green Giant

Cut spears asparagus, 50% less sodium, canned, 1/2 cup	0
Cut spears asparagus, canned, 1/2 cup	0
Extra long asparagus spears, canned, 5 spears	0

Green Giant Simply Steam

Asparagus cuts, 2/3 cup	0

Hanover

Asparagus cuts and tips, 3/4 cup	0

Hanover The Gold Line

Petite asparagus spears, 14 spears	0

Kounty Kist

Cut spears asparagus, 1/2 cup	0
Long green asparagus spears, 5	0
Long green xl asparagus spears, 3	0

LeSueur

Extra large asparagus spears, canned, 3 spears	0

Market Day

Asparagus spears, 19 pieces	0

Schwan's LiveSmart

Asparagus spears, 6	0

Triton International

Gourmet asparagus spears, 5 spears	0
Gourmet asparagus tips and cuts, 1/2 cup	0

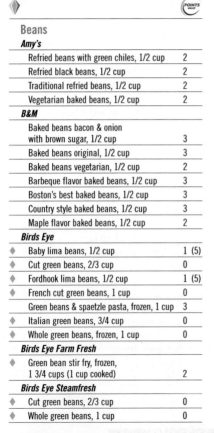

Beans

Amy's

	POINTS VALUE
Refried beans with green chiles, 1/2 cup	2
Refried black beans, 1/2 cup	2
Traditional refried beans, 1/2 cup	2
Vegetarian baked beans, 1/2 cup	2

B&M

	POINTS VALUE
Baked beans bacon & onion with brown sugar, 1/2 cup	3
Baked beans original, 1/2 cup	3
Baked beans vegetarian, 1/2 cup	2
Barbeque flavor baked beans, 1/2 cup	3
Boston's best baked beans, 1/2 cup	3
Country style baked beans, 1/2 cup	3
Maple flavor baked beans, 1/2 cup	2

Birds Eye

	POINTS VALUE
Baby lima beans, 1/2 cup	1 (5)
Cut green beans, 2/3 cup	0
Fordhook lima beans, 1/2 cup	1 (5)
French cut green beans, 1 cup	0
Green beans & spaetzle pasta, frozen, 1 cup	3
Italian green beans, 3/4 cup	0
Whole green beans, frozen, 1 cup	0

Birds Eye Farm Fresh

	POINTS VALUE
Green bean stir fry, frozen, 1 3/4 cups (1 cup cooked)	2

Birds Eye Steamfresh

	POINTS VALUE
Cut green beans, 2/3 cup	0
Whole green beans, 1 cup	0

Bush's

	POINTS VALUE
Baby butter beans, 1/2 cup	1
Black beans, 1/2 cup	1 (5)
Boston baked beans, 1/2 cup	3
Cannellini beans, 1/2 cup	1 (5)
Chili beans - hot (red beans), 1/2 cup	1
Chili beans - medium (red beans), 1/2 cup	1
Chili beans - mild (pinto bean), 1/2 cup	1
Dark red kidney beans, 1/2 cup	1 (5)
Garbanzo beans, drained, 1/2 cup	3 (5)
Great northern beans, 1/2 cup	1 (5)
Homestyle baked beans, 1/2 cup	2
Large butter beans, 1/2 cup	1
Light red kidney beans, 1/2 cup	1 (5)
Mixed beans (pinto & great northern), 1/2 cup	1 (5)
Navy beans, 1/2 cup	1 (5)
Onion baked, 1/2 cup	2
Original baked beans, 1/2 cup	2
Pinto beans, 1/2 cup	1 (5)
Pinto beans with seasoned bacon, 1/2 cup	1
Red beans, 1/2 cup	1 (5)
Speckled butter beans, 1/2 cup	1

Cascadian Farm

	POINTS VALUE
Green beans (cut), 3/4 cup	0
Green beans (petite whole), 1 cup	0
Green beans with toasted almonds (French-cut), 2/3 cup	1

Beans (con't) (POINTS VALUE)

Del Monte

Cut, Italian green beans, 1/2 cup	0
Cut, no salt added green beans, 1/2 cup	0
Dilled green beans, 1/2 cup	1
French style green beans, 1/2 cup	0
French style, no salt added green beans, 1/2 cup	0
Green & wax beans, 1/2 cup	0
Lima beans, 1/2 cup	1 (5)
Organic cut green beans, 1/2 cup	0
Seasoned green beans, 1/2 cup	0
Whole green beans, 1/2 cup	0

Eden Organic

Aduki beans, 1/2 cup	1
Baked beans (navy) with sorghum, 1/2 cup	2
Black beans, 1/2 cup	1 (5)
Black eyed peas, 1/2 cup	1 (5)
Black soybeans, 1/2 cup	2 (5)
Butter beans, 1/2 cup	1
Cannellini (white kidney) beans, 1/2 cup	1 (5)
Chili beans (dark red kidney), 1/2 cup	2
Garbanzo beans (chick peas), 1/2 cup	2 (5)
Great northern beans, 1/2 cup	1 (5)
Navy beans, 1/2 cup	1 (5)
Pinto beans, 1/2 cup	1 (5)
Small red beans, 1/2 cup	1 (5)
Spicy pinto beans, 1/2 cup	2

(POINTS VALUE)

Fantastic World Foods

Instant black beans, 1/4 cup	2

Faraon

Black beans, canned, 1/2 cup	1 (5)
Black beans, uncooked, 1/2 cup	1 (5)
Garbanzo beans, canned, 1/4 cup	2 (5)
Garbanzo beans, uncooked, 1/2 cup	1 (5)
Great northern beans, uncooked, 1/4 cup	1 (5)
Lima beans, uncooked, 1/4 cup	1 (5)
Mayocoba beans, uncooked, 1/4 cup	0
Mexican haba beans, uncooked, 1/4 cup	3
Pink beans, uncooked, 1/4 cup	1 (5)
Pinto beans, canned, 1/2 cup	1 (5)
Pinto beans, uncooked, 1/4 cup	0 (5)
Red kidney beans, uncooked, 1/4 cup	1 (5)
Refried pinto beans, 1/2 cup	2
Small red beans, uncooked, 1/4 cup	0 (5)

Goya

Black beans, 1/2 cup	1 (5)
Cannellini, 1/2 cup	1 (5)
Chick peas, 1/2 cup	1 (5)
Dark kidney beans, 1/2 cup	1 (5)
Great northern beans, 1/2 cup	1 (5)
Navy beans, 1/2 cup	1 (5)
Pink beans, 1/2 cup	1 (5)
Pinto beans, 1/2 cup	1 (5)

	POINTS VALUE
Red kidney beans, 1/2 cup	1 (5)
Small red beans, 1/2 cup	1 (5)
Small white beans, 1/2 cup	1 (5)
Green Giant	
Black beans (frijoles negro), canned, 1/2 cup	1 (5)
Butter beans, canned, 1/2 cup	1
Cut green beans, 50% less sodium, canned, 1/2 cup	0
Cut green beans, canned, 1/2 cup	0
Cut green beans, frozen, 3/4 cup	0
French style green beans, canned, 1/2 cup	0
Garbanzo beans (chick peas), canned, 1/2 cup	1 (5)
Great northern beans, canned, 1/2 cup	1
Green bean casserole, 2/3 cup	3
Kidney (dark) red beans, canned, 1/2 cup	1 (5)
Kidney (light) red beans, canned, 1/2 cup	1 (5)
Kitchen sliced green beans 1/2" diagonal cut, 1/2 cup	0
Kitchen sliced green beans, canned, 1/2 cup	0
Pinto beans, canned, 1/2 cup	1 (5)
Red beans, canned, 1/2 cup	1 (5)
Select whole green beans, frozen, 1 cup	0
Spicy chili beans, canned, 1/2 cup	1
Green Giant Butter Sauce Vegetables	
Baby lima beans, frozen, 2/3 cup	2 (5)

	POINTS VALUE
Green Giant Simply Steam	
Baby lima beans, 1/2 cup	1 (5)
Green beans & almonds, 2/3 cup	1
Hanover	
Canned black beans in brine, 1/2 cup	2 (5)
Canned cut and whole green beans, 1/2 cup	0
Cut golden beans, 3/4 cup	0
Cut green beans, 3/4 cup	0
Cut Italian green beans, 3/4 cup	0
Fordhook lima beans, 1/2 cup	1 (5)
French style green beans, 1 cup	0
Garbanzo beans in brine (chick peas), 1/2 cup	1 (5)
Great Northern beans "9" brine, 1/2 cup	1 (5)
Light & dark red kidney beans "9" brine, 1/2 cup	1 (5)
Pinto beans in "9" sauce, 1/2 cup	1
Whole green beans, 1 cup	0
Hanover The Gold Line	
Baby lima beans, 1/2 cup	1 (5)
Petite green beans, 3/4 cup	0
Heinz	
Vegetarian beans, 1 cup	4
Vegetarian beans, no meat, 1/2 cup	2
Joan of Arc	
Black beans, 1/2 cup	1 (5)
Butter beans, 1/2 cup	1

VEGETABLES

Beans, Joan of Arc (con't)

	POINTS VALUE
Dark red kidney beans, 1/2 cup	1 (5)
Garbanzo beans, 1/2 cup	2 (5)
Light red kidney beans, 1/2 cup	1 (5)
Red beans, 1/2 cup	1 (5)
Spicy chili beans, 1/2 cup	2

Market Day

Gourmet green beans, 1 cup	0

Old El Paso

Refried beans with green chillies, 1/2 cup	1

Progresso

Black beans, 1/2 cup	1 (5)
Cannellini beans, 1/2 cup	1 (5)
Chick peas, 1/2 cup	1 (5)
Dark red kidney beans, 1/2 cup	1 (5)
Fava beans, 1/2 cup	1
Garbanzo beans, 1/2 cup	1 (5)
Pinto beans, 1/2 cup	1 (5)
Red kidney beans, 1/2 cup	1 (5)

Schwan's LiveSmart

Green beans, 2/3 cup	0

Season Brand

Bean sprouts, 1/2 cup	0

Tree of Life

Organic cut green beans, 2/3 cup	0

Zapata

Black beans, 1/2 cup	1 (5)
Garbanzo beans, 2/3 cup	2 (5)

Broccoli and Cauliflower

Birds Eye

	POINTS VALUE
Baby broccoli, 1 cup	0
Baby broccoli spears, frozen, 4 spears	0
Broccoli & cheese sauce, frozen, 1/2 cup	2
Broccoli florets, 1 cup	0
Cauliflower, frozen, 4 pieces	0
Chopped broccoli, frozen, 3/4 cup	0

Birds Eye Steamfresh

Broccoli cuts, 1 cup	0
Broccoli florets, 1 cup	0
Garlic cauliflower, 1 cup	1

Cascadian Farm

Broccoli & cheese sauce, 2/3 cup	1
Broccoli cuts, 2/3 cup	0
Broccoli florets, 1 1/3 cups	0

Dole

Broccoli, 1 stalk	0
Cauliflower, 1 serving (1/6 medium head)	0

Green Giant

Broccoli & cheese sauce, frozen, 2/3 cup	1
Broccoli & cheese sauce, frozen, 1 tray	1
Broccoli & three cheese sauce, frozen, 1 cup	1
Broccoli & three cheese sauce, frozen, 1 1/4 cup	1
Broccoli & white cheddar cheese sauce, frozen, 3/4 cup	1

	POINTS VALUE
Broccoli & zesty cheese sauce, frozen, 3/4 cup	1
Broccoli cuts (no sauce), 2/3 cup	0
Broccoli cuts, frozen, 1 cup	0
Broccoli spears and butter sauce, frozen, 4 oz	1
Cauliflower & three cheese sauce, frozen, 1 cup	1
Cauliflower and cheese sauce, frozen, 1/2 cup	1
Chopped broccoli, frozen, 3/4 cup	0
Select broccoli florets, frozen, 1 1/3 cups	0
Green Giant Just for One	
Broccoli & cheese sauce, frozen, 1 tray	1
Hanover	
Broccoli florets, 4 florets	0
Cauliflower, 3/4 cup	0
Cut broccoli, 1 cup	0
Hanover The Gold Line	
Broccoli mini florets (petit), 1 cup	0
Market Day	
Broccoli florets, 1/2 cup	0
Schwan's LiveSmart	
Broccoli & cheese, 1 cup	1
Broccoli florets, 1 cup	0
California blend, 1 cup	0

	POINTS VALUE
Tree of Life	
Organic broccoli cuts, 1 cup	0
Organic broccoli cuts, 1 cup	0
Veggie Patch	
Broccoli bites with real cheddar cheese, 3	3
Brussels Sprouts	
Birds Eye	
Brussels sprouts, 10	0
Birds Eye Steamfresh	
Baby brussels sprouts, 10	0
Dole	
Brussels sprouts, 4	0
Green Giant	
Baby brussels sprouts & butter sauce, 1 cup	1
Green Giant Butter Sauce Vegetables	
Baby brussels sprouts, frozen, 1/2 cup	1
Hanover The Gold Line	
Brussels sprouts, 1/2 cup	0
Cabbage	
Dole	
Shredded red cabbage, 3 oz	0
Carrots	
Birds Eye	
Carrots, sliced, 2/3 cup	0
Del Monte	
Carrots, 1/2 cup	0
Carrots, organic, 1/2 cup	0

Carrots (con't)

	POINTS VALUE

Dole

Carrots, 1 (7" long, 1-1/4" diameter)	0
Peeled mini carrots, 3 oz	0
Shredded carrots, 3 oz	0

Green Giant

Honey glazed carrots, frozen, 1 cup	1

Hanover

Frozen sliced carrots, 1/2 cup	0

Hanover The Gold Line

Baby whole carrots, 2/3 cup	0

LeSueur

Tender baby whole carrots, canned, 1/2 cup	0

Celery

Dole

Celery, 2 stalks	0

Corn

Birds Eye

Baby gold & white corn, 2/3 cup	2 (6)
Baby white corn, 2/3 cup	1 (6)
Super sweet kernel corn, 2/3 cup	1 (6)
Sweet corn & bacon in a creamy cheese sauce, 1/2 cup	3
Sweet corn & butter sauce, 1/2 cup	3
Sweet corn on the cob, frozen, 1 ear	3 (6)
Sweet corn, frozen, 2/3 cup	2 (6)

	POINTS VALUE

Birds Eye Steamfresh

Gold & white corn, 2/3 cup	1 (6)
Super sweet corn, 2/3 cup	1 (6)
Sweet mini corn on the cob, 1 ear	2 (6)

Cascadian Farm

Super sweet corn, 3/4 cup	1 (6)

Del Monte

Cream style corn - supersweet, no salt added, 1/2 cup	1
Fiesta corn, whole kernel supersweet, 1/2 cup	1 (6)
Gold & white, whole kernel supersweet, 1/2 cup	1 (6)
Golden, cream style, 1/2 cup	1
Golden, cream style supersweet, 1/2 cup	1
Golden, cream style, no salt added, 1/2 cup	1
Golden, whole kernel, 1/2 cup	1 (6)
Golden, whole kernel supersweet/ vac pack, 1/2 cup	1 (6)
Golden, whole kernel supersweet/ vac pack NSA, 1/2 cup	1 (6)
Organic whole kernel golden corn, 1/2 cup	1 (6)
Organic whole kernel golden corn super sweet, 1/2 cup	1 (6)
Santa Fe corn, 1/2 cup	1
White, cream style, 1/2 cup	2
White, whole kernel, 1/2 cup	1 (6)
Whole kernel golden corn - no salt added, 1/2 cup	1 (6)

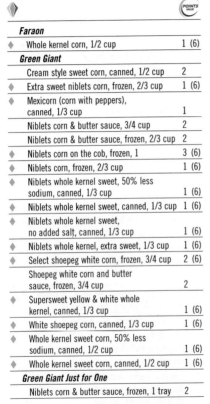

	POINTS VALUE
Faraon	
◆ Whole kernel corn, 1/2 cup	1 (6)
Green Giant	
Cream style sweet corn, canned, 1/2 cup	2
◆ Extra sweet niblets corn, frozen, 2/3 cup	1 (6)
◆ Mexicorn (corn with peppers), canned, 1/3 cup	1
Niblets corn & butter sauce, 3/4 cup	2
Niblets corn & butter sauce, frozen, 2/3 cup	2
Niblets corn on the cob, frozen, 1	3 (6)
◆ Niblets corn, frozen, 2/3 cup	1 (6)
◆ Niblets whole kernel sweet, 50% less sodium, canned, 1/3 cup	1 (6)
◆ Niblets whole kernel sweet, canned, 1/3 cup	1 (6)
◆ Niblets whole kernel sweet, no added salt, canned, 1/3 cup	1 (6)
◆ Niblets whole kernel, extra sweet, 1/3 cup	1 (6)
◆ Select shoepeg white corn, frozen, 3/4 cup	2 (6)
Shoepeg white corn and butter sauce, frozen, 3/4 cup	2
◆ Supersweet yellow & white whole kernel, canned, 1/3 cup	1 (6)
◆ White shoepeg corn, canned, 1/3 cup	1 (6)
◆ Whole kernel sweet corn, 50% less sodium, canned, 1/2 cup	1 (6)
◆ Whole kernel sweet corn, canned, 1/2 cup	1 (6)
Green Giant Just for One	
Niblets corn & butter sauce, frozen, 1 tray	2

	POINTS VALUE
Green Giant Simply Steam	
◆ Niblets corn, 2/3 cup	1 (6)
◆ Shoepeg white corn, 1/2 cup	1 (6)
Hanover	
◆ Sweet corn, 2/3 cup	1 (6)
Hanover The Gold Line	
◆ Shoepeg corn, 2/3 cup	1 (6)
◆ White sweet corn, 2/3 cup	1 (6)
Kounty Kist	
◆ Whole kernel golden sweet corn, 1/3 cup	1 (6)
◆ Whole kernel sweet corn, 1/2 cup	1 (6)
Market Day	
◆ Supersweet corn, 1/2 cup	1 (6)
Schwan's LiveSmart	
◆ Mini super sweet corn on the cob, 1	1 (6)
◆ Super sweet cut corn, 2/3 cup	2 (6)
Season Brand	
◆ Cut baby corn, 1/2 cup	0 (6)
◆ Flower cut corn, 1/2 cup	0 (6)
Tree of Life	
◆ Organic sweet corn, 2/3 cup	2 (6)
Veggie Patch	
Sweet corn bites with real cheese, 3	3
Lentils	
Eden Organic	
◆ Lentils (green) with onion & bay leaf, 1/2 cup	1

VEGETABLES

Lentils (con't)	POINTS VALUE
Faraon	
◆ Lentils, uncooked, 1/4 cup	2 (5)
Goya	
◆ Lentils, 1/2 cup	1 (5)

Lettuce/Leafy Greens
Birds Eye

Creamed spinach with a real cream sauce, frozen, 1/2 cup	2
◆ Cut leaf spinach, 1 cup	0
Boston Market Home Style Meals	
Creamed spinach, 1/2 cup	4
Cascadian Farm	
◆ Spinach (cut), 1/3 cup	0
Del Monte	
◆ Chopped spinach, 1/2 cup	0
◆ Spinach, no salt added, 1/2 cup	0
◆ Spinach, organic baby leaf, 1/2 cup	0
Dole	
◆ Classic & romaine blend, 3 oz	0
◆ Iceberg lettuce, 3 oz	0
◆ Lettuce (iceburg), 1 serving (1/6 medium head)	0
◆ Lettuce (leaf), 1 1/2 cups (shredded)	0
◆ Lettuce (Romaine), 6 leaves	0
◆ Spinach, 1 1/2 cups (shredded)	0

	POINTS VALUE
Green Giant	
Creamed spinach, frozen, 1/2 cup	1
Cut leaf spinach & butter sauce, frozen, 1/2 cup	0
Green Giant Harvest Fresh	
◆ Spinach, frozen, 1/2 cup	0
Hanover The Gold Line	
◆ Spinach, 1 cup	0
Tree of Life	
◆ Organic chopped spinach, 1 cup	0
◆ Organic chopped spinach, 1 cup	0
Veggie Patch	
Bistro au naturel - spinach & three cheese bites, 3	3
Spinach bites with three cheese, 3	3

Mushrooms
Alexia

Mushroom bites, 2 oz	2
Eden	
◆ Maitake mushrooms, dried sliced, 10 pieces	0
◆ Shiitake mushrooms, dried sliced, 6 slices	0
◆ Shiitake mushrooms, whole dried, 3	0
Fanci Food	
◆ Pickled cocktail mushrooms, 1 serving (1 oz)	0
Green Giant	
◆ Pieces & stems, canned, 1/2 cup	0
Sliced mushrooms broiled in butter, canned, 1/2 cup	0

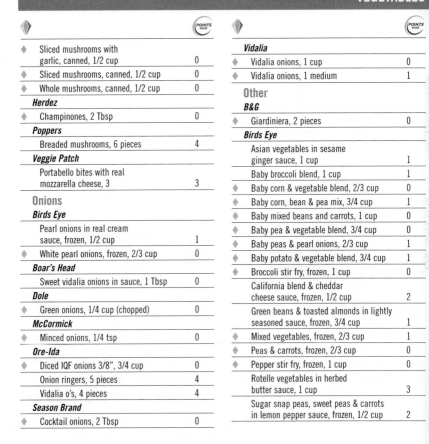

	POINTS VALUE
Sliced mushrooms with garlic, canned, 1/2 cup	0
Sliced mushrooms, canned, 1/2 cup	0
Whole mushrooms, canned, 1/2 cup	0
Herdez	
Champinones, 2 Tbsp	0
Poppers	
Breaded mushrooms, 6 pieces	4
Veggie Patch	
Portabello bites with real mozzarella cheese, 3	3
Onions	
Birds Eye	
Pearl onions in real cream sauce, frozen, 1/2 cup	1
White pearl onions, frozen, 2/3 cup	0
Boar's Head	
Sweet vidalia onions in sauce, 1 Tbsp	0
Dole	
Green onions, 1/4 cup (chopped)	0
McCormick	
Minced onions, 1/4 tsp	0
Ore-Ida	
Diced IQF onions 3/8", 3/4 cup	0
Onion ringers, 5 pieces	4
Vidalia o's, 4 pieces	4
Season Brand	
Cocktail onions, 2 Tbsp	0

	POINTS VALUE
Vidalia	
Vidalia onions, 1 cup	0
Vidalia onions, 1 medium	1
Other	
B&G	
Giardiniera, 2 pieces	0
Birds Eye	
Asian vegetables in sesame ginger sauce, 1 cup	1
Baby broccoli blend, 1 cup	1
Baby corn & vegetable blend, 2/3 cup	0
Baby corn, bean & pea mix, 3/4 cup	1
Baby mixed beans and carrots, 1 cup	0
Baby pea & vegetable blend, 3/4 cup	0
Baby peas & pearl onions, 2/3 cup	1
Baby potato & vegetable blend, 3/4 cup	1
Broccoli stir fry, frozen, 1 cup	0
California blend & cheddar cheese sauce, frozen, 1/2 cup	2
Green beans & toasted almonds in lightly seasoned sauce, frozen, 3/4 cup	1
Mixed vegetables, frozen, 2/3 cup	1
Peas & carrots, frozen, 2/3 cup	0
Pepper stir fry, frozen, 1 cup	0
Rotelle vegetables in herbed butter sauce, 1 cup	3
Sugar snap peas, sweet peas & carrots in lemon pepper sauce, frozen, 1/2 cup	2

Other, Bird's Eye (con't)	POINTS VALUE
◆ Sugar snap stir fry, frozen, 1 cup	0
Szechuan vegetables in a sesame sauce, frozen, 1 cup	1
Tender peas & pearl onions in lightly seasoned sauce, frozen, 2/3 cup	1
Tuscan vegetables in herbed tomato sauce, 1 cup	1
Vegetables & shells in garlic butter sauce, frozen, 1 package	6
◆ Vegetables for soup, frozen, 2/3 cup	1
◆ Winter blend, 1 1/4 cups	0
◆ Zucchini & squash mixture, 3/4 cup	0
Birds Eye Farm Fresh	
◆ Broccoli & cauliflower, 1 cup	0
◆ Broccoli, carrots & water chestnuts, 1 cup	0
◆ Broccoli, cauliflower & peppers, 1 cup	0
◆ Broccoli, cauliflower, carrots, frozen, 1 cup	0
◆ Broccoli, corn, & peppers, frozen, 3/4 cup	1
◆ Broccoli, green beans, onions, peppers, 1 cup	0
◆ Broccoli, peppers, onions, & mushrooms, 1 cup	0
◆ Brussels sprouts, cauliflower & carrots, 3/4 cup	0
◆ Cauliflower, carrots, snow pea pods, 1 cup	0
◆ Italian blend, 3/4 cup	0

	POINTS VALUE
Birds Eye Steamfresh	
Asian medley, 1 cup	1
Asian vegetables with roasted cashews, 1 cup	3
◆ Asparagus, gold & white corn, baby carrots, 2/3 cup	1
Beans with a twist, 1 cup	2
◆ Broccoli & cauliflower, 1 cup	0
◆ Broccoli, carrots, sugar snap peas & water chestnuts, 3/4 cup	0
◆ Broccoli, cauliflower & carrots, 3/4 cup	0
Carrots & cranberries, 1 cup	2
Garlic baby peas & mushrooms, 3/4 cup	1
Italian herb harvest vegetables, 1 1/4 cups	2
Lemon pepper vegetables, 1 cup	2
◆ Mixed vegetables, 2/3 cup	1
Spring vegetables in citrus sauce, 1 1/4 cups	1
Brooks	
◆ Slimcado, 1/3 cup	1
Cascadian Farm	
Organic purely steam broccoli & carrots lightly seasoned, 1 1/2 cups	1
◆ Premium gardener's blend, 3/4 cup	1
◆ Premium mixed vegetables: carrots, corn, peas, 2/3 cup	1 (6)
◆ Premium peas & carrots, 2/3 cup	0

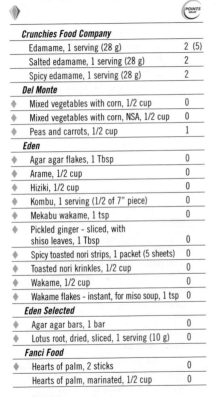

	POINTS VALUE
Crunchies Food Company	
Edamame, 1 serving (28 g)	2 (5)
Salted edamame, 1 serving (28 g)	2
Spicy edamame, 1 serving (28 g)	2
Del Monte	
Mixed vegetables with corn, 1/2 cup	0
Mixed vegetables with corn, NSA, 1/2 cup	0
Peas and carrots, 1/2 cup	1
Eden	
Agar agar flakes, 1 Tbsp	0
Arame, 1/2 cup	0
Hiziki, 1/2 cup	0
Kombu, 1 serving (1/2 of 7" piece)	0
Mekabu wakame, 1 tsp	0
Pickled ginger - sliced, with shiso leaves, 1 Tbsp	0
Spicy toasted nori strips, 1 packet (5 sheets)	0
Toasted nori krinkles, 1/2 cup	0
Wakame, 1/2 cup	0
Wakame flakes - instant, for miso soup, 1 tsp	0
Eden Selected	
Agar agar bars, 1 bar	0
Lotus root, dried, sliced, 1 serving (10 g)	0
Fanci Food	
Hearts of palm, 2 sticks	0
Hearts of palm, marinated, 1/2 cup	0

	POINTS VALUE
Faraon	
Frozen yuca, 1/2 cup	4
Mixed vegetables, 1/2 cup	1
Tender cactus, 1/2 cup	0
White hominy, 1/2 cup	1
Green Giant	
Alfredo vegetables, frozen, 1 cup	1
Baby vegetable medley, seasoned, frozen, 3/4 cup (frozen, 1/2 cup prepared)	0
Broccoli & carrots with garlic & herbs, frozen, 1 1/4 cups	0
Broccoli, carrots, cauliflower & cheese sauce, frozen, 1 cup	1
Broccoli, cauliflower & carrots and cheese sauce, frozen, 2/3 cup	1
Garden medley vegetables, canned, 1/2 cup	1
Garden vegetable medley: peas, potatoes, peppers & herbs, frozen, 1 cup	1
Italian-style vegetables, seasoned, frozen, 1 cup (frozen, 1/2 cup prepared)	1
Mixed vegetables, frozen, 2/3 cup	1
Parmesan asiago sauce: select peas, cauliflower, pepper, frozen, 1/2 cup	1
Pasta, broccoli, carrots, sugar snap peas & garlic sauce, 1 cup	4
Roasted garlic & herb sauce: select broccoli & cauliflower, frozen, 1 1/4 cups	1

Other, Green Giant (con't)

	POINTS VALUE
Roasted potatoes with broccoli & cheese sauce, frozen, 1 cup (frozen, 1.2 cup prepared)	2
Super sweet corn, peas & herb butter sauce, frozen, 3/4 cup	1
◆ Sweet peas with tiny pearl onions, canned, 1/2 cup	1
Tuscan herb sauce: select cauliflower, broccoli, beans, carrots, low-fat sauce, frozen, 1 1/4 cups	1

Green Giant Just for One
Broccoli, carrots & Italian seasoning, 1 tray	1

Green Giant Simply Steam
Broccoli & carrots (lightly seasoned with garlic & herbs), 3/4 cup	1
◆ Garden medley, 1/2 cup	1
◆ Sweet peas & pearl onions, 1/2 cup	1

Hanover
◆ 5-way mixed vegetables, 2/3 cup	1
◆ Crinkle cut yellow & zucchini squash blend, 2/3 cup	0
◆ Garden medley, 3/4 cup	0
◆ Green & red peppers & onion strips, 2/3 cup	0
◆ Latino blend, 1/2 cup	1
◆ Oriental blend, 3/4 cup	0
◆ Soup vegetables, 2/3 cup	1
◆ Succotash, 2/3 cup	1

Hanover The Gold Line
	POINTS VALUE
◆ Petite green beans, petite golden beans, baby whole carrot blend, 3/4 cup	0
◆ Shoepeg corn & petite peas, 1/2 cup	1
◆ White corn, asparagus, red peppers, 3/4 cup	1
◆ White sweet corn, petite broccoli florets, red peppers, 3/4 cup	1

LeSueur
◆ Early peas with mushrooms & pearl onions, canned, 1/2 cup	1

Market Day
Gemelli pasta & vegetable blend, 1 cup	1
◆ Prince Edward vegetable medley, 1 cup	0
◆ Stir fry blend, 1 cup	1

Milpas
◆ Nixtamal hominy, 1 cup	2

Port Arthur
◆ Water chestnuts, sliced and peeled, 1/2 cup	1
◆ Water chestnuts, whole, peeled, 1/2 cup	1

Sabra
Caponata, 1 serving (1 oz)	1

Sardo
◆ Pickled mild mixed vegetables, 1 oz	0

Schwan's LiveSmart
Fire roasted vegetable blend, 3/4 cup	1
Grilled onions and mushrooms, 3/4 cup	1
Mediterranean vegetable blend, 1 cup	1

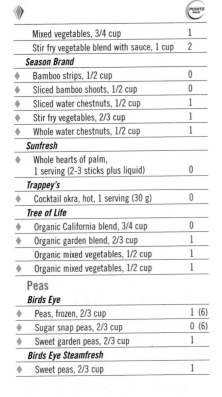

Mixed vegetables, 3/4 cup	1	
Stir fry vegetable blend with sauce, 1 cup	2	
Season Brand		
Bamboo strips, 1/2 cup	0	
Sliced bamboo shoots, 1/2 cup	0	
Sliced water chestnuts, 1/2 cup	1	
Stir fry vegetables, 2/3 cup	1	
Whole water chestnuts, 1/2 cup	1	
Sunfresh		
Whole hearts of palm, 1 serving (2-3 sticks plus liquid)	0	
Trappey's		
Cocktail okra, hot, 1 serving (30 g)	0	
Tree of Life		
Organic California blend, 3/4 cup	0	
Organic garden blend, 2/3 cup	1	
Organic mixed vegetables, 1/2 cup	1	
Organic mixed vegetables, 1/2 cup	1	

Peas

Birds Eye		
Peas, frozen, 2/3 cup	1 (6)	
Sugar snap peas, 2/3 cup	0 (6)	
Sweet garden peas, 2/3 cup	1	
Birds Eye Steamfresh		
Sweet peas, 2/3 cup	1	

Bush's		
Blackeye peas, 1/2 cup	1 (5)	
Blackeye peas with bacon, 1/2 cup	1	
Blackeye peas with bacon & jalapeño, 1/2 cup	1	
Dry blackeye peas, 1 oz	1 (5)	
Cascadian Farm		
Peas (garden), 2/3 cup	1 (6)	
Peas (petite sweet), 2/3 cup	0 (6)	
Peas (sweet), 2/3 cup	1 (6)	
Del Monte		
Organic peas, 1/2 cup	0 (6)	
Peas, sweet, no salt added, 1/2 cup	0 (6)	
Peas, sweet, very young small, 1/2 cup	0 (6)	
Dole		
Sugar peas, 1/2 cup	0	
Faraon		
Black eye peas, uncooked, 1/4 cup	1 (5)	
Split peas, uncooked, 1/4 cup	2 (5)	
Whole green peas, uncooked, 1/4 cup	2 (6)	
Goya		
Blackeye peas, 1/2 cup	1 (5)	
Whole green peas, 1/2 cup	1 (6)	
Green Giant		
Select sugar snap peas, frozen, 3/4 cup	0 (6)	
Sweet peas, 50% less sodium, 1/2 cup	1 (6)	
Sweet peas, 50% less sodium, young tender, canned, 1/2 cup	1 (6)	

Peas, Green Giant (con't)

	POINTS VALUE
Sweet peas, frozen, 2/3 cup	1 (6)
Sweet peas, very young small early, canned, 1/2 cup	1 (6)
Sweet peas, young tender, canned, 1/2 cup	1 (6)

Green Giant Simply Steam

Baby sweet peas, 2/3 cup	0 (6)
Sugar snap peas, 2/3 cup	0 (6)

Hanover

Blackeye peas, 2/3 cup	1 (5)
Sweet peas, 2/3 cup	0 (6)

Hanover The Gold Line

Petite peas, 1/2 cup	1 (6)
Snow peas, 1 cup	0 (6)
Sugar snap peas, 3/4 cup	0 (6)

Kounty Kist

Very young small early June peas, 1/2 cup	1 (6)

LeSueur

50% less sodium very young small early peas, canned, 1/2 cup	0 (6)
Baby sweet peas & butter sauce, frozen, 3/4 cup	1
Baby sweet peas, frozen, 2/3 cup	0 (6)
Early June peas & butter sauce, frozen, 3/4 cup	1
Peas small early June, 1/2 cup	1 (6)
Very young small early peas, canned, 1/2 cup	1 (6)

	POINTS VALUE
Market Day	
Extra young tiny peas, 2/3 cup	0 (6)
Minnesota Valley	
Small early June peas, 1/2 cup	1 (6)
Schwan's LiveSmart	
Green peas, 2/3 cup	1 (6)
Sugar snap peas, 2/3 cup	0 (6)
Tree of Life	
Organic green peas, 2/3 cup	1
Peas, wasabi, 1/4 cup	2

Peppers
B&G

Hot jalapeno slices, 7 pieces	0
Roasted peppers, 1 oz	0

B&G Sandwich Toppers

Hot peppers, 7 pieces	0

Cherchies

Pretty hot peppers, 2 Tbsp	1
Pretty peppers, 2 Tbsp	1
Roasted peppers 'n garlic, 2 Tbsp	1

Chi-Chi's

Green chilies diced, 2 Tbsp	0
Green chilies whole, 1	0
Green jalapeno wheels, 1/4 cup	0
Green jalapenos whole peppers, 2	0
Red jalapeno wheels, 1/4 cup	0

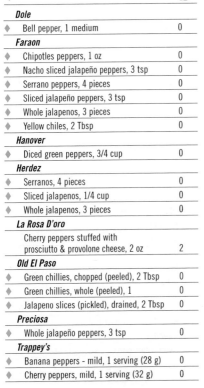

	POINTS VALUE
Dole	
Bell pepper, 1 medium	0
Faraon	
Chipotles peppers, 1 oz	0
Nacho sliced jalapeño peppers, 3 tsp	0
Serrano peppers, 4 pieces	0
Sliced jalapeño peppers, 3 tsp	0
Whole jalapenos, 3 pieces	0
Yellow chiles, 2 Tbsp	0
Hanover	
Diced green peppers, 3/4 cup	0
Herdez	
Serranos, 4 pieces	0
Sliced jalapenos, 1/4 cup	0
Whole jalapenos, 3 pieces	0
La Rosa D'oro	
Cherry peppers stuffed with prosciutto & provolone cheese, 2 oz	2
Old El Paso	
Green chillies, chopped (peeled), 2 Tbsp	0
Green chillies, whole (peeled), 1	0
Jalapeno slices (pickled), drained, 2 Tbsp	0
Preciosa	
Whole jalapeño peppers, 3 tsp	0
Trappey's	
Banana peppers - mild, 1 serving (28 g)	0
Cherry peppers, mild, 1 serving (32 g)	0

	POINTS VALUE
Jalapeno peppers - sliced, 1 serving (28 g)	0
Tabasco peppers in vinegar, 1 serving (28 g)	0
Tempero peppers - golden green pepperoncini, 1 serving (28 g)	0
Torrido peppers - Santa fe grande, 1 serving (36 g)	0
Zapata	
Diced green chili peppers, 2 Tbsp	0
Diced jalapeños, 4 Tbsp	0
Whole green chili peppers, 1	0
Potatoes	
Alexia	
Hashed browns, 1 serving (3 oz)	1
Betty Crocker Specialty Potatoes	
Sweet potato casserole, prepared, 2/3 cup	6
Boston Market Home Style Meals	
Mashed potatoes, 1/2 cup	4
Cascadian Farm	
Country style potatoes, 3/4 cup	1
Hash browns, 1 cup	1
Spud puppies, 10 pieces	3
Del Monte	
Sliced, new potatoes, 2/3 cup	1 (6)
Whole, new potatoes, 1 serving (approx 2 medium w/ liquid)	1 (6)
Dole	
Potato, 1 medium	1 (6)

VEGETABLES

Potatoes (con't)

	POINTS VALUE
Green Giant	
Roasted potatoes with garlic & herb sauce, frozen, 3/4 cup	2
Sweet potato casserole, 1 1/4 cup	4
Sweet potato casserole, 1 1/4 cups	4
Ian's	
Super tots, 1 serving (3.5 oz)	3
Sweet potato fries, 1 serving (2.5 oz)	1
Market Day	
Baby baked potatoes, 1 serving (3 oz)	2
Cheesy hashbrown casserole, 1 serving (4 oz)	4
Mashed potato patties, 1 patty	3
Triple cheese stuffed potatoes, 1	3
Ore-Ida	
Country style hashbrowns, 1 1/4 cups	1
Extra crispy tater tots, 12 pieces	4
Golden patties, 1	3
Hash browns, 1 patty	1
Mashed potatoes, prepared, 2/3 cup	2
Mini tater tots, 19 pieces	4
Onion tater tots, 9 pieces	3
Potato wedges with skin, 9 pieces	2
Potatoes O'Brien, 3/4 cup	1
Southern style hashbrowns, 3/4 cup	1
Tater tots, 9 pieces	3

	POINTS VALUE
Toaster hash browns, 2 patties	5
Twice baked potatoes, butter, 1 piece	4
Twice baked potatoes, cheddar cheese, 1 piece	4
Twice baked potatoes, sour cream & chives, 1 piece	4
Tree of Life	
Organic sweet potato puree, 1/2 cup	2

Pumpkin
Libby's
Pumpkin pie mix, 1/3 cup	1
♦ Solid pack pumpkin, 1/2 cup	0

Tree of Life
Organic pumpkin puree, 1/2 cup	0

Root Vegetables
Del Monte
♦ Sliced beets, 1/2 cup	0
Sliced, pickled beets, 1/2 cup	1

Dole
♦ Red radishes, 7	0

Eden
♦ Daikon - dried & shredded, 2 Tbsp	0
♦ Pickled daikon radish, 2 slices	0

Market Day
Sweet potato medley, 1 serving (3 oz)	2

POINTS VALUE

Squash and Zucchini

Birds Eye

Cooked winter squash, 1/2 cup	1

Cascadian Farm

Winter squash, 1/2 cup	1

Del Monte

Zucchini with Italian style tomato sauce, 1/2 cup	0

Sabra

Classic babaganoush, 1 oz	2
Flame roasted eggplant with sweet red peppers, 1 oz	1
Grilled natural eggplant with onions, 1 oz	1
Open flame roasted eggplant, 1 oz	1
Sauteed (Mediterranean) eggplant, 1 serving (1 oz)	2

Tomatoes

Contadina

Crushed tomatoes in tomato puree, 1/4 cup	0
Crushed tomatoes with Italian herbs, 1/4 cup	0
Crushed tomatoes with roasted garlic, 1/4 cup	0
Diced tomatoes, 1/2 cup	0
Diced tomatoes - Italian, 1/2 cup	1
Diced tomatoes with roasted garlic, 1/2 cup	1
Diced tomatoes with sauteed onions, 1/2 cup	1

	POINTS VALUE
Peeled whole tomatoes, 1/2 cup	0
Stewed tomatoes, 1/2 cup	1
Stewed tomatoes - Italian style, 1/2 cup	1

Del Monte

Chunky tomatoes, chili style, 1/2 cup	0
Chunky tomatoes, pasta style, 1/2 cup	1
Diced tomatoes in brine, 1/2 cup	0
Diced tomatoes in brine, seasoned with basil, garlic & oregano, 1/2 cup	0
Diced, tomatoes with garlic & onion, 1/2 cup	1
Diced, tomatoes with green pepper & onion, 1/2 cup	0
Diced, tomatoes with jalapenos, 1/2 cup	0
Organic crushed tomatoes in rich, thick puree, 1/4 cup	0
Organic diced tomatoes seasoned with basil, garlic & oregano, 1/2 cup	1
Organic diced tomatoes, in tomato juice, no salt added, 1/2 cup	0
Organic peeled diced tomatoes in tomato juice, 1/2 cup	0
Organic whole peeled tomatoes, 1/2 cup	0
Petite diced tomatoes in brine, 1/2 cup	0
Petite diced tomatoes in brine, seasoned with basil, garlic & oregano, 1/2 cup	0
Sliced tomatoes in brine, 1/2 cup	0
Stewed, Cajun recipe, 1/2 cup	0

Tomatoes, Del Monte (con't)	POINTS VALUE
Stewed, Italian recipe, 1/2 cup	0
Stewed, Mexican recipe, 1/2 cup	0
Stewed, original recipe, 1/2 cup	0
Stewed, original recipe, no salt added, 1/2 cup	0
Tomato wedges, 1/2 cup	0
Eden Organic	
Crushed tomatoes, 1/4 cup	0
Crushed tomatoes with basil, 1/4 cup	0
Crushed tomatoes with onion & garlic, 1/4 cup	0
Diced tomatoes, 1/2 cup	0
Diced tomatoes with basil, 1/2 cup	0
Diced tomatoes with green chilies, 1/2 cup	0
Diced tomatoes with roasted onion, 1/2 cup	0
Whole tomatoes with basil, peeled, 1/2 cup	0
Whole tomatoes, peeled, 1/2 cup	0
Fanci Food	
Diced Italian tomatoes, 1/2 cup	0
Muir Glen Organic	
Diced tomatoes with basil & garlic, 1/2 cup	0
Diced tomatoes with garlic & onion, 1/2 cup	0
Diced tomatoes with Italian herbs, 1/2 cup	0
Premium diced tomatoes, 1/2 cup	0
Premium diced tomatoes no salt added, 1/2 cup	0

	POINTS VALUE
Premium ground peeled tomatoes, 1/4 cup	0
Premium stewed tomatoes, 1/2 cup	0
Premium whole peeled tomatoes, 1/2 cup	0
Premium whole peeled tomatoes with basil, 1/2 cup	0
Whole peeled plum tomatoes, 1/2 cup	0
Whole peeled tomatoes, 1/2 cup	0
Muir Glen Organic Farm Select	
Fire roasted crushed tomatoes, 1/4 cup	0
Fire roasted diced tomatoes, 1/2 cup	0
Fire roasted diced tomatoes with medium green chilies, 1/2 cup	0
Fire roasted whole tomatoes, 1/2 cup	0
Progresso	
Crushed tomatoes with added puree, 1/4 cup	0
Diced tomatoes, 1/2 cup	0
Diced tomatoes with Italian herbs, 1/2 cup	1
Fire roasted crushed tomatoes with added puree, 1/4 cup	0
Fire roasted diced tomatoes, 1/2 cup	0
Whole tomatoes peeled with basil, Italian, 1/2 cup	0
Sardo	
Sundried tomatoes, 1 oz	2

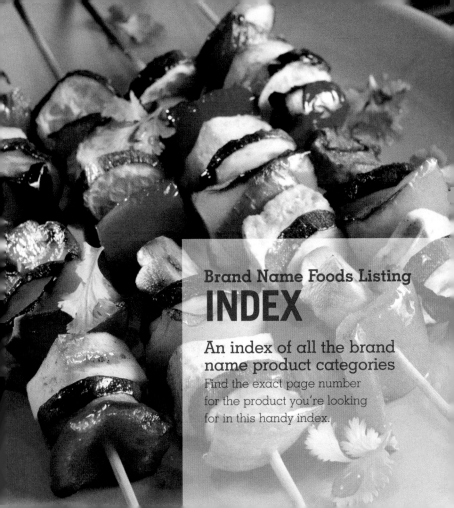

Brand Name Foods Listing
INDEX

An index of all the brand name product categories

Find the exact page number for the product you're looking for in this handy index.

INDEX TO BRAND NAME FOODS LISTING

INDEX TO BRAND NAME FOODS LISTING

INDEX TO BRAND NAME FOODS LISTING